Prevention of Myocardial Infarction

PREVENTION OF MYOCARDIAL INFARCTION

Edited by

JoAnn E. Manson,
MD, DrPH
Co-Director of Women's Health
Division of Preventive Medicine
Brigham and Women's Hospital
Harvard Medical School

Paul M. Ridker,
MD, MPH
Director of Clinical Trials
Division of Preventive Medicine
Brigham and Women's Hospital
Harvard Medical Schoool

J. Michael Gaziano,
MD, MPH
Director of Cardiovascular Research
Division of Preventive Medicine
Brigham and Women's Hospital
Harvard Medical School

Charles H. Hennekens,
MD, DrPH
Chief, Division of Preventive Medicine
Brigham and Women's Hospital
Harvard Medical School

New York   Oxford
OXFORD UNIVERSITY PRESS
1996

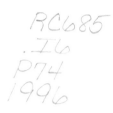

Oxford University Press

Oxford   New York
Athens   Auckland   Bangkok   Bombay
Calcutta   Cape Town   Dar es Salaam   Delhi
Florence   Hong Kong   Istanbul   Karachi
Kuala Lumpur   Madras   Madrid   Melbourne
Mexico City   Nairobi   Paris   Singapore
Taipei   Tokyo   Toronto

and associated companies in
Berlin   Ibadan

Copyright © 1996 by Oxford University Press, Inc.

Published by Oxford University Press, Inc.,
198 Madison Avenue, New York, New York 10016

Oxford is a registered trademark of Oxford University Press

Library of Congress Cataloging-in-Publication Data
Prevention of myocardial infarction/
edited by JoAnn E. Manson . . . [et al.].
p. cm.   Includes bibliographical references and index.
ISBN 0-19-508582-5
1. Myocardial infarction—Prevention.
2. Myocardial infarction—Epidemiology.
3. Coronary heart disease—Prevention.
4. Coronary heart disease—Epidemiology.
I. Manson, JoAnn E.
[DNLM: 1. Myocardial Infarction—prevention & control.
WG 300 P9456] RC685.I6P74 1996
616.1'23705—dc20 DNLM/DLC for Library of Congress 94-49176

2 4 6 8 9 7 5 3 1

Printed in the United States of America
on acid-free paper

This book is dedicated to our families

Foreword

Acute myocardial infarction, perhaps more than any other condition, may be considered the quintessential "twentieth century disease." When the century began, acute myocardial infarction was uncommon and the pathogenesis not clear. Early in the century the clinical-pathologic correlations between coronary atherosclerosis, coronary thrombosis and myocardial infarction were established, opening the door to much of the research that was to follow. The prevalence of coronary artery disease grew at an alarming rate, and by mid-century it had reached epidemic proportions and had become the most common cause of death in industrialized nations. Soon thereafter, however, the development and application of newly developed monitoring, pharmacologic, surgical and catheter-based techniques reduced both death and disability in individual patients. Clues to the pathogenesis of myocardial infarction also emerged in the middle of the century, and suggested that this condition could be prevented. The idea of identifying coronary risk factors and attempting to reverse them has been one of the most powerful in clinical medicine and has been primarily responsible for the massive—more than thirty percent—reduction in coronary artery disease mortality which has occurred during the past three decades. Thus, the tide against this dread condition has finally turned.

Dr. Manson and her colleagues have made a signal contribution to this important field by preparing this superb book. *Prevention of Myocardial Infarction* is up-to-date, comprehensive, yet eminently readable. A team of distinguished editors and authors have summarized and placed into perspective the enormous literature in this rapidly growing field. Some of the effective preventive measures such as aspirin and lifestyle changes are relatively inexpensive. Others, such as lowering arterial pressure or cholesterol, may be more costly. A unique feature of this book is that it deals explicitly with the cost-effectiveness of each intervention. *Prevention of Myocardial Infarction* will be of interest to cardiologists, to specialists in preventive medicine and public health as well as to individuals responsible for health policy.

It is especially exciting to contemplate the future. Further reductions in coronary mortality clearly are possible through the wider application of established preventive measures. Moreover, as summarized in this book, a number of new risk factors have been identified, and their reversal could offer immense additional benefit. If we take advantage of the enormous amount of information and the concepts presented in *Prevention of Myocardial Infarction*, then we will have come full circle and should be able to enter the next century as we came into this one—with coronary artery disease low on the list of mankind's fatal, disabling illnesses.

Eugene Braunwald, MD
Chief of Medicine
Brigham and Women's Hospital
Harvard Medical School
Boston, Massachusetts

Preface

Despite substantial reductions in death rates from acute myocardial infarctions in the United States during the past quarter-century, coronary heart disease remains the leading cause of death in both men and women in the United States and most other industrialized countries. Available evidence from epidemiologic and clinical studies indicates that coronary heart disease is largely preventable. Traditional risk factors such as cigarette smoking, hypercholesterolemia, hypertension, sedentary lifestyle, obesity, and glucose intolerance explain a major proportion of coronary events. Recent evidence also suggests important preventive and adjunctive roles for hormone replacement therapy and low-dose aspirin. A promising role for dietary factors, including folate, antioxidants, and other micronutrients, in the prevention of myocardial infarction is also suggested by recent data. Although physicians and other health care providers recognize that major benefits can be realized for their patients and the population as a whole by modifications in behavior and lifestyle, the implementation of available strategies to modify risk factors has been limited. Given current demographic and economic trends, widespread application of cost-effective preventive strategies will be increasingly important. The totality of clinical and epidemiologic evidence supporting prevention of myocardial infarction, as well as the feasibility and cost-effectiveness of risk-reduction strategies, has not been previously synthesized and made widely available to health care providers in office and community settings.

Prevention of Myocardial Infarction attempts to fill these gaps by providing a compendium of the scientific evidence on the efficacy of coronary disease prevention, while focusing on developing intervention skills to help clinicians utilize available knowledge. The quality of available data, estimated risk reduction, comparability of effect in men and women, and cost-effectiveness are addressed explicitly for each intervention. Chapters by leading authorities in cardiovascular epidemiology, clinical cardiology, cost-effectiveness analysis, and public health provide valuable insights and strategies to translate the theory of preventive cardiology into practice. The counseling and other intervention strategies detailed in this textbook, in addition to having documented clinical efficacy, are cost-efficient and require little time to learn or to implement. Patient education and health promotion appendices are also provided. The textbook is written primarily for health care providers, including general internists, family physicians, gynecologists, and nurse practitioners, as well as medical subspecialists such as cardiologists and endocrinologists. Valuable insights and tools will also be afforded to dietitians, psychologists, epidemiologists, as well as students, practitioners, and researchers in preventive medicine and public health.

JoAnn E. Manson, MD, DrPH
Paul M. Ridker, MD, MPH
J. Michael Gaziano, MD, MPH
Charles H. Hennekens, MD, DrPH

Acknowledgments

Cardiovascular epidemiology owes an enormous debt of gratitude to the dedicated women and men who volunteer their time and energy as participants in medical research studies. The frontiers of epidemiology, and medical science in general, have been greatly extended by their commitment and altruism. In particular, we thank the participants in the Nurses' Health Study, Physicians' Health Study, Health Professionals' Follow-up Study, Women's Health Study, Women's Antioxidant and Cardiovascular Study, and the Women's Health Initiative, for their ongoing commitment to our prevention research; we add to this our gratitude to the hundreds of thousands of participants in other research studies throughout the United States and worldwide.

We have been privileged to have as mentors the giants in epidemiology and cardiology. We especially thank Sir Richard Doll and Professor Eugene Braunwald for their inspiration, vision, and leadership.

We are also indebted to our outstanding professional colleagues and staff, who have provided support and encouragement for this effort. We are particularly grateful to Sherry Mayrent and Michael Jonas, whose dedication, talents, and outstanding efforts helped bring this project to fruition.

Finally, and above all, we thank our families for their tireless support, devotion, patience, and inspiration throughout this endeavor.

J.E.M.
P.M.R.
J.M.G.
C.H.H.

Contents

Contributors

Robert Allan, PhD
Division of Cardiology
The New York Hospital
Cornell Medical Center
New York, New York

Lawrence J. Appel, MD
Johns Hopkins Health Institutions
Baltimore, Maryland

Eugene Braunwald, MD
Chief of Medicine
Brigham and Women's Hospital
Harvard Medical School
Boston, Massachusetts

Jan L. Breslow, MD
Professor of Biochemical Genetics
Rockefeller University
New York, New York

Julie E. Buring, ScD
Co-Director of Women's Health
Division of Preventive Medicine
Brigham and Women's Hospital
Harvard Medical School
Boston, Massachusetts

Lowell C. Dale, MD
Nicotine Dependence Center
Mayo Clinic
Rochester, Minnesota

Patricia A. Daly, MD
Department of Endocrinology
New England Deaconess Hospital
Harvard Medical School
Boston, Massachusetts

Marilyn Dammerman, PhD
Professor of Biochemical Genetics
Rockefeller University
New York, New York

J. Michael Gaziano, MD, MPH
Director of Cardiovascular Research
Division of Preventive Medicine
Brigham and Women's Hospital
Harvard Medical School
Boston, Massachusetts

Lee Goldman, MD, MPH
Professor and Chairman
Department of Medicine
University of California, San Francisco
San Francisco, California

Francine Grodstein, ScD
Channing Laboratory
Brigham and Women's Hospital
Harvard Medical School
Boston, Massachusetts

J. Taylor Hays, MD
Nicotine Dependence Center
Mayo Clinic
Rochester, Minnesota

Jiang He, MD
Johns Hopkins Health Institutions
Baltimore, Maryland

Charles H. Hennekens, MD, DrPH
Chief, Division of Preventive Medicine
Brigham and Women's Hospital
Harvard Medical School
Boston, Massachusetts

Richard D. Hurt, MD
Professor of Medicine
Nicotine Dependence Center
Mayo Clinic
Rochester, Minnesota

Steven H. Kelder, PhD
Department of Pediatrics
Medical College of Georgia
Augusta, Georgia

I-Min Lee, MBBS, ScD
Division of Preventive Medicine
Brigham and Women's Hospital
Harvard Medical School
Boston, Massachusetts

Elizabeth B. Lenart, PhD
Department of Nutrition
Harvard School of Public Health
Boston, Massachusetts

JoAnn E. Manson, MD, DrPH
Co-Director of Women's Health
Division of Preventive Medicine
Brigham and Women's Hospital
Harvard Medical School
Boston, Massachusetts

Christopher J. O'Donnell, MD
Division of Preventive Medicine
Brigham and Women's Hospital
Harvard Medical School
Boston, Massachusetts

Ralph S. Paffenbarger, Jr., MD, DrPH
Professor of Epidemiology (Emeritus, active)
Stanford University School of Medicine
Stanford, California

Paul M. Ridker, MD
Director of Clinical Trials
Division of Preventive Medicine
Brigham and Women's Hospital
Harvard Medical School
Boston, Massacusetts

Frank M. Sacks, MD
Department of Nutrition
Harvard School of Public Health
Boston, Massachusetts

Stephen Scheidt, MD
Professor of Clinical Medicine
Division of Cardiology
The New York Hospital
Cornell Medical Center
New York, New York

Peter Sleight, MD, FRCP
Professor Emeritus of Cardiovascular
  Medicine
John Radcliffe Hospital
University of Oxford
Oxford, England

Caren G. Solomon, MD
Endocrinology Division
Brigham and Women's Hospital
Harvard Medical School
Boston, Massachusetts

Angela Spelsberg, MD, MPH
Division of Preventive Medicine
Brigham and Women's Hospital
Harvard Medical School
Boston, Massachusetts

Meir J. Stampfer, MD, DrPH
Professor of Epidemiology
Harvard School of Public Health
Boston, Massachusetts

Daniel Steinberg, MD, PhD
Professor of Medicine
Department of Medicine
University of California, San Diego
LaJolla, California

Peter H. Stone, MD
Director, Clinic Trials
Cardiovascular Division
Brigham and Women's Hospital
Harvard Medical School
Boston, Massachusetts

William B. Strong, MD
Chief of Pediatric Cardiology
Department of Pediatrics
Medical College of Georgia
Augusta, Georgia

Nanette K. Wenger, MD
Professor of Medicine, Cardiology
Emory University School of Medicine
Atlanta, Georgia

Paul K. Whelton, MD, MSc
Professor of Epidemiology and Medicine
Johns Hopkins Health Institutions
Baltimore, Maryland

Walter C. Willett, MD, DrPH
Chair, Professor of Nutrition
Harvard School of Public Health
Boston, Massachusetts

I

BACKGROUND

1

Myocardial Infarction:
Epidemiologic Overview

JoAnn E. Manson, J. Michael Gaziano, Paul M. Ridker,
and Charles H. Hennekens

Coronary heart disease (CHD) remains the leading cause of death in the United States and most western countries despite a dramatic decline in CHD mortality in the past quarter-century. While the former observation underscores the tremendous public health burden that heart disease continues to exact in industrialized countries, the latter suggests that CHD mortality rates can be modified. Advances in the medical treatment of CHD have contributed significantly to the decline in mortality, but preventive measures—both lifestyle changes and improvements in the medical management of coronary risk factors—have been estimated to account for most of the decrease in heart disease mortality (Goldman 1984).

In this chapter we discuss (1) the current burden of heart disease in the United States; (2) some of the evidence from cross-cultural investigations and studies of population migration that provides support for the now widely accepted conclusion that CHD risk may be altered by lifestyle changes; (3) temporal trends in CHD mortality that have occurred over the past several decades in the United States and in other industrialized countries; (4) the current prevalence of the major CHD risk factors in the United States and the changes in these factors that have occurred over the past several decades; and, finally, (5) the role of various epidemiologic research strategies in elucidating determinants of CHD and effective preventive interventions.

Public Health Impact of Coronary Heart Disease in the United States

In 1990, CHD was responsible for approximately 490,000, or nearly 1 of every 4, of the 2.2 million deaths in the United States (American Heart Association 1992, 1993). Myocardial infarction (MI) accounts for the majority of all CHD and thus is the single leading cause of death. Before age 60, heart disease rates are substantially higher in men than in women; however, heart disease increases markedly in women after menopause, and is the leading cause of death for both sexes, with women accounting for nearly half of the approximately 500,000 CHD deaths annually (Manson 1992). Heart disease also exacts a tremendous financial burden from society. In 1993, the economic costs associated with heart disease, including medical care, drug costs, and lost productivity in the work force, were estimated to be $51.6 billion (American Heart Association 1994).

Cross-Cultural Differences

Comparison of disease rates in different populations has provided evidence of tremendous variation in the worldwide occurrence of CHD. The Seven Countries Study was one of the earliest, most comprehensive efforts to record systematically the occurrence of cardiovascular disease in different populations. From 1958 to 1964, an international collaboration of investigators enrolled a total of 12,763 men, aged 40–59, living in 16 different population regions in seven countries (Keys 1980). Striking differences in disease rates were apparent after 10 years of follow-up (Table 1.1). The age-adjusted incidence of CHD ranged from 26 per 10,000 among men on the Mediterranean island of Crete to 1,074 per 10,000 among men in East Finland, the area with the highest recorded heart disease rates in the world. Within Europe, a general pattern emerged: the CHD death rates in northern European countries were more than $2\frac{1}{2}$ times greater than those of southern European populations. Baseline blood pressure and serum cholesterol measurements from the 16 populations were strongly correlated with CHD risk, while the other risk factors measured were not clearly linked to sub-

Table 1.1. Ten-Year Incidence of Coronary Heart Disease Among Men Free of Cardiovascular Disease at Entry (Age-Standardized Rate per 10,000)

Cohort	N	CHD		
		N	Rate	SE
Dalmatia	662	13	185	52
Slavonia	680	18	253	60
Tanushimaru	504	8	148	54
East Finland	728	71	1,074	115
West Finland	806	45	539	80
Crevalcore	956	43	450	67
Montegiorgio	708	22	353	69
Zutphen	845	45	513	76
Ushibuka	496	11	204	63
Crete	655	2	26	20
Corfu	525	17	337	79
Rome railroad	736	25	357	68
Velika Krsna	487	6	132	52
Zrenjanin	476	12	239	70
Belgrade	516	13	317	77
Total	9,780	351	369.9	19.1

Source: From Keys (1980), with permission.

sequent disease risk (Keys 1980). Figure 1.1 shows 1985 CHD death rates for middle-aged men and women in 27 countries.

Migrant Studies

Investigations of migrant populations are a second type of descriptive study that supports the conclusion that CHD risk may have environmental determinants. Migrant studies compare disease rates between an indigenous defined population and members of the population who have migrated to other regions. Unlike cross-cultural comparisons, in which differences in both environmental factors and genetics could be postulated to play a role in observed variations in disease rates, migrant studies compare rates among genetically similar populations.

The best-known study of migration and disease focused on three populations of Japanese men: those living in (1) the Japanese cities of Hiroshima and Nagasaki, (2) the Honolulu area on the Hawaiian island of Oahu, and (3) the San Francisco Bay area. The Ni-Hon-San Study (the name derived from the three locations: Nippon, Honolulu, and San Francisco) revealed substantial differences in CHD mortality rates between the three groups, with men in Japan having the lowest rates, those in Hawaii somewhat higher rates, and men in the San Francisco area having the highest rates (Figure 1.2). Since studies have shown that migrant populations tend to adopt dietary and other lifestyle habits prevalent in the region to which they immigrate, findings

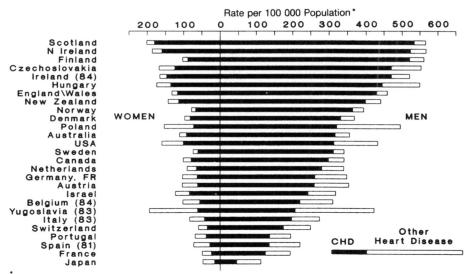

*
Rates are age–adjusted and coded to the Ninth Revision of the ICD except in Finland, Norway, Denmark, Sweden, and Switzerland (8th Revision)

Fig. 1.1. Death rates in 1985 for coronary heart disease and other heart disease by sex, for persons ages 45–64, in 27 countries. [From Thom TJ (1989), with permission.]

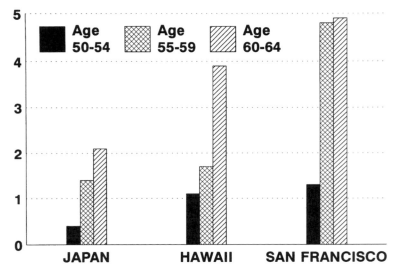

Fig. 1.2. Annual CHD death rates per 1,000 among Japanese men in Japan, Hawaii, and San Francisco. [Adapted from Worth RM et al. (1975), with permission.]

such as those from the Ni-Hon-San Study have implicated such environmental factors as significant determinants of coronary disease risk.

Studies have also been carried out to assess the possible effect of migration on specific disease risk factors, such as blood pressure. Although age-related increases in blood pressure are seen in most populations, more than 30 populations have been identified in which little change is seen in blood pressure levels with increasing age (Shaper 1974). These populations tend to live in isolated rural areas and have lifestyle characteristics very different from those now prevalent in developed countries, including low sodium intake, high levels of strenuous physical labor, and an absence of obesity.

One such population is the Yi people, who are subsistence farmers in a mountainous region of southwestern China. A migrant study was carried out to assess blood pressure levels and environmental variables among Yi farmers, Yi migrants to urban areas in Puge County, China, and the Han natives of the urban centers in Puge County (He 1991). As shown in Figure 1.3, Yi men and women farmers show only a very modest increase in systolic blood pressure with age, while their migrant counterparts exhibit the steep, age-related increase in blood pressure seen in most populations. The study provided striking evidence of changes in the relationship of blood pressure with age associated with migration from a rural to an urban environment.

Temporal Trends

As infectious diseases declined as the major cause of death, heart disease rates rose in the United States from the turn of the century until the mid-1960s. At its peak in

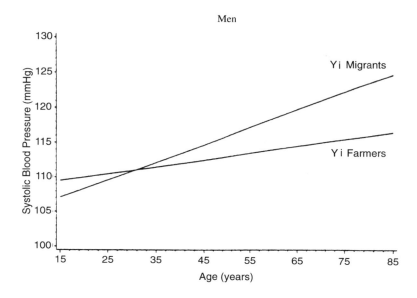

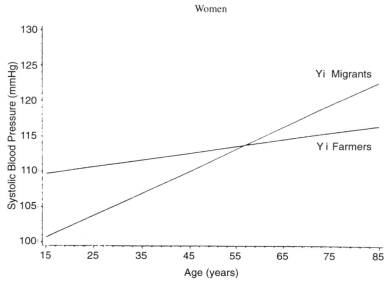

Fig. 1.3. Estimates of the effect of migration on change in systolic blood pressure with age among Yi farmers and migrants, adjusted for body mass index, heart rate, alcohol use, and smoking. [From He J et al. (1991), with permission.]

1965, age-adjusted CHD mortality in the United States was approximately 240 per 100,000. Since that time, however, a dramatic decrease has occurred, with rates declining approximately 2% each year since the mid-1960s (Figure 1.4). This decline has occurred in men and women, blacks and whites, and across all adult age groups.

Most western European countries and Japan have also experienced marked declines in CHD over the past several decades (Thom 1989). Figure 1.5 illustrates the percent change in CHD death rates for 27 countries over two time periods, 1969–1978 and 1979–1985. By the later time period, CHD death rates among men were declining in all western European countries surveyed, and among women in all but two. Eastern European countries, in contrast, are experiencing substantial increases in CHD death rates. These countries have more recently adopted western lifestyle habits and are now exhibiting CHD mortality patterns seen in western European countries several decades ago.

Prevalence and Secular Trends in Coronary Risk Factors in the United States

Blood Pressure

As is the case in most societies, in the United States blood pressure and the prevalence of hypertension tend to rise with age. Beginning with the initiation in 1972 by the

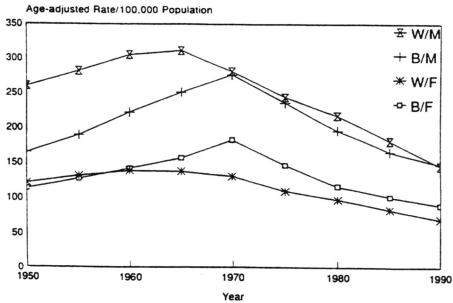

Fig. 1.4. Decline in coronary heart disease mortality in the U.S., 1950–1990. W/M = white males; B/M = black males; W/F = white females; B/F = black females. [From US Department of Health and Human Services. National Heart, Lung, and Blood Institute Report of the Task Force on Research in Epidemiology and Prevention of Cardiovascular Disease. US PHS, 1994.]

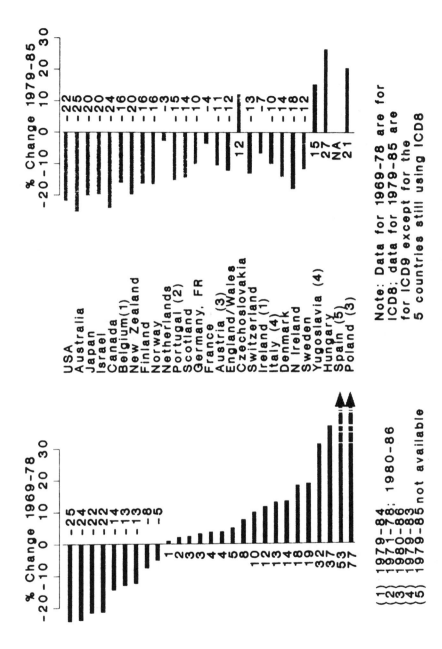

Fig. 1.5A. Percent change in death rates for coronary heart disease, 1969–78 and 1979–85, for men in 27 countries. [From Thom TJ (1989), with permission.]

9

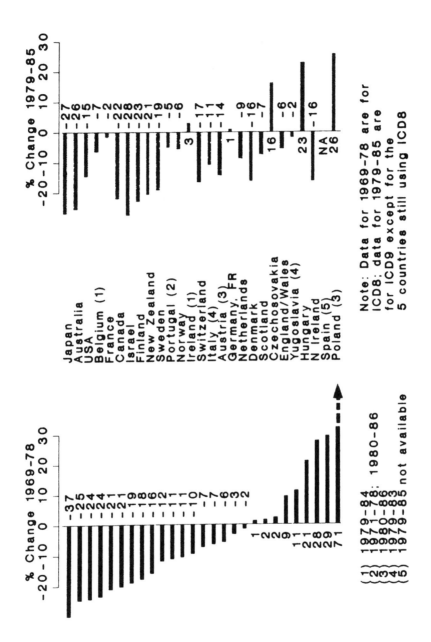

Fig. 1.5B. Percent change in death rates for coronary heart disease, 1969–78 and 1979–85, for women in 27 countries. [From Thom TJ (1989), with permission.]

National Institutes of Health of the National High Blood Pressure Education Program, a major focus of public health efforts has been the detection and treatment of high blood pressure. These campaigns were prompted by blood pressure population data that has become known as the "rule of halves." These data indicated that about half of all people with hypertension had not been detected and diagnosed, that half of those in whom a diagnosis had been made were not being treated, and, finally, that blood pressure levels were not adequately controlled in about half of those patients receiving treatment (Stamler 1993).

Current data on the prevalence of hypertension derive from the Third National Health and Nutrition Examination Survey (NHANES III), the most recent in a series of five national probability sample surveys that have been conducted since 1960 by the National Center for Health Statistics. NHANES III data, based on blood pressure measurements taken in a national sample from 1988 through 1991, indicate that one in four adults in the United States, or approximately 50 million people, have high blood pressure (National High Blood Pressure Education Program Working Group 1993). Individuals screened for NHANES III were classified as hypertensive if they met one or more of the following three criteria: systolic blood pressure (SBP) ≥ 140 mmHg, diastolic blood pressure (DBP) ≥ 90 mmHg, or currently under treatment with antihypertensive medication. Based on data indicating a continuous and graded association between blood pressure and cardiovascular disease risk, these cut-points reflect the trend toward defining hypertension at lower levels than in the past. In the earlier NHANES reports, for example, hypertension was defined as current SBP ≥ 160 and DBP ≥ 95 and/or receiving current antihypertensive medication. The prevalence of hypertension by age in NHANES III, using the newer definition, is shown in Table 1.2.

While complete NHANES III data are not yet available on demographic subgroups, in NHANES II data based on the more restrictive cut-points, the prevalence of hypertension was more than $1\frac{1}{2}$ times higher in blacks than whites (25.7% vs 16.8%) (DHHS 1986). Among young and middle-aged adults, the prevalence of hy-

Table 1.2. Hypertension[a] Prevalence by Age in Civilian, Noninstitutionalized Population, 1988–1991

Age	% Hypertensive
18–29	4
30–39	11
40–49	21
50–59	44
60–69	54
70–79	64
80+	65

Source: From National High Blood Pressure Education Program, 1993, with permission.

[a]Defined as the average of three blood pressure measurements of 140/90 mmHg or more on a single occasion or reported taking of antihypertensive medication. Source: Centers for Disease Control and Prevention, National Center for Health Statistics, National Health and Nutrition Examination Survey III (1988 through 1991).

pertension was greater in men, but this pattern was reversed in the older age categories (55–64 and 65–74), where the prevalence was greater in women.

Because complete blood pressure data are not yet available from NHANES III, comparisons of changes over time can only be made from the national surveys conducted between 1960 and 1980. These data indicate that mean SBP levels decreased significantly over the 20-year period covered by these surveys: In the 1960–1962 survey, the mean SBP level was 131, in 1971–1974, it was 129, and in 1976–1980, it was 124 (Dannenberg 1987). The declines were greater for women than men and for blacks than whites, but were nonetheless significant across all four groups (Figure 1.6). Diastolic blood pressure levels, in contrast, showed no consistent overall change, with age-adjusted mean levels for the total adult population of 78 in 1960–1962, 81 in 1971–1974, and 79 in 1976–1980. Among race-sex subgroups, however, white men experienced a statistically significant increase in mean DBP from 79 mmHg in 1960–1962 to 83 mmHg in 1976–1980 (Dannenberg 1987).

Targeted efforts aimed at those with highest blood pressure levels would be expected to affect population mean levels and the upper percentiles of the blood pressure distribution curve, but not the median value. In contrast, downward shifts across the entire range of blood pressures, due to improvement in lifestyle habits or other prevention measures, would lower both median and mean blood pressure levels. Both factors appear to have played a role in the changes in blood pressure levels between 1960 and 1980, but the effect of detection and treatment of those with the highest blood pressure values has been identified as the more important force (Dannenberg 1987). The 95th percentile of SBP values decreased from 168 mmHg in 1960–1962 to 158 mmHg in 1976–1980. However, the median SBP value decreased as well, from 129 mmHg in 1960–1962 to 124 mmHg in 1976–1980.

The age-adjusted prevalence of hypertension among adults (defined as blood pressure ≥160 SBP or 95 DBP or receiving medical antihypertensive treatment) increased slightly from 1960 to 1980 for white men and women, but decreased for black men and women. Nonetheless, prevalence rates at each survey period were higher in blacks than whites. It is difficult to draw firm conclusions from secular trend data on hypertension prevalence. On the one hand, apparent increases in the prevalence of hypertension may reflect secular changes predisposing the population to higher blood pressure levels, such as increased body mass index or decreased physical activity levels. However, this period of time has also witnessed heightened blood pressure awareness, which may have led to more frequent screening and the identification of individuals with labile hypertension. Because all persons receiving pharmacologic therapy are categorized as hypertensive, regardless of blood pressure level, the increased tendency during this period to treat those with modest blood pressure elevations is likely to have artificially increased the proportion of adults classified as hypertensive (Dannenberg 1987).

Figure 1.7 provides an assessment of hypertension detection, treatment, and control effects over the 31-year period from 1960 to 1991: The right-hand column indicates the percentage of those with hypertension who were aware of their condition before taking part in the population screening survey; the middle column indicates the percentage of those with hypertension receiving pharmacologic treatment; the left-hand column indicates the percentage of those with previously diagnosed hypertension in

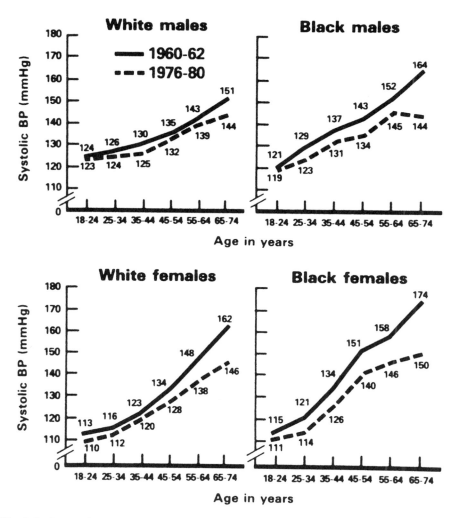

Fig. 1.6. Comparison of mean systolic blood pressure by race, sex and age in the US for two time periods, 1960–62 and 1976–80. [From Dannenberg AL et al. (1987), with permission.]

whom the condition is being controlled effectively with medication (defined as SBP <160 mmHg and DBP <95 mmHg). By the 1988–1991 survey, based on the stricter definition used in the earlier NHANES reports, 84% of those defined as hypertensive were aware of their condition, 73% were receiving treatment, and in 55% the condition was controlled (defined as blood pressure <160/95 among those currently taking medication) (Whelton 1993). These data indicate substantial gains in detection, treatment, and control of high blood pressure levels in the last three decades. Nevertheless,

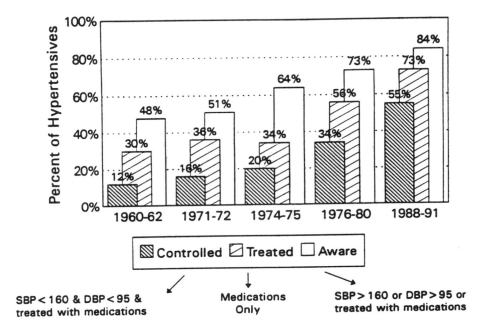

Fig. 1.7. Trends in hypertension awareness, treatment and control among US adults, ages 18–74, from 1960 to 1991. [From Whelton PK, Brancati FL (1993), with permission.]

considerable room is left for continued aggressive efforts. If the currently favored lower cut-points are used (Figure 1.8), for example, about one-third of all adults with hypertension remained unaware of their condition in the late 1980s and early 1990s, and hypertension was effectively controlled in only one in five hypertensive adults (Whelton 1994).

Cholesterol

Although the presence of cholesterol in atherosclerotic plaque was noted as early as the mid-nineteenth century (Epstein 1990), the hypothesis that dietary fat intake— and its consequent effect on serum cholesterol level—may be an important risk factor for coronary heart disease began to gain widespread support based on the pioneering international comparison studies of Ancel Keys in the late 1940s and early 1950s.

Since the first National Health Examination Survey (NHES) from 1960 through 1962, population-wide cholesterol levels have been tracked by the federal government for the noninstitutionalized adult population. Data from the first phase of NHANES III provide the most current information on cholesterol levels. In this report, based on measurements taken between 1988 and 1991, the mean serum cholesterol level for adults of age 20 and older was 206 mg/dl (5.33 mmol/l), with mean levels of 205 mg/dl (5.30 mmol/l) and 207 mg/dl (5.35 mmol/l) in men and women, respectively (Figure 1.9) (Johnson 1993).

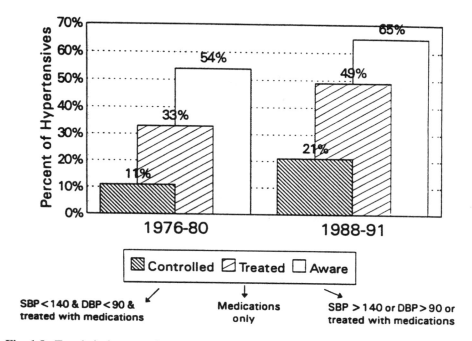

Fig. 1.8. Trends in hypertension awareness, treatment and control among US adults, ages 18–74, 1976 to 1991. [From Whelton PK, Brancati FL (1993), with permission.]

As in the earlier NHANES reports, NHANES III data indicate that mean cholesterol levels increase in men and women with succeeding age groups until the 55–64 age group, after which mean levels decline (Table 1.3). While men exhibit higher cholesterol levels than women at younger ages, starting with the 55–64 age group a crossover occurs, and women have higher mean levels in succeeding age categories.

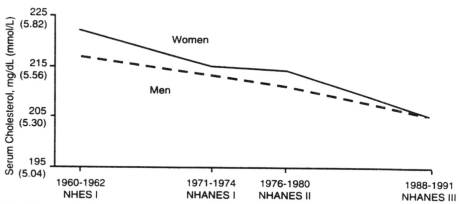

Fig. 1.9. Trends in age-adjusted mean serum total cholesterol levels, US men and women, ages 20–74, 1960–1991. [From Johnson CL et al. (1993), with permission.]

Table 1.3. Mean Serum Total, Lipoprotein Cholesterol, and Triglyceride Levels, U.S. Population, 1988–1991, Aged 20 Years and Older

	Serum Cholesterol, mg/dL (mmol/L)[a]				Serum Triglycerides[b]
Population Group: Sex/age	Total	LDL	HDL	VLDL	mg/dl (mmol/l)
Men					
≥20	205 (5.30)	131 (3.39)	47 (1.22)	26 (0.67)	143 (1.61)
20–34	189 (4.89)	120 (3.10)	47 (1.22)	22 (0.57)	112 (1.26)
35–44	207 (5.35)	134 (3.47)	46 (1.19)	26 (0.67)	141 (1.59)
45–54	218 (5.64)	138 (3.57)	47 (1.22)	29 (0.75)	199 (2.25)
55–64	221 (5.72)	142 (3.67)	46 (1.19)	30 (0.78)	164 (1.85)
65–74	218 (5.64)	141 (3.65)	45 (1.16)	31 (0.80)	159 (1.80)
≥75	205 (5.30)	132 (3.41)	47 (1.22)	26 (0.67)	134 (1.51)
Women					
≥20	207 (5.35)	126 (3.26)	56 (1.45)	24 (0.62)	126 (1.42)
20–34	185 (4.78)	110 (2.84)	56 (1.45)	19 (0.49)	101 (1.14)
35–44	195 (5.04)	117 (3.03)	54 (1.40)	21 (0.54)	113 (1.28)
45–54	217 (5.61)	132 (3.41)	57 (1.47)	24 (0.62)	126 (1.42)
55–64	237 (6.13)	145 (3.75)	56 (1.45)	30 (0.78)	168 (1.90)
65–74	234 (6.05)	147 (3.80)	56 (1.45)	29 (0.75)	155 (1.75)
≥75	230 (5.95)	147 (3.80)	57 (1.47)	28 (0.72)	157 (1.77)

Source: From Johnson et al., (1993), with permission.

[a]LDL indicates low-density lipoprotein cholesterol; HDL, high-density lipoprotein cholesterol; and VLDL, very low-density lipoprotein cholesterol. LDL was estimated from the equation: LDL cholesterol = (total cholesterol − HDL) − (triglycerides/5); VLDL was calculated as (triglycerides/5). LDL and VLDL were calculated for persons in the morning fasting subsample who fasted 9 hours or more and whose triglyceride levels were ≤400 mg/dl (4.52 mmol/l). The sum of LDL, HDL, and VLDL may not equal the value for total cholesterol due to the approximation of LDL and VLDL using the above equation.

[b]Persons in the morning fasting sample who fasted 9 hours or more.

With respect to low-density lipoprotein (LDL) cholesterol, overall mean level was 128 mg/dl (3.30 mmol/l), with higher mean levels in men (131 mg/dl [3.39 mmol/l]) than women (126 mg/dl [3.26 mmol/l]). The overall mean high-density lipoprotein (HDL) level was 51 mg/dl (1.32 mmol/l). There was a large sex difference in HDL levels, with mean values of 56 mg/dl (1.45 mmol/l) for women and 47 mg/dl (1.22 mmol/l) for men.

Substantial improvement has occurred in population-wide cholesterol levels over the 31-year period covered by NHES and NHANES. As shown in Figure 1.9, mean cholesterol among adults decreased over this period by 15 mg/dl (0.39 mmol/l). This decrease reflects a population-wide downward shift in values. While the decrease was present for every sex-age group, women experienced greater decreases than men (17 mg/dl [0.44 mmol/l] versus 12 mg/dl [0.31 mmol/l]). The decrease in women's cholesterol levels was greater with each succeeding age category, with women aged 65–74 experiencing the largest change, a decrease in mean cholesterol of 32 mg/dl (0.83 mmol/l) from the 1960–1962 period to 1988–1991.

With respect to categories of cholesterol level, the proportion of adults in NHANES III with cholesterol levels ≥240 mg/dl (6.21 mmol/l) was 19% and 20% for men and women, respectively. These figures have decreased since the NHANES

II data from 1976 to 1980, at which time the proportions were 25% and 28%, respectively (Figure 1.10).

Regional surveys have reported similar findings. In the Minnesota Heart Survey, for example, which has assessed cholesterol levels in adults aged 25–74 in the Minneapolis-St. Paul area, mean serum cholesterol decreased 5–6 mg/dl (0.13–0.16 mmol/l) in both men and women from 1980–1982 to 1985–1987 (Burke 1991). As in the NHANES data, there was an overall shift toward lower values, indicating that the decreased mean levels are not solely the result of lowered cholesterol among those with the highest levels.

Population-wide health goals for the year 2000 have been established by the U.S. Department of Health and Human Services (DHHS 1991). Among these are the goal of reducing mean cholesterol levels among adults to 200 mg/dl (5.17 mmol/l) or lower and reducing the proportion of adults with cholesterol levels ≥240 mg/dl (6.21 mmol/l) to no more than 20%. The latter goal has already been achieved, and the former goal appears attainable, given the current mean level of 206 mg/dl (5.33 mmol/l) and the impressive 8 mg/dl (0.21 mmol/l) decrease that occurred since the 1976–1980 NHANES II survey.

Meeting the year 2000 goal of mean population cholesterol level of no more than 200 mg/dl (5.17 mmol/l) would represent an important public health victory. However, because there is a continuous, graded association between cholesterol levels and CHD risk at all levels, even if the year 2000 goal is met, continued efforts through promotion of lifestyle changes to further reduce population cholesterol levels may yield further public health benefits. Indeed, in follow-up data from the Framingham Heart Study, approximately 30% of all MIs occurred among individuals with cholesterol levels below 200 mg/dl (5.17 mmol/l). This finding underscores the fact that the overall distribution of cholesterol levels in the United States is skewed toward higher values in relation to countries with very low coronary disease rates, such as Japan and China,

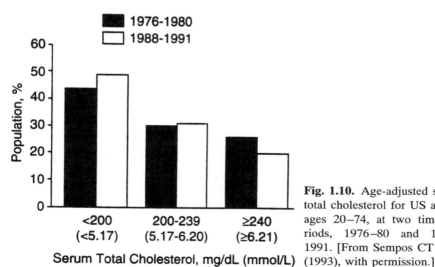

Fig. 1.10. Age-adjusted serum total cholesterol for US adults, ages 20–74, at two time periods, 1976–80 and 1988–1991. [From Sempos CT et al. (1993), with permission.]

where mean levels are substantially less than 200 mg/dl (5.17 mmol/l). However, this finding also highlights the importance of assessing other lipid measurements in addition to total cholesterol in developing population-wide risk profiles as well as those for individual patients. In particular, HDL cholesterol levels show a strong inverse relation with CHD risk, and the ratio of total:HDL cholesterol has been shown to provide a more accurate measure of coronary risk than total cholesterol alone. Current National Cholesterol Education Project (NCEP) guidelines call for measurement of total as well as HDL cholesterol as part of the initial cholesterol screening recommended for all adults 20 and older (Expert Panel 1993).

Cigarette Smoking

Cigarette smoking, which constitutes a major risk factor for the development of CHD, was a relatively uncommon behavior in the United States before the turn of the century (Fiore 1992). However, cigarette smoking rates rose throughout the first part of this century, peaking in the mid-1960s; since that time, rates have declined.

In 1990, approximately 25% of the adult population smoked: 28% of adult men and 23% of adult women (CDC 1992a). This represents a significant decrease from 1965, when 42% of the adult population smoked. Although the decrease in the overall smoking rate is encouraging, troubling patterns have emerged in certain subgroups, notably adolescent females and young adult women as well as those of lower educational level.

Although smoking rates in women remain lower than those for men, they have declined more slowly than rates in men. For example, while male smoking rates decreased by 46% from 1965 to 1990 (from 52% to 28%), the rate among women decreased by 32% during this period (from 34% to 23%). With regard to adolescent smoking behavior, rates among teenagers have historically mirrored those of adults, with higher rates among males than females. However, since 1990, the prevalence of daily smoking among high-school seniors has been greater for females than males (DHHS 1992). Based on current trends, it has been estimated that smoking rates among men and women will converge during the 1990s, after which rates will be higher for women than men (Figure 1.11). By the year 2000, it is estimated that rates among women will remain at their present level of 23%, whereas the smoking rate among men will have fallen to 20% (Pierce 1989). Since this crossover is being driven largely by unfavorable smoking patterns among younger women, unless reversed over coming decades, these changing demographics of smoking may contribute substantially to the future burden of CHD, as well as other smoking-related illnesses, among women (Peto 1992).

At the peak of smoking rates in the United States in the mid-1960s, there were only small differences in smoking rates among adults of varying levels of educational background. Based on data from the 1966 National Health Interview Survey, smoking rates were 36% among those without a high school diploma, 41% among high-school graduates, 42% among those with some college education, and 34% among college graduates. By 1990, however, the smoking rate among college graduates had decreased by more than 50%, from 34% to 14%, while the rate among those without a high-school diploma decreased only slightly over this 25-year period, from 36% to 32%.

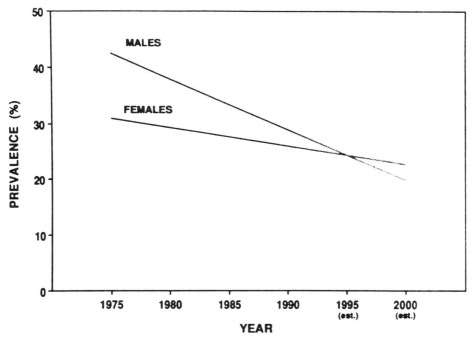

Fig. 1.11. Trends in the prevalence of cigarette smoking among US men and women, ages 20 and older, with projections to the year 2000. [From Fiore MC (1992), with permission.]

Table 1.4 shows the trend in smoking rates from 1970 to 1991 according to sex, race, and education level. Projections for the year 2000 based on National Health Interview Survey (NHIS) data through the mid-1980s suggest that the smoking rate among those who have not completed high school will remain at least 30%, while less than 10% of college graduates will be regular cigarette smokers (Pierce 1989).

Table 1.4. Cigarette Smoking (%) By Sex, Race, and Educational Attainment

Characteristics	1970	1978	1983	1988	1991
Sex					
Male	44.3	39.0	35.5	30.9	28.1
Female	30.8	29.6	28.7	25.3	23.5
Race					
White	36.5	33.6	31.4	27.5	25.5
Black	41.4	38.2	36.6	32.3	29.2
Educational attainment					
Less than high school	34.8	35.3	34.7	32.8	32.0
High school graduate	38.3	36.5	35.6	32.6	30.0
Some college	36.7	32.7	30.0	25.4	23.4
College graduate	28.1	23.8	19.9	15.6	13.6

Source: From U.S. Department of Health and Human Services (1989); *MMWR* (1993); and unpublished data.

Obesity

Obesity is associated with several coronary risk factors, including hypertension, diabetes, and hypercholesterolemia, and is an important predictor of CHD events in both men and women. Data from NHANES III indicate that dramatic increases in the prevalence of overweight have occurred among the United States population over the past two decades (Kuczmarski 1994). NHANES uses body mass index (calculated as weight in kilograms divided by height in meters squared) as a measure of obesity, defining overweight as body mass index values ≥27.8 for men and ≥27.3 for women. These cut-points correspond to the 85th percentile values for men and women aged 20–29 in NHANES II, and are approximately 124% of desirable weight for men and 120% of desirable weight for women, based on 1983 Metropolitan Life Insurance height and weight tables.

Overall in NHANES III, one-third of adults (31% of men and 35% of women) were estimated to be overweight, representing approximately 58 million adults (26 million men and 32 million women). These prevalence estimates from NHANES III represent a dramatic change from the rates recorded in three previous national surveys (Figure 1.12). Overweight prevalence estimates from those surveys showed strikingly little change over time, with the prevalence of overweight estimated to be 24.3% during the NHES in 1960–1962, 25.0% at the NHANES I in 1971–1974, and 25.4% at NHANES II in 1976–1980. In all surveys the prevalence of obesity has been substantially higher for black, as compared to white, women.

The federal Healthy People 2000 goal for reducing the burden of obesity is to decrease the prevalence of overweight to no more than 20% of the adult population. Based on the recent NHANES III data, the United States is moving farther from, not closer to, this goal. The trend toward increased prevalence of obesity is cause for particular concern because, in contrast to those risk factors for which gains have been made—either through more aggressive detection and treatment, as with hypertension, or through successful education efforts, as with cigarette smoking—no current approaches to weight loss thus far have been demonstrated to have widespread, long-term efficacy.

Diabetes

Diabetes mellitus is an important risk factor for the development of coronary heart disease. The incidence and prevalence of diabetes have been estimated annually since 1959 through the NHIS, a population-based household survey conducted by the Centers for Disease Control and Prevention among approximately 120,000 noninstitutionalized residents. In the 1989 NHIS, about 2.7% of the population (~6.7 million people) reported that they had diabetes (Geiss 1993). However, data based on self-reports substantially underrepresent the true prevalence of diabetes. The NHANES II, conducted from 1976 to 1980, collected information on self-reported diagnoses of diabetes and administered glucose tolerance tests to a representative subset of the group in order to assess the prevalence of undiagnosed diabetes in the population. The survey estimated that 6.6% of the population aged 20–74 (more than 8 million people) suf-

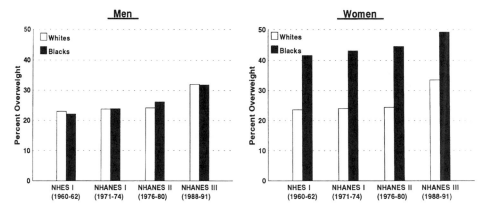

Prevalence of Obesity Among US Adults

Fig. 1.12. Prevalence of obesity among US men and women, ages 20–75, at four intervals. (Defined as body mass index [weight in kilograms divided by height in meters, squared] ≥27.8 for men and ≥27.3 for women). [Adapted from Kuczmarski RJ et al. (1994), with permission.]

fered from diabetes (Harris 1987). The prevalence of previously undiagnosed diabetes (3.2%) was nearly as great as the prevalence of diagnosed diabetes (3.4%). Based on current prevalence estimates, approximately 12–14 million individuals in the United States have diabetes.

The self-reported prevalence of diabetes has risen substantially since the first NHIS in 1959. The prevalence increased 67% from 1959 through 1966, rose by 41% from 1966 through 1973, and by 21% from 1973 through 1980. From 1980 through 1989, self-reported prevalence of diabetes increased by only 4% (Geiss 1993). Secular increases in the prevalence of obesity, which is associated with increased risk of diabetes, may be contributing to an increase in the prevalence of diabetes. However, because of increased attention to screening for diabetes, it remains unclear to what extent there has been a true increase in diabetes that is not explained by more aggressive screening (Jarrett 1989). Among population subgroups, as shown in Figure 1.13, the prevalence of diabetes is substantially higher among black men and women than among white men and women. Prevalence of diabetes is also high in the Hispanic population.

Physical Activity

Increasing levels of leisure-time physical activity are associated with decreased risks of coronary heart disease in numerous studies (Berlin 1990). Data on levels of physical activity among the U.S. population are available for the years 1986 through 1991 from the Behavioral Risk Factor Surveillance System (Siegel 1991; CDC 1993b). Sedentary

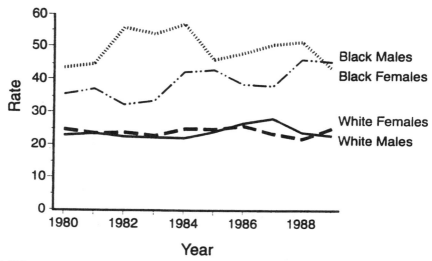

*Per 1,000 persons.

Fig. 1.13. Age-standardized prevalence of diabetes per 1,000 in the US by race and sex, 1980–1988. [From Geiss LS et al. (1993), with permission.]

lifestyle was defined in these surveys as engaging in no or only irregular physical activity. There was no change in the prevalence of sedentary lifestyle over this period, with nearly 60% of adults defined as sedentary in each of five annual surveys. Figure 1.14 shows the prevalence of sedentary lifestyle by sex, race, and age group. A small

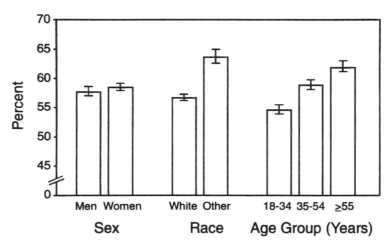

Fig. 1.14. Prevalence of sedentary lifestyle by sex, race and age group for US adults, ages 18 and older, 1991. (Bars indicate 95% confidence intervals.) [From CDC (1993), with permission.]

decrease was recorded in the percentage of adults who engage in no leisure-time activity, with prevalence rates decreasing from 31.9% in 1986 to 28.7% in 1990. As with cigarette smoking rates, striking differences in the prevalence of sedentary life-style are present according to level of education (Figure 1.15). Because these surveys measured only leisure-time activity, they may overestimate somewhat the extent of sedentary behavior among those with lower education levels, who may be more likely to engage in occupation-related physical activity. The prevalence of no leisure-time activity remains nearly twice as great as the Healthy People 2000 objective, which is to reduce to 15% the proportion of Americans 6 years of age and older who engage in no leisure-time physical activity.

Postmenopausal Estrogen Therapy

Postmenopausal estrogen replacement therapy is associated with a decreased risk of coronary heart disease in several observational epidemiologic studies (Stampfer 1991). Many women currently taking postmenopausal estrogen have primary indications other than prevention of CHD, which is not presently an approved prescription indication for this drug. Nevertheless, since estrogen is used during the peri- and post-menopausal years—the time period when CHD risk in women begins to rise—significant changes in the prevalence of women receiving estrogen replacement therapy could, at least in theory, influence CHD rates among women.

A survey of retail prescriptions containing estrogen shows a steady increase in the number of prescriptions dispensed from 1966 through the mid-1970s. In 1975, a steep 5-year decline began in the number of prescriptions dispensed, after which time the number of prescriptions began to rise again (Kennedy 1985). Estimates of dispensed prescriptions for the time period from 1982–1992 indicate a marked increase in the number of prescriptions for oral estrogen and transdermal estrogen, which was first

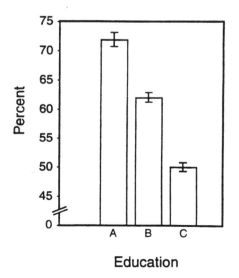

Fig. 1.15. Prevalence of sedentary lifestyle by education for US adults, ages 18 and older, 1991. A = less than high school graduate; B = high school or technical school graduate; C = college attendee or graduate [From CDC (1993), with permission.]

introduced in 1986. (Wysowski 1995). (Figure 1.16). The number of annual prescriptions for estrogen preparations more than doubled, from 13.6 million in 1982 to 31.7 million in 1992 (Wysowski 1995). These temporal trends may have been influenced by reports linking estrogen use to increased risk of uterine and breast cancer, as well as to a protective relationship with coronary heart disease and osteoporosis (Johannes 1994).

In the Nurses' Health Study, a prospective study of 121,700 female U.S. registered nurses in 11 large states, 35% of postmenopausal women were current users of postmenopausal estrogen in 1976 (Stampfer 1985). In a survey of postmenopausal estrogen use conducted in two southeastern New England communities for the period from 1981 through 1990, the overall prevalence of estrogen therapy among 2,215 postmenopausal women increased from 5.3% in 1981–1982 to 10.9% in 1989–1990 (Derby 1993). The prevalence of postmenopausal estrogen use was substantially higher among women with surgical menopause than natural menopause (Figure 1.17).

Pronounced regional differences in the rate of estrogen use make it difficult to extrapolate these data to the overall U.S. population. Further, women of higher socioeconomic status may be disproportionately represented in these cohorts. Since postmenopausal estrogen therapy may be associated with socioeconomic status, data from these study populations may substantially overestimate the prevalence of estrogen use in the overall population.

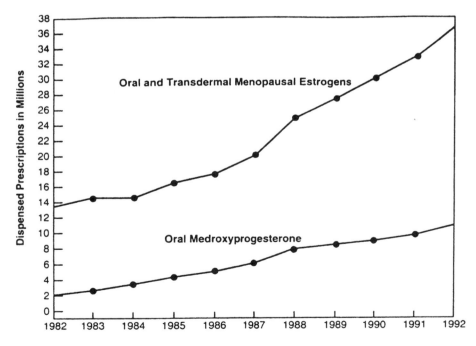

Fig. 1.16. Estimated number of dispensed prescriptions of oral and transdermal menopausal estrogens and medroxyprogesterone in the US, 1982–1992. [From Wysowski DK et al. (1995), with permission.]

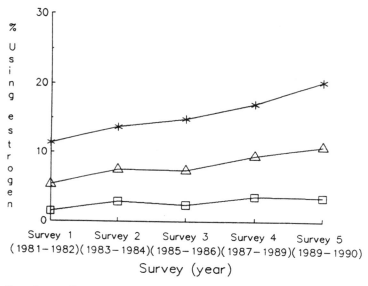

Fig. 1.17. Prevalence of postmenopausal estrogen use in women aged 40–64 in two south-eastern New England communities, by type of menopause, 1981–1990. (*, surgical menopause; △, all postmenopause; □, natural menopause) [From Derby CA et al. (1993), with permission.]

Public Health Impact of Coronary Risk Factors

As the summaries above have illustrated, despite favorable trends in some areas, such as cigarette smoking, serum cholesterol levels, and blood pressure, risk factors for CHD remain widely prevalent among the U.S. adult population. Data from the 1992 Behavioral Risk Factor Surveillance System were used to examine the prevalence of adults with no major CHD risk factors (MMWR 1994). The survey collected data from 91,428 adults of age 18 or older on six major coronary risk factors: current cigarette smoking, sedentary lifestyle (no or irregular leisure-time physical activity), obesity, hypertension, elevated blood cholesterol, and diabetes. Only 18% of those surveyed reported having none of the six major CHD risk factors; 35% of respondents reported having one risk factor; 29% reported two risk factors; 13% reported three risk factors; and 5% reported four to six risk factors. The prevalence of no risk factors increased with increasing level of education. Because the survey was based on self-reports, the prevalence of most risk factors is likely to have been underestimated. In particular, prevalence estimates will be underreported for risk factors with low awareness levels, such as cholesterol measurement (MMWR 1994).

With respect to the public health burden of coronary risk factors, using National Center for Health Statistics mortality data for 1986, the number of coronary heart disease deaths attributable to five major coronary risk factors has been estimated (Hahn 1990). As shown in Table 1.5, each of the five risk factors contributes substantially to CHD mortality in the United States. Each estimate considers the maximum potential impact of the factor, without controlling for the effects of other CHD risk factors.

Table 1.5. Number of Deaths and Proportions of Deaths (%) Attributable to Risk Factors for CHD: United States—1986

Risk Factor	Coronary Heart Disease
Total no. of deaths	593,111
Current/former smoking, (%)	148,879 (25.1)
Cholesterol level ≥5.20 mmol/L. (%)	253,194 (42.7)
Hypertension (systolic blood pressure ≥ 140 mmHg), (%)	171,121 (28.9)
Obesity (≥110/130% of desirable weight), (%)	190,456 (32.1)
No regular exercise, (%)	205,254 (34.6)
Diabetes, (%)	77,709 (13.1)

Adapted from Hahn et al. (1990), with permission.

CHD risk factors are highly correlated with one another, so the numbers of deaths and proportions are not additive.

The Role of Epidemiologic Studies: Complementary Approaches to Elucidating Determinants of Coronary Heart Disease and Effective Preventive Measures

The difficulty in quantifying the proportion of CHD deaths due to any one factor underscores the complex nature of atherogenesis as a multifactorial process. Potential determinants of atherosclerotic disease include nonmodifiable factors, such as age, sex, and race; behavioral characteristics, such as smoking and exercise; constitutional traits, such as blood pressure and body weight; and biochemical markers, such as serum cholesterol level. The correlations and complex interactions between factors can lead to difficulties in the establishment of associated risk. The situation is further complicated by imprecision in the definition of some potential risk factors.

Techniques in multivariate analysis allow epidemiologists to consider simultaneously a multiplicity of factors in very large databases. A risk factor that is causally linked to a particular disease should be strongly and consistently associated with disease. However, the strength of the association may depend on whether or not other related factors are controlled for. Inadequate control for related factors may result in either underestimation or overestimation of the true relationship of any factor with disease. Control for factors in the causal pathway would tend to underestimate any association. For example, obesity is clearly associated with increased risk of CHD, but the association appears to be mediated, at least in part, by hypertension, lipoprotein abnormalities, and diabetes mellitus. The apparent strength of the association of obesity with CHD will be attenuated by the degree to which one or more of these other factors are controlled for in the model.

The role of epidemiology in the development of preventive strategies involves a number of complementary methodologies (Hennekens 1987). These include descriptive studies, observational analytic studies (case-control studies and prospective cohort studies), randomized trials, meta-analyses, and cost- and risk-benefit analyses.

Descriptive studies, which have been the source of data used in this chapter, include case reports, case series, cross-sectional surveys, cross-cultural studies, and studies of population-based temporal trends. Case reports and case series describe characteristics associated with a particular disease, usually at the time of presentation. In cross-sectional surveys the prevalence of both disease and exposure variables are assessed at the same time among a group of individuals. Cross-cultural studies describe differences between populations in disease rates and the prevalence of potential risk factors, while population-based temporal trends describe changes in disease rates and potential risk factors within a population over time. The value of these studies is in the generation of hypotheses that can be tested in more analytic epidemiologic studies, such as case-control and prospective cohort studies as well as randomized trials.

The major contribution of descriptive studies, particularly cross-cultural and temporal trend, has been the strong suggestion that environmental factors play an important role in the development of atherosclerotic disease. As described earlier in this chapter, the relatively high rates of heart disease in northern, compared to southern, Europe, the differences in cardiovascular disease rates among industrialized and less developed nations, and changing heart disease rates over the past three decades in the United States and other westernized nations, strongly implicate environmental components in the pathogenesis of atherosclerotic disease. Migration studies such as the Ni-Hon-San study, which show increasing heart disease rates as Japanese men migrated from Japan to Honolulu and San Francisco, indicate that genetic factors can not explain a large portion of the cross-cultural differences in heart disease rates (Worth 1975).

The weakness of descriptive studies derives from the inability to control adequately for potential factors that may confound any apparent association, thus making it difficult to causally link any single factor with disease. Potential confounders include behavioral, dietary, and other lifestyle characteristics, differences in availability of health care resources, and genetics. For example, worldwide heart disease rates are correlated with the number of television sets per capita. This does not imply a causal relationship; the number of television sets per capita is merely a marker for other risk factors.

In contrast to descriptive studies, observational analytic studies (case-control and prospective cohort studies) enable researchers to attempt to control for potential confounders. Case-control studies are designed to identify cases of a particular disease and appropriately matched controls, and compare exposure status of potential risk factors obtained at the time disease status is established. Although case-control studies tend to be more efficient and less costly than prospective cohort studies, selection and recall bias may have an impact on risk estimates, since exposure status is ascertained after disease occurrence. Selection of both cases and matched controls may introduce bias, since selected cases or controls may not adequately represent the intended source populations. Cases may recall information regarding exposure status in a systematically different way in contrast to controls.

In prospective cohort studies, researchers ascertain exposure status at the beginning of the study and follow individuals for subsequent events. Like case-control studies, prospective studies are less subject to the biases of descriptive studies because the outcome as well as the exposure data are available for each individual in the study population, thus enabling control for many potential confounders. Furthermore, in contrast to case-control studies, the exposure is measured in prospective cohort studies before the development of clinically apparent disease, thereby minimizing the impact of recall and selection bias.

Case-control and prospective cohort studies are quite useful in establishing risk attributable to a single factor, particularly when the effect of a given risk factor is large. When the effect size is large it is often not necessary or feasible to conduct randomized trials. The observational data on cigarette smoking and increased risk of lung cancer was so overwhelming that it would have been unethical to randomize individuals to cigarette smoking. On the other hand, when searching for small to moderate effects, the amount of uncontrolled confounding in observational studies may be as large as the likely risk reduction itself. In this case, randomized trials may be necessary to establish an association and quantify reliably its magnitude. In addition, when there are competing risks and benefits, randomized trials may be needed to determine the net effect of any given intervention. Estrogen replacement therapy, for example, appears to confer a protective effect on risk of CHD and osteoporosis, but such benefits must be weighed against the potential risks of breast and uterine cancer. In randomized trials, investigators allocate subjects to various treatment groups and observe subsequent effects of each treatment. Large randomized trials overcome some of the limitations of observational epidemiologic studies by equally distributing the known as well as the unknown confounders among treatment groups.

In some instances, data from individual observational studies or randomized trials are not sufficient to establish a clear risk or benefit of a factor or intervention. Therefore, it may be helpful to pool data from several studies in an overview or meta-analysis. Pooling data from either observational studies or randomized trials may be difficult if there are major differences in study design, interventional strategies, or definitions of exposure variables or outcome measures. Meta-analyses must be interpreted cautiously because the results may depend on how the data are summarized or the underlying assumptions that dictate the studies to be included in any analysis.

Once reasonable estimates of risk and benefit for a particular risk factor or intervention have been established, cost:- and risk:benefit analyses can be helpful in establishing guidelines for intervention. Similar to estimates derived from meta-analyses, those from cost:- and risk:benefit analyses are often quite dependent on the underlying assumptions for a given analysis.

Summary

This chapter has utilized descriptive studies to summarize trends in coronary heart disease rates and CHD risk factors. While such studies have provided strong support for the hypothesis that there are modifiable determinants of CHD, descriptive studies alone rarely provide sufficient evidence to demonstrate a causal link between a particular factor and disease occurrence. The following chapters review the data from analytic observational studies as well as randomized trials that provide direct quantitative evidence on the relationship of coronary risk factors to disease occurrence. Each chapter also provides a detailed assessment of the current clinical approach to reducing CHD risk through the control or elimination of specific risk factors or through the use of preventive interventions. Cost-effectiveness analyses are provided, where data are available. The strength of the evidence on the effect of modification of each factor is also graded in each chapter and summarized in a table in the final chapter.

In addition to chapters focusing on those risk factors and interventions that have been described in this chapter, the role of stress, anger, and psychosocial factors is explored. Preventive interventions are reviewed in Section II, with chapters on aspirin prophylaxis, antioxidant vitamins, and other promising nutritional interventions. Gender differences in CHD risk and risk factors as well as postmenopausal hormone therapy, are examined in Section III on prevention of heart disease in women. The recognition that atherosclerosis begins early in life has led to increased attention to the issue of risk factor surveillance and intervention in childhood and adolescence. These issues are explored in Section IV. Half of all coronary events occur among individuals with a history of coronary disease. Section V reviews current strategies in secondary prevention of CHD. Finally, several promising new areas of research in the prevention of MI are explored in Section VI, and a table summarizes achievable risk reductions in the last chapter. Patient education and health promotion appendices are provided throughout the textbook.

References

American Heart Association. 1993 Heart and Stroke Facts. Dallas: American Heart Association, 1992.

American Heart Association. Heart and Stroke Facts: 1994 Statistical Supplement. Dallas: American Heart Association, 1993.

Berlin JA, Colditz GA. A meta-analysis of physical activity in the prevention of coronary heart disease. Am J Epidemiol 1990;132:639–46.

Burke GL, Sprafka JM, Folsom AR, et al. Trends in serum cholesterol levels from 1980 to 1987: the Minnesota Heart Survey. N Engl J Med 1991;324:941–6.

Centers for Disease Control (CDC). Cigarette smoking among adults: United States, 1990. MMWR 1992;41:354, 355, 361, 362.

Centers for Disease Control (CDC). Cigarette smoking among adults–United States 1993, MMWR 1993;42:230–33.

Centers for Disease Control. Prevalence of sedentary lifestyle–Behavioral Risk Factor Surveillance, United States, 1991. MMWR 1993;42:576–79.

Dannenberg AL, Drizd T, Horan MJ, et al. Progress in the battle against hypertension: changes in blood pressure levels in the United States from 1960 to 1980. Hypertension 1987; 10:226–33.

Department of Health and Human Services. Blood pressure levels in persons 18–74 years of age in 1976–80, and trends in blood pressure from 1960 to 1980 in the United States.

Hyattsville, MD: National Center for Health Statistics, DHHS Publication (PHS) 86-1684, 1986.

Department of Health and Human Services. Healthy People 2000: national health promotion and disease prevention objectives for the nation. Washington, DC: Public Health Service, 1991.

Department of Health and Human Services. Health United States, 1991. Hyattsville, MD: National Center for Health Statistics, 1992.

Department of Health and Human Services. Reducing the health consequences of smoking: 25 years of progress. DHHS Publication (CDC) 89-8411, 1989.

Derby CA, Hume AL, Barbour MM, et al. Correlates of postmenopausal estrogen use and trends through the 1980s in two southeastern New England communities. Am J Epidemiol 1993;137:1125–35.

Epstein FH. Die historische Entwicklung des Cholesterin-Atherosklerose-Konzepts. Ther Umsch 1990;47:435–42.

Expert Panel on Detection, Evaluation, and Treatment of High Blood Cholesterol in Adults. Summary of the Second Report of the National Cholesterol Education Program (NCEP) Expert Panel on Detection, Evaluation, and Treatment of High Blood Cholesterol in Adults (Adult Treatment Panel II). JAMA 1993;269:3015–23.

Fiore MC. Trends in cigarette smoking in the United States. Med Clin North Am 1992;76:289–303.

Geiss LS, Herman WH, Goldschmid MG, et al. Surveillance for diabetes mellitus: United States, 1980–1989. MMWR 1993;42:1–20.

Goldman L. Cook EF. The decline in ischemic heart disease mortality rates. Ann Intern Med 1984;101:825–36.

Hahn RA, Teutsch SM, Rothenberg RB, Marks JS. Excess deaths from nine chronic diseases in the United States, 1986. JAMA 1990;264:2654–9.

Harris MI, Hadden WC, Knowler WC, Bennett PH. Prevalence of diabetes and impaired glucose tolerance and plasma glucose tolerance levels in U.S. population aged 20–74 years. Diabetes 1987;36:523–34.

He J, Klag MJ, Whelton PK, et al. Migration, blood pressure pattern, and hypertension: the Yi Migrant Study. Am J Epidemiol 1991;134:1085–101.

Hennekens CH, Buring JE. Epidemiology in medicine. Boston: Little, Brown, 1987.

Jarrett RJ. Epidemiology and public health aspects of non-insulin-dependent diabetes mellitus. Epidemiol Rev 1989;11:151–71.

Johannes CB, Crawford SL, Posner JG, McKinlay SM. Longitudinal patterns and correlates of hormone replacement therapy use in middle-aged women. Am J Epidemiol 1994;140:439–52.

Johnson CL, Rifkind BM, Sempos CT, et al. Declining serum total cholesterol levels among US adults: the National Health and Nutrition Examination Surveys. JAMA 1993;269:3002–8.

Kennedy DL, Baum C, Forbes MB. Noncontraceptive estrogens and progestins: use patterns over time. Obstet Gynecol 1985;65:441–6.

Keys A. Seven countries. Cambridge, MA: Harvard University Press, 1980.

Kuczmarski RJ, Flegal KM, Campbell SM, Johnson CL. Increasing prevalence of overweight among US adults: the National Health and Nutrition Examination Surveys, 1960 to 1991. JAMA 1994;272:205–11.

Manson JE, Tosteson H, Ridker PM, et al. Medical Progress: Primary prevention of myocardial infarction. N Engl J Med 1992;326:1406–16.

Morbidity and Mortality Weekly Report. Prevalence of adults with no known major risk factors for coronary heart disease: behavioral risk factor surveillance system, 1992. MMWR 1994;43:61–3,69.

National Center for Health Statistics, Hadden WC, Harris MI. Prevalence of diagnosed diabetes, undiagnosed diabetes, and impaired glucose tolerance in adults 20–74 years of age, United States, 1976–80. Hyattsville, MD: National Center for Health Statistics. Vital and Health Statistics, Series 11, No. 237, 1987.

National High Blood Pressure Education Program Working Group. National High Blood Pressure Education Program Working Group Report on Primary Prevention of Hypertension. Arch Intern Med 1993;153:186–208.

Peto R, Lopez AD, Broeham J, et al. Mortality from tobacco in developed countries: indirect estimates from national vital statistics. Lancet 1992;339:1268–78.

Pierce JP, Fiore MC, Novotny TE, et al. Trends in cigarette smoking in the United States: projections to the year 2000. JAMA 1989;261:61–5.

Shaper AG. Communities without hypertension. In: Shaper AG, Hutt MSR, Feifar Z, eds. Cardiovascular disease in the tropics. London: British Medical Association, 1974, pp. 77–83.

Siegel PZ, Brackbill RM, Frazier EL, et al. Behavioral risk factor surveillance, 1986–1990. MMWR 1991; 40(No. SS-4):1–23.

Stamler J, Stamler R, Neaton JD. Blood pressure, systolic and diastolic, and cardiovascular risks. Arch Intern Med 1993;153:598–615.

Stampfer MJ, Willett WC, Colditz GA, et al. A prospective study of postmenopausal estrogen therapy and coronary heart disease. N Engl J Med 1985;313:1044–9.

Stampfer MJ, Colditz GA. Estrogen replacement therapy and coronary heart disease: a quantitative assessment of the epidemiologic evidence. Prev Med 1991;20:47–63.

Thom TJ. International mortality from heart disease: rates and trends. Int J Epidemiol 1989;18: S20–8.

Whelton PK. Epidemiology of hypertension. Lancet 1994;344:101–6.

Whelton PK, Brancati FL. Hypertension management in populations. Clin Exp Hypertens 1993; 15:1147–56.

Worth RM, Kata H, Rhoads GG, et al. Epidemiologic studies of coronary heart disease and stroke in Japanese men living in Japan, Hawaii and California: mortality. Am J Epidemiol 1975;102:481–90.

Wysowski DK, Golden L, Burke L. Use of menopausal estrogens and medroxyprogesterone in the United States, 1982–1992. Obstet Gynecol 1995;85:6–10.

2

The Pathogenesis of Atherosclerosis and Acute Thrombosis: Relevance to Strategies of Cardiovascular Disease Prevention

Paul M. Ridker

Understanding current concepts in the etiology and pathogenesis of atherosclerosis is fundamental for practitioners concerned with the primary prevention of coronary heart disease (CHD). Research completed during the past decade indicates that complex interactions between vascular injury, inflammatory response, oxidation of lipids, hemodynamic shear stress, and endogenous fibrinolytic activation are all involved in the initiation, progression, and acute rupture of the atherosclerotic plaque. Thus, the century-old ''incrustation'' and ''lipid'' hypotheses of atherogenesis first presented by Rokitansky (1852) and Virchow (1856) have been radically modified by recent findings. These modifications have led to a separation of *atherogenic* from *thrombotic* risk factors, to a broader understanding of both the chronic and acute phases of vascular occlusion, and to new concepts of plaque stabilization and regression. These concepts form the basis for understanding accepted preventive strategies as well as the framework for novel approaches to the prevention of CHD.

In the first part of this chapter, current concepts in the pathogenesis of atherosclerosis and thrombosis are reviewed with an emphasis on how these principles are related to cardiovascular prevention. In the second part, a series of important hemostatic and thrombotic markers of risk and their potential use in cardiovascular screening are examined.

Pathogenesis of Atherosclerosis

Initiation of Atherosclerosis

In the broadest terms, atherosclerosis is the result of an exaggerated inflammatory response to injury of the endothelial and smooth muscles cells of the arterial wall (Munro 1988; Libby 1991; Ross 1993). The earliest pathologic lesion of atherosclerosis, the ''fatty streak,'' represents the accumulation of lipid-laden macrophages and lymphocytes within the arterial intima. Autopsy studies among both Korean (Enos 1953) and Vietnamese (McNamara 1971) war casualties indicate that these precursor lesions are common among young men in the United States. Recent and detailed work from the Pathological Determinants of Atherosclerosis in Youth (PDAY) Research Group (PDAY Research Group 1990) indicates that as early as age 15, male subjects with coronary risk factors have over 30% of their abdominal aorta involved with lesions, as compared with 10% in age-matched subjects without traditional risk factors. Further, these precursor lesions of atherosclerosis do not occur randomly but have a predictable topographic distribution, suggesting that local shear stresses may be a critical factor in the initiation of vascular injury (Cornhill 1990; Strong 1992).

A clear relationship exists between early atherosclerosis and traditional "adult" coronary risk factors. In the PDAY study, the extent of atherosclerosis in the aorta and right coronary artery in young men was positively associated with low density (LDL) and very low density (VLDL) lipoprotein cholesterol and negatively correlated with serum high density lipoprotein cholesterol (HDL). Similarly, the serum thiocyanate concentration, a strong marker for recent smoking, was associated with prevalence of raised atherosclerotic lesions in the abdominal aorta of young men (PDAY Research Group 1990).

The finding of a correlation between LDL cholesterol and early fatty streak lesions is consistent with the hypothesis that oxidation of LDL plays a central role in atheroma formation. Oxidized LDL is a potent attractant for local monocyte adhesion to the arterial intimal surface as well as invasion into the underlying media (Steinberg 1989). A series of studies employing hypercholesterolemic animals indicate that, once inside, these migrating monocytes become macrophages, locally accumulate lipid, transform into foam cells, and then—with accompanying smooth muscle proliferation—form the earliest fatty streaks (Ross 1993). This process of cellular transformation appears consistently to follow intimal vascular injury, whether chronic and mild (the classical explanation of spontaneous atherosclerosis) or due to toxic or mechanical denudation (Ip 1990). Transition of the fatty streak into a palpable lipid-rich plaque surrounded by fibrotic cap has been characterized as occurring in five distinct phases (Stary I to Stary V), which reflect complex interactions between smooth muscles cells, platelets, the endothelium, and growth factors derived from these sources (Stary 1989).

Progression of Atherosclerosis and Acute Coronary Occlusion

Early hypotheses concerning atherogenesis assumed that small atheromatous lesions, once formed, grew inevitably inward to yield vascular occlusion. Several paradoxical findings, however, strongly challenged these initial assumptions.

First, the prevalence of early atherosclerosis does not correlate closely with the incidence of myocardial infarction (MI). For example, data from the International Atherosclerosis Project (McGill 1968) indicate that fatty streaks are common in countries with both high and low incidence rates for infarction, suggesting that the rate of progression of atherosclerosis—not its initiation—may be the major difference between high- and low-risk populations. Indeed, contrary to the widely held opinion that more atherosclerosis is linearly associated with higher risk of MI, it has been argued that the risk of infarction rises sharply only after a threshold level of atherosclerosis has been reached (Gofman 1969).

Second, despite the presence of fatty streaks, there appear to be "lesion-prone" and "lesion-resistant" arteries, suggesting that local anatomic and hemodynamic forces play a significant role in atherosclerotic progression independent of fatty streak initiation (Gertz 1990). While the mechanisms underlying these differences remain unclear, differential rates of atherosclerotic progression in the internal mammary as compared with the coronary arteries have been exploited for great clinical benefit in patients undergoing coronary artery bypass surgery.

Finally, a series of prospective clinical studies indicate that the artery with the tightest stenosis is not necessarily the artery most likely to occlude. Specifically, it is becoming increasingly apparent that MI occurs more often in vessels with stenoses of 70% or less rather than in vessels with tighter obstructions (Ambrose 1988; Little 1988; Webster 1990; Little 1991; Giroud 1992). In one study of patients suffering acute infarction who were treated with thrombolytic therapy, the severity of underlying atherosclerotic stenoses in the infarct-related artery was measured to be less than 50% in one-third of cases and between 50% and 60% in another third (Brown 1986). At the same time, severe stenoses tend to progress to near-total occlusion at rates almost threefold that of less severe stenoses (Webster 1990).

At least in part as a response to these paradoxical findings, an evolving concept in the pathogenesis of atherosclerosis is that factors involved in the initiation of atherosclerosis may well be different from factors involved in the progression of prevalent lesions. Moreover, rather than being a simple continuation of the underlying inflammatory response, rapid progression of plaque appears to occur in a process of plaque fissuring, rupture, acute thrombus formation, and subsequent fibrotic organization. This process, distinct from that involved in the initiation of atherosclerosis, appears related more the thrombogenic risk than to usual atherogenic risk factors (Figure 2.1)

Although only recently accepted, the concepts that acute thrombus formation is the final common pathway for most vascular occlusions (DeWood 1980) and that this thrombus formation usually results from "rupture" of the underlying atherosclerotic plaque (Constantinides 1966; Davies 1985) are not new. Recent reviews have described in detail the process of plaque rupture and repair that characterizes the fast progressing complex atherosclerotic plaque (Schwartz 1991; Fuster 1992). In brief, as demonstrated in autopsy studies of patients with atheromatous disease (Davies 1988), fissures appear to occur on a regular basis in prevalent atherosclerotic plaques. These fissures or "ruptures" acutely disrupt the intima underlying plaque, a process leading to rapid platelet aggregation, which, if unchecked, can lead to complete vessel occlusion and subsequent infarction (Figure 2.2). More often than not, complete occlusion does not ensure. Rather, in response to activation of the endogenous fibrinolytic system, recanalization occurs with restoration of anterograde flow. Along with resealing of the fissure, local inflammation, and fibrosis, an increase in the absolute size and volume of the plaque can be observed.

The plaque rupture hypothesis of atherosclerotic progression is critical to evolving strategies of cardiovascular prevention. First, the concept that plaque rupture acutely leads to coronary occlusion helps to explain the clinical observation that "triggers" of vascular occlusion exist and that these triggers are a primary mechanism leading

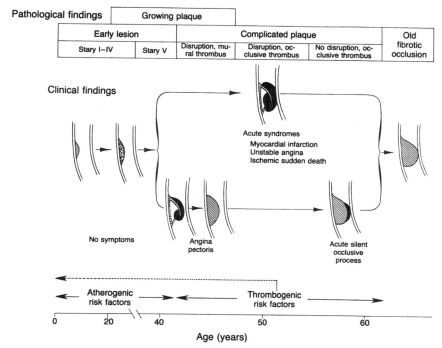

Fig. 2.1. Atherosclerotic initiation and progression. [From Fuster et al. (1992), with permission.]

to the circadian variation of MI and sudden death (Muller 1985, 1987; Ridker 1990). Second, because an important immediate result of plaque rupture is the activation of platelet function and subsequent platelet/fibrin deposition, the plaque rupture hypothesis helps to explain the clinical efficacy of aspirin in both the primary and secondary prevention of cardiovascular disease (Hennekens 1990) and is consistent with the observation that the clinical effect of prophylactic aspirin appears to result from inhibition of thrombosis rather than a slowing of atherogenesis (Ridker 1991).

The plaque rupture theory of vascular occlusion is also critical to prevention strategies because it implies that certain plaques are more likely to rupture than others and that strategies designed to decrease the probability of rupture may be of great clinical utility (Falk 1992). Current data indicate that the risk of plaque rupture depends more on plaque type than plaque volume and that "rupture-prone" plaques tend to be rich in soft extracellular lipids (Falk 1989; Richardson 1989). Specifically, it appears that smaller, less sclerotic plaques are more likely to rupture than are larger fibrotic plaques. In addition, plaque rupture is not a random process but one that occurs in a predictable manner dependent in part on hemodynamic shear stresses and local characteristics of the plaque ultrastructure (Figure 2.3) (Loree 1994; Cheng 1993). Recent studies suggest that inflammation itself plays a role in destabilizing the fibrous cap that overlies atherosclerotic lesions, a finding that indicates the initially reparative

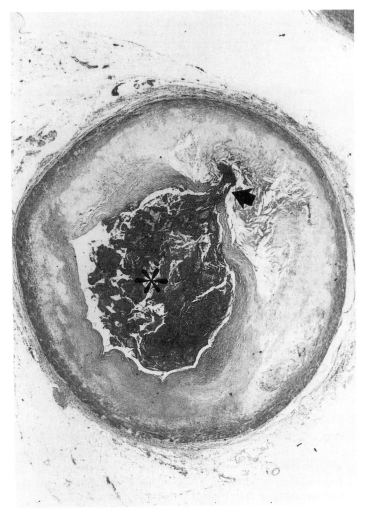

Fig. 2.2. Histologic cross section of human coronary artery showing evidence of plaque fissuring and rupture. (Courtesy of Dr. Frederick Schoen.)

inflammatory process may also mediate future plaque rupture (Buja 1994; van Der Waal 1994).

It is intriguing to speculate that several currently employed prevention practices may be effective in part because they reduce the probability of acute plaque rupture. For example, beta-blockers, which have proven so effective in secondary prevention (Yusuf 1985), may alter plaque vulnerability by reducing the cumulative hemodynamic strain placed on unstable plaque. (See Chapter 18 for further discussion.) Similarly, antiplatelet therapy may be effective by limiting the aggregation of platelets following plaque rupture (Antiplatelet Trialists' Collaboration 1994). Further, the observation

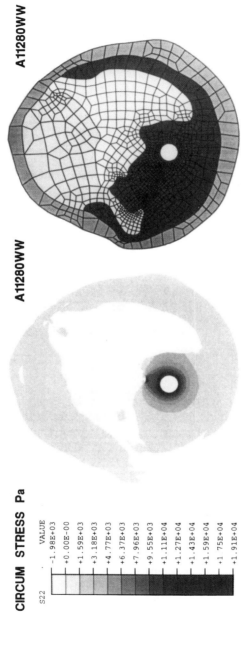

Fig. 2.3. Cross sectional structure-function map of human coronary artery showing sites of predicted plaque rupture. (Courtesy of Dr. Richard Lee.)

Table 2.1. Principal Results of Major Angiographic Lipid–Lowering Trials

			Stenosis Progression		Stenosis Regression	
			Treatment Group (%)	Control Group (%)	Treatment Group (%)	Control Group (%)
Study	Reference	Year				
NHLBI II	Brensike	1984	32	49	7	7
CLAS I	Blankenhorn	1987	39	61	16	2
POSCH	Buchwald	1990	37	65	14	6
Lifestyle	Ornish	1990	14	32	41	32
FATS	Brown	1990	23	46	36	11
CLAS II	Cashin-Hemphill	1990	30	83	18	6
UC-SCOR	Kane	1990	20	41	33	13
SCRIP	Aldermann	1991	—	—	21	10
STARS	Watts	1992	13	46	35	4
Heidelberg	Schuler	1992	23	47	28	6

Source: Adapted from Brown et al. (1993), with permission.

Data shown are percent progression and regression for treatment and control groups, respectively. See text for details of interventions.

that the increased risk of coronary occlusion associated with smoking declines soon after quitting raises the possibility that cigarette consumption has a direct effect on plaque stability, independent of any effect on fatty streak initiation (Rosenberg 1985, 1990).

Plaque Stabilization and Regression

The most important preventive strategy to arise from the plaque rupture hypothesis is related to the evolving concepts of plaque stabilization and regression. Given that it is the *type* rather than the *size* of plaque that is related to rupture, the possibility has been raised that strategies designed to convert soft, lipid-laden plaques into mature fibrotic plaques may reduce the occurrence of future rupture (Blankenhorn 1989). In the laboratory, the ability to effect such a change has been demonstrated with the use of several lipid-lowering strategies that preferentially "leech" mobile soft lipid from vulnerable plaques, a process resulting in a firmer and less vulnerable fibrotic structure (Small 1988; Wissler 1990). This process of lipid depletion is selective in that soft cholesterol esters in foam cells and lipoproteins are more mobile than are the cholesterol monohydrate crystals of the core lipid zone (Small 1984). Histologic measurements of lesions clearly indicate in animal models that plaque size is reduced during "regression" therapy.

From the perspective of the prevention-oriented clinician, the hypothesis that lipid reduction may delay or even inhibit plaque rupture has gained substantial support with the presentation of data from nine lipid-lowering clinical trials in which angiographic studies were performed before and after experimental interventions (Table 2.1) (Brown 1993). These studies used different comparative approaches to lipid reduction:

1. Dietary therapy alone with diet plus cholestyramine (Brensike 1984)
2. Diet alone with diet plus combinations of niacin, colestipol, and lovastatin (Blankenhorn 1987; Brown 1990; Cashin-Hemphill 1990; Kane 1990; Watts 1992
3. Usual care with partial ileal bypass (Buchwald 1990)
4. Usual care with vegetarian diet, exercise, and relaxation (Ornish 1990)
5. Usual care with a risk reduction program including blood pressure control, lipid reduction, weight loss, smoking cessation, and counseling (Alderman 1991)
6. Usual care with a low-fat diet plus regular exercise (Schuler 1992).

These studies included a wide spectrum of patients with and without hyperlipidemia or known coronary disease.

Despite substantial differences in inclusion criteria, angiographic definitions, and interventional approach, each of these studies demonstrated a net benefit associated with treatment; overall, 8% of the control group patients demonstrated coronary regression as compared with 24% among treated patients (Brown 1993). In what is perhaps the most tightly controlled of these trials, the Familial Atherosclerosis Treatment Study, mean coronary stenosis severity increased by 3% in the control group, while decreasing 1% to 2% in the treatment groups (Brown 1990).

It is important to point out that the absolute change in lesion size in all of these trials is exceptionally small, usually <0.1 mm. Nonetheless, angiographic stabilization of plaque size was a consistent finding in treated patients as compared with control patients in these lipid-lowering trials. Further, a trend toward decreasing rates of vascular events was also found, although as a group these studies were not designed with adequate power to assess clinical outcomes adequately.

Taken together, available data indicate that stenoses subjected to lipid-lowering strategies *progress* less rapidly and *regress* more often than do control lesions. To date, the angiographic and histologic changes observed in association with lipid reduction have not been linked to significant reductions in coronary events. However, these angiographic and pathologic findings are consistent with clinical data from the Lipid Research Clinics (LRC 1984) and Helsinki Heart Trial (Manninen 1988) results, which indicate reduced rates of total cardiac events (although not mortality) associated with long-term cholesterol reduction.

Endothelial Dysfunction and Atherosclerosis

The development of atherosclerosis has deleterious effects that extend beyond plaque growth and luminal occlusion. In particular, emerging evidence indicates that atherosclerosis may adversely interact with several functions of the vascular endothelium, a process that often leads to further myocardial ischemia.

Traditionally, the vascular endothelium has been regarded as a permeable but relatively inert nonthrombogenic barrier, which served to separate blood elements from underlying vascular smooth muscle. This view has been radically altered by experimental studies, indicating that the vascular endothelium directly interacts with hemostasis and thrombosis through several antiplatelet, antithrombotic, and fibrinolytic functions. Of particular importance with regard to myocardial ischemia is the finding that the endothelium synthesizes several important coronary vasodilators, including endothelium-derived relaxing factor (EDRF), a substance related to nitric oxide radicals, which has potent vasodilatory effects (Furchgott 1980; Palmer 1987). Indeed, emerging evidence suggests that endothelium-dependent vasodilation is a critical function of the normal intact vascular wall.

It is now apparent that atherosclerosis often renders dysfunctional the underlying endothelium, impairing the production and secretion of factors like endothelium-derived relaxing factor (Meridith 1993). Such endothelial dysfunction not only inhibits the ability of the artery to dilate in response to stress, but actually can lead to paradoxical vasoconstriction in the presence of substances like acetycholine, which normally dilate coronary segments (Ludmer 1986). Important endothelial dysfunction does not appear to be limited to advanced or stenotic coronary lesions but can be observed in arteries with minimal atherosclerosis (Werns 1989). In fact, loss of normal endothelial relaxation appears to correlate with the presence of coronary risk factors (Vita 1990), particularly with systemic hypertension (Treasure 1992). A major component of the premature coronary narrowing commonly found in cardiac transplant patients also appears mediated by endothelial dysfunction.

As our understanding of endothelium-dependent vasodilitation evolves, it is probable that entirely new strategies for coronary disease prevention will develop that focus on the restoration of normal vascular relaxation. In this regard, experimental data suggest that cholesterol reduction using dietary and pharmacologic methods can in some situations reverse endothelial dysfunction (Harrison 1987; Osborne 1989). Promising data also suggest that administration of *l*-arginine, the precursor to nitric oxide, may also restore endothelial function (Drexler 1991). Several on-going clinical trials should determine whether such effects can be translated into lowered rates of vascular occlusion.

Hemostatic and Thrombotic Risk Factors

While lipid lowering and its effects on plaque stability represent one approach to prevention directly related to the atherosclerotic process, a second approach involves the identification and early treatment of subjects at increased risk for acute coronary thrombosis. Until recently, most efforts to identify high-risk patients have focused on atherogenic risk factors, particularly total and HDL cholesterol. Unfortunately, these markers of atherogenic initiation and progression fail to identify the majority of subjects at risk for future coronary thrombosis. For example, in the United Kingdom Heart Disease Prevention Project, high-risk patients identified by elevated blood pressure, smoking, and hyperlipidemia accounted for only 32% of all future infarctions (Heller 1984). Similarly, in recent data from the British United Provident Association Study (Wald 1994) where the false-positive screening rate was set at 5%, detection rates for future cardiovascular deaths were only 12% using total cholesterol alone and 30% for the most efficient combination of total cholesterol, HDL cholesterol, apolipoproteins, blood pressure, smoking status, and family history.

Blood Rheology, Fibrinogen, and Viscosity

In an effort to identify individuals at high risk for acute thrombosis, several investigations have examined whether hemostatic and thrombotic markers of risk are predictive of future cardiovascular disease. Of these potential markers, serum fibrinogen level and plasma viscosity—the two primary determinants of blood rheology—have been the best studied.

With regard to fibrinogen, observational data indicate that patients with angina have increased fibrinogen levels (Rainer 1987) and that plasma fibrinogen increases with severity of coronary artery disease (Lowe 1980; Broadhurst 1990). At least six well-controlled prospective cohort studies have demonstrated a positive association between plasma fibrinogen level and cardiovascular risk, even among otherwise healthy individuals. In the Northwick Park Heart Study, for example, higher baseline fibrinogen (and factor VII) levels were found among individuals who subsequently died of cardiovascular disease or suffered a nonfatal vascular event (Figure 2.4) (Meade 1986). Similarly, in the Leigh Clinical Research Unit study in which a cohort of 297 men were followed for seven years, plasma fibrinogen was found to be the strongest independent predictor of future coronary occlusion (Stone 1985). These associations have subsequently been confirmed in the Goteborg (Wilhelmsen 1984), Framingham (Kannel 1987), and Caerphilly (Yarnell 1991) populations. Taken together, these studies indicate a 1.6-fold increase in incidence of cardiovascular disease for each standard deviation increase fibrinogen level, independent of usual atherogenic factors.

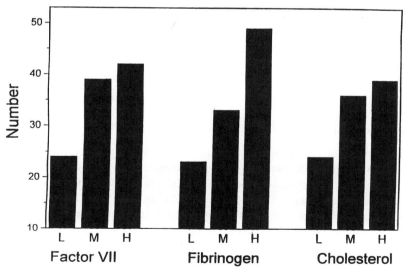

Fig. 2.4. The relationship of factor VII, fibrinogen, and total cholesterol to incidence of future ischemic heart disease: principal findings of the Northwick Park Heart Study. *L*, lowest, *M*, middle, and *H*, highest tertile. [Adapted from Meade et al. (1986), with permission.]

While plasma fibrinogen appears to be an independent cardiovascular risk factor, it is related to other known predictors of coronary occlusion. Fibrinogen levels increase with age and body mass index and are positively correlated with serum cholesterol. Smoking appears to elevate fibrinogen in a dose-dependent and reversible manner. Reduced fibrinogen levels have been reported among individuals who regularly exercise, eat vegetarian diets, and consume moderate levels of alcohol (Ernst 1990).

While blood viscosity and fibrinogen are closely related, the Caerphilly and Speedwell studies (Yarnell 1991) demonstrated that these hemorheologic factors—while not entirely independent of traditional risk factors—were as predictive of future ischemic heart disease as were a combination of cholesterol, body mass, age, and blood pressure. Overall, men with the highest levels of either blood viscosity or plasma fibrinogen had age-adjusted risks of ischemic heart disease more than four times that of men with the lowest levels. Confirmatory studies indicate that blood viscosity is a strong marker of risk both in healthy individuals (Moller 1991) and in those with unstable angina (Neumann 1991).

Plasma fibrinogen also appears to be a marker of risk for stroke. In the major prospective study conducted to date, baseline fibrinogen level was associated with future stroke, but the relationship was substantially attenuated when smoking, cholesterol, and blood pressure were accounted for (Wilhelmsen 1984). Case-control studies of patients with recent stroke are difficult to interpret, as fibrinogen is an acute-phase reactant. Thus, only those studies in which fibrinogen is assessed well after the index event provide interpretable data. In one such analysis (Qizilbash 1991), fibrinogen levels higher than 3.6 g/L were associated with a twofold increase in risk of ischemic stroke, an effect that persisted after controlling for other cardiovascular risk factors.

Smoking cessation is the single most effective intervention to reduce fibrinogen level. In addition, evidence is accumulating that regular exercise may favorably alter fibrinogen levels (Stratton 1991). However, no pharmacologic regimen is currently recommended that can effectively reduce fibrinogen without unacceptable side effects. Of equal importance, no prospective data are available from which to assess whether reducing fibrinogen on a preventive basis yields any net health benefits.

Platelet Size, Function, and Aggregation

As platelets and platelet-derived growth factors play a major role in thrombosis, it is not surprising that baseline platelet function has also emerged as a potential independent risk factor for acute coronary occlusion (Wilhelmsen 1991). This hypothesis has gained considerable strength from four recent studies of platelet function and acute thrombosis. In the first of these, platelet hyperreactivity as measured by spontaneous platelet aggregation (SPA) was found to be a useful marker for survival and secondary coronary events among a cohort of patients followed for five years after their index MI (Trip 1990). Specifically, postinfarction patients who were SPA-positive had a relative risk of death more than five times that of the SPA-negative group. Although these results are based upon small samples and few events (6 deaths among 94 SPA-negative and 9 deaths among 26 SPA-positive patients), they are consistent with earlier studies indicating a link between platelet reactivity and complications of coronary artery disease. Indeed, a shortened bleeding time—the best clinical marker of heightened platelet reactivity—is often seen in acute infarction patients.

The second important study evaluating platelet function and risks of cardiovascular disease derives from cross-sectional data from the Caerphilly Collaborative Heart Disease Study, in which platelet aggregation was measured in blood obtained from nearly 2,000 men with no history of recent aspirin or nonsteroidal antiinflammatory drug use (Elwood 1991). For ADP-induced aggregation, a strong relationship was found between platelet function and a past history of MI, particularly when the analysis was restricted to the extreme upper and lower quintiles of induced platelet aggregation.

Third, data are now available that indicate that platelet size measured several months after a first MI may be a sensitive marker of future thrombotic risk; among 1,716 men who had platelet studies performed six months after their first infarction, mean platelet volume was greater among those individuals who suffered a recurrent infarction and among those who died. This effect was largely independent of usual coronary risk factors (Figure 2.5) (Martin 1991).

Finally, strong epidemiologic data linking platelet concentration and function to subsequent vascular disease has been provided by the publication of the first prospective study to evaluate these issues. Among 487 apparently healthy Norwegian men followed over a decade for the occurrence of vascular disease, a significantly

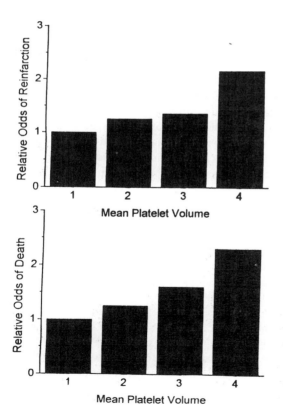

Fig. 2.5. Relative odds of reinfarction and death associated with increasing quintiles of platelet volume and platelet count among 1,700 British men. [Adapted from Martin et al. (1991), with permission.]

higher rate of cardiovascular mortality was observed among subjects with the highest platelet counts (RR = 2.5 for individuals in the top quartile, p = .0025) (Thaulow 1991). As in earlier case-control studies, part of the increase in platelet concentration was due to concurrent cigarette smoking, although control for this factor in multivariate analysis did not materially alter the strength and independence of the association.

While the prognostic importance of platelet size and concentration is relatively new, the efficacy of antiplatelet agents in treatment of cardiovascular disease and, more recently, in primary prevention, is widely appreciated. At least 25 trials have consistently demonstrated the efficacy of low-dose aspirin in both the primary and secondary prevention of CHD (Hennekens 1990; Antiplatelet Trialists' Collaboration 1994a). (See Chapter 12 for detailed discussion.) Recent overviews also indicate the efficacy of aspirin in the prevention of deep venous thrombosis and pulmonary embolism as well as in the long-term maintainence of vascular grafts (Antiplatelet Trialists' Collaboration 1994a, 1994c). In addition to aspirin, other pharmacologic, dietary, and behavioral interventions alter platelet function. Organic nitrates have antiplatelet properties in addition to effects on vascular smooth muscle and arteriolar dilation (Stamler 1991). Diets with high ratios of polyunsaturated to saturated fats (Beswick 1991) and those with increased n-3 fatty acids (Nelson 1991) have been associated with reduced platelet aggregability. Smoking cessation may also change platelet reactivity, although prospective data on this interaction are not currently available.

Endogenous Fibrinolytic Capacity: The Role of Plasminogen Activators and Plasminogen Activator Inhibitors

Abnormalities of endogenous fibrinolysis have long been thought to increase the risk of acute thrombosis. In large part, the systemic fibrinolytic balance between thrombosis and hemorrhage is mediated by two proteins, endogenous tissue-type plasminogen activator (tPA) and its fast-acting inhibitor, plasminogen activator inhibitor-type one (PAI-1). With the development of commercially available assays for these factors, data have begun to accumulate describing the association between fibrinolytic state and vascular occlusion.

With respect to venous thromboembolism, an overview of available studies suggests that the acceptance of impaired fibrinolysis as a clinical risk factor may be premature (Prins 1991). In large part, this conclusion is based on the absence of appropriately controlled studies in which otherwise healthy individuals were prospectively followed for the occurrence of deep venous thrombosis or pulmonary embolism. Such skepticism—despite a wide range of case reports and retrospective studies to the contrary (Wiman 1991)—appears to be warranted. In the only controlled prospective study in which baseline tPA and PAI-1 levels have been analyzed with respect to future risks of venous thrombosis, no evidence of an association between baseline fibrinolytic state and future venous thrombosis was found (Ridker 1992).

In contrast, several observations support a causal role for abnormalities of tPA and/ or PAI-1 in the etiology of acute thrombosis in the arterial circulation. First, recent work has demonstrated a circadian variation in tPA activity and PAI-1, which mimics that demonstrated for the onset of several acute thrombotic disorders (Angleton 1989;

Andreotti 1991). In addition, hereditary deficiencies of PAI-1 appear to result in bleeding diathesis (Schleef 1989), while high plasma concentrations of PAI-1 are associated with frank arterial thrombosis (Erickson 1990). Most importantly, clinical data are now available regarding endogenous tPA and PAI-1 as predictors of future acute thrombosis. Since the report by Hamsten and colleagues (1985) that increased plasma levels of PAI-1 are present among young survivors of MI, a series of retrospective studies have described abnormal levels of PAI-1 and/or tPA among patients with stable and unstable angina, severe coronary artery disease, and recurrent ischemia (Paramo 1985; Azner 1988; Olofsson 1989; Huber 1990; Jansson 1991; Zalewski 1991). In aggregate, these findings suggest that abnormalities of tPA and/or PAI-1 may represent early preclinical markers for endothelial dysfunction. However, as most of these early studies were retrospective, it is impossible to determine from them whether alterations of fibrinolytic state were a consequence or a cause of vascular thrombosis.

Recently, prospective data regarding endogenous fibrinolytic capacity and the risks of future cardiovascular disorders have become available, making it possible to answer this question directly. In plasma samples collected prospectively from 15,000 apparently healthy men participating in the Physicians' Health Study, higher mean levels of endogenous tPA concentration have been reported among those who went on to suffer a first MI (Ridker 1993a) or stroke (Ridker 1994a) as compared with men who remained free from vascular disease. In fact, in the Physicians' Health Study, the relative risk of future MI for men with the highest tPA antigen concentrations was almost three times that of men with the lowest plasma levels (Figure 2.6). Interestingly, the relative risk of first MI was attenuated in analyses controlling for usual cardiovascular risk factors, suggesting that elevations of tPA are a response to the presence of preclinical atherosclerosis rather than an etiologic risk factor. In contrast, the risk

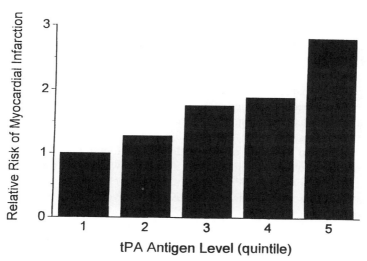

Fig. 2.6. Relative risk of first myocardial infarction associated with increasing quintiles of tPA antigen among participants in the Physicians' Health Study. [Adapted from Ridker et al. (1993), with permission.]

of future stroke associated with tPA antigen elevation was independent of total and HDL cholesterol. Similar analyses of data from this cohort did not show a relationship between PAI-1 and risk of MI. Confirmation of these findings regarding tPA and PAI-1 have recently come from both the ECAT Study Group (Thompson 1995) and from a prospective study of 213 patients with prevalent angina pectoris (Jansson 1993).

The hypothesis that activation of the endogenous fibrinolytic system may be a marker for future cardiovascular disease also is supported by other studies of hemostatic parameters. For example, levels of D-dimer, the breakdown product of fibrinogen, have been reported to be elevated among men with high risk of future infarction (Figure 2.7) (Fowkes 1993; Ridker 1994b). On the other hand, prospective data from Northwick Park using a global marker of fibrinolytic capacity suggest that low fibrinolytic capacity is associated with higher risk (Meade 1993). Further studies are required to clarify the net risks and benefits of altering endogenous fibrinolytic capacity so that preventive strategies aimed at this mechanism can be explored. Early findings suggest that changes in tPA and or PAI-1 may be possible using strategies as diverse as angiotensin-converting enzyme inhibitors (Ridker 1993b), gemfibrozil (Fugii 1992), and moderate alcohol consumption (Ridker 1994c).

Lipoprotein(a)

Lipoprotein(a) [Lp(a)] represents a unique group of lipoprotein particles having as a protein moiety apolipoprotein B-100 disulfide linked to apoprotein(a). Since its initial description over thirty years ago, Lp(a) has been extensively studied as a potential cardiovascular risk factor for many reasons (Loscalzo 1990; Scanu 1992). First, because of the suggestion from several retrospective studies that individuals with MI and stroke have elevated levels of Lp(a), this lipid marker is often considered an independent risk factor. Second, Lp(a) levels are in large part genetically determined such that levels measured in childhood track closely with those later in life. Third, and most importantly, Lp(a) shares several structural similarities with plasminogen and therefore has been hypothesized to be a critical link between lipoproteins and thrombosis.

Despite recommendations for screening, prospective data describing the predictive value of Lp(a) as a marker of risk among healthy populations have been inconsistent. To date, seven prospective studies of plasma Lp(a) concentration and one study of Lp(a) evaluated by electrophoresis have been presented (Ridker 1993, Schaefer 1994, Rosengren 1990, Bostom 1994; Cremer 1994, Jauhiainen 1991, Ridker 1995); of these, three found no evidence of association while four reported modest positive results. In addition, two studies report associations between apo(a) and vascular risk (Wald 1994, Sigurdsson 1992). When examined from a clinical perspective, these data indicate that Lp(a) assessment has low positive predictive value in terms of screening for underlying coronary disease.

Conclusions

Many current and promising strategies for cardiovascular disease prevention relate directly to evolving concepts in the pathogenesis of atherosclerosis. It is now clear

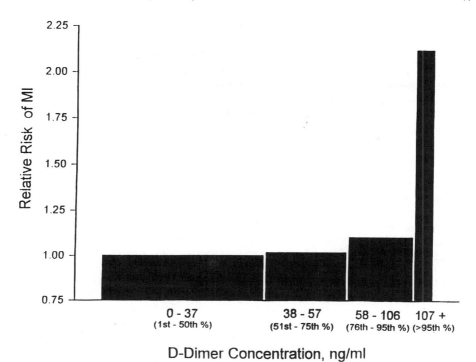

Fig. 2.7. Relative risk of first myocardial infarction associated with increasing levels of baseline D-dimer concentration among participants in the Physicians' Health Study. [Adapted from Ridker et al. (1994), with permission.]

that the initiation and progression of atherosclerosis is not an inexorable process, but rather is highly modifiable and can be slowed and often reversed using dietary as well as pharmacologic approaches to risk factor modification. Prevention strategies related to lipid reduction, antioxidant repletion, fibrinolytic enhancement, and restoration of endothelial function are all undergoing intense clinical investigation and likely will make their way into standard practice within a few years. Similarly, as evidence accumulates regarding the predictive value of hemostatic and thrombotic risk factors, population-based screening strategies are likely to develop that will allow for specific targeting of high-risk individuals. In this regard, the identification of genetic markers may prove exceptionally valuable and become as routine in the future as cholesterol screening is today.

For the prevention-oriented physician, the chief immediate task must be translating our current understanding of the etiology of cardiovascular disease into a rational clinical prevention practice. This goal is the primary focus of chapters to follow, which are concerned with the techniques of risk factor modification as well as their expected clinical benefits.

References

Alderman E, Haskell WL, Fain JM, et al. Beneficial angiographic and clinical response to multifactor modification in the Stanford Coronary Risk Intervention Project (SCRIP). [Abstract]. Circulation 1991;85(Suppl II):II–140.

Ambrose J, Tannenbaum M, Alexopoulos D, et al. Angiographic progression of coronary artery disease and the development of myocardial infarction. J Am Coll Cardiol 1988;12: 56–62.

Andreotti F, Kluft C. Circadian variation of fibrinolytic activity in blood. Chronobiol Int 1991; 8:336–51.

Angleton P, Chandler WL, Schmer G. Diurnal variation of tissue-type plasminogen activator and its rapid inhibitor (PAI-1). Circulation 1989;79:101–6.

Antiplatelet Trialists' Collaboration. Collaborative overview of randomised trials of antiplatelet therapy. I: Prevention of death, myocardial infarction, and stroke by prolonged antiplatelet therapy in various categories of patients. Br Med J 1994a;308:81–106.

Antiplatelet Trialists' Collaboration. Collaborative overview of randomised trials of antiplatelet therapy. II: Maintenance of vascular graft or arterial patency by antiplatelet therapy. Br Med J 1994b;308:159–68.

Antiplatelet Trialists' Collaboration. Collaborative overview of randomised trials of antiplatelet therapy. III: Reduction in venous thrombosis and pulmonary embolism by antiplatelet prophylaxis among surgical and medical patients. Br Med J 1994c;308:235–46.

Azner J, Estelles A, Tormo G, et al. Plasminogen activator inhibitor activity and other fibrinolytic variables in patients with coronary artery disease. Br Heart J 1988;59:535–41.

Beswick AD, Fehily AM, Sharp DS, et al. Long-term diet modification and platelet activity. J Intern Med 1991;229:511–15.

Blankenhorn DH, Nessim SA, Johnson RL, et al. Beneficial effects of colestipol niacin therapy on coronary atherosclerosis and coronary venous bypass grafts. JAMA 1987;257: 3233–40.

Blankenhorn DH, Dramsch DM. Reversal of atherosis and sclerosis: the two components of atherosclerosis. Circulation 1989;79:1–7.

Bostom A, Gagnon DR, Cupples LA, et al. Sinking prebeta lipoprotein predicts incident cardiovascular disease in women: the Framingham Study. Circulation 1993;88:2438(A).

Bostom AG, Gagnon DR, Cupples A, et al. A prospective investigation of elevated lipoprotein(a) detected by electrophoresis and cardiovascular disease in women. The Framingham Heart Study. Circulation 1994;90:1688–95.

Brensike JF, Levy RI, Kelsey SF, et al. Effects of therapy with cholestryramine on progression of coronary atherosclerosis: results of the NHLBI type II coronary intervention study. Circulation 1984;69:313–24.

Broadhurst P, Kelleher C, Hughes L, et al. Fibrinogen, factor VII clotting activity and coronary artery disease severity: atherosclerosis 1990;85:169–73.

Brown BG, Gallery CA, Badger RS, et al. Incomplete lysis of thrombus in the moderate underlying atherosclerotic lesion during intracoronary infusion of streptokinase for acute myocardial infarction: quantitative angiographic observations. Circulation 1986;73:653–61.

Brown BG, Albers JJ, Fisher LD, et al. Regression of coronary artery disease as a result of intensive lipid-lowering therapy in men with high levels of apolipoprotein B. N Engl J Med 1990;323:1289–98.

Brown BG, Zhao X-Q, Sacco DE, Albers JJ. Lipid lowering and plaque regression: new insights into prevention of plaque disruption and clinical events in coronary disease. Circulation 1993;87:1781–91.

Buchwald H, Varco RL, Matts JP, et al. Effect of partial ileal bypass on mortality and morbidity from coronary heart disease in patients with hypercholesterolemia: report of the Program on Surgical Control of the Hyperlipidemias (POSCH). N Engl J Med 1990;323:946–55.

Buja LM, Willerson JT. Role of inflammation in coronary plaque disruption. Circulation 1994; 89:503–5.

Cashin-Hemphill L, Mack WJ, Pogoda MJ, et al. Beneficial effects of colestipol-niacin on coronary atherosclerosis. JAMA 1990;264:3013–17.

Cheng GC, Loree HM, Kamm RD, et al. Distribution of circumferential stress in ruptured and stable atherosclerotic lesions: a structural analysis with histopathological correlation. Circulation 1993;87:1179–87.

Constantinides P. Plaque fissures in human coronary thrombosis. J Atheroscler Res 1966;6: 1–7.

Cornhill JF, Hererick EE, Starey HD. Topography of human aortic sudanophilic lesions. Monogr Atheroscler 1990;15:13–19.

Cremer P, Nagel D, Labrot B, Mann H, Muche R, Elster H, Seidel D. Lipoprotein Lp(a) as predictor of myocardial infarction in comparison to fibrinogen, LDL cholesterol and other risk factors: results from the prospective Gottingen Risk Incidence and Prevalence Study (GRIPS). Eur J Clin Invest 1994;24:444–53.

Davies MJ, Thomas AC. Plaque fissuring: the cause of acute myocardial infarction, sudden ischaemic death, and crescendo angina. Br Heart J 1985;53:363–73.

Davies MJ, Woolf N, Rowles PM, Pepper J. Morphology of the endothelium over atherosclerotic plaques in human coronary arteries. Br Heart J 1988;60:459–64.

DeWood MA, Spores J, Notske R, et al. Prevalence of total coronary occlusion during the early hours of transmural myocardial infarction. N Engl J Med 1980;303:897–902.

Drexler H, Zeiher AM, Meinzer K, Just H. Correction of endothelium dysfunction in coronary microcirculation of hypercholesterolemic patients by *l*-arginine. Lancet 1991;338: 1546–50.

Elwood PC, Renaud S, Sharp DS, et al. Ischemic heart disease and platelet aggregation: the Caerphilly Collaborative Heart Disease Study. Circulation 1991;83:38–44.

Enos WF, Holmes RH, Beyer J. Coronary disease among United States soldiers killed in action in Korea: preliminary report. JAMA 1953;152:1090–3.

Erickson LA, Fici GJ, Lund JE, Boyle TP, Polites HG, Marotti KR. Development of venous occlusions in mice transgenic for the plasminogen activator inhibitor-1 gene. Nature 1990;346(6279):74–6.

Ernst E. Plasma fibrinogen: an independent cardiovascular risk factor. J Intern Med 1990;27: 365–72.

Falk E. Morphologic features of unstable atherothrombotic plaques underlying acute coronary syndromes. Am J Cardiol 1989;63:114E–20E.

Falk E. Why do plaques rupture? Circulation 1992;86(Suppl III):III30–42.

Fowkes FGR, Lowe GDO, Housley E, et al. Cross-linked fibrin degradation products, progression of peripheral arterial disease, and risk of coronary heart disease. Lancet 1993;342: 84–6.

Fugii S, Sobel BE. Direct effects of gemfibrozil on the fibrinolytic system: diminution of synthesis of plasminogen activator inhibitor type 1. Circulation 1992;85:1888–93.

Furchgott RF, Zawadski JV. The obligatory role of endothelial cells in the relaxation of arterial smooth muscle by acetylcholine. Nature 1980;288:373–6.

Fuster V, Badimon L, Badimon JJ, Chesebro JH. The pathogenesis of coronary artery disease and the acute coronary syndromes. N Engl J Med 1992;326:242–50, 310–18.

Gertz SD, Roberts WC. Hemodynamic sheer force in rupture of coronary arterial atherosclerotic plaques. Am J Cardiol 1990;66:1368–71.

Giroud D, Li JM, Urban P, Meier B, Rutishauser W. Relation of the site of acute myocardial infarction to the most severe coronary arterial stenosis at prior angiography. Am J Cardiol 1992;69:729–32.

Gofman JW. The quantitative nature of the relationship of coronary artery atherosclerosis and coronary heart disease risk. Cardiol Digest 1969;4:28–38.

Hamsten A, Wiman B, de Fai, Blomback M. Increased plasma levels of a rapid inhibitor of tissue plasminogen activator in young survivors of myocardial infarction. N Engl J Med 1985;313:1557–63.

Heller RF, Chinn S, Tunstall Pedoe HD, Rose G. How well can we predict coronary heart disease? Findings in the United Kingdom Heart Disease Prevention Project. Br Med J 1984;288:1409–11.

Hennekens CH, Buring JE, Sandercock P, et al. Aspirin and other antiplatelet agents in the secondary and primary prevention of cardiovascular disease. Circulation 1989;80: 749–756.

Huber K, Resch I, Stefenelli T, et al. Plasminogen activator inhibitor-1 levels in patients with chronic angina pectoris with or without angiographic evidence of coronary sclerosis. Thromb Haemost 1990;63:336–9.

Ip JH, Fuster V, Badimon L, et al. Syndromes of accelerated atherosclerosis: role of vascular injury and smooth muscle cell proliferation. J Am Coll Cardiol 1990;15:1667–87.

Jansson JH, Nilsson TK, Olofsson BO. Tissue plasminogen activator and other risk factors as predictors of cardiovascular events in patients with severe angina pectoris. Eur Heart J 1991;12:157–61.

Jansson JH, Olofsson BO, Nilsson TK. Predictive value of tissue plasminogen activator mass concentration on long term mortality in patients with coronary artery disease: a seven-year follow-up. Circulation 1993;88:2030–4.

Jauhiainen M, Koskinen P, Ehnholm C, et al. Lipoprotein(a) and coronary heart disease risk: a nested case-control study of the Helsinki Heart Study participants. Atherosclerosis 1991; 89:59–67.

Kane JP, Malloy MJ, Ports TA, et al. Regression of coronary atherosclerosis curing treatment of familial hypercholesterolemia with combined drug regimens. JAMA 1990;264: 3007–12.

Kannel WB, Wolf PA, Castelli WP, D'Agostino RB. Fibrinogen and risk of cardiovascular disease: the Framingham Study. JAMA 1987;258:1183–6.

Libby P, Hansson GK. Involvement of the immune system in human atherogenesis: current knowledge and unanswered questions. Lab Invest 1991;64:5–15.

Lipid Research Clinics Program. The Lipid Research Clinics Coronary Prevention Trial results: reduction in incidence of coronary heart disease. JAMA 1984;251:351–64.

Little W, Constantinescu M, Applegate R, et al. Can coronary angiography predict the site of a subsequent myocardial infarction in patients with mild-to-moderate coronary artery disease? Circulation 1988;78:1157–66.

Little W, Downes T, Applegate R. The underlying coronary lesion in myocardial infarction: implications for coronary angiography. Clin Cardiol 1991;14:868–74.

Loree HM, Tobias BJ, Gibson LJ, et al. Mechanical properties of model atherosclerotic lesion lipid pools. Arterioscler Thromb 1993; 1994;14:230–234.

Loscalzo J. Lipoprotein(a): a unique risk factor for atherothrombotic disease. Arteriosclerosis 1990;10:671–9.

Lowe GDO, Drummond MM, Lorimer AR. Relation between extent of coronary artery disease and blood viscosity. Br Med J 1980;1:674–674.

Ludmer PL, Slewyn AP, Shook TL, et al. Paradoxical vasoconstriction induced by acetycholine in atherosclerotic coronary arteries. N Engl J Med 1986;315:1046–51.

Manninen V, Elo MO, Frick MH, et al. Lipid alterations and decline in the incidence of coronary heart disease in the Helsinki Heart Study. JAMA 1988;260:641–51.

Martin JF, Bath PMW. Burr ML. Influence of platelet size on outcome after myocardial infarction. Lancet 1991;338:1409–11.

McGill HC. Introduction to the geographic pathology of atherosclerosis. Lab Invest 1968;18: 465–7.

McNamara JJ, Molot MA, Stremple JF, Cutting RT. Coronary artery disease in combat casualties in Vietnam. JAMA 1971;216:1186–7.

Meade TW, Mellows S, Brozovic M, et al. Haemostatic function and ischaemic heart disease: principle results of the Northwick Park Heart Study. Lancet 1986;2:533–7.

Meade TW, Ruddock V, Stirling Y, et al. Fibrinolytic activity, clotting factors, and long term incidence of ischaemic heart disease in the Northwick Park Heart Study. Lancet 1993; 342:1076–9.

Meridith IT, Yeung AC, Weidinger FF, et al. Role of impaired endothelium-dependent vasodilation in ischemic manifestations of coronary artery disease. Circulation 1993;87(Suppl V):V-56–66.

Moller L, Kristensen TS. Plasma fibrinogen and ischemic heart disease risk factors. Arterioscler Thromb 1991;11:344–50.

Muller JE, Stone PH, Turi ZG, et al., and the MILIS Study Group: circadian variation in the frequency of onset of acute myocardial infarction. N Engl J Med 1985;313:1315–22.

Muller JE, Ludmer PL, Willich SN, et al. Circadian variation in the frequency of sudden cardiac death. Circulation 1987;5:131–8.

Munro JM, Cotran RS. The pathogenesis of atherosclerosis: atherogenesis and inflammation. Lab Invest 1988;58:249–261.

Nelson GJ, Schmidt PC, Corash L. The effect of a salmon diet on blood clotting, platelet aggregation and fatty acids in normal adult men. Lipids 1991;26:87–96.

Neumann FJ, Katus HA, Hoberg E, et al. Increased plasma viscosity and erythrocyte aggregation: indicators of an unfavourable clinical outcome in patients with unstable angina pectoris. Br Heart J 1991;66:425–30.

Olofsson BO, Dahlen G, Nilsson TK. Evidence for increased levels of plasminogen activator inhibitor and tissue plasminogen activator in plasma of patients with angiographically verified coronary artery disease. Eur Heart J 1989;10:77–82.

Ornish D, Brown SE, Scherwitz LW, et al. Can lifestyle changes reverse coronary heart disease? Lancet 1990;336:129–33.

Osborne JA, Lento PH, Seigfried MR, et al. Cardiovascular effects of acute hypersholesterolemia in rabbits: reversal with lovastatin treatment. J Clin Invest 1989;84:465–73.

Palmer RM, Ferrige AG, Moncada S. Nitric oxide release accounts for the biological activity of endothelium-derived relaxing factor. Nature 1987;327:524–6.

Paramo JA, Colucci M, Collen D. Plasminogen activator inhibitor in the blood of patients with coronary artery disease. Br Med J 1985;291:573–4.

PDAY Research Group. Relationship of atherosclerosis in young men to serum lipoprotein cholesterol concentrations and smoking: a preliminary report from the Pathobiological Determinants of Atherosclerosis in Youth (PDAY) Research Group. JAMA 1990;264: 3018–24.

Prins MH, Hirsh J. A critical review of the evidence supporting a relationship between impaired fibrinolytic activity and venous thromboembolism. Arch Intern Med 1991;151:1721–31.

Qizilbash N, Jones L, Warlow C, Mann J. Fibrinogen and lipid concentrations as risk factors for transient ischaemic attacks and minor ischaemic strokes. Br Med J 1991;303: 605–9.

Rainer C, Kawanishi DT, Chandraratna AN, et al. Changes in blood rheology in patients with stable angina pectoris as a result of coronary artery disease. Circulation 1987;76:15Jj20.

Richardson PD, Davies MJ, Born GVR. Influence of plaque configuration and stress distribution on fissuring of coronary atherosclerotic plaques. Lancet 1989;2:941–4.

Ridker PM, Manson JE, Buring JE, et al. Circadian variation of acute myocardial infarction and the effect of aspirin in a randomized trial of physicians. Circulation 1990;82: 897–902.

Ridker PM, Manson JE, Buring JE, et al. The effect of chronic platelet inhibition with low-dose aspirin on atherosclerotic progression and acute thrombosis: clinical evidence from the Physicians' Health Study. Am Heart J 1991;122:1588–92.

Ridker PM, Vaughan DE, Stampfer MJ, et al. Baseline fibrinolytic state and the risk of venous thrombosis: a prospective study of endogenous tissue-type plasminogen activator and plasminogen activator inhibitor. Circulation 1992;85:1822–7.

Ridker PM, Vaughan DE, Stampfer MJ, et al. Endogenous tissue-type plasminogen activator and risk of myocardial infarction. Lancet 1993a;341:1165–8.

Ridker PM, Gaboury CL, Conlin PR, et al. Stimulation of plasminogen activator inhibitor in vivo by infusion of angiotensin II: evidence of a potential interaction between the renin angiotensin system and fibrinolytic function. Circulation 1993b;87:1969–73.

Ridker PM, Hennekens CH, Stampfer MJ. A prospective study of lipoprotein(a) and the risk of myocardial infarction. JAMA 1993c;270:2195–9.

Ridker PM, Hennekens CH, Stampfer MJ, et al. A prospective study of endogenous tissue plasminogen activator and the risk of stroke. Lancet 1994a;343:940–3.

Ridker PM, Hennekens CH, Cerskus A, Stampfer MJ. Plasma concentration of cross linked fibrin degradation product (D-dimer) and the risk of future myocardial infarction. 1994b; Circulation 1994;90:2236–2240.

Ridker PM, Vaughan DE, Stampfer MJ, Hennekens CH. Association of moderate alcohol consumption and plasma concentration of endogenous tissue plasminogen activator. 1994c; JAMA 1994;272:919–933.

Ridker PM, Stampfer MJ, Hennekens CH. Plasma concentration of lipoprotein(a) and risk of future stroke. JAMA 1995;273:1269–73.

Rokitansky C von. A manual of pathological anatomy, Vol. 4. (Translated by GE Day). London: Sydenham Society, 1982:261.

Rosenberg L, Kaufman DW, Helmrich SP, Shapiro S. The risk of myocardial infarction after quitting smoking in men under 55 years of age. N Engl J Med 1985;313:1511–14.

Rosenberg L, Palmer JR, Shapiro S. Decline in the risk of myocardial infarction among women who stop smoking. N Engl J Med 1990;322:213.

Rosengren A, Wilhelmsen L, Eriksson E, et al. Lipoprotein(a) and coronary heart disease: a prospective case-control study in a general population of middle aged men. Br Med J 1990;301:1248–51.

Ross R. The pathogenesis of atherosclerosis: a perspective for the 1990s. Nature 1993;362: 801–9.

Scanu AM. Lipoprotein(a): a genetic risk factor for premature coronary heart disease. JAMA 1992;267:3326–9.

Schaefer EJ, Lamon-Fava S, Jenner JL, et al. Lipoprotein(a) levels and risk of coronary heart disease in men. The Lipid Research Clinics Coronary Primary Prevention Trial. JAMA 1994;271:999–1003.

Schleef RR, Higgins DL, Pillemer E, Levitt LJ. Bleeding diathesis due to decreased functional activity of type 1 plasminogen activator inhibitor. J Clin Invest 1989;83:1747–52.

Schuler G, Hambrecht R, Schlierf G, et al. Regular physical exercise and low-fat diet: effects on progression of coronary artery disease. Circulation 1992;86:1–11.

Schwartz CJ, Valente AJ, Sprague EA, et al. The pathogenesis of atherosclerosis: an overview. Clin Cardiol 1991;14:11–16.

Sigurdsson G, Baldursdottir A, Sigvaldsonason H, et al. Predictive value of apolipoproteins in a prospective study of coronary artery disease in men. Am J Cardiol 1992;69:1251–54.

Small DM, Bond MG, Waugh D, et al. Physicochemical and histological changes in the arterial wall of nonhuman primates during progression and regression of atherosclerosis. J Clin Invest 1984;73:1590–605.

Small DM. Progression and regression of atherosclerotic lesions: insights from lipid physical biochemistry. Arteriosclerosis 1988;8:103–29.

Stamler JS, Loscalzo J. The antiplatelet effects of organic nitrates and related nitroso compounds in vitro and in vivo and their relevance to cardiovascular disorders. J Am Coll Cardiol 1991;18:1529–36.

Stary HC. Evolution and progression of atherosclerotic lesions in coronary arteries of children and young adults. Arteriosclerosis 1989;99(Suppl I):I19–32.

Steinberg D, Parthasarathy S, Carew TE, et al. Beyond cholesterol: modifications of low-density lipoprotein that increase its atherogenicity. N Engl J Med 1989;320:915–24.

Stone MC, Thorpe JM. Plasma fibrinogen: a major coronary risk factor. J R Coll Gen Pract 1985;35:565–9.

Stratton JR, Chandler WL, Schwartz RS, et al. Effects of physical conditioning on fibrinolytic variables and fibrinogen in young and old healthy adults. Circulation 1991;83:1692–7.

Strong JP. Atherosclerotic lesions: natural history, risk factors, and topography. Arch Pathol Lab Med 1992;116:1268–75.

Thaulow E, Erikssen J, Sandvik L, et al. Blood platelet count and function are related to total and cardiovascular death in apparently healthy men. Circulation 1991;84:613–617.

Treasure CB, Manoukian SV, Klein JL, et al. Epicardial coronary artery responses to acetylcholine are impaired in hypertensive patients. Circ Res 1992;71:776–81.

Trip MD, Manger Cats V, van Capelle FJL, Vreeken J. Platelet hyperreactivity and prognosis in survivors of myocardial infarction. N Engl J Med 1990;322:1549–54.

Thompson SG, Kienast J, Pyke SDM, et al. Hemostatic factors and the risk of myocardial infarction or sudden death in patients with angina pectoris. N Engl J Med 1995;332:635–41.

van der Waal AC, Becker AE, van der Loos CM, Das PK. The site of intimal rupture or erosion of thrombosed coronary atherosclerotic plaques is characterized by an inflammatory process irrespective of the dominant plaque morphology. Circulation 1994;89:36–44.

Virchow R. Phlogose und Thrombose in Gefässystem, gesammelte Abhandlungen zur wissenschaftlichen Medicin. Frankfurt-am-Main: Meidinger Sohn, 1856:458.

Vita JA, Treasure CB, Nabel EG, et al. The coronary vasomotor response to acetycholine relates to risk factors for coronary artery disease. Circulation 1990;81:491–7.

Wald NJ, Law M, Watt HC, et al. Apolipoproteins and ischaemic heart disease: implications for screening. Lancet 1994;343:75–9.

Watts GF, Lewis B, Brunt JNH, et al. Effects on coronary artery disease of lipid-lowering diet, or diet plus cholestyramine, in the St. Thomas' Atherosclerosis Regression Study (STARS). Lancet 1992;339:563–9.

Webster M, Chesebro J, Smith H, et al. Myocardial infarction and coronary artery occlusion: a prospective 5-year angiographic study. J Am Coll Cardiol 1990;15:218A.

Werns SW, Walton JA, Hsia HH, et al. Evidence of endothelial dysfunction in angiographically normal coronary arteries of patients with coronary artery disease. Circulation 1989;79:287–91.

Wilhelmsen L, Svardsudd K, Korsan-Bengtsen K, et al. Fibrinogen as a risk factor for stroke and myocardial infarction. N Engl J Med 1984;311:501–5.

Wiman B, Hamsten A. Impaired fibrinolysis and risk of thromboembolism. Prog Cardiovasc Dis 1991;34:179–92.

Wissler RW, Vesselinovitch D. Can atherosclerotic plaques regress? anatomic and biochemical evidence from nonhuman animal models. Am J Cardiol 1990;65:33F–40F.

Yarnell JWG, Baker IA, Sweetnam PM, et al. Fibrinogen, viscosity, and white blood cell count are major risk factors for ischemic heart disease: the Caerphilly and Speedwell Collaborative Heart Disease Studies. Circulation 1991;83:836–844.

Yusuf S, Peto J, Lewis J, et al. Beta blockage during and after myocardial infarction: an overview of the randomized trials. Prog Cardiovasc Dis 1985;27:335–71.

Zalewski A, Shi Y, Nardone D, et al. Evidence for reduced fibrinolytic activity in unstable angina at rest: clinical, biochemical, and angiographic correlates. Circulation 1991;83:1685–91.

3

Genetic Determinants of Myocardial Infarction

Marilyn Dammerman and Jan L. Breslow

Until recently, there has been little need to discuss in detail genetic issues related to cardiovascular disease prevention, except to state that a family history of premature atherosclerosis constitutes an independent risk factor and that several lipid abnormalities appear to be related to specific inherited defects. In recent years, however, there has been a remarkable increase in information on the role of genetics in a wide variety of cardiovascular diseases. As genetic testing becomes widely available, clinicians and their patients will be faced for the first time with critical information likely to have major importance for personal risk factor modification as well as reproductive decision-making. Thus, detailed discussions of genetic issues in cardiovascular disease prevention are now required so that the prevention-oriented physician can begin to integrate this developing field into daily practice.

In this chapter, several important cardiovascular disorders that have been linked to specific genes are discussed, while particular attention is given to the genetics of lipoprotein metabolism, diabetes, obesity, and hypertension. In addition, genetic issues surrounding new markers of hemostatic and thrombotic risk are presented. While the utility of genetic screening for coronary heart disease in the general population is currently unknown, the information in this chapter should form a basis for deciding when to screen patients who have presented with premature atherosclerosis. In turn, identification of such genetically high-risk individuals provides a critical mechanism to single out families for whom early intervention and lifestyle changes should have disproportionate benefit.

Genetic Perspectives on Coronary Artery Disease

Coronary artery disease (CAD) and the conditions predisposing to it are, in their common forms, complex disorders with multiple genetic and environmental components. For example, a family history of myocardial infarction (MI), especially MI at an early age, is a potent risk factor for CAD. The risk increases with the number of first-degree relatives affected and is inversely related to the age at which they became affected (Roncaglioni 1992). While some of this increased risk is due to shared environment, genetic factors appear to predominate (Nora 1980). Monozygotic (identical) twins are significantly more likely to be concordant for CAD than are dizygotic (fraternal) twins (Goldbourt 1986). Dyslipidemia, diabetes mellitus, hypertension, and obesity, the major metabolic risk factors for CAD, are in large measure genetically determined. In addition, a family history of MI confers increased risk in both genders independent of other known risk factors (Colditz 1986; Colditz 1991; Roncaglioni 1992). However, such disorders are difficult to study genetically due to late age of onset, the likelihood that not all individuals with a genetic predisposition will develop the disease, and the probability that multiple genes—and different genes in different families—are involved. Nevertheless, clues to the genetic factors underlying CAD have been obtained from studies of single-gene disorders. Considerable progress has been made in elucidating the genetic basis of lipoprotein abnormalities. The genes for many proteins involved in lipid metabolism have been isolated, and relatively common as well as rare mutations have been found (Breslow 1991; Zannis 1993; Dammerman 1995). Single genes causing rare forms of diabetes have been identified (Steiner 1990; van den Ouweland 1992; Taylor 1992; Froguel 1993), and common susceptibility genes for hypertension and MI have been proposed (Cambien 1992; Jeneumaitre 1992).

Two major investigative strategies in human genetics are association studies and linkage studies. Both assess the involvement of a candidate gene in a disorder of interest using DNA sequence polymorphisms. These are sites of genetic variation within the population that result in alternative forms (alleles) of the same gene. In association studies, a candidate gene is tested for association with a trait in a sample population of unrelated subjects. The frequencies of two or more alleles may be compared in an affected and a normal group (case-control study), or carriers of a particular allele may be compared to noncarriers with respect to a quantitative trait. In classical linkage analysis, the coinheritance in families of a disorder with a particular allele of a gene is assessed. This method has been used to identify single genes responsible for a large number of disorders. A related method, sib pair analysis, has recently been used to assess the contribution of a particular gene to a disease by determining whether affected siblings have inherited the same alleles from their parents more frequently than would be expected by chance. Strategies for investigating complex disorders are still evolving, but complementary use of association, linkage, and sib pair studies is a common approach.

Understanding the molecular basis of genetically mediated disorders is critical to the development of improved treatments. However, the use of genetic methods to predict clinical outcomes with respect to CAD is at an early stage. The most common single-gene disorder resulting in CAD is familial hypercholesterolemia (FH), which is associated with very significant premature morbidity and mortality. While the genetic basis of FH has been extensively investigated, a mass genetic screening effort to detect FH is impractical due to the large number of different mutations that cause the disorder. Genetic testing has, however, facilitated development of more accurate cholesterol criteria for identifying potential FH heterozygotes (Williams RR 1993), and clinical trials of gene replacement therapy for FH homozygotes have yielded promising initial results (Grossman 1994). In the general population, genetic variation in apolipoprotein E (apo E) is associated with modest differences in low density lipoprotein (LDL) cholesterol levels and atherosclerosis susceptibility. However, the recently discovered association between the apo E4 allele and Alzheimer's disease has made the use of this marker ethically problematic, particularly in settings in which a board-certified genetic counselor is not available. Plasma levels of lipoprotein(a) [Lp(a)], a highly heritable trait, are strongly associated with CAD in case-control studies, but recent negative prospective studies have called this relationship into question, and further work is needed to determine the appropriate use of this marker. It is not clear to what extent the recently proposed susceptibility genes for hypertension and MI will be useful from a predictive standpoint.

In the vast majority of individuals, the genetic basis of CAD is likely to lie in multiple subtly abnormal genes, and it is clear that adverse lifestyle choices can lead to expression of this genetic potential. It is probable that the development of appropriate genetic markers will facilitate identification of those members of CAD-prone families, and perhaps members of the general public as well, who are likely to develop CAD or its predisposing disorders. This information would presumably take the form of a genetic profile specifying the alleles carried at genes known to strongly influence CAD risk. Devising a means of assuring the confidentiality of such profiles remains an important problem.

In the future, intensive preventive efforts with respect to modifiable CAD risk factors may focus on carriers of high-risk alleles. At present, all patients with a family history of CAD or related disorders should receive special attention with respect to modifiable risk factors.

Genetic Factors Predisposing to Atherosclerosis

Lipoprotein Disorders

Lipoprotein disorders result from abnormal synthesis, processing, or catabolism of plasma lipoprotein particles. These particles consist of a core of cholesterol ester and triglyceride enclosed in a coat of phospholipids and apolipoproteins. More than half of patients with angiographically confirmed CAD before age 60 have a familial lipoprotein disorder (Genest 1992). The association is most striking among younger patients and declines with increasing age at first MI. This suggests the presence of genetic factors that accelerate age-associated cardiovascular changes seen in the general population (Bierman 1991). Severe hyperlipidemia (total cholesterol above 300 mg/dl or triglycerides above 500 mg/dl) usually indicates a genetic disorder, and xanthomas almost always signal an underlying genetic defect. These findings warrant examination of the patient's first-degree relatives (Bierman 1991). Four types of lipoprotein abnormality are observed (Table 3.1): elevated LDL cholesterol; reduced high density lipoprotein (HDL) cholesterol, usually with increased triglycerides and very low density lipoprotein (VLDL) cholesterol; elevated levels of chylomicron remnants and intermediate density lipoproteins (IDL); and elevated levels of Lp(a) particles (Breslow 1991).

Table 3.1. Genetic Factors in Lipoprotein Abnormalities

Lipoprotein Profile	Gene(s) Implicated
↑ LDL cholesterol	Apolipoprotein B
	Apolipoprotein E
	LDL receptor
	Lysosomal acid lipase
↓ HDL cholesterol	Apolipoprotein AI
↑ Triglyceride (VLDL)	Apolipoprotein CII
	Apolipoprotein CIII
	Lecithin: cholesterol acyltransferase
	Lipoprotein lipase
↑ Remnants and IDL	Apolipoprotein E
↑ Lipoprotein(a)	Apolipoprotein(a)

LDL, low density lipoprotein; HDL, high density lipoprotein; IDL, intermediate density lipoprotein; VLDL, very low density lipoprotein.
Source: From Dammerman and Breslow, 1995, with permission of Circulation. Copyright 1995 American Heart Association.

Elevated LDL Cholesterol. Family and twin studies indicate that half the population variance in LDL cholesterol is genetic. Approximately 7% of the variance is explained by known mutations in the genes for the LDL receptor, apolipoprotein B (apo B) and apo E (Table 3.2), with the preponderance of the variance unexplained (Breslow 1991). Individuals differ in their responses to dietary fat and cholesterol, and genes controlling diet response may explain much of the variation in LDL cholesterol. These genes may influence such processes as cholesterol absorption and synthesis, bile acid syn-

Table 3.2. Genes Affecting LDL Cholesterol Levels

Disorder	Gene	Chromosome	LDL-C	CAD	Frequency
Familial hypercholesterolemia	LDL receptor	19	↑	↑	
Heterozygotes					1/500
Homozygotes					1/1,000,000
Familial defective apo B[a]	Apolipoprotein B	2	↑	↑	1/500–1/700
Hypobetalipoproteinemia[a]	Apolipoprotein B	2	↓	↓?	1/1000
Abetalipoproteinemia[b]	Microsomal triglyceride transfer protein	4	↓	—	~15 cases
Familial combined hyperlipidemia	?	?	↑	↑	1/100
Cholesterol ester storage disease[b]	Lysosomal acid lipase	10	↑	↑	~30 cases
Variation in LDL-C in the population	Apolipoprotein E4[a,b]	19	↑	↑	1/4
	Apolipoprotein E2[a]	19	↓	↓	1/7

[a]Heterozygotes.

[b]Homozygotes.

LDL-C, low density lipoprotein cholesterol; Apo, apolipoprotein; CAD, coronary artery disease.
Source: From Dammerman and Breslow, 1995, with permission of Circulation. Copyright 1995 American Heart Association.

thesis, and LDL receptor synthesis and catabolism (Brown 1991). Disorders characterized by elevation of LDL cholesterol alone are classified as Frederickson type IIa hyperlipoproteinemia.

Familial hypercholesterolemia (Table 3.3) is a relatively common cause of elevated LDL cholesterol and is present in approximately 5% of patients with MI (Brown 1991). An autosomal dominant disorder, FH is due to a defective LDL receptor gene on chromosome 19. As in other dominant disorders, 50% of first-degree relatives are affected. Since there is a gene-dosage effect, patients inheriting a defective gene from both parents are severely affected. Reduction in or absence of functional cell surface LDL receptor molecules impairs LDL catabolism, and failure to carry out receptor-mediated IDL uptake results in enhanced IDL conversion to LDL.

FH homozygotes typically have sixfold elevations in LDL cholesterol, with total cholesterol levels of 650 to 1,000 mg/dl, and they can be identified at birth by markedly elevated cholesterol in umbilical cord blood (Goldstein 1989). CAD is often clinically apparent before age 10, with MI as early as 18 months of age (Brown 1991), and most homozygotes suffer fatal MI by age 30. A unique type of planar cutaneous xanthoma is present at birth or develops in childhood, often between the thumb and index finger, and many patients are first identified by dermatologists. However, diagnosis may be delayed until the appearance of angina pectoris or until an episode of syncope due to xanthomatous aortic stenosis (Brown 1991). A diagnosis of pediatric FH often serves as the impetus for further case-finding in the family.

FH heterozygotes have LDL cholesterol levels approximately 140 mg/dl higher than family members with two normal genes. By age 30, 5% of males have had an MI; by age 50, 25% have died of MI; and by age 60, 50% have died (Goldstein 1989). Onset is typically delayed by 10 years in women. Heterozygous FH may be distinguishable from most other hypercholesterolemias by the presence of nodular xanthomas of the Achilles and other tendons, seen in up to 75% of heterozygotes (Brown 1991). Diabetes and obesity are not associated with FH, and a slender physique is typical (Brown 1991). Clinical presentation may, however, be influenced by other genetic and lifestyle factors.

At least 150 different LDL receptor mutations have been described. In families in which the specific mutation is known, genetic testing (including prenatal testing) can be used to identify additional affected individuals. In certain ethnic groups, including French Canadians, Lebanese Christians, Jews of Lithuanian origin, Finns, and South

Table 3.3. Familial Hypercholesterolemia: LDL Receptor Mutations

	Heterozygotes	Homozygotes
Frequency	1/500	1/1,000,000
LDL cholesterol ↑	2x	5–7x
Clinical CAD onset	40–60 years	0–30 years
Xanthomas	75%	100%

LDL, low density lipoprotein; CAD, coronary artery disease.
Source: From Dammerman and Breslow, 1995, with permission of Circulation. Copyright 1995 American Heart Association.

African Afrikaners, FH is unusually common, and one or a few mutations predominate due to a founder effect, making genetic screening feasible. At present, however, genetic testing for FH is available only from specialized laboratories, and most patients are identified on the basis of lipoprotein profile and clinical findings. Cholesterol guidelines based on genetic testing have recently been developed for identifying possible FH heterozygotes (Williams RR 1993), as noted previously. Among first-degree relatives of known FH patients, a total cholesterol >220 mg/dl for patients under age 40 or >290 mg/dl for age 40+ suggests FH. In the general population, total cholesterol >270 mg/dl under age 40 or >360 mg/dl for age 40+ suggests FH. In the past, FH has been overdiagnosed among the general population and underdiagnosed within FH families (Williams RR 1993). Patients with FH and other well-defined hereditary disorders should receive genetic counseling.

Drug therapy is required to reduce cholesterol levels in FH heterozygotes. HMG CoA reductase inhibitors lower LDL cholesterol by 30% to 50% by reducing cholesterol synthesis and by increasing LDL receptor synthesis from the normal gene (Brown 1991). While most homozygotes are treated by plasma exchange, liver transplantation has been used successfully in recent years.

Clinical trials of gene therapy for homozygous FH are in progress in a few patients, as noted previously. In the first reported case, hepatocytes derived from a section of the patient's liver were genetically repaired in culture and then returned to the liver via cell infusions into the portal circulation. This resulted in stable engraftment of a small number of LDL receptor-synthesizing hepatocytes and conferred responsiveness to lovastatin (Grossman 1994). The patient's LDL cholesterol dropped from a mean of 448 mg/dl on lovastatin prior to gene therapy to a mean of 366 mg/dl on lovastatin after the procedure, a highly significant decline. Together with a small increase in HDL cholesterol, this resulted in a decline in the LDL/HDL cholesterol ratio from the 10–13 range before gene therapy to 5–8 following the procedure. While these modest improvements may not translate into an improved clinical outcome, they demonstrate the feasibility of the strategy (Grossman 1994). More efficient methods of gene replacement are under development, and these may result in enhanced LDL receptor synthesis and more dramatic improvement.

A second relatively common single-gene disorder causing elevated LDL cholesterol, familial defective apo B100 (FDB), is due to a mutation in the apo B gene on chromosome 2 (Breslow 1991; Zannis 1993). The resulting amino acid substitution disrupts binding of apo B, present on the surface of LDL particles, to the LDL receptor, impairing LDL uptake. Heterozygosity for this disorder increases LDL cholesterol levels by at least 50% (60 to 80 mg/dl) relative to unaffected family members. In general FDB may be clinically milder than FH, but many patients have tendon xanthomas, and cholesterol levels may fall within the FH range. In some cases the two disorders are distinguishable only by genetic tests, and the approach to treatment is the same.

In the general population, genetic variation in apo E accounts for 3% to 5% of the variance in LDL cholesterol levels (Table 3.4). Apo E mediates hepatic uptake of chylomicron remnants as well as IDL particles. While liver-derived VLDL particles are the primary carriers of endogenously synthesized fats, intestinally derived chylomicrons are the primary carriers of dietary fats. Following synthesis, chylomicrons

Table 3.4. Common Variation in Apolipoprotein E

Apolipoprotein E genotype	E 4/3	E 3/3	E 3/2
Caucasian frequency	23%	59%	12%
LDL cholesterol	110%	100%	90%
Coronary artery disease	↑	↔	↓
Longevity	↓	↔	↑

LDL, low density lipoprotein.
Source: From Dammerman and Breslow, 1995, with permission of Circulation. Copyright 1995 American Heart Association.

pass into lymph and then into plasma for transport to adipose tissue and skeletal muscle, where their core triglycerides are hydrolyzed by lipoprotein lipase (LPL) to yield free fatty acids and chylomicron remnants. Cholesterol ester- and apo E-enriched remnants travel to the liver for uptake by the remnant receptor. Efficiency of apo E-mediated uptake of both IDL and chylomicron remnants is thought to influence LDL cholesterol levels.

Apo E is encoded by a gene cluster on chromosome 19 that also encodes apolipoproteins CI and CII. Apo E genotyping, available only from specialized laboratories, has revealed three common alleles in the population: E3, E4, and E2 (Caucasian frequencies 77%, 15%, and 8%, respectively). Individuals with the E4/3 genotype (the E4 protein is synthesized from one parental allele and E3 from the other) have mean LDL cholesterol levels 5–10 mg/dl higher than subjects with the most common genotype, E3/3, while individuals with E3/2 have LDL cholesterol levels 10–20 mg/dl lower than E3/3 subjects. Several mechanisms have been proposed to account for this (Breslow 1991). Hepatic clearance of IDL and chylomicron remnants is faster in individuals with E4/3 and slower in those with E3/2 relative to those with E3/3. This may cause E4/3 subjects to synthesize fewer LDL receptor molecules, reducing LDL clearance, while E3/2 subjects may synthesize more LDL receptors, increasing LDL clearance. In addition, in vitro evidence suggests that apo E is necessary for conversion of IDL to LDL and that E2 functions less well than E3 in this regard.

Apo E genetic variation also influences atherosclerosis progression in the general population, as noted previously. In an autopsy study of more than 500 young male trauma victims, E3/2 was associated with reduced atherosclerosis relative to E3/3 (Hixson 1991). This was observed in both whites and blacks and was only partially explained by apo E-associated differences in cholesterol levels. Apo E genotypes accounted for 6% to 7% of the variance in aortic lesion extent. While the apo E4 allele was not strongly associated with increased atherosclerosis in this study, several other studies have shown an association of this allele with CAD.

Familial combined hyperlipidemia (FCHL), a complex disorder of unknown etiology, is the most common genetic hypercholesterolemia and one of the most frequent causes of premature CAD (Table 3.5). FCHL (type IIb hyperlipoproteinemia) is characterized by elevations of LDL cholesterol and VLDL triglyceride (>95th percentile for age and gender) within the same family. Affected subjects may have one or both abnormalities, and the lipid profile may vary over time. Xanthomas are uncommon. VLDL and apo B are overproduced in FCHL, and this may lead to elevated plasma VLDL and hypertriglyceridemia in some family members, while in others with more

Table 3.5. Familial Combined Hyperlipidemia

Frequency
   1% among the general population
   10% among myocardial infarction patients
↑ Apolipoprotein B, ↑ LDL cholesterol, and/or ↑ VLDL triglyceride
Premature coronary artery disease; xanthomas rare
Genetically heterogeneous
Candidate genes
   Apolipoprotein AI/CIII/AIV gene cluster
   Lipoprotein lipase

LDL, low density lipoprotein; VLDL, very low density lipoprotein.
Source: From Dammerman and Breslow, 1995, with permission of Circulation. Copyright 1995 American Heart Association.

efficient lipolysis the consequence is elevated LDL. Hyperlipidemia appears in 10% to 20% of patients in childhood, usually as hypertriglyceridemia (Kane 1989). Patients usually have a strong family history of premature CAD, and hypertriglyceridemic family members seem to be at the same increased risk as those with hypercholesterolemia (Bierman 1991). FCHL accounts for 10% of individuals with LDL cholesterol >95th percentile and is present in approximately 10% of patients with MI (Brown 1991). The disorder is exacerbated by obesity, diabetes, hypothyroidism, exogenous estrogen, and alcohol. Patients are often responsive to low-fat diet and exercise, but drug therapy may be necessary.

When elevated cholesterol and triglycerides are considered as a single trait, an autosomal dominant pattern is often observed for FCHL (Brown 1991). The disorder appears to be genetically heterogeneous, however, and other patterns are also observed. There is evidence favoring a role, in some families, for a chromosome 11 region that includes the genes for apolipoproteins AI, CIII, and AIV (Wojciechowski 1991). Heterozygosity for mutations in the LPL gene on chromosome 8 has been documented in a few cases (Babirak 1989). It is likely that as yet unknown genes responsible for increased apo B levels are also involved.

Elevated apo B levels (above 130 mg/dl) are present in one-third of patients with confirmed premature CAD (Kwiterovich 1993). In one study, LDL cholesterol levels >95th percentile were present in 15% of patients with MI prior to age 60, while LDL apo B levels >95th percentile were present in 35% (Sniderman 1990). Plasma apo B levels are measured by commercial laboratories, and some investigators support the use of this test, especially for patients with hypertriglyceridemia or known CAD. It has been argued that elevated apo B in such patients is an indication for more aggressive treatment (Sniderman 1990). Small dense LDL particles are frequently observed in, although not unique to, patients with FCHL. These particles are associated with increased triglycerides and elevated apo B, as well as with reduced HDL cholesterol (Austin 1988). A single gene appears to have a major influence on LDL particle size, although this trait is also diet-responsive (Austin 1993). Small dense LDL particles are highly susceptible to oxidation, which may make them highly atherogenic. In one study, this trait was found in 50% of MI victims but in only 26% of controls, although this was not independent of triglyceride level (Austin 1988).

Reduced HDL Cholesterol and Elevated Triglycerides. Approximately half the population variance in HDL cholesterol is likely to be attributable to genetic factors (Table 3.6). Several studies have documented a 1.5- to 2-fold greater concordance for HDL cholesterol levels in monozygotic versus dizygotic twins (Breslow 1989). In an inpatient study of monozygotic twins on identical metabolic diets, HDL cholesterol showed the highest concordance of the lipid parameters measured (de Oliveira e Silva 1991).

There are two major HDL particle size classes in plasma, HDL_3 and the larger HDL_2. Nascent HDL particles produced by the liver and small intestine consist primarily of complexes of phospholipid and apolipoprotein AI (apo AI), and remodeling of these particles occurs as they circulate in plasma (Breslow 1989). HDL particles attract excess free cholesterol from extrahepatic cells and from other types of lipoprotein particles. The cholesterol is esterified by the enzyme lethicin:cholesterol acyltransferase (LCAT), using apo AI as a cofactor, and the resulting cholesterol ester enters the HDL core, enlarging the particle. HDL particles may also become smaller as a result of the action of cholesteryl ester transfer protein (CETP), which exchanges the cholesterol ester in HDL for triglycerides in VLDL and IDL. Hepatic lipase can then hydrolyze HDL triglycerides, reducing particle size. Excess cholesterol in peripheral tissues can thus be transferred from HDL to other lipoprotein particles, which are cleared from plasma by hepatic receptors. This process, termed *reverse cholesterol transport*, may account in part for the protective effect of HDL.

A small number of patients with defective HDL production due to mutations in the apo AI gene on chromosome 11 have been described. These mutations preclude

Table 3.6. Genes Affecting HDL Cholesterol Levels

Genetic Defect or Variant	Chromosome	HDL-C	CAD	Frequency
Apolipoprotein AI deficiency[a]	11	↓	↑	7 families
Apolipoprotein AI amino acid substitutions:	11			
Arg 173 → Cys (Apoliprotein AI$_{Milano}$)[b]		↓	↓	1 Italian village
Pro 165 → Arg[b]		↓	—	4 families, 12 cases
Lecithin: cholesterol[a] acyltransferase deficiency	16	↓	↑	~30 families, >50 cases
Lipoprotein lipase deficiency	8	↓	↓[a]	
Heterozygotes				<1/500
Homozygotes				<1/1,000,000
Apolipoprotein CII deficiency[a]	19	↓	↓?	11 families, >30 cases
Cholesterol ester transfer protein deficiency[a,b]	16	↑	↓?	>1/50 in Japan[b]
Hepatic lipase deficiency[a]	15	↑	↑	3 families

[a]Homozygotes.

[b]Heterozygotes.

HDL-C, high density lipoprotein cholesterol; CAD, coronary artery disease.
Source: From Dammerman and Breslow, 1995, with permission of Circulation. Copyright 1995 American Heart Association.

synthesis of the protein and, in the homozygous state, are characterized by very low or undetectable HDL cholesterol (Breslow 1989). Most of these patients develop planar xanthomas and CAD between the ages of 25 and 50. Deficiency of the LCAT enzyme results in abnormal lipoprotein particles of all types due to inability to esterify free cholesterol, large quantities of which accumulate in plasma and tissues (Zannis 1993). This rare disorder is caused by homozygosity for mutations in the LCAT gene on chromosome 16. HDL cholesterol may be markedly reduced, and patients may have premature CAD as well as renal damage due to the lipoprotein disorder.

Several disorders have been described that result in low HDL cholesterol but not in premature CAD. These include Tangier disease, characterized by abnormally rapid HDL clearance; dyslipidemia due to certain apo AI amino acid substitutions; and homozygous LPL deficiency.

Two deficiencies of proteins involved in HDL processing have been found to raise HDL cholesterol levels (Breslow 1991; Zannis 1993). In hepatic lipase deficiency, which causes hypertriglyceridemia, there is premature CAD despite elevated HDL cholesterol. This rare disorder is characterized by a failure to remodel HDL_2 to HDL_3 due to a mutation in the hepatic lipase gene on chromosome 15. The second disorder, CETP deficiency, is due to mutations in the CETP gene on chromosome 16. These result in elevated apo AI and HDL cholesterol levels and reduced apo B and LDL cholesterol levels, a profile associated with protection against CAD and with longevity. CETP mutations occur frequently among Japanese and in this population are a common cause of high HDL cholesterol (Tall 1993). Apart from cases of CETP deficiency, families with unusually high HDL cholesterol and apo AI levels have been reported. Simple mendelian inheritance is generally not observed, and the genetic factors responsible have yet to be identified (Breslow 1989).

Single-gene syndromes probably account for a very small fraction (perhaps 1%) of the variance in HDL cholesterol levels. A large number of studies have failed to demonstrate a major single-gene effect on HDL cholesterol in the general population (Breslow 1989). Based on computer modeling of data from family studies, however, a very significant proportion of the variance (40–60%) appears attributable to polygenic inheritance. This could result from common sequence variations in a small number of genes, and it seems likely that genes regulating HDL particle size, including those influencing the activity of HDL-processing proteins, may play an important role. The LPL gene was shown to influence HDL_3 cholesterol levels in a recent study of families of CAD victims (Coresh 1993).

HDL cholesterol levels are moderately responsive to exercise and weight loss, as well as to some drugs that lower LDL cholesterol and/or triglycerides. Increasing HDL cholesterol should be a therapeutic goal in patients with low HDL levels and with CAD, but treatment of otherwise normal patients with no family history of CAD is controversial.

Elevated triglycerides are generally found together with low HDL cholesterol and these appear to be causally linked. In relatives of CAD patients with familial lipoprotein disorders, an elevated triglyceride level with reduced HDL cholesterol was nearly fourfold more common than reduced HDL cholesterol alone (Genest 1992). In some, but not all, studies, elevated triglycerides have been shown to be an independent CAD risk factor (Austin 1991). Nearly 25% of patients with CAD prior to age 60 had hypertriglyceridemia in a recent study (Genest 1992). These cases were more often familial than sporadic and were almost always associated with low HDL cholesterol. Among diabetics, hypertriglyceridemia constitutes a major CAD risk factor (Chait 1990).

Elevated triglycerides are common in the population. Among males aged 35–39, for example, approximately 10% have triglycerides ≥250 mg/dl (Lipid Research Clinics 1980). Genetic hypertriglyceridemia may present as elevated triglycerides in the absence of secondary causes or as unusual triglyceride sensitivity to alcohol, exogenous estrogen, weight gain, hyperglycemia, or hypothyroidism. While moderate triglyceride elevations may be secondary to other metabolic abnormalities or to exogenous agents, severe hypertriglyceridemia (>1,000 mg/dl) generally reflects a genetic propensity.

VLDL and chylomicrons are the principal triglyceride-rich lipoproteins. Type IV hyperlipoproteinemia is characterized by elevated VLDL, with triglycerides of 250–500 mg/dl, while type V hyperlipoproteinemia is characterized by elevated VLDL and fasting chylomicronemia, with triglycerides >500 mg/dl. Families with isolated hypertriglyceridemia are less common than those with FCHL, and triglycerides tend to be higher. In severe hypertriglyceridemia, cholesterol is often elevated, since it is a constituent of VLDL. This may be important, since the cholesterol ester content of triglyceride-rich lipoproteins may determine their atherogenicity. Some individuals with high VLDL levels also have markedly elevated LDL cholesterol, and these patients may be at especially high risk for CAD. Hypertriglyceridemic patients with elevated apo B appear to be substantially more likely to develop CAD than those with normal apo B levels (Sniderman 1990).

Familial hypertriglyceridemia is genetically heterogeneous, and in most cases the genetic basis is unknown. In some families the disorder appears to be inherited in an autosomal dominant manner, while in others recessive or nonmendelian patterns are observed. Hypertriglyceridemia is strongly associated with hyperinsulinemia, hyperglycemia, and hypertension, a constellation of features known as syndrome X (Reaven 1988). Hypertriglyceridemia may be due to VLDL overproduction, impaired catabolism, or both. A genetic defect in the ability to catabolize VLDL triglycerides may be expressed in the presence of exacerbating factors. When VLDL is overproduced, as in obesity or diabetes, or as a result of alcohol or estrogen use, affected patients may be unable to increase VLDL catabolism proportionately (Brown 1991).

Among Caucasians and in west Japan, hypertriglyceridemia is strongly associated with the minor (less common) allele of a two-allele polymorphism near the coding sequence for apolipoprotein CIII (apo CIII) on chromosome 11 (Rees 1983; Zeng 1995). In one study, this marker was present in 44% of Caucasian patients with severe hypertriglyceridemia and in 17% of controls (Dammerman 1993). Association of this and other polymorphisms in the apo AI/CIII/AIV gene cluster with CAD among subjects with a family history of CAD has been reported (Price 1989). Genetic factors conferring protection against hypertriglyceridemia also reside in this region (Dammerman 1993). Apo CIII is a major protein constituent of chylomicrons and VLDL particles. Normolipidemic subjects carrying the minor allele of the apo CIII polymorphism have higher apo CIII levels than noncarriers (Shoulders 1991), and apo CIII and triglyceride levels are strongly correlated. Apo CIII inhibits LPL in vitro and may also inhibit hepatic uptake of triglyceride-rich particles and their remnants. Transgenic mice overexpressing the human apo CIII gene have severe hypertriglyceridemia (Breslow 1993), making this the strongest candidate gene in this region with respect to regulation of triglycerides. Apo E4 carriers and heterozygotes for LPL mutations are also at increased risk of hypertriglyceridemia (Ghiselli 1982; Babirak 1989; Wilson 1990).

Triglycerides should be measured in patients with CAD or a family history of CAD, as well as in those with diabetes, hypertension, obesity, chronic renal disease, or peripheral vascular disease. Moderate hypertriglyceridemia (250–750 mg/dl) that persists after secondary causes have been eliminated may respond to low-fat diet, exercise, and weight loss, while severe hypertriglyceridemia often requires drug therapy. Triglycerides >1,500 mg/dl may lead to pancreatitis and require immediate treatment with a low-fat diet.

Elevated Chylomicron Remnants and IDL Cholesterol. Type III hyperlipoproteinemia is characterized by plasma accumulation of chylomicron remnants and IDL particles due to impaired catabolism. Both cholesterol and triglycerides are elevated, with mean levels of 450 mg/dl and 700 mg/dl, respectively (Mahley 1989). LDL cholesterol is generally low due to reduced conversion of VLDL to LDL and/or to upregulation of LDL receptors. Patients are susceptible to severe premature CAD, strokes, and peripheral vascular disease.

Chylomicron remnants and IDL particles are normally cleared by hepatic remnant and LDL receptors, which recognize apo E on the surface of these particles, as described previously. A common impairment of this pathway is due to the apo E2 allele, which encodes a protein with only 1–2% of normal receptor binding activity. About 1% of the population is homozygous for E2 (E2/2 genotype). These individuals do not generally exhibit fasting hyperlipidemia but have difficulty clearing chylomicron remnants from plasma postprandially (Brown 1991). Approximately 1 in 50 E2/2 individuals is unable to compensate for the defective apo E protein and develops the fasting lipid elevations characteristic of type III hyperlipoproteinemia. Xanthoma striata palmaris, orange or yellow discolorations of the palmar and digital creases, are pathognomonic of type III disease (Mahley 1989). The diagnosis is supported by the results of lipoprotein electrophoresis, available from commercial laboratories. The difference between E2/2 individuals with and without fasting hyperlipidemia is presumably due to factors that affect IDL metabolism. These may include aging, exogenous estrogen, obesity, glucose intolerance, and hypothyroidism, as well as heterozygosity for another genetic defect, such as FH (Mahley 1889; Brown 1991). Type III hyperlipoproteinemia has been reported in several patients with the apo E2/2 genotype who are also heterozygous for an LPL mutation (Ma 1993), and there are almost certainly other mutant genes that can serve as a ''second hit,'' resulting in type III disease. Type III patients are highly responsive to dietary modification and weight loss, but drug therapy is often required.

Homozygous apo E mutations resulting in very low to undetectable levels of plasma apo E have recently been described (Zannis 1993). Apo E deficiency is associated with very high plasma levels of VLDL plus IDL cholesterol and with atherosclerosis. In mice, germline ablation of both copies of the apo E gene results in advanced atherosclerotic lesions similar to those observed in human CAD (Breslow 1993).

Elevated Lipoprotein(a). In case-control studies, elevated plasma levels of Lp(a) have been found to be an independent risk factor for CAD (Berg 1992). Levels of Lp(a), an LDL-like particle, vary greatly in the population (from <0.1 to >200 mg/dl) and are almost entirely genetically determined. Plasma Lp(a) concentrations >20 mg/dl have been reported to confer increased risk of CAD, as well as cerebrovascular and peripheral vascular disease. Lp(a) >39 mg/dl was the most common familial dyslipidemia in a study of patients with confirmed CAD before age 60, accounting for 19% of patients with a familial dyslipidemia (Genest 1992). Among Hawaiian men of Japanese ancestry, 14% of all cases of MI and 28% of cases prior to age 60 were attributed to elevated Lp(a) (Rhoads 1986). In contrast to case-control studies, prospective studies of Lp(a) and CAD have produced inconsistent results. While two small Swedish studies detected an association (Berg 1992), a prospective analysis of Helsinki Heart Study participants found no relationship between Lp(a) levels and future coronary events (Jauhiainen 1991). Similarly, no association between Lp(a) levels and future MI in men was detected in the Physicians' Health Study (296 cases, 296 controls) (Ridker 1993a). Blacks have higher Lp(a) levels than Caucasians, but this does not appear to translate into increased CAD risk (Sorrentino 1992).

The protein component of the Lp(a) particle consists of one molecule of apo B disulfide-bonded to one molecule of apolipoprotein(a) [apo (a)], a very large protein of unknown function. Apo(a) bears a striking resemblance to the fibrinolytic enzyme precursor plasminogen, and the genes for these two proteins are closely linked on chromosome 6 (Berg 1992). Plasminogen consists of five pretzel-shaped domains, called *kringles*, and a protease domain, while apo(a) consists of multiple tandem copies of a sequence resembling the plasminogen kringle IV domain, plus single copies of plasminogenlike kringle V and protease domains. The protease domain of apo(a) is unable to degrade fibrin. Both the apo(a) gene and protein vary widely in size within the population due to differing numbers of copies of the kringle IV sequence (Berg 1992).

Approximately 90% of the variability in Lp(a) levels in the population is attributable to the apo(a) gene (Boerwinkle 1992). Lp(a) levels are inversely correlated with apo(a) size, and individuals with smaller apo(a) isoforms are therefore presumed to be at greater risk of CAD (Berg 1992). Size polymorphisms account for nearly 70% of the variance in Lp(a) levels (Boerwinkle 1992). Apo(a) alleles of the same size are heterogeneous at the DNA sequence level, and it has been estimated that there may be more than 100 alleles in total (Cohen 1993). Alleles of the same size but differing sequence are coinherited with different Lp(a) levels in families (Cohen 1993), and variation in regions of the apo(a) gene that regulate messenger RNA levels are likely to make an independent contribution to variability in Lp(a) levels. Sequence heterogeneity in the apo(a) gene may contribute to genetic variation in CAD risk not only via effects on Lp(a) levels but also via qualitative differences in the apo(a) molecule.

Lp(a) may participate in both thrombogenic and atherogenic processes due to the plasminogenlike properties of apo(a) and the LDL-like properties of Lp(a) (Scanu 1990). Fibrinolysis by plasmin requires the conversion of plasminogen to plasmin by tissue-type plasminogen activator (tPA). In vitro studies suggest that Lp(a) may inter-fere with this process. In addition, apo(a) can compete with plasminogen for binding to fibrin and to plasminogen receptors on cultured endothelial cells, preventing assem-bly of the fibrinolytic system on cell surfaces (Berg 1992). A relationship between elevated plasma Lp(a) and increased thrombosis or reduced thrombolysis has not been established in humans but has been demonstrated in primates following arterial injury (Williams JK 1993). Apo(a), much of it in the form of cholesterol-rich Lp(a), is a tightly bound constituent of human atherosclerotic plaques (Berg 1992), and transgenic mice expressing human apo(a) develop early atherosclerotic lesions on a high-fat diet (Breslow 1993).

Measurement of Lp(a) levels, available from commercial laboratories, has been recommended in patients with premature CAD, and elevated levels may warrant test-ing and counseling of first-degree relatives (Berg 1992). Since known treatments fail to normalize Lp(a), intervention focuses on reduction of coexisting risk factors, es-pecially elevated LDL cholesterol. Further studies are required to reconcile the results of the prospective and case-control studies.

Diabetes Mellitus

The familial nature of diabetes is well-known. Hyperglycemia is a feature of at least 60 rare genetic syndromes, demonstrating that mutations in many different genes can produce diabetes (Shohat 1992). While genetic factors play a role in insulin-dependent diabetes mellitus (IDDM), they appear to be a very strong determinant of non-insulin-dependent diabetes mellitus (NIDDM) susceptibility (Table 3.7).

Insulin-Dependent Diabetes Mellitus. A widely held view of IDDM posits the coin-cidence of a genetic predisposition with a viral infection or other environmental insult, leading to T cell-mediated destruction of pancreatic beta cells (Shohat 1992; Thorsby 1993). IDDM is a potent risk factor for premature CAD. Cardiovascular mortality among IDDM patients aged 30–34 has been estimated at 32 times the U.S. population rate for this age group (Shohat 1992). Having a first-degree relative with IDDM was an independent CAD risk factor in one study (Nora 1980), suggesting common un-derlying genetic factors. The inheritance pattern of IDDM is complex, apparently involving multiple genes. Concordance in monozygotic twins is only 35% to 50% (Thorsby 1993), confirming the importance of environmental factors.

The human leukocyte antigen (HLA) gene complex on chromosome 6, which encodes highly polymorphic molecules of the immune system, accounts for 60% to 70% of the genetic susceptibility to IDDM (Shohat 1992). The HLA D (or class II) region contains the genes for the cell-surface molecules DP, DQ, and DR, which are expressed on B lymphocytes, monocytes, macrophages, and endothelial cells. The function of these proteins is to present foreign antigen fragments to helper T cells (Thorsby 1993). Approximately 95% of Caucasians with IDDM carry the DR3 or DR4 alleles or both, compared with 50% of nondiabetic controls, while DR2 is as-sociated with resistance to IDDM (Shohat 1992). Attention has recently focused on the DQ genes, which are adjacent and tightly linked to the DR genes (Thorsby 1993). The relative importance of the DR and DQ genes in IDDM is controversial, and the

Table 3.7. Genetic Factors in Diabetes Mellitus

Disorder	Gene(s)	Chromosome	Frequency	Comment
IDDM			1/250	
	HLA[a,b]	6		Susceptibility region
	Insulin[b]	11		Susceptibility gene
NIDDM (rare forms)				
	Insulin[a]	11	10 families	Known causative mutations
	Insulin receptor[a,b]	19	1/1000	Known causative mutations
	Glucokinase[a]	7	1/2500	Known MODY mutations; ~60% of MODY cases
	?[a]	20	1 family	Known MODY region
	Mitochondrial mutation (tRNA-leu) or deletion	Mt DNA	>30 families	Known causative mutation or deletion
NIDDM (common form)			1/15	
	Glycogen synthase minor allele[a,b]	19	1/3 diabetics, 1/12 controls in Finland	Candidate susceptibility region in Finns

[a]Heterozygotes.

[b]Homozygotes.

IDDM, insulin-dependent diabetes mellitus; NIDDM, non-insulin-dependent diabetes mellitus; HLA, human leukocyte antigens; MODY, maturity-onset diabetes of the young; tRNA, transfer RNA; MtDNA, mitochondrial DNA.

precise molecular bases of HLA-mediated susceptibility and resistance to IDDM are unknown.

Polymorphisms near the insulin gene on chromosome 11 are associated with IDDM in population studies, and some but not all family studies have shown linkage of IDDM to this gene (Julier 1991). The insulin amino acid sequence does not differ between IDDM-associated and other alleles, suggesting that genetic variation may instead affect regulation of insulin synthesis. There is some evidence for HLA and insulin gene interaction in IDDM (Julier 1991).

Non-Insulin-Dependent Diabetes Mellitus. While simple mendelian inheritance of NIDDM is generally not observed and a polygenic etiology is likely, the concordance rate for monozygotic twins is approximately 90% (Shohat 1992). For individuals with a diabetic sibling, the lifetime risk of developing NIDDM is approximately 40% (Kobberling 1982). NIDDM is more prevalent among blacks and Hispanics than among Caucasians. Diabetes is especially common among the Pima Indians of Arizona, with a prevalence of 40%–50% and an early onset (mid-30s to mid-40s). Obesity is also common among the Pima, and obese individuals have nearly three times the incidence of NIDDM as the nonobese (Saad 1988).

Insulin gene mutations are a rare cause of NIDDM (Steiner 1990). Certain insulin amino acid substitutions have been shown to cause greatly reduced affinity for the insulin receptor, resulting in hyperinsulinemia and glucose intolerance or mild diabetes, with autosomal dominant inheritance. Other insulin mutations resulting in hyperproinsulinemia and mild diabetes have also been described.

Some single-gene disorders cause NIDDM by disrupting the complex process of insulin release. Glucose entering the beta cell is phosphorylated by glucokinase, in the rate-limiting step in glycolysis, to form glucose 6-phosphate. The subsequent oxidation of glucose results in a rising ATP/ADP ratio. This is thought to trigger closure of ATP-sensitive potassium channels, membrane depolarization, and opening of voltage-dependent calcium channels. The resulting rise in intracellular calcium, along with other second messengers, leads to recruitment and extrusion of insulin-containing vesicles (Leahy 1992).

Maturity-onset diabetes of the young (MODY) is an autosomal dominant form of NIDDM with an early onset, usually before age 25. MODY is not associated with obesity and generally has a mild course. One form of MODY is caused by a defective glucokinase gene on chromosome 7 (Froguel 1993), while a second form has been mapped via family studies to chromosome 20 (Bell 1991). More than 25 different glucokinase mutations have been identified. Such mutations have been found in most of the MODY families studied and account for approximately 6% of familial NIDDM in France (Froguel 1993).

Heritable mutations of mitochondrial DNA have been shown to cause diabetes in a small number of families (Ballinger 1992; van den Ouweland 1992). The circular mitochondrial genome, present in thousands of copies per cell, is inherited only from the mother, and maternal inheritance of diabetes is observed in these families. In one family, diabetes with deafness is due to a mitochondrial DNA deletion affecting 16 of the 22 mitochondrial transfer RNA (tRNA) genes and the genes for 12 of the 13 respiratory chain enzyme subunits (Ballinger 1992). In the other families, this syndrome is due to a single nucleotide substitution in the gene encoding the tRNA for leucine, which lies outside the region of the large deletion (van den Ouweland 1992). This mutation causes mitochondrial myopathy, encephalopathy, lactic acidosis and strokelike episodes (MELAS) in some families and diabetes with deafness in others; the former appears to be associated with a higher proportion of mutant mitochondrial DNA molecules in muscle (van den Ouweland 1992). Diabetes caused by mitochondrial mutations may present as IDDM (early onset, low to undetectable insulin levels, ketoacidosis) or as NIDDM (late onset, normal to high insulin levels, without ketoacidosis).

Glucokinase is believed to act as the glucose sensor for beta cells (Froguel 1993). Much of the glucokinase is attached to the mitochondrial membrane, and detection of high glucose concentrations may involve glucose phosphorylation using mitochondrial ATP. This may explain why mutations affecting either glucokinase or mitochondrial DNA can cause diabetes (Ballinger 1994).

Impaired beta-cell function is believed to be necessary but not sufficient for the development of NIDDM, which also requires impaired response to insulin (DeFronzo 1992). In normal individuals, the binding of insulin to its cell-surface receptor activates the receptor tyrosine kinase, resulting in receptor autophosphorylation. This initiates a cascade of intracellular phosphorylations that mediate the many actions of insulin. Reduced response to insulin is often present in first-degree relatives of diabetics, suggesting a genetic component, and insulin resistance is commonly the first sign of abnormal glucose metabolism (DeFronzo 1992). Obesity is believed to be an independent contributor to insulin resistance, and obese diabetics are more insulin-resistant than lean diabetics. The major manifestation of insulin resistance is defective insulin-stimulated glycogen storage in muscle (DeFronzo 1992).

Mutations in the insulin receptor gene on chromosome 19 result in several rare syndromes characterized by insulin resistance, hyperinsulinemia, glucose intolerance or frank diabetes, and acanthosis nigricans; in females, hyperandrogenism may also be present (Taylor 1992). More than 40 insulin receptor mutations are known (Leahy 1993). Some result in decreased receptor number, while others reduce receptor affinity for insulin or impair tyrosine kinase activity. While patients with two mutant alleles generally have extreme insulin resistance, heterozygotes may have a clinical presentation similar to common NIDDM.

Single-gene disorders characterized to date are likely to account for only a small fraction of the cases of NIDDM. In a Finnish study, an association between common NIDDM and a polymorphism in the glycogen synthase gene on chromosome 19 has been reported (Groop 1993). The minor allele for this polymorphism, which does not affect the amino acid sequence of the protein, was found in 30% of NIDDM patients, compared with 8% of controls (Groop 1993). This allele is associated with marked insulin resistance, hypertension, and a strong family history of NIDDM.

The glycogen synthase gene has been viewed as a promising potential candidate gene for NIDDM because of the central role of defective glycogen synthesis in insulin resistance. Glucose clearance is carried out to a large extent by skeletal muscle (DeFronzo 1992). After entering a muscle cell and undergoing phosphorylation by hexokinase, glucose that does not enter the glycolytic pathway is stored as glycogen in a reaction catalyzed by glycogen synthase, which is activated by both glucose 6-phosphate and insulin. Glucose clearance is reduced by 30% to 50% in NIDDM, and this has been attributed to an impairment of insulin-stimulated glycogen synthase activation (DeFronzo 1992). Reduced glycogen synthase activity has also been observed in normoglycemic first-degree relatives of diabetics.

In the Finnish study, the rate of insulin-stimulated glycogen synthesis was reduced by 50% in diabetic carriers of the glycogen synthase minor allele relative to diabetic noncarriers, and the former were nearly twice as likely to be hypertensive as the latter. In addition, both first-degree relatives of NIDDM patients and normoglycemic controls carrying the minor allele were three to four times more likely to be hypertensive than were noncarriers (Groop 1993). Normoglycemic subjects with hypertension are insulin-resistant following insulin infusion, and this finding is associated with impaired glycogen synthesis. It should be noted, however, that association of the glycogen synthase polymorphism with NIDDM has not been observed in several other ethnic groups studied, and additional work is needed to determine the significance of the Finnish study.

Obesity

Obesity reflects an imbalance between caloric intake and energy expenditure. It has been proposed that there is an inherent set-point for body weight and adipose stores that is regulated by the central nervous system, primarily the hypothalamus (Leibel 1984; Friedman 1992). Reduction of body weight below the set-point appears to be accompanied by compensatory metabolic changes, notably reduced calorie requirements, that make it very difficult to maintain the new lower weight (Leibel 1984). Lesions of the ventromedial nucleus of the hypothalamus lead to obesity, while lesions in other hypothalamic regions have the opposite effect, indicating the presence of both stimulatory and inhibitory centers with respect to weight gain. Lesions producing obesity are accompanied by increased parasympathetic activity and decreased sympathetic tone, leading to reduced energy expenditure and increased insulin release (Friedman 1992).

Obesity and insulin resistance, together with hyperandrogenism, are features of polycystic ovary disease, a relatively common disorder that in some families appears to be autosomal dominant. Obesity is also a feature of several rare genetic disorders characterized by hypogonadism and often by diabetes. The common form of obesity is a consequence of a genetic predisposition together with environmental factors. Studies of twins reared apart indicate that genetic factors predominate, accounting for up to 70% of the variance in body mass index (BMI) (Stunkard 1990). The results of several studies indicate that BMI is strongly influenced by a major recessive gene. Genetic factors are also thought to play a role in abdominal adiposity, which is associated with increased glucocorticoid levels and, in women, with increased androgens (Despres 1992).

Efforts to find human genes predisposing to obesity have focused largely on single-gene rodent models of obesity, notably *ob* (obese) and *db* (diabetes), which act in a recessive manner (Friedman 1992). The *ob* and *db* mice are hyperphagic and hypometabolic, and both may become diabetic, depending on the mouse strain onto which the mutations are bred. The mice have abnormalities of several hypothalamic functions, including gonadotrophin secretion, leading to infertility. Glucocorticoids appear to play a role in expression of obesity in these animals. Similar metabolic abnormalities are present in *ob* and *db* mice with the same genetic background, and it has been proposed that the *ob* and *db* genes encode two proteins in the same pathway. Thus, *ob* mice may be deficient in a circulating satiety factor, while *db* mice may be refractory to the effects of this factor, perhaps due to a defective receptor. The *ob* and *db* genes have been mapped to mouse chromosomal regions similar to regions of human chromosomes 7 and 1, respectively (Friedman 1992). Both the mouse and the human *ob* genes have recently been isolated (Zhang 1994).

Obesity affects 75% of Pima Indians, and it has been proposed that the Pima and other ethnic groups with a high prevalence of obesity harbor a "thrifty" gene. This gene (or set of genes) is thought to confer a selective advantage in times of famine but to predispose to obesity and diabetes when calorie intake is high and energy expenditure is low (Neel 1962). Such a gene may confer a low relative metabolic rate and/or favor fat storage, with reduced fat oxidation and depletion of carbohydrate stores. The expression of the "thrifty" trait appears most pronounced in societies undergoing a rapid shift from an agrarian way of life to a more sedentary Western lifestyle. This shift is likely to account for the sharp rise in the prevalence of obesity and NIDDM observed worldwide, most notably in rapidly developing countries (Diamond 1992). Similar factors may explain the rising prevalence of obesity in the United States, especially among the less educated, who consume more calories and fat than more educated individuals (Stamler 1993). These trends illustrate the importance of the interaction between lifestyle and common genetic factors.

Hypertension

Essential hypertension, which accounts for over 90% of cases, is a heterogeneous group of disorders. The renin-angiotensin system is central to blood pressure home-ostasis, and the complexity of this system as a mediator of blood pressure is under-scored by the fact that patients with essential hypertension may have low, normal, or high renin levels. Sodium sensitivity is a feature of approximately 60% of cases of hypertension (Williams 1991). Salt-sensitive hypertensives with normal or high renin have been described as "nonmodulators," since the response of the renin-angiotensin system to salt-loading is abnormal in these patients, leading to impaired sodium ex-cretion (Williams 1991).

Blood pressure is known to be influenced by genetic factors (Table 3.8), although the observed strength of this influence has differed widely among various studies, accounting for between 20% and 60% of the variance (Kurtz 1993). Individuals with essential hypertension are twice as likely to have a hypertensive parent than are nor-motensives (Burke 1992). The blood pressure correlations observed between mono-zygotic twins (0.6 for diastolic and 0.55–0.7 for systolic) are at least twofold greater than those observed between dizygotic twins (Burke 1992). Several lines of evidence indicate that nonmodulating hypertension has a strong genetic component (Williams GH 1993). A family history of hypertension can be elicited from 85% of nonmodu-lators, compared with 25% to 30% of other normal- or high-renin hypertensives. In

Table 3.8. Genetic Factors in Hypertension

Disorder	Gene(s)	Chromosome(s)	Frequency	Comment
Polycystic kidney disease (PKD)[a]			1/1000	
	PKD1	16		Known PKD gene
	PKD2	4		Known PKD region
Glucocorticoid-remediable aldosteronism[a]	11β-Hydroxylase/ aldosterone synthase	8	<100 cases	Known causative DNA rearrangement (1 family)
11β-Hydroxylase deficiency[b]	11β-Hydroxylase [cytochrome P450(11)]	8	1/100,000	Known causative mutations
17α-Hydroxylase deficiency[b]	17α-Hydroxylase [cytochrome P450(17)]	10	~40 cases	Known causative mutations
Familial dysautonomia (FD)[a]	?	9	1/3600 Ashkenazi Jews	Known FD region
Essential hypertension			~1/2 Caucasians >140/90 mmHg	
	Angiotensinogen minor allele[a,b]	1	76% of severe cases; 59% of controls	Candidate susceptibility gene
Preeclampsia			1/15–1/20 pregnancies	
	Angiotensinogen minor allele[a,b]	1	92% of cases (primigravidas); 63% of controls	Candidate susceptibility gene

[a]Heterozygotes.

[b]Homozygotes.

addition, a high degree of sibling concordance has been observed for the nonmodulating trait. Multiple genes are presumed to interact with obesity, sedentary lifestyle, high salt intake, noise, crowding, and stress to influence blood pressure (Burke 1992).

Single-gene disorders leading to neurogenic, renal, or endocrine hypertension have been described (Williams 1991). The most common is autosomal dominant polycystic kidney disease, a genetically heterogeneous disorder that results in hypertension in 75% of cases. Glucocorticoid-remediable aldosteronism (GRA), a rare autosomal dominant disorder causing hypertension, has been mapped to the adjacent 11β-hydroxylase and aldosterone synthase genes on chromosome 8 (Lifton 1992).

Variation in the angiotensinogen gene on chromosome 1 may influence susceptibility to essential hypertension and preeclampsia in the general population. Angiotensinogen is the precursor of angiotensin I and II, and the latter has multiple actions that promote blood pressure elevation. In studies of subjects from France and Utah, an association has been demonstrated between hypertension and the minor allele of an angiotensinogen polymorphism, and hypertension has been shown to be linked to this gene via analysis of affected sibling pairs (Jeunemaitre 1992). The polymorphism results in a methionine to threonine amino acid substitution in angiotensinogen, with a Caucasian allele frequency of 35%. The threonine allele was found to be associated with elevated plasma angiotensinogen, especially in women (Jeunemaitre 1992), and conferred a relative risk of 1.85 for severe hypertension. Plasma angiotensinogen levels are strongly correlated with blood pressure and are elevated in hypertensive families. Blood pressure in rodents is increased by injection of angiotensinogen and decreased by injection of antibodies to angiotensinogen (Jeunemaitre 1992). It has been proposed that overexpression of angiotensinogen in carriers of the threonine allele may result in a small increase in angiotensin II levels, causing hyperreactivity of the renin-angiotensin system in response to salt or other environmental factors. This may lead to hyperaldosteronism with sodium retention, as well as vascular hypertrophy and increased peripheral vascular resistance (Jeunemaitre 1992).

Subsequent to the initial report on the angiotensinogen polymorphism among populations from Utah and France, the threonine allele was also found to be enriched in Japanese hypertensive subjects (Hata 1994). It should be noted, however, that a large Finnish study was negative (Kiema 1994), and a British sib pair study which implicated the angiotensinogen gene in essential hypertension nevertheless failed to detect an association with the threonine allele (Caulfield 1994). Further work is clearly needed to resolve the role of the angiotensinogen gene in essential hypertension.

The threonine allele has also been implicated in preeclampsia in both Caucasian and Japanese women (Ward 1993). In normal pregnancy, renin-angiotensin stimulation is responsible for a physiologic hypervolemia of 40% to 50%. Preeclamptic women fail to develop hypervolemia but have increased vascular resistance, and normal pregnancy-induced refractoriness to the pressor effects of infused angiotensin II is not observed in preeclampsia (Ward 1993). Several studies have suggested a genetic link between essential hypertension and preeclampsia. Preeclamptic women are more likely than other women to have a family history of essential hypertension (Lindeberg 1988). Some, but not all, studies have shown that preeclamptic women are themselves more likely to develop essential hypertension (Sibai 1986); in addition, their offspring have higher blood pressures than the offspring of normotensive women (Seidman 1991).

Preeclampsia is a heterogeneous disorder and susceptibility to at least some forms appears to be due to a single gene. In Caucasians, the threonine-encoding allele of the angiotensinogen gene conferred a relative risk of primigravida preeclampsia of 2.8 compared with the methionine-encoding allele. Preeclamptic carriers of the threonine allele have higher angiotensinogen levels than noncarriers, and it has been suggested that preeclampsia may result from threonine allele-associated vascular hypertrophy (Ward 1993).

The renin-angiotensin system appears to play a role in MI apart from its role in hypertension. The gene for angiotensin-converting enzyme (ACE) on chromosome 17 has been implicated as a common contributor to MI in men. An ACE gene polymorphism is associated, in the homozygous state, with MI in both Caucasian and Japanese men (Cambien 1992; Ohishi 1993). Subjects carrying the MI-associated allele have higher plasma ACE levels than noncarriers. ACE cleaves angiotensin I to generate angiotensin II and also degrades bradykinin. Angiotensin II and bradykinin have opposing effects on smooth muscle cells and on vascular tone. Angiotensin II promotes growth of myocardial and vascular smooth muscle cells and promotes neointimal hyperplasia after arterial wall injury, while bradykinin appears to be a growth inhibitor. It has been proposed that the ACE polymorphism may influence MI risk by modulating levels of angiotensin II and bradykinin in coronary arteries (Cambien 1992). Angiotensin II may also reduce fibrinolysis by increasing plasma levels of plasminogen activator inhibitor-1 (PAI-1), which inhibits endogenous tPA (Ridker 1993b). While ACE genetic variation affects blood pressure in rodents, no such association has been observed in humans.

The MI-associated ACE allele has a frequency of over 50% in Caucasians. In the initial study, the homozygous state was associated with a modest overall increase in MI susceptibility (relative risk: 1.1–2.1). Among subjects defined as low-risk (normal BMI and apo B levels, not under treatment for hyperlipidemia), homozygosity for this allele conferred a relative risk of 3 (Cambien 1992). The percentage of cases of MI attributable to this genotype was estimated to be 8% in the general population and 35% in the otherwise low-risk group (Cambien 1992). Several subsequent studies have supported and extended these findings in men (Ludwig 1993; Ohishi 1993), although negative studies have also been reported, including a large prospective study (Bohn 1993; Lindpaintner 1994). One study found an association between the MI-related allele and low BMI but did not replicate the initial finding of a stronger association between the ACE polymorphism and MI among otherwise low-risk men (Ludwig 1993). Among Japanese heart attack victims, homozygosity for the MI-associated allele conferred a relative risk of approximately 4 for restenosis following emergency angioplasty (Ohishi 1993). This allele was not significantly increased among patients selected on the basis of CAD, whether or not they had suffered an MI (Kreutz 1993; Ludwig 1993). This suggests that the polymorphism may be a predictor of MI-related events independent of and/or subsequent to the development of atherosclerosis.

An association has been reported between homozygosity for the MI-associated ACE allele and left ventricular hypertrophy (LVH) (Schunkert 1994). This allele conferred a relative risk for LVH of over 3 among middle-aged men in one study. Experimentally induced aortic stenosis leading to LVH increases ACE activity in rat cardiac tissue (Schunkert 1990), and the ACE system in tissues may have an important pathophysiologic role in the development of hypertrophy and congestive heart failure (Dzau 1993). It is possible that the MI-associated ACE allele is hyperresponsive to the cardiac stresses that lead to LVH.

In addition to lowering blood pressure, ACE inhibitors retard atherosclerosis progression in animals and reduce the risk of heart failure and second MI in heart attack patients (Beckwith 1993). It has been suggested that cardiac patients homozygous for the MI-associated ACE allele may benefit most from ACE inhibitors (Ohishi 1993), but this has not been established. The properties of the ACE polymorphism provide further evidence that activities of the renin-angiotensin system other than blood pressure regulation play a role in cardiovascular disease.

Syndrome X

Dyslipidemia, glucose intolerance, and hypertension cluster in individuals and families to a greater extent than would be expected based on the frequency of each in the population (Reaven 1988; Burke 1991; Shohat 1992), suggesting common underlying causes and a genetic predisposition. This constellation of metabolic abnormalities has been termed syndrome X (Reaven 1988). Hyperuricemia, impaired fibrinolysis and small dense LDL particles are also associated with syndrome X (Reaven 1993a, 1993b). Syndrome X and related disorders markedly increase MI susceptibility, since CAD risk increases continuously as glucose and blood pressure rise and as HDL cholesterol falls (Ginsberg 1993).

It has been proposed that the underlying defect in syndrome X is insulin resistance (Reaven 1988). Quantitative measures of insulin resistance are directly correlated with glucose levels, triglycerides, and, among Caucasians, blood pressure (Ginsberg 1993). The degree of insulin sensitivity varies widely in the normoglycemic population, with the least insulin-sensitive quartile demonstrating insulin resistance comparable to that seen in glucose intolerance or frank NIDDM (Reaven 1988). Insulin resistance is overcome by increased insulin secretion, and hyperglycemia develops only in those who cannot maintain hyperinsulinemia because of deficient beta-cell function. Impaired insulin action results in failure to store glucose as glycogen and in failure to suppress both gluconeogenesis in the liver and lipolysis in adipose tissue.

Glucose-intolerant subjects and hyperinsulinemic subjects with normal glucose tolerance have increased triglycerides relative to controls (Reaven 1988). Enhanced adipose tissue lipolysis results in increased mobilization of free fatty acids, leading to increased VLDL secretion, while clearance of VLDL and chylomicrons declines due to reduced lipoprotein lipase activity. The resulting hypertriglyceridemia may depress HDL cholesterol levels. Increased fatty acid flux stimulates gluconeogenesis and favors fatty acid oxidation at the expense of insulin-stimulated glucose disposal (DeFronzo 1992). Many investigators have emphasized the role of obesity, especially abdominal adiposity, in metabolic disorders predisposing to CAD. Obesity both increases insulin resistance and provides a larger adipose store, augmenting fatty acid flux.

Glucose-intolerant patients have higher blood pressures than those with normal glucose tolerance (Zavaroni 1991), and untreated hypertensives are more likely to be insulin-resistant, hyperinsulinemic, and hypertriglyceridemic than are normotensive controls (Reaven 1988). Insulin promotes renal sodium and water resorption and activates the sympathetic nervous system, increasing vascular resistance (Reaven 1988). The role of insulin resistance in hypertension is controversial, however, since an association has not been demonstrated in all studies, particularly after adjustment for confounding variables (Jarrett 1992). A study which confirmed an association between insulin resistance and blood pressure in Caucasians found no such relationship in blacks or in the highly insulin-resistant Pima Indians (Saad 1991). Animal studies have been inconsistent, and induction of hyperinsulinemia in humans has been found to cause vasodilation rather than vasoconstriction (Mark 1992). Hyperinsulinemia does not invariably lead to hypertension, since patients with insulinomas are not generally hypertensive (Jarrett 1992). Thus, hyperinsulinemia and insulin resistance are associated with hypertension in a subset of patients; further work is required to clarify the significance of this finding.

Based on epidemiologic and cell culture studies, it has been argued that hyperinsulinemia may be directly atherogenic (Reaven 1988). Two large prospective studies found elevated plasma insulin levels to be an independent CAD risk factor in men, and some, but not all, case-control studies have shown an association between insulin levels and atherosclerosis in NIDDM (Shohat 1992). The prospective studies did not take into account the effect of HDL cholesterol levels on CAD risk, however, and long-term insulin treatment of NIDDM patients does not appear to increase CAD mortality (Jarrett 1988). The Pima Indians, with a very high prevalence of hyperinsulinemia and NIDDM, do not have a high prevalence of CAD, demonstrating that among some ethnic groups even NIDDM is not a strong predictor of CAD.

The role of genetic factors in syndrome X has been investigated only recently. First-degree relatives of glucose-intolerant or NIDDM patients have an increased prevalence of insulin resistance, hyperinsulinemia, hypertension, and hypertriglyceridemia (Zavaroni 1991). A study of over 2,500 male twins aged 56 to 68 found that concordance rates for hypertension, diabetes, obesity, and the confluence of these traits were higher in monozygotic than in dizygotic twins (Carmelli 1993). The estimated contribution of genetic factors to the variance in susceptibility to these disorders was 56% for hypertension, 72% for NIDDM, and 65% for obesity. Multivariate analysis supported a common underlying factor, influenced by both genes (59%) and environment (41%), explaining the clustering of these abnormalities in individuals (Carmelli 1993). Diabetes and hypertriglyceridemia were found to be inherited independently in families with both traits, although untreated diabetics with hypertriglyceridemia had the highest triglyceride levels (Brunzell 1975). A large family in which a heterozygous lipoprotein lipase mutation was found to cosegregate with dyslipidemia and hypertension in individuals over age 40 has been described; these abnormalities were especially common in family members with hyperinsulinemia and obesity (Wilson 1990). The previously described apo CIII marker associated with hypertriglyceridemia was not associated with diabetes, hypertension or increased BMI among subjects with triglycerides $\geq 1,000$ mg/dl (D. Buyer, M. Dammerman, and J. Breslow, unpublished results, 1994). There is unlikely to be a single genetic etiology for most cases of syndrome X and related disorders. These conditions probably represent a confluence of several common susceptibility genes with relevant environmental factors. Each of the genes may confer an abnormality that in isolation appears mild but that, in combination with other such genes or with adverse lifestyle choices, can cause major metabolic disturbances.

Non-traditional Risk Factors and New Classes of Candidate Genes

In addition to the traditional metabolic risk factors, attention has focused recently on other factors found to be correlated with CAD in population studies. These include plasma homocyst(e)ine and several plasma proteins involved in coagulation and fibrinolysis. The investigation of genetic influences on these risk factors is at a relatively early stage.

Homocyst(e)ine

Moderately elevated plasma levels of homocyst(e)ine have received considerable attention as a CAD risk factor. Homocyst(e)ine levels are sharply elevated in the autosomal recessive disorder homocystinuria, which is characterized in part by premature occlusive vascular disease (Mudd 1989). This rare disorder is due to mutations in the cystathionine β-synthase gene on chromosome 21 (Kozich 1992); several different mutations have been reported. This enzyme catalyzes the condensation of homocysteine with serine to form cystathionine (Mudd 1989). Since the alternative fate of homocysteine is methylation to form methionine, both homocyst(e)ine and methionine accumulate in plasma and tissues in cystathionine β-synthase deficiency, and homocystine is excreted in urine (Mudd 1989). The associated vascular lesions have been attributed to abnormalities of platelets, vascular endothelium, and/or clotting factors (Mudd 1989). In addition, homocysteine enhances binding of Lp(a) to fibrin, a potentially atherogenic interaction (Harpel 1992). In one study, thromboembolic events among patients with homocystinuria included phlebothrombosis (51%) and stroke (32%); only 4% were classified as MI (Mudd 1989). At autopsy, thrombi and emboli have been reported in almost every major artery or vein and in many smaller vessels of affected patients.

Several studies, including a large prospective study, have found an association between moderately elevated plasma homocyst(e)ine levels and CAD, independent of traditional risk factors. In the prospective study, 7% of cases of MI were attributed to elevated plasma homocyst(e)ine (Stampfer 1992). In another study, 28% of CAD patients had homocyst(e)ine levels above the 90th percentile for controls (Genest 1991). Familial segregation of elevated homocyst(e)ine was observed in half of these cases, and this was attributed to both genetic and environmental factors (Genest 1991). Reduced fibroblast cystathionine β-synthase activity has been reported in CAD, and in one study 21% of CAD patients had an abnormal response to an oral methionine load (Dudman 1993).

Several issues remain to be resolved with respect to the role of moderately elevated homocyst(e)ine in CAD. Increased risk of MI has not been observed among obligate heterozygotes for cystathionine β-synthase deficiency, and several early studies failed to detect elevated homocyst(e)ine among CAD patients after methionine loading (Mudd 1989). Metabolic events associated with elevated plasma homocyst(e)ine in

CAD patients may be quite different from those in patients with classic homocystin-uria. Elevated homocyst(e)ine may often be due to folic acid deficiency, and this is easily corrected by folate supplementation (Stampfer 1992). Serum homocysteine lev-els are determined by commercial laboratories.

Hemostatic Factors

Three proteins involved in coagulation or fibrinolysis have been implicated in CAD: factor VII, fibrinogen, and PAI-1. Activated factor VII is a protease that activates factor X, which in turn cleaves prothrombin to generate thrombin. Thrombin cleaves fibrinogen to generate fibrin, which polymerizes to form the fibrin clot. During fibri-nolysis, tPA cleaves plasminogen to form plasmin, which in turn degrades fibrin. PAI-1 regulates this process by inhibiting tPA. Factor VII, fibrinogen, and PAI-1 are pos-itively correlated with triglycerides, and high levels of these proteins are also associated with glucose intolerance, hyperinsulinemia, and obesity (Andersen 1992). Present evidence suggests that elevations of factor VII, fibrinogen, and PAI-1 may play an etiologic role in CAD. Levels of tPA, which are inversely correlated with HDL cholesterol levels, were a strongly associated with MI in a prospective study and may therefore prove useful as a predictive marker (Ridker 1993c). Elevated tPA is believed to be a result rather than a cause of CAD, however. Plasma factor VII and fibrinogen assays are available from commercial laboratories.

Increased factor VII coagulant activity (VIIc) was found to be an independent CAD risk factor in a large prospective study. An increase of one standard deviation in plasma VIIc was associated with a 62% increase in the risk of an episode of ischemic heart disease within a 5-year follow-up period (Francis 1992). Increased factor VIIc may predispose to thrombosis at sites of vessel narrowing and may con-tribute to atherosclerosis by promoting fibrin deposition at sites of endothelial injury. The gene for factor VII is on chromosome 13, and the gene for a protein that regulates factor VII is present on chromosome 8 (Francis 1992). An amino acid substitution of glutamine for arginine in factor VII is associated with reduced levels of coagulant activity (Humphries 1992). Carriers of this polymorphism (approximately 20% of the population) have 20% to 25% lower VIIc than noncarriers. VIIc is positively corre-lated with triglycerides, as noted previously, and this relationship is weaker in carriers of the glutamine allele (Humphries 1992). VIIc is also correlated with dietary fat, and a reduction in fat intake has been observed to cause a rapid decline in coagulant activity, providing a rationale for a low-fat diet even among patients with advanced atherosclerosis (Connelly 1993).

Elevated plasma fibrinogen levels have been found to be an independent CAD risk factor in at least four prospective studies, conferring a relative risk ranging from 1.8 to over 4 (Francis 1992). Plasma fibrinogen concentration is an important deter-minant of the rate of fibrin formation and is a major determinant of blood viscosity (Scarabin 1993), which itself has been proposed as a CAD risk factor. In addition, elevated fibrinogen levels may increase platelet aggregation. Atherosclerotic lesions have been found to contain high fibrinogen concentrations. Cigarettes and oral con-traceptives raise plasma fibrinogen, while aerobic exercise reduces it. Fibrinogen con-sists of three pairs of polypeptides (alpha, beta, and gamma) encoded by adjacent genes on chromosome 4. While the correlation in fibrinogen levels between mono-zygotic twins was quite low (0.27) in one study, genetic factors were estimated to account for half the variance in plasma fibrinogen in another study (Francis 1992). A β-fibrinogen polymorphism is associated with elevated fibrinogen levels but not with increased risk of MI (Scarabin 1993). This polymorphism lies in the region of the gene that controls the amount of fibrinogen synthesized.

PAI-1 is a key determinant of plasma fibrinolytic activity. Increased PAI-1 levels have been observed in patients with CAD relative to healthy controls, and elevated PAI-1 levels following coronary angioplasty are correlated with restenosis. While PAI-1 levels have not yet been assessed as a CAD risk factor in a large prospective study, increased PAI-1 was associated with recurrent MI in a small prospective study (Francis 1992). Increased PAI-1 gene expression has been demonstrated in atherosclerotic human arteries (Schneiderman 1992). The available data suggest that PAI-1 may contribute to CAD primarily in concert with other risk factors, notably obesity, NIDDM, hyperinsulinemia, and hypertriglyceridemia. While low PAI-1 heritability was found in a twin study (Francis 1992), sequence variation in the PAI-1 gene on chromosome 7 is associated with variation in plasma PAI-1 activity (Humphries 1992). At least part of this effect is due to a polymorphism in the region of the gene that regulates the amount of PAI-1 synthesized. PAI-1 activity correlates with triglyceride levels, as noted previously, and this relationship was found to be genotype-specific, as was PAI-1 response to insulin during an oral glucose tolerance test. Polymorphisms associated with variation in PAI-1 activity have not been found to differ in frequency between patients with premature CAD and controls, however, and further studies are required to clarify this issue (Humphries 1992).

Future Prospects

Intensive efforts are under way to elucidate the pathogenesis of atherosclerosis, as described in the previous chapter, and important advances are likely to result from the development of new animal models based on transgenic and gene ablation technologies. The ability to express a human gene in transgenic mice, or to ablate an endogenous gene in "knock-out" mice, affords an unprecedented opportunity to establish the functions of specific genes and to test new therapies, including gene therapy (Breslow 1993). In addition, new strategies have recently been developed for identifying rodent genes controlling quantitative traits such as plasma cholesterol, triglycerides, glucose, and blood pressure. In many cases, this is likely to lead to the identification of corresponding human genes. Improved understanding of the genetic and cellular processes underlying atherosclerosis will suggest new interventions to inhibit or reverse these processes.

Our growing awareness of the strongly familial nature of CAD and predisposing metabolic disorders should encourage primary care physicians to focus additional attention on the younger members of affected families, particularly the families of patients with MI under age 55. This should take the form of patient education and follow-up with respect to hygienic measures of proven efficacy and aggressive treatment of metabolic disorders that prove resistant to changes in lifestyle.

Acknowledgments

We thank the following colleagues for helpful comments on the manuscript: Drs. Noah Robbins, Mark Rabinovitch, Neal Azrolan, Markus Stoffel, Wendy Chung, Rudolph Leibel, Peter Weinstock, and Chithranjan Nath. We also thank Andrew Arsham and Cristina Alfaro, who provided expert research assistance, and Marjan Kamali, who assisted in manuscript preparation.

References

Andersen P. Hypercoagulability and reduced fibrinolysis in hyperlipidemia: relationship to the metabolic cardiovascular syndrome. J Cardiovasc Pharmacol 1992;20:S29–31.

Austin MA, Breslow JL, Hennekens CH, et al. Low-density lipoprotein subclass patterns and risk of myocardial infarction. JAMA 1988;260:1917–21.

Austin MA. Plasma triglyceride and coronary heart disease. Arterioscler Thromb 1991;11:2–14.

Austin MA. Genetics of low-density lipoprotein subclasses. Curr Opin Lipidol 1993;4:125–32.

Babirak SP, Iverius P-H, Fujimoto WY, Brunzell JD. Detection and characterization of the heterozygote state for lipoprotein lipase deficiency. Arteriosclerosis 1989;9:326–34.

Ballinger SW, Shoffner JM, Hedaya EV, et al. Maternally transmitted diabetes and deafness associated with a 10.4kb mitochondrial DNA deletion. Nature Genet 1992;1:11–15.

Ballinger SW, Shoffner JM, Gebhart S, et al. Mitochondrial diabetes revisited. [Letter]. Nature Genet 1994;7:458–9.

Beckwith C, Munger MA. Effect of angiotensin-converting enzyme inhibitors on ventricular remodeling and survival following myocardial infarction. Ann Pharmacother 1993;27:755–66.

Bell GI, Xiang K-S, Newman MV, et al. Gene for non-insulin-dependent diabetes mellitus (maturity-onset diabetes of the young subtype) is linked to DNA polymorphism on human chromosome 20q. Proc Natl Acad Sci USA 1991;88:1484–8.

Berg K. Lp(a) lipoprotein: an important genetic risk factor for atherosclerosis. Monogr Hum Genet 1992;14:189–207.

Bierman EL. Atherosclerosis and other forms of arteriosclerosis. In: Wilson JD, Braunwald E, Isselbacher KJ, et al., eds. Harrison's principles of internal medicine, 12th ed. New York: McGraw-Hill, 1991:992–1001.

Boerwinkle E, Leffert CC, Lin J, et al. Apolipoprotein(a) gene accounts for greater than 90% of the variation in plasma lipoprotein(a) concentrations. J Clin Invest 1992;90:52–60.

Bohn M, Berge KE, Bakken A, et al. Insertion/deletion (I/D) polymorphism at the locus for angiotensin I-converting enzyme and myocardial infarction. Clin Genet 1993;44:292–7.

Breslow JL. Familial disorders of high density lipoprotein metabolism. In: Scrivner CR, Beaudet AL, Sly WS, Valle D, eds. The metabolic basis of inherited disease, 6th ed, Vol. I. New York: McGraw-Hill, 1989:1251–66.

Breslow JL. Lipoprotein transport gene abnormalities underlying coronary heart disease susceptibility. Annu Rev Med 1991;42:357–71.

Breslow JL. Transgenic mouse models of lipoprotein metabolism and atherosclerosis. Proc Natl Acad Sci USA 1993;90:8314–8.

Brown MS, Goldstein JL. The hyperlipoproteinemias and other disorders of lipid metabolism. In: Wilson JD, Braunwald E, Isselbacher KJ, et al., eds. Harrison's principles of internal medicine, 12th ed. New York: McGraw-Hill, 1991:1814–25.

Brunzell JD, Hazzard WR, Motulsky AG, Bierman EL. Evidence for diabetes mellitus and genetic forms of hypertriglyceridemia as independent entities. Metabolism 1975;24:1115–21.

Burke GL, Savage PJ, Sprafka JM, et al. Relation of risk factor levels in young adulthood to parental history of disease: the CARDIA study. Circulation 1991;84:1176–87.

Burke W, Motulsky AG. Molecular genetics of hypertension. Monogr Hum Genet 1992;14:228–36.

Cambien F, Poirier O, Lecerf L, et al. Deletion polymorphism in the gene for angiotensin-converting enzyme is a potent risk factor for myocardial infarction. Nature 1992;359:641–4.

Carmelli D, Cardon LR, Fabsitz R. Clustering of hypertension, diabetes, and obesity in adult male twins: same genes or same environment? Circulation 1993;88:Suppl:I-451.

Caulfield M, Lavender P, Farrall M, et al. Linkage of the angiotensinogen gene to essential hypertension. N Engl J Med 1994;330:1629–33.

Chait A, Brunzell JD. Acquired hyperlipidemia (secondary dyslipoproteinemias). Endocrinol Metab Clin North Am 1990;19:259–78.

Cohen JC, Chiesa G, Hobbs HH. Sequence polymorphisms in the apolipoprotein(a) gene: evidence for dissociation between apolipoprotein(a) size and plasma lipoprotein(a) levels. J Clin Invest 1993;91:1630–6.

Colditz GA, Stampfer MJ, Willett WC, et al. A prospective study of parental history of myocardial infarction and coronary heart disease in women. Am J Epidemiol 1986;123:48–58.

Colditz GA, Rimm EB, Giovannucci E, et al. A prospective study of parental history of myocardial infarction and coronary artery disease in men. Am J Cardiol 1991;67:933–8.

Connelly JB, Roderick PJ, Cooper JA, et al. Positive association between self-reported fatty food consumption and factor VII coagulant activity, a risk factor for coronary heart disease, in 4246 middle-aged men. Thromb Haemost 1993;70:250–2.

Coresh J, Svenson KL, Beaty TH, et al. Sib-pair linkage analysis of the lipoprotein lipase gene and lipoprotein levels: the Johns Hopkins Coronary Artery Disease Family Study. Am J Hum Genet 1993;53:Suppl:Abstract 788.

Dammerman M, Sandkuijl LA, Halaas JL, et al. An apolipoprotein CIII haplotype protective against hypertriglyceridemia is specified by promoter and 3' untranslated region polymorphisms. Proc Natl Acad Sci USA 1993;90:4562–6.

Dammerman M, Breslow JL. Genetic basis of lipoprotein disorders. Circulation 1995;9:505–12.

DeFronzo RA, Bonadonna RC, Ferrannini E. Pathogenesis of NIDDM: a balanced overview. Diabetes Care 1992;15:318–68.

De Oliveira e Silva ER, Brinton EA, Cundey K, Breslow JL. Heritability of HDL turnover parameters. Circulation 1991;84:Suppl:II-339.

Despres J-P, Moorjani S, Lupien PJ, et al. Genetic aspects of susceptibility to obesity and related dyslipidemias. Mol Cell Biochem 1992;113:151–69.

Diamond JM. Diabetes running wild. Nature 1992;357:362–3.

Dudman NPB, Wilcken DEL, Wang J, et al. Disordered methionine/homocysteine metabolism in premature vascular disease: its occurrence, cofactor therapy, and enzymology. Arterioscler Thromb 1993;13:1253–60.

Dzau VJ. Tissue renin-angiotensin system in myocardial hypertrophy and failure. Arch Intern Med 1993;153:937–42.

Francis RB Jr. Hemostatic factors in ischemic heart disease and stroke: pathophysiologic significance and molecular genetics. Monogr Hum Genet 1992;14:237–52.

Friedman JM, Leibel RL. Tackling a weighty problem. Cell 1992;69:217–20.

Froguel P, Zouali H, Vionnet N, et al. Familial hyperglycemia due to mutations in glucokinase: definition of a subtype of diabetes mellitus. N Engl J Med 1993;328:697–702.

Genest JJ Jr, McNamara JR, Upson B, et al. Prevalence of familial hyperhomocyst(e)inemia in men with premature coronary artery disease. Arterioscler Thromb 1991;11:1129–36.

Genest JJ Jr, Martin-Munley SS, McNamara JR, et al. Familial lipoprotein disorders in patients with premature coronary artery disease. Circulation 1992;85:2025–33.

Ghiselli G, Schaefer EJ, Zech LA, et al. Increased prevalence of apolipoprotein E4 in type V hyperlipoproteinemia. J Clin Invest 1982;70:474–7.

Ginsberg HN. Syndrome X: what's old, what's new, what's etiologic? J Clin Invest 1993;92:3.

Goldbourt U, Neufeld HN. Genetic aspects of arteriosclerosis. Arteriosclerosis 1986;6:357–77.

Goldstein JL, Brown MS. Familial hypercholesterolemia. In: Scrivner CR, Beaudet AL, Sly WS, Valle D, eds. The metabolic basis of inherited disease, 6th ed, Vol I. New York: McGraw-Hill, 1989:1215–50.

Groop LC, Kankuri M, Schalin-Jantti C, et al. Association between polymorphism of the glycogen synthase gene and non-insulin-dependent diabetes mellitus. N Engl J Med 1993;328:10–14.

Grossman M, Raper SE, Kozarsky K, et al. Successful ex vivo gene therapy directed to liver in a patient with familial hypercholesterolemia. Nature Genet 1994;6:335–41.

Harpel PC, Chang VT, Borth W. Homocysteine and other sulfhydryl compounds enhance the binding of lipoprotein(a) to fibrin: a potential biochemical link between thrombosis, atherogenesis, and sulfhydryl compound metabolism. Proc Natl Acad Sci USA 1992;89:10193–7.

Hata A, Namikawa C, Sasaki M, et al. Angiotensinogen as a risk factor for essential hypertension in Japan. J Clin Invest 1994;93:1285–7.

Hixson JE. Pathobiological Determinants of Atherosclerosis in Youth (PDAY) Research Group. Apolipoprotein E polymorphisms affect atherosclerosis in young males. Arterioscler Thromb 1991;11:1237–44.

Humphries SE, Lane A, Dawson S, Green FR. The study of gene-environment interactions that influence thrombosis and fibrinolysis: genetic variation at the loci for factor VII and plasminogen activator inhibitor-1. Arch Pathol Lab Med 1992;116:1322–9.

Jarrett RJ. Is insulin atherogenic? Diabetologia 1988;31:71–5.

Jarrett RJ. In defence of insulin: a critique of syndrome X. Lancet 1992;340:469–71.

Jauhiainen M, Koskinen P, Ehnholm C, et al. Lipoprotein (a) and coronary heart disease risk: a nested case-control study of the Helsinki Heart Study participants. Atherosclerosis 1991;89:59–67.

Jeunemaitre X, Soubrier F, Kotelevtsev YV, et al. Molecular basis of human hypertension: role of angiotensinogen. Cell 1992;71:169–80.

Julier C, Hyer RN, Davies J, et al. Insulin-IFG2 region on chromosome 11p encodes a gene implicated in HLA-DR4-dependent diabetes susceptibility. Nature 1991;354:155–9.

Kane JP, Havel RJ. Disorders of the biogenesis and secretion of lipoproteins containing the B apolipoproteins. In: Scrivner CR, Beaudet AL, Sly WS, Valle D, eds. The metabolic basis of inherited disease, 6th ed, Vol I. New York: McGraw-Hill 1989:1139–64.

Kiema T, Rantala AO, Kauma H, et al. Polymorphisms in renin-angiotensin cascade genes and hypertension. Circulation 1994;90:Suppl:I-130.

Kobberling J, Tillil H. Empirical risk figures for first degree relatives of non-insulin dependent diabetics. In: Kobberling J, Tattersall R, eds. The genetics of diabetes mellitus. London: Academic Press, 1982:201−9.

Kozich V, Kraus JP. Screening for mutations by expressing patient cDNA segments in *E. coli*: Homocystinuria due to cystathionine β-synthase deficiency. Hum Mutat 1992;1:113−23.

Kreutz R, Lindpaintner K, Pfeffer MA, et al. Angiotensin-converting enzyme genotype and risk for coronary heart disease. Circulation 1993;88:Suppl:I-510.

Kurtz TW. Genetics of essential hypertension. Am J Med 1993;94:77−84.

Kwiterovich PO Jr. Genetics and molecular biology of familial combined hyperlipidemia. Curr Opin Lipidol 1993;4:133−43.

Leahy JL, Bonner-Weir S, Weir GC. β-cell dysfunction induced by chronic hyperglycemia: current ideas on mechanism of impaired glucose-induced insulin secretion. Diabetes Care 1992;15:442−55.

Leahy JL, Boyd AE III. Diabetes genes in non-insulin-dependent diabetes mellitus. N Engl J Med 1993;328:56−7.

Leibel RL, Hirsch J. Diminished energy requirements in reduced-obese patients. Metabolism 1984;33:164−70.

Lifton RP, Dluhy RG, Powers M, et al. A chimaeric 11 β-hydroxylase/aldosterone synthase gene causes glucocorticoid-remediable aldosteronism and human hypertension. Nature 1992;355:262−5.

Lindeberg S, Axelsson O, Jorner U, et al. A prospective controlled five-year follow-up study of primiparas with gestational hypertension. Acta Obstet Gynecol Scand 1988;67:605−9.

Lindpaintner K, Kreutz R, Stampfer MJ, et al. A prospective case-control study of angiotensin-converting enzyme genotype and the risk for myocardial infarction. Circulation 1994;90:Suppl:I-472.

Lipid Research Clinics. Population Studies data book: the prevalence study, Vol I. Bethesda: US Dept Health Human Serv, 1980:39.

Ludwig EH, Comeli PS, Anderson JL, et al. The ACE insertion/deletion polymorphism is independently associated with myocardial infarction and body mass index but not with stenosis. Circulation 1993;88:Suppl:I-364.

Ma Y, Zhang H, Liu M-S, et al. Type III hyperlipoproteinemia in apo E2/2 homozygotes: possible role of mutations in the lipoprotein lipase gene. Circulation 1993;88:Suppl:I-179.

Mahley RW, Rall SC Jr. Type III hyperlipoproteinemia (dysbetalipoproteinemia): the role of apolipoprotein E in normal and abnormal lipoprotein metabolism. In: Scrivner CR, Beaudet AL, Sly WS, Valle D, eds. The metabolic basis of inherited disease, 6th ed, Vol I. New York: McGraw-Hill, 1989:1195−213.

Mark AL. 'Syndrome X': is it a significant cause of hypertension? negative. Hosp Pract 1992;27:Suppl 1:41−4.

Mudd SH, Levy HL, Skovby F. Disorders of transsulfuration. In: Scrivner CR, Beaudet AL, Sly WS, Valle D, eds. The metabolic basis of inherited disease, 6th ed, Vol I. New York: McGraw-Hill, 1989:693−734.

Neel JV. Diabetes mellitus: A "thrifty" genotype rendered detrimental by "progress"? Am J Hum Genet 1962;14:353−62.

Nora JJ, Lortscher RH, Spangler RD, et al. Genetic-epidemiologic study of early-onset ischemic heart disease. Circulation 1980;61:503−8.

Ohishi M, Fujii K, Minamino T, et al. A potent genetic risk factor for restenosis. [Letter]. Nature Genet 1993;5:324−5.

Price WH, Kitchin AH, Burgon PRS, et al. DNA restriction fragment length polymorphisms as markers of familial coronary heart disease. Lancet 1989;i:1407–11.

Reaven GM. Role of insulin resistance in human disease. Diabetes 1988;37:1595–607.

Reaven GM, Chen Y-DI, Jeppesen J, et al. Insulin resistance and hyperinsulinemia in individuals with small, dense, low density lipoprotein particles. J Clin Invest 1993a;92:141–6.

Reaven GM. Role of insulin resistance in human disease (syndrome X): an expanded definition. Annu Rev Med 1993b;44:121–31.

Rees A, Shoulders CC, Stocks J, Galton DJ, Baralle FE. DNA polymorphism adjacent to the human apoprotein AI gene: relation to hypertriglyceridemia. Lancet 1983;i:444–6.

Rhoads GG, Dahlen G, Berg K, et al. Lp(a) lipoprotein as a risk factor for myocardial infarction. JAMA 1986;256:2540–4.

Ridker PM, Hennekens CH, Stampfer MJ. A prospective study of lipoprotein(a) and the risk of myocardial infarction. JAMA 1993a;270:2195–9.

Ridker PM, Gaboury CL, Conlin PR, et al. Stimulation of plasminogen activator inhibitor in vivo by infusion of angiotensin II: evidence of a potential interaction between the renin-angiotensin system and fibrinolytic function. Circulation 1993b;87:1969–73.

Ridker PM, Vaughan DE, Stampfer MJ, et al. Endogenous tissue-type plasminogen activator and risk of myocardial infarction. Lancet 1993c;341:1165–8.

Roncaglioni MC, Santoro L, D'Avanzo B, et al. Role of family history in patients with myocardial infarction: an Italian case-control study. Circulation 1992;85:2065–72.

Saad MF, Knowler WC, Pettitt DJ, et al. The natural history of impaired glucose tolerance in the Pima Indians. N Engl J Med 1988;319:1500–6.

Saad MF, Lillioja S, Nyomba BL, et al. Racial differences in the relation between blood pressure and insulin resistance. N Engl J Med 1991;324:733–9.

Scanu AM, Fless GM. Lipoprotein(a). Heterogeneity and biological relevance. J Clin Invest 1990;85:1709–15.

Scarabin P-Y, Bara L, Ricard S, et al. Genetic variation at the β-fibrinogen locus in relation to plasma fibrinogen concentrations and risk of myocardial infarction: the ECTIM study. Arterioscl Thromb 1993;13:886–91.

Schneiderman J, Sawdey MS, Keeton MR, et al. Increased type 1 plasminogen activator inhibitor gene expression in atherosclerotic human arteries. Proc Natl Acad Sci USA 1992; 89:6998–7002.

Schunkert H, Dzau VJ, Tang SS, et al. Increased rat cardiac angiotensin converting enzyme activity and mRNA expression in pressure overload left ventricular hypertrophy: effects on coronary resistance, contractility, and relaxation. J Clin Invest 1990;86:1913–20.

Schunkert H, Hense HW, Holmer SR, et al. Association between a deletion polymorphism of the angiotensin-converting-enzyme gene and left ventricular hypertrophy. N Engl J Med 1994;330:1634–8.

Seidman DS, Laor A, Gale R, et al. Pre-eclampsia and offspring's blood pressure, cognitive ability and physical development at 17 years of age. Br J Obstet Gynecol 1991;98: 1009–14.

Shohat T, Raffel LF, Vadheim CM, Rotter JI. Diabetes mellitus and coronary heart disease genetics. Monogr Hum Genet 1992;14:272–310.

Shoulders CC, Harry PJ, Lagrost L, et al. Variation at the apo AI/CIII/AIV gene complex is associated with elevated plasma levels of apo CIII. Atherosclerosis 1991;87:239–47.

Sibai BM, El-Nazer A, Gonsalez-Ruiz A. Severe preeclampsia-eclampsia in young primigravid women: subsequent pregnancy outcome and remote prognosis. Am J Obstet Gynecol 1986;155:1011–6.

Sniderman AD, Silberberg J. Is it time to measure apolipoprotein B? Arteriosclerosis 1990;10: 665–7.

Sorrentino MJ, Vielhauer C, Eisenhart JD, et al. Plasma lipoprotein(a) protein concentration and coronary artery disease in black patients compared with white patients. Am J Med 1992;93:658–62.

Stamler J. Epidemic obesity in the United States. Arch Intern Med 1993;153:1040–3.

Stampfer MJ, Malinow MR, Willett WC, et al. A prospective study of plasma homocyst(e)ine and risk of myocardial infarction in US physicians. JAMA 1992;268:877–81.

Steiner DF, Tager HS, Chan SJ, et al. Lessons learned from molecular biology of insulin-gene mutations. Diabetes Care 1990;13:600–9.

Stunkard AJ, Harris JR, Pedersen NL, McClearn GE. The body-mass index of twins who have been reared apart. N Engl J Med 1990;322:1483–7.

Tall AR. Plasma cholesteryl ester transfer protein. J Lipid Res 1993;34:1255–74.

Taylor SI. Lilly Lecture: Molecular mechanisms of insulin resistance: lessons from patients with mutations in the insulin-receptor gene. Diabetes 1992;41:1473–90.

Thorsby E, Ronningen KS. Particular HLA-DQ molecules play a dominant role in determining susceptibility or resistance to type 1 (insulin-dependent) diabetes mellitus. Diabetologia 1993;36:371–7.

Van den Ouweland JMW, Lemkes HHPJ, Ruitenbeek W, et al. Mutation in mitochondrial tRNA$^{Leu(UUR)}$ gene in a large pedigree with maternally transmitted type II diabetes mellitus and deafness. Nature Genet 1992;1:368–71.

Ward K, Hata A, Jeunemaitre X, et al. A molecular variant of angiotensinogen associated with preeclampsia. Nature Genet 1993;4:59–61.

Williams GH. Hypertensive vascular disease. In: Wilson JD, Braunwald E, Isselbacher KJ, et al., eds. Harrison's principles of internal medicine, 12th ed. New York: McGraw-Hill 1991:1001–15.

Williams GH, Hollenberg NK. Derangements in renin-angiotensin regulation in the pathogenesis of hypertension. In: Raizada MK, Phillips MI, Sumners C, eds. Cellular and molecular biology of the renin-angiotensin system. Boca Raton: CRC Press, 1993:515–36.

Williams JK, Bellinger DA, Nichols TC, et al. Occlusive arterial thrombosis in cynomolgus monkeys with varying plasma concentrations of lipoprotein(a). Arterioscler Thromb 1993;13:548–54.

Williams RR, Hunt SC, Schumacher MC, et al. Diagnosing heterozygous familial hypercholesterolemia using new practical criteria validated by molecular genetics. Am J Cardiol 1993;72:171–6.

Wilson DE, Emi M, Iverius P-H, et al. Phenotypic expression of heterozygous lipoprotein lipase deficiency in the extended pedigree of a proband homozygous for a missense mutation. J Clin Invest 1990;86:735–50.

Wojciechowski AP, Farrall M, Cullen P, et al. Familial combined hyperlipidemia linked to the apolipoprotein AI-CIII-AIV gene cluster on chromosome 11q23-q24. Nature 1991;349: 161–4.

Zannis VI, Kardassis D, Zanni EE. Genetic mutations affecting human lipoproteins, their receptors, and their enzymes. Adv Hum Genet 1993;21:145–319.

Zavaroni I, Reaven G. Insulin-resistance and associated risk factors for coronary heart disease as seen in families. Diabetes Metab 1991;17:109–11.

Zeng Q, Dammerman M, Takada Y, et al. An apolipoprotein CIII marker associated with hypertriglyceridemia in Caucasians also confers increased risk in a west Japanese population. Hum Genet 1995;95:371–5.

Zhang Y, Proenca R, Maffei M, et al. Positional cloning of the mouse *obese* gene and its human homologue. Nature 1994;372:425–32.

II

Modifiable Determinants of Myocardial Infarction and Intervention Strategies

4

Coronary Health Promotion: An Overview

CHRISTOPHER J. O'DONNELL, PETER SLEIGHT, AND JOANN E. MANSON

Coronary health promotion is the summation of efforts by health care organizations and providers to identify as well as prevent and treat risk factors for coronary heart disease (CHD). Since acute myocardial infarction (MI) is the leading cause of mortality and morbidity from CHD in the developed world, the effective promotion of behaviors known to decrease coronary risk may lead to substantial reductions in the burden of MI worldwide. Population and patient-based health promotion approaches represent complementary strategies that have been developed for intervention in individual coronary risk factors and are often implemented simultaneously. While most risk factors predisposing to acute MI and other adverse CHD events can be identified and modified, solid evidence for significant benefits from health promotion interventions, in overall populations or in specific patient subtypes, often derives from randomized trials and prospective observational studies. When available, data from well-designed randomized trials provide the strongest qualitative and quantitative evidence for a causal link between intervention and reduced risk of CHD. Because the quality and strength of data concerning different interventions are not uniform, we advocate an evidence-based health promotion strategy. Consideration of the quality and strength of evidence when calculating the benefits, risks, and costs of individual interventions aids clinicians in selecting and implementing the most optimal risk reduction strategy for individual patients.

In this chapter we describe the rationale for elevating coronary health promotion to a high priority in clinical practice. The evidence is compelling for a strong and consistent association between modifiable coronary risk factors and CHD, for overall benefit from individual interventions, and for the possibility of sizeable reductions in CHD morbidity and mortality from coronary health promotion. This chapter describes a system for grading the quality of evidence to be used by clinicians when assessing whether individual components of the coronary health promotion strategy confer net benefit, net risk, or an unclear balance of benefits to risks. Finally, we offer a framework for clinicians and policymakers to effectively incorporate the information in this textbook into a practical coronary health promotion strategy.

Rationale for Coronary Health Promotion

Relative Risk, Attributable Risk, and the Link Between Coronary Risk Factors and CHD

As the leading cause of death for both women and men and for both blacks and whites in the United States, CHD accounted for 478,530 deaths in 1991 (American Heart Association 1993). Prospective observational studies have consistently demonstrated a significant association between modifiable risk factors and CHD risk. As discussed in detail in this textbook, this evidence includes compelling data that cigarette smoking (Bartecchi 1994), an elevated cholesterol level (Lipid I 1984a; Davis 1990), and an elevated diastolic and/or systolic blood pressure (Joint National Committee 1993; Stamler 1993; Whelton 1994) are associated with an increased likelihood of developing CHD. Moreover, a dose-response effect has been identified for exposure to each of these risk factors, such that a cumulative increase in numbers of cigarettes smoked (Bartecchi 1994), increasing levels of cholesterol (Lipid I 1984a, 1984b), and increasing levels of diastolic and/or systolic blood pressure (Stamler 1993; Whelton 1994) are associated with higher rates of MI and of coronary death. Indeed, the American Heart Association has considered these risk factors to be well established for many years. Further, the overall evidence now suggests that a sedentary lifestyle increases CHD risk (Berlin 1990), and the American Heart Association has recently added physical inactivity to the list of established CHD risk factors (American Heart Association 1993). Emerging evidence supports a role of obesity, diabetes, alcohol, diet, as well as pharmacologic agents, such as aspirin and exogenous estrogens, in the genesis or prevention of CHD.

To understand the magnitude of hazard conferred by any given CHD risk factor, it is important to clearly distinguish between attributable risk and relative risk. Observational studies and trials often describe their findings in terms of a relative risk, a ratio that describes the likelihood of developing disease in the exposed group relative to those who are not exposed (Hennekens 1987). Thus, the relative risk is a measure of the strength of the association between an exposure (e.g., the presence of a CHD risk factor) and a disease, and it provides information that can be used to judge whether an observed association is causal. In contrast, the attributable risk is a measure of the public health impact of an exposure, and it is calculated on the assumption that an association exists. The attributable risk is often described as a percent reduction or increase in disease risk, but an alternative easily understood measure of attributable risk is the population attributable risk, which is the actual number of cases of disease that occur due to the harmful exposure (Hennekens 1987). A small relative risk does not necessarily imply that the attributable risk is small. For example, an exposure may lead to a 10-fold relative risk of death, but if the exposure or disease is uncommon, the resulting number of total deaths caused (population attributable risk) may be very small. Conversely, an exposure associated with a small (e.g., 1.5-fold) relative risk of disease incidence may still lead to substantial numbers of cases if the exposure and disease are quite common.

The concept of attributable CHD risk can be applied to cross-sectional data, which reveal that many potentially modifiable CHD risk factors are highly prevalent in the United States. For example, nearly 150,000 deaths from CHD in 1986 were attributable to cigarette smoking alone, not to mention an additional 200,000 deaths from cerebrovascular disease, cancers, and respiratory diseases attributed to cigarette tobacco (CDC 1993). Likewise, 33,280 deaths were attributable to hypertension in 1991 (American Heart Association 1993). Since there is a remarkably high prevalence of cigarette smoking (26%) and hypertension (18%), as well as elevated serum cholesterol (37%), diabetes (6.6%), physical inactivity (58%), and obesity (33%), a substantial proportion of CHD deaths has been attributed to each of these factors (Table 4.1) (CDC 1993). While the prevalence of each of these risk factors is well characterized, the precise proportion of overall CHD morbidity and mortality attributable to the presence of one or more of these risk factors is difficult to ascertain. However, it is known that only 18% of adult men and women in the United States, in a representative cross section, reported none of the risk factors listed in Table 4.1, but nearly half had at least two risk factors (CDC 1994). Thus, most American adults carry an elevated CHD risk due to the presence of one or more modifiable risk factors.

Evidence for Net Benefit from Interventions to Modify CHD Risk

In addition to identifying the magnitude of attributable CHD risk, research has focused on interventions that reduce rates of CHD morbidity and mortality. Indeed, it is clear that targeted behavioral and pharmacologic interventions can reduce or normalize levels of individual risk factors. For example, effective strategies exist for achieving short-term cigarette smoking cessation (Tonneson 1991; Transdermal 1991; Hurt 1994), though they are less effective in maintaining long-term abstinence. Likewise, substantial and sustained reductions in levels of blood pressure or serum cholesterol are clearly achievable by dietary and pharmacologic interventions.

While small randomized trials have clearly demonstrated that levels of such risk factors as blood pressure and serum cholesterol can be favorably reduced, large randomized trials are required to assess reliably the net balance of clinical benefits and

Table 4.1. Attributable Risk of CHD Deaths and Estimated Societal Costs, by Selected Risk Factors in the US Population

Risk Factor	Prevalence (%)	Attributable Risk (%)	Estimated Cost[c] (billions)
Physical inactivity	58.0	34.6	$5.7
Elevated serum cholesterol	37.0	42.7	$7.0
Smoking	25.5	25.1	$4.1
Obesity	33.0[a]	32.1	$5.3
Hypertension	18.0	28.9	$4.7
Diabetes mellitus[b]	6.6	13.1	Not available

Source: Adapted from CDC 1993, except where noted.

[a]Prevalence estimate recently upgraded from 23% to 33% (see Kuczmarski 1994).

[b]Prevalence rates from Hadden (1987), and attributable risk from Hahn (1990).

[c]These are conservative estimates reflecting CHD related costs not costs of other risk factor related illnesses.

risks associated with these interventions. To detect a small but clinically important risk reduction requires large-scale trials often including tens of thousands of participants. For example, multiple trials of antihypertensive drug therapy in mild to moderate hypertension have demonstrated an unequivocal benefit on stroke in patients with mild to moderate hypertension (Hebert 1993). In only two of these studies was there a significant benefit on CHD (Hypertension 1988; SHEP 1991). However, the majority of these trials appear to have been performed in a sample size too small to exclude reliably the possibility of a small but significant treatment benefit. In fact, in an overview of 17 randomized controlled trials of mild to moderate hypertension, including 23,847 participants, there was a significant reduction in the rate of both fatal and total MI (Hebert 1993).

Similarly, randomized trials of serum cholesterol reduction demonstrate a clear benefit from dietary or pharmacologic reduction of cholesterol in individuals with known coronary heart disease. However, nutritional or pharmacologic primary prevention interventions lead to a less clear overall benefit on CHD endpoints or mortality (Expert 1993), although a benefit appears for those with markedly elevated cholesterol or with multiple risk factors, such as the presence of both increased cholesterol and hypertension. Similarly, the benefit:risk ratio is unclear for universal screening, so preventive task forces have recommended that screening be restricted to certain subpopulations, such as men between the ages of 30 and 59 (Canadian 1993).

Thus, while measurable reductions in levels of risk factors are readily achieved, they should be viewed as surrogate markers for clinically relevant reductions in incident CHD and other cardiovascular events. Since any given health promotion strategy is expected to be only modestly effective over short time intervals, costly and time-consuming randomized trials in large numbers of patients are often required to reliably demonstrate a clear benefit. An overview of several trials may be needed to provide a reliable estimate of the magnitude of benefit and of the balance of benefits and risks.

Why Coronary Health Promotion Should be a Priority in Clinical Practice

While CHD risk attributable to modifiable risk factors in the United States is great, and there is substantial evidence that screening and intervention can reduce CHD risk, implementation of effective coronary health promotion is still not a high priority among U.S. clinicians. This may in part be due to a continued emphasis in both practice and education on treatment rather than prevention of CHD, as well as a false complacency fostered by the declining rates of CHD.

Since patients traditionally seek care after the first manifestation of disease, it is understandable that clinicians have evolved a practice style in which effective treatment of disease is a priority. Dramatic accomplishments in the therapy of CHD are numerous, and they include the institution of life-saving practices such as cardiopulmonary resuscitation, defibrillation, and coronary care units. Randomized controlled trials have demonstrated a benefit from treatments such as coronary artery bypass surgery in those with three-vessel coronary artery disease (Coronary 1983), as well as from aspirin (ISIS-2 1988), thrombolytic therapy (Fibrinolytic 1994), beta-adrenergic blockers (ISIS-1 1986), and angiotensin-converting enzyme inhibitors (SAVE 1992; ISIS-4 1994) in those with acute myocardial infarction. Indeed, many medical school curricula have traditionally focused upon therapeutics, but curricula in the fields of "preventive medicine" and "epidemiology" have only recently become established in many medical schools.

While therapeutic advances have been demonstrated to be highly effective in randomized trials, rough correlations suggest that these practices have had only a modest impact upon observed population-wide mortality trends. One recent cross-sectional analysis of the decline in CHD mortality between 1968 and 1976 suggested that only about a third of the decline in CHD mortality was attributable to prehospital care, inpatient care, and bypass surgery, while the remainder of the mortality reduction was attributed to lifestyle changes such as smoking cessation, cholesterol reduction, and the treatment of hypertension (Goldman 1984). Thus, even in a past era when coronary health promotion was not a priority in many clinicians' practices, lifestyle changes appear to have played a major role in reducing rates of CHD death.

Indeed, despite the observed association between preventive practices and mortality reduction, it is not surprising that some clinicians may have become complacent about prevention, given the impressive secular decline in CHD mortality as well as in prevalence of several CHD risk factors. Yet, in the United States, CHD remains the leading cause of adult death in both blacks and whites, regardless of gender. Further examination of the epidemiology of acute myocardial infarction suggests that improvements in the therapy of acute MI will continue to be of modest benefit compared to the potential of preventive strategies (Figure 4.1). While therapies for acute MI are available to hospitalized survivors, it appears that the majority of those who sustain an acute MI or who die from acute MI never reach the hospital. Estimates of the numbers of "silent" myocardial infarction indicate that perhaps 33% or more of all MIs may be silent, with the incidence of unrecognized MI being higher in women than in men (Kannel 1984; Grimm 1987; Sigurdsson 1995). Survivors who do not receive immediate treatment are at increased risk of further CHD morbidity as well as death. Sudden cardiac death due to acute MI often occurs prior to hospital presentation, and the availability of prehospital resuscitation has made only a minor impact on the high death rates among these victims (American Heart Association 1993). Thus, while a therapy that improves survival by 20% for hospitalized patients could prevent 10,000 to 20,000 deaths, a similar magnitude of benefit in primary prevention of MI would save over 100,000 lives in the United States each year (see Figure 4.1).

In summary, the overall decrease in CHD mortality, while impressive, leaves no room for complacency, since CHD remains the leading cause of death in the United States. It is hoped that a significant number of deaths may be prevented by wider utilization of the entire armamentarium of acute therapies for acute MI and unstable angina. However, because of the high prevalence of modifiable determinants of coronary risk, all of which have been associated with an elevated incidence of coronary events and deaths, future declines in CHD incidence and mortality are likely to require further development and widespread implementation of preventive interventions. Promotion of both primary and secondary coronary prevention remains a high priority for U.S. adults.

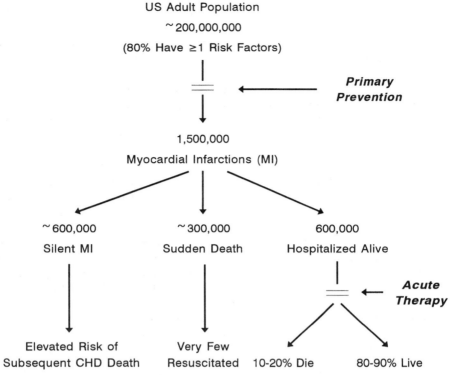

Fig. 4.1. Comparison of the potential benefit of acute versus preventive therapies for acute myocardial infarction. An *acute therapy* that improves survival by 20% for hospitalized patients could prevent 10,000 to 20,000 deaths, while a similar magnitude of benefit in *primary prevention* of myocardial infarction would save over 100,000 lives per year in the United States.

Evidence-Based Rationale for Tailoring Coronary Health Promotion Strategies to the Individual Patient

We advocate identifying, prioritizing, and treating risk factors in either populations or in individual patients according to the quality and strength of available evidence. With the large and growing body of animal, laboratory, and clinical data regarding CHD prevention, there is an ever-increasing need for a sound and rational basis for selecting appropriate diagnostic and therapeutic approaches. While certain coronary health promotion strategies may have strong intuitive appeal, we recommend that practice be based upon the best available scientific evidence. In this regard, studies with minimal risk of bias provide stronger and more reliable data than studies in which there may be considerable bias. For example, much of medical practice fifty years ago was based upon opinions of experts or data from descriptive studies. However, there may have been substantial bias in these recommendations, since referred patients, who tend to be more ill, were the source of much of the descriptive data. Cohort and case-control study designs represented a marked improvement in the quality of clinical data available, since these methods allowed at least an attempt at controlling for confounding and other sources of bias (Hennekens 1987). However, these methods are also not completely without risk of bias or confounding. Controlled trials, preferably with randomization, have become the gold standard for proof of a benefit from preventive or other interventions, and large-scale trials allow reliable comparison of benefits versus risks. Proper randomization in a sample of adequate size virtually eliminates the chance that baseline differences among treatment groups will play any meaningful role in the study outcome, and blinding, if possible, further reduces the risk that any observed differences could be attributed to nontrial treatments that differed after randomization (Hennekens 1987). Thus, the quality of evidence in preventive interventions is strongest if derived from properly designed randomized controlled trials, less strong if derived from cohort or case-control studies, and weakest if derived from descriptive studies or from the clinical experience of one or a few experts. Recognizing the importance of evidence-based decision-making, the US Preventive Services Task Force has employed such a grading system for the quality of evidence for many of its recommendations in its *Guide to Clinical Preventive Services* (US 1989) (Table 4.2).

Given this background, we recommend that an evidence-based system dictate the clinician's choice of a strategy for screening and intervening in individual patients (Manson 1992). In practice, many CHD risk factors can be identified by a simple medical history or blood pressure measurement, although there is still controversy regarding the effectiveness of cholesterol, lipoprotein, and glucose screening. Once the patient's CHD risks have been identified by an appropriate screening strategy, the clinician may then further prioritize the risk factor profile by magnitude of attributable risk and by degree to which effective therapy is expected to reduce risk. Particularly for preventive drug therapies, such as aspirin or exogenous estrogen therapy, clinicians require good quality evidence on which to base the decision to treat. Clearly, the individual clinician's judgment plays an important role, particularly in assessing psychological, social, and other factors that are less easily measured but may strongly determine the expected ease with which a risk reduction strategy might be implemented in an individual patient.

Developing a Comprehensive Clinical Strategy for Coronary Health Promotion

To facilitate clinicians in implementing an evidence-based program for coronary health promotion, we provide a summary of the quality of evidence and magnitude of expected benefit for each intervention. At the end of each chapter in this section, there is a summary of the quality of available evidence for modification of the specific risk factor, an estimate of the risk reduction (a measure of attributable CHD risk) to be expected from each intervention, and an assessment of the gender comparability for specific guidelines. The quality scale is described above and in Table 4.2, and it allows the clinician to rapidly assess whether a potential intervention is supported by well-designed research. Estimates of the magnitude of benefit to be expected from a given

Table 4.2. Grading of Quality of Evidence for Preventive Interventions (in Decreasing Order of Quality)

1. Evidence obtained from at least one properly designed randomized controlled trial
2. Evidence obtained from well-designed controlled trials without randomization
3. Evidence obtained from well-designed cohort or case-control analytic studies, preferably from more than one center or research group
4. Evidence obtained from multiple time series with or without the intervention; dramatic results in uncontrolled experiments as well
5. Opinions of respected authorities based on clinical experience, descriptive studies, or reports of expert committees

Source: Adapted from *Guide to Clinical Preventive Services* (US 1989), Appendix A, page 388.

intervention are provided for the clinician to begin to formulate a ratio of benefits: risk based upon the specific patient's underlying risk factors and comorbidities. Gender comparability has been included, since most studies of coronary risk and risk reduction have been in males, and clinicians require an assessment of the appropriateness of extrapolating results to their female patients. These simple and clear summaries of the available evidence are intended to facilitate the implementation of coronary health promotion for patients and to serve as groundwork for modifying health promotion practices in light of the rapid growth of knowledge expected in the coming years.

In addition, a table summarizing the available evidence and achievable risk reductions for each intervention is provided in the final chapter of the textbook, and patient education materials are provided throughout the book.

References

American Heart Association. Heart and stroke facts; 1994 statistical supplement. Dallas: American Heart Association, 1993.

Bartecchi CE, MacKenzie TD, Schrier TW. The human costs of tobacco use. N Engl J Med 1994;330:907–12,975–80.

Berlin JA, Colditz GA. A meta-analysis of physical activity in the prevention of coronary heart disease. Am J Epidemiol 1990;132:612–28.

Canadian Task Force on the Periodic Health Examination. Periodic health examination, 1993 update: 2. Lowering blood total cholesterol level to prevent coronary heart disease. Can Med Assoc J 1993;148:521–38.

Coronary Artery Surgery Study (CASS). A randomized trial of coronary artery bypass surgery: survival data. Circulation 1983;68:939–50.

CDC. Public health focus: physical activity and the prevention of coronary heart disease. MMWR 1993;42:669–72.

CDC. Prevalence of adults with no known major risk factors for coronary heart disease: behavioral risk factor surveillance system, 1992. MMWR 1994;43:61–3,69.

Davis CE, Rifkind BM, Brenner H, Gordon DJ. A single cholesterol measurement underestimates the risk of coronary heart disease. JAMA 1990;264:3044–6.

Expert Panel on Detection, Evaluation, and Treatment of High Blood Cholesterol in Adults. Summary of the Second Report of the National Cholesterol Education Program (NCEP) Expert Panel on Detection, Evaluation, and Treatment of High Blood Cholesterol in Adults (Adult Treatment Panel II). JAMA 1993;269:3015–23.

Fibrinolytic Therapies Trialists: Collaborative Group. Indications for fibrinolytic therapy in suspected acute myocardial infarction: collaborative overview of mortality and major morbidity results from all randomised trials of more than 1000 patients. Lancet 1994;343:311–22.

Grimm RH, Tillinghast S, Daniels K, et al. Unrecognized myocardial infarction: experience in the multiple risk factor intervention trial (MRFIT). Circulation 1987;75(suppl II):II-6–8.

Goldman L, Cook EF. The decline in ischemic heart disease mortality rates: an analysis of the comparative effects of medical interventions and changes in lifestyles. Ann Intern Med 1984;101:825–36.

Hadden WC, Knowler WC, Bennett PH. Prevalence of diabetes and impaired glucose tolerance and plasma glucose levels in U.S. population aged 20–74 yr. Diabetes 1987;36:523–34.

Hahn RA, Teutsch SM, Rothenberg RB, Marks JS. Excess deaths from nine chronic diseases in the United States, 1986. JAMA 1990;264:2654–9.

Hebert P, Moser M, Mayer J, et al. Recent evidence on drug therapy of mild to moderate hypertension and decreased risk of coronary heart disease. Arch Intern Med 1993;153:578–81.

Hennekens CH, Buring JE. Epidemiology in medicine. Boston: Little, Brown, 1987.

Hurt RD, Dale LC, Fredrickson PA, et al. Nicotine patch therapy for smoking cessation combined with physician advice and nurse follow-up: one-year outcome and percentage of nicotine replacement. JAMA 1994;271:595–600.

Hypertension Detection and Follow-up Program Cooperative Group. Persistence of reduction in blood pressure and mortality of participants in the Hypertension Detection and Follow-up Program. JAMA 1988;259:2113–22.

ISIS 1 (First International Study of Infarct Survival) Collaborative Group. Randomised trial of intravenous atenolol among 16,027 cases of suspected acute myocardial infarction: ISIS-1. Lancet 1986;ii:57–66.

ISIS-2 (Second International Study of Infarct Survival) Collaborative Group. Randomised trial of intravenous streptokinase, oral aspirin, both or neither among 17,187 cases of suspected acute myocardial infarction. Lancet 1988;ii:349–60.

ISIS-4 (Fourth International Study of Infarct Survival) Collaborative Group. A randomised trial comparing oral captopril versus placebo, oral mononitrate versus placebo, and intravenous magnesium sulphate versus control among 58,043 patients with suspected acute myocardial infarction. Lancet 1995 (in press).

Joint National Committee on Detection, Evaluation, and Treatment of High Blood Pressure. The fifth report of the Joint National Committee on detection, evaluation, and treatment of high blood pressure (JNC V). Arch Intern Med 1993;153:154–83.

Kannel WB, Abbott RD. Incidence and prognosis of unrecognized myocardial infarction: an update from the Framingham Study. N. Engl J Med 1984;311:1144–7.

Kuczmarski RJ, Flegal KM, Campbell SM, Johnson CL. Increasing prevalence of overweight among US adults: the National Health and Nutritional Examination Surveys, 1960 to 1991. JAMA 1994;272:205–11.

Lipid Research Clinics Program: the Lipid Research Clinics Coronary Primary Prevention Trial results: I. Reduction in incidence of coronary heart disease. JAMA 1984a;251:351–64.

Lipid Research Clinics Program: the Lipid Research Clinics Coronary Primary Prevention Trial results: II. The relationship of reduction in incidence of CHD to cholesterol lowering. JAMA 1984b;251:365–74.

Manson JE, Tosteson H, Ridker PM, et al. The primary prevention of myocardial infarction. N Engl J Med 1992;326:1406–16.

The SAVE Investigators. Effect of captopril on mortality in patients with left ventricular dysfunction after myocardial infarction: results of the Survival and Ventricular Enlargement Trial. N Engl J Med 1992;327:669–77.

SHEP Cooperative Research Group. Prevention of stroke by antihypertensive drug treatment in older persons with isolated systolic hypertension: final results of the Systolic Hypertension in the Elderly Program (SHEP). JAMA 1991;265:3255–64.

Sigurdsson E, Thurgeirsson G, Signaldason H, Sigfusson N. Unrecognized myocardial infarction: epidemiology, clinical characteristics, and the prognostic role of angina pectoris. The Roykjavik Study. Ann Intern Med 1995;122:96–102.

Stamler J, Stamler R, Neaton JD. Blood pressure, systolic and diastolic, and cardiovascular risks: US population data. Arch Intern Med 1993;153:598–615.

Tonneson P, Norregaard J, Simonsen K, Sawe U. A double-blind trial of a 16-hour transdermal nicotine patch in smoking cessation. N Engl J Med 1991;325:311–5.

Transdermal Nicotine Study Group. Transdermal nicotine for smoking cessation: six-month results from two multicenter controlled clinical trials. JAMA 1991;266:3133–8.

US Preventive Services Task Force. Guide to clinical preventive services. Baltimore: Williams and Wilkins, 1989.

Whelton PK. Epidemiology of hypertension. Lancet 1994;344:101–6.

5

Smoking Cessation

J. TAYLOR HAYS, RICHARD D. HURT, AND LOWELL C. DALE

Evidence For or Against Benefit

Tobacco has been used in the Americas in various forms for centuries. The first references to tobacco smoking are found in the accounts of New World explorers during the sixteenth century (US DHSS 1992). During the seventeenth and eighteenth centuries, tobacco was a major cash crop in the American colonies, with expansion of tobacco product manufacturing in the United States through the beginning of the Civil War. The manufactured cigarette is a recent phenomenon, having been introduced in the 1880s. During the early part of the twentieth century, manufactured cigarettes became the predominant form of tobacco consumed in the United States. The consumption of cigarettes has increased rapidly during this century; the greatest increase was noted during World War II (US DHSS 1989). By 1963, annual per capita cigarette consumption reached its maximum at 4,300 per adult but has steadily declined since then.

Smoking prevalence among different groups has also changed dramatically in recent decades. In 1955 approximately 39% of all American adults were smoking and a peak prevalence of 41% was reached in 1965 (Fiore 1992a). In 1955 twice as many men were smoking as women (53% and 24%, respectively), but by 1965 the smoking prevalence among women had increased to 34%, while the prevalence among men remained stable. Since 1965, there has been a steady decline in smoking prevalence in both sexes, although the rate of decline in men has been about three times that in women. In 1991 approximately 26% of American adults were smokers, including 28% of all men and 24% of women (CDC 1993a). Smoking prevalence was highest among lower socioeconomic groups and among those with high-school education or less. The changing demographics of smokers is most dramatically illustrated by the smoking prevalence among college graduates (13.6%) compared to those with high-school education or less (30%) in 1991 (CDC 1993a).

The trend in declining prevalence of smoking has been accompanied by a slight decline in overall smoking-attributable mortality from 1988 to 1990. In spite of this, smoking attributable mortality and years of potential life lost remain substantial. In

1990 over 400,000 deaths were attributed to smoking (McGinnis 1993), and there were more than 5 million years of potential life lost (CDC 1993b) (see Table 5.1). Although cardiovascular disease mortality is steadily declining, it continues to account for 43% of all smoking-attributable mortality, with 55% of cardiovascular deaths due to coronary heart disease (CHD) (CDC 1993b).

Cigarette smoking has been recognized as a risk factor for the development of CHD for 40 years. The first studies to link smoking and CHD were published by Doll and Hill (1956) in Great Britain and by Hammond and Horn (1958) in the United States. The 1964 Surgeon General's Report (US PHS 1964) expanded this epidemiologic link. By 1983 the Surgeon General's Report concluded that cigarette smoking was the most important of the known modifiable risk factors for CHD (US DHHS 1983). Although the epidemiologic evidence correlating smoking and CHD is convincing, there are many confounding variables such as obesity, dietary habits, exercise level, and others that obscure the link between smoking and the mechanisms of coronary atherosclerosis and acute coronary syndromes. There are, however, several lines of evidence that link smoking to many of the proposed mechanisms of CHD.

Smoking and Coronary Heart Disease: Proposed Mechanisms

CHD and the clinical syndromes of angina pectoris, acute myocardial infarction (MI), and sudden cardiac death are not simply the result of coronary atherosclerosis, but are due to a complex interplay of several processes, which can be exacerbated or caused by smoking (Figure 5.1). The earliest lesion in coronary atherosclerosis results from injury to the arterial endothelium and progresses via lipid accumulation, platelet adhesion, smooth muscle proliferation, and thrombus formation to an occlusive lesion (Fuster 1992). Animal studies have demonstrated intimal injury (Zimmerman 1987) and increased endothelial permeability to large molecules such as fibrinogen (Allen 1989) in arteries exposed to nicotine. In humans, umbilical vessels from smoking mothers show ultrastructural changes in the endothelium distinct from those in nonsmokers (Asmussen 1984). In addition to endothelial injury, other effects of acute and chronic cigarette smoking that may promote atherosclerosis include decreased HDL cholesterol levels (Mjos 1988), imbalance between prostacycline and thromboxane in the arterial wall (Jeremy 1990), and platelet activation (Murray 1990).

Acute coronary syndromes, such as acute MI, are thought to be a result of thrombus formation at the site of atherosclerotic plaque disruption (Fuster 1992). Thrombogenic effects of smoking include activation of the coagulation system and platelet

Table 5.1. The Human Cost of Smoking: 1990

Total smoking-attributable mortality	418,690
Cardiovascular disease-specific smoking-attributable mortality	
All cardiovascular disease	179,820
Ischemic heart disease	98,921
Smoking-attributable years of potential life lost (total)	5,048,740
Smoking-attributable years of potential life lost before age 65	1,152,635

Source: From CDC (1993b).

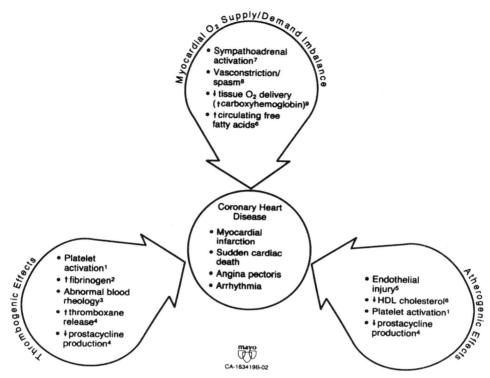

Fig. 5.1. Smoking and proposed mechanisms of coronary heart disease. *1*, Murray 1990, FitzGerald 1988; *2*, Feher 1990, O'Connor 1984; *3*, Ernst 1990; *4*, Jeremy 1990; *5*, Pitillo 1990, Asmussen 1984, Zimmerman 1987, Allen 1989; *6*, Mjos 1988; *7*, Robertson 1988; *8*, Klein 1990, Moreyra 1992; *9*, U.S. DHHS 1983.

activation (Fitzgerald 1988), as well as increased circulating fibrinogen (O'Connor 1984; Fitzgerald 1988). Nicotine causes sympathetic nervous system stimulation, which acutely raises blood pressure and heart rate (Robertson 1988). These changes in turn increase coronary vessel wall stress (Caro 1990) and may promote plaque disruption and vessel occlusion.

The thrombogenic and atherogenic effects of smoking are the major mechanisms involved in CHD found in smokers. Imbalance between myocardial oxygen demand and delivery mediated by several different mechanisms is also likely playing a significant role in CHD pathogenesis (Figure 5.1). Clinical correlates of these effects include angiographic evidence of coronary artery narrowing after smoking (Moreyra 1992) and demonstration of ''silent'' ischemia after a single cigarette (Deanfield 1986). The acute and chronic effects of smoking are mediated not only by nicotine, but also by carbon monoxide and over 4,000 other constituents of tobacco smoke (US DHHS 1989).

In spite of the experimental evidence linking smoking to CHD, the reported attempts to develop an animal model of atherosclerosis from smoke inhalation have failed. This is probably due to the inability of animal models to duplicate the dose, depth of inhalation, or duration of exposure of a human smoker. Moreover, no randomized or controlled experiment in humans has demonstrated this connection. Consequently, the strongest evidence for the causal link between smoking and CHD comes from observational data in cohort and case-control studies.

Smoking and Increased CHD Risk

Observational studies of the possible association of CHD and cigarette smoking have consistently shown that smoking increases the risk for CHD morbidity and mortality (US DHHS 1983; US DHHS 1989). Concern over this association was expressed in the 1964 Surgeon General's Report (US PHS 1964); however, a causal link was not suggested. Early information on this association was reported by Hammond and Horn (1958). They noted a 52% excess mortality from CHD in smokers and a definite dose-response relationship between number of cigarettes smoked per day and CHD mortality in a cohort of 187,783 men. Similar findings were reported for a cohort of U.S. veterans (Rogot 1980), where the mortality ratio for CHD in smokers versus nonsmokers was 1.58 after 16 years of observation. There was also a consistent dose-response phenomenon between CHD mortality and number of cigarettes smoked. Mortality data from a British study involving over 34,000 men again showed a marked excess mortality among smokers from CHD, especially in those under 45 years of age (Doll 1976). The population-based cohort in the Framingham Heart Study has exhibited similar rates of excess CHD mortality in smokers (Gordon 1974). CHD mortality has also been shown to be consistently higher in smokers versus nonsmokers among various ethnic groups and among international cohorts (US DHHS 1983).

Most of the studies noted previously either did not include women or numbers of women were so small that conclusions could not be reached. However, recent evidence has confirmed the association of CHD and smoking in women. The largest cohort of women has been followed in the Nurses' Health Study, where the 6-year follow-up revealed a relative risk of 5.5 for fatal CHD among the heaviest smokers (Willet 1987). Risk for CHD mortality increased in a dose-dependent fashion with increasing numbers of cigarettes smoked. Relative risk of nonfatal MI increased similarly. In a case-control study of women experiencing first MI, the relative risk of MI was 3.6 in smokers versus nonsmokers (Rosenberg 1990). La Croix and colleagues (1991) found that the increased risk of CHD mortality extended to women who were over 65 years old. This prospective cohort study found a relative risk of total cardiovascular mortality to be 1.8, with CHD mortality of 1.5 in smokers versus nonsmokers. In the Rochester Coronary Heart Disease Project, a population-based, case-control study, 64% of all CHD events in women aged 40–59 were attributable to smoking (Beard 1989).

Prospective studies have also found strong correlations between smoking and nonfatal CHD events (US DHHS 1983). The Pooling Project Research Group (1978) reported a 3.2 times greater risk of a first CHD event in smokers versus nonsmokers for a cohort of over 8,000 men. The absolute risk of an event increased progressively with age and with increasing cigarette consumption. Similar conclusions have come from studies in various ethnic groups (US DHHS 1983) and among women (Willet 1987; Rosenberg 1990). The increase in relative risk for CHD appears to extend to those smokers over 65 as well (Benfante 1991).

Other study methods also support the association between smoking and CHD. Auerback and coworkers (1976) found significantly greater amounts of coronary atherosclerosis in smokers versus nonsmokers in a cross-sectional autopsy study, and smokers had more extensive microscopic evidence of intimal thickening in myocardial arterioles. Protocol autopsies in the Honolulu Heart Study found significant increases in coronary atherosclerosis in smokers versus nonsmokers (Reed 1990). Weintraub (1990) has also reported a significant association between angiographic evidence of CHD and smoking.

Smoking appears to interact with other CHD disease risk factors in a multiplicative fashion. In a cohort of over 300,000 men, elevated blood pressure (systolic and diastolic) and serum cholesterol interacted with smoking to increase risk of CHD mortality significantly (Neaton 1992). The relative risk for smokers at the highest levels of systolic blood pressure and cholesterol was over 20 times that in nonsmokers who were at the lowest levels for systolic blood pressure and cholesterol. The Pooling Project Research Group (1978) also showed similar interactions between blood pressure, cholesterol, and smoking.

Although a causal link between smoking and CHD cannot be proven by the data cited, several observations can be made which do support causality. The association between smoking and increased risk for CHD is strong and consistent across studies and groups of subjects. There is a consistent dose-dependent relationship between cigarettes consumed and risk for disease. The association is also biologically plausible, with multiple links between smoking and proposed mechanisms of CHD. The temporal element is the weakest link in this chain of causality. However, one recent study showed that length of time exposed to cigarettes was an important factor in determining CHD risk (Kawachi 1994). Thus, a relatively long latent period between smoking initiation and evidence of significant CHD is to be expected.

Smoking Cessation and Decreased Risk of CHD

Goldman and Cook (1984) analyzed the reasons for the striking decline in CHD mortality noted since 1968 and determined that over half of the decline could be attributed to reductions in cholesterol levels and cigarette smoking. Smoking cessation alone was estimated to account for 24% of the overall decline in CHD mortality from 1968 to 1976. Improvement in risk factors accounted for the 60% decline in cardiovascular mortality noted in the Framingham Heart Study (Sytkowski 1990). These studies only demonstrate that improvement in risk factor status, and smoking cessation in particular, has accompanied declining cardiovascular mortality. Causality is implied by the temporal association between the observed decline in smoking prevalence and declining cardiovascular mortality.

Smoking cessation may bring about improvement in CHD mortality via several possible scenarios, depicted in Figure 5.2. If no reversible effects of smoking exist, then improvement in relative risk of CHD mortality would occur slowly by removing

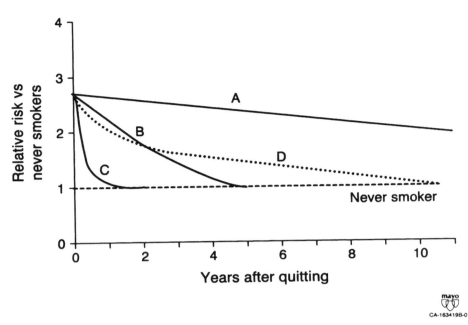

Fig. 5.2. Risk reduction for coronary heart disease following smoking cessation. (**A**) Gradually declining risk if the effects of smoking are irreversible. Risk declines because of elimination of ongoing tobacco-induced injury. (**B**) Slowly reversible effects of smoking. (**C**) Immediate and complete reversibility of smoking effects. (**D**) The approximate, actual rate of risk reduction based on observational studies.

ongoing tobacco-induced injury. In this case the risk for the former smoker may never reach the risk level of the never-smoker. However, if the effects of smoking are reversible, the time needed for CHD risk reduction might be quite short (immediate and completely reversible effects) or somewhat longer (slowly reversible effects). Several studies of both healthy individuals and those with established CHD have clarified these issues.

Prospective cohort studies have provided the bulk of the evidence for the benefits of smoking cessation (US DHHS 1990). A summary of the findings from some of the large cohorts is shown in Table 5.2. These studies include over 1.5 million men and women and span four decades of experience. They indicate a fairly uniform pattern of declining CHD mortality following smoking cessation. One of the studies revealed an increased mortality for smokers who had recently stopped smoking (within one year of quitting), probably indicating new onset of symptomatic CHD as the reason for their smoking cessation (Hammond 1958). These studies also indicate that 30–50% of the reduction in risk of CHD mortality occurs relatively early (within 2 years of cessation) and that there is a gradual decline in risk for the next 10–20 years until levels of risk similar to those of nonsmokers are achieved. These results are consistent with the proposed mechanisms noted previously, that is, the thrombogenic effects of smoking are reversed quickly, accounting for the early risk reduction, while the rapid

Table 5.2. Relative Risk of Coronary Heart Disease Mortality Related to Time Since Quitting: Cohort Studies

Smoking Status	9-State Study[a]	ACS-CPS II[b]*	Nurse Health Study[c]**	CASS[d]
Current	1.75	2.02	4.0	1.73
Quit				
<1–2 years	2.09	1.57	3.1	1.56
2–10 years	1.54	1.41	2.04	1.37
>10 years	1.09	0.99	1.04	1.28
Never smoked	1.0	1.0	1.0	1.0

[a]Hammond (1958); [b]US DHHS (1990); [c]Kawachi (1994); [d]Omenn (1990).

ACS-CPS II, American Cancer Society-Cancer Prevention Project II; CASS, Coronary Artery Surgery Study.

*Data for men who smoked > or = 21 cigarettes per day.

**Includes both fatal and nonfatal CHD events.

progression of atherosclerosis is slowed or halted. It is also noteworthy that the beneficial effects of smoking cessation are not confined to apparently disease-free people, but also extend to those with known CHD, as demonstrated in the Coronary Artery Surgery Study cohort (Omen 1990). In fact, the benefits of coronary revascularization in this cohort were negated in those subjects who continued to smoke (Cavender 1992), while among individuals over 65 years of age there was a salutary effect of smoking cessation (Hermanson 1988).

The time interval for reduction of acute MI risk appears to be somewhat shorter than for reduction of overall CHD mortality to levels seen in nonsmoking patients. Hospital-based, case-control studies in both men (Rosenberg 1985) and women (Rosenberg 1990) have shown reduction of risk to levels of nonsmokers within three years. These studies are summarized in Table 5.3.

Only one randomized intervention study has tried to assess the effect of smoking cessation advice without intervening on other CHD risk factors (Rose 1982). Mortality from CHD declined by 18% in the intervention group, but this risk reduction did not reach statistical significance. The difference in smoking prevalence between the intervention and control groups was relatively small at the 10-year follow-up (45% and 59%, respectively). One-third of those who quit cigarettes continued to use tobacco in the form of cigars or pipe, but were counted as "nonsmokers."

The Multiple Risk Factor Intervention Trial (MRFIT) was a randomized primary prevention trial to test the effect of multifactor intervention on CHD mortality among

Table 5.3. Relative Risk of Myocardial Infarction After Smoking Cessation: Case-Control Studies

Time since quitting	Current	1–23 months	24–35 months	>35 months	Never smoked
Men*	2.9	2.0	1.1	1.0	1.0
Women[†]	3.6	2.6	1.3	0.9	1.0

Source: *Rosenberg (1985); [†]Rosenberg (1990).

men who were at increased risk of death for CHD. After 10.5 years of follow-up, there was a reduction of 10.6% in CHD mortality in the intervention group as compared with the controls (MRFIT Research Group 1990). Most of this reduction was due to a 24% lower death rate from MI in the intervention group. At the end of 6 years of intervention smoking prevalence in the intervention group was 32% compared with 45% in the controls. Kuller and colleagues (1991) reported a 37% reduction in CHD mortality for those randomized MRFIT participants who reported quitting during the first year of the trial.

Intervention Strategies

Increasing awareness of the harmful effects of cigarette smoking is one of the primary reasons for the declining smoking prevalence over the past 30 years. However, the rate for decline in smoking appears to be slowing as overall prevalence rates fall. This phenomenon may be due to an increasing proportion of more highly addicted smokers and/or smoking initiation equal to the number of smokers who quit each year. This means that a substantial number of people will be smoking for years to come and makes smoking cessation intervention a continuing need.

It is estimated that 90% of Americans who successfully quit smoking do so using individual methods of smoking cessation rather than organized programs (Fiore 1990). This does not imply that other types of smoking intervention are not necessary. Fiore (1990) noted that about one-third of smokers who successfully quit had been advised by their physicians to do so. In addition, smokers who consumed 25 or more cigarettes per day and those who had made 5 or more attempts to quit were twice as likely to have used an assisted cessation method when compared to other smokers. Organized smoking cessation programs serve an important role in this population of heavier smokers who are at the greatest risk of tobacco-related morbidity and mortality.

Self-Help

Schwartz has extensively reviewed self help materials available through books, pamphlets, kits, and both audio and video tapes (Schwartz 1987). The median 1-year cessation rate of self-help programs is 18% (Schwartz 1987). This rate may seem unusually high, but probably indicates that those smokers who are able to quit using self-help methods are highly motivated to change. Several studies of self-help/minimal intervention programs are underway, but results are pending (Glynn 1990a). Resources for obtaining self-help materials are noted in Appendix A.

Most smokers who quit using self-help strategies will relapse (Fiore 1990; Orleans 1991). However, rather than being viewed as failure, serious attempts to quit are useful in the process of self-change described by Prochaska (1991) and DiClemente (1991). Energy should be focused on motivating more smokers to make serious attempts to quit smoking while directing heavier, more severely addicted smokers to organized cessation programs (Glynn 1990a). The largest number of smokers will continue to be reached through the provision of self-help materials. If existing self-help materials are more widely disseminated, smokers may be motivated to quit. This method of smoking cessation would appear to be the most cost-effective, although this has not yet been proven.

Physician Advice to Quit

In 1991 approximately 70% (35.8 million) of the 51 million smokers in the United States reported at least one outpatient visit to a health-care professional during the preceding 12 months, and over two-thirds of these individuals reported multiple visits (CDC 1993c). Only 37% of these smokers reported receiving any advice to quit smoking from a health-care professional. A study by Frank and coworkers (1991) from a cross-sectional population survey indicated that only 49% of current smokers had ever been advised by their physicians to quit. These studies point out that physicians are in a position to have a great impact on reducing smoking prevalence, and that they must improve efforts to deliver effective smoking cessation advice.

Ockene (1987) has extensively reviewed physician-delivered intervention studies. A number of randomized trials through 1986 revealed one-year cessation rates from 5% to 18%. The types of interventions varied among studies, with some intervention groups receiving adjuvant nicotine gum treatment. Randomized intervention groups that received advice to stop only and for whom one-year cessation rates are reported, had a mean one-year cessation rate of approximately 6% (Ockene 1987). Schwartz (1987) reported an identical mean one-year cessation rate when he reviewed 28 intervention trials of physician cessation advice/counseling.

Recently the National Cancer Institute supported five randomized trials to determine the efficacy of physician training in smoking cessation intervention and whether or not smoking cessation rates of patients are improved because of the physician training. These studies are summarized in Table 5.4. The investigation by Ockene and colleagues (1991) had the best levels of physician compliance with delivering the

Table 5.4. Randomized Trials of Physician Intervention for Smoking Cessation (Percent)[a]

| | Control vs. Intervention[b] | | | | |
| | Physician Outcomes | | | Smoking Cessation | |
Reference	Discussed Smoking	Advised Quitting	Quit Date Suggested	6 months	12 months
Wilson 1988	31	24	2	—	4.4
	85	84	54	—	8.8
Ockene 1991	—	—	—	9.1	—
	99	91	85	17.4	—
Cummings 1989[a]	50	—	11	—	1.5
	45	—	38	—	2.6
Cohen 1987, 1989	41	27	2	0.9	1.5
	95	84	58	3.8	5.2
Kottke 1989	51	40	5	—	5.0
	58	54	19	—	5.5

[a]Results are reported for the most intense intervention group in each study.
[b]Control group results in first row and intervention group in second row for each study.

smoking cessation message. Correspondingly, the patients in this study reported the highest abstinence rates at six months. However, the nonsmoking status of these patients was not biochemically verified as it was in each of the other studies. Biochemically verified abstinence in these studies ranged from 2.6% to 8.8% at six to 12 months. Important conclusions from these investigations are as follows:

1. Physicians trained in smoking cessation intervention will deliver stop smoking advice.
2. Patients who receive smoking cessation intervention are more likely to quit smoking than patients receiving ''usual care.''
3. The use of nicotine-containing gum for nicotine replacement may improve cessation rates.
4. Chart reminders improve physician compliance with delivering a smoking cessation message.

One of the trials noted in Table 5.4 suggested an improved smoking cessation rate with increasing follow-up visits (Wilson 1988); however, in a companion study, no significant improvement in smoking cessation at one year was noted in a group of smokers who received scheduled follow-up versus a control group who did not receive follow-up (Gilbert 1992). Ockene (1991) also noted no effect for scheduled telephone counseling follow-up in improving smoking cessation at six months, although others have found that telephone counseling increases the smoking cessation rate (Orleans 1991). Furthermore, a metanalysis of 39 controlled smoking cessation trials showed that the number of contacts between subject and therapist and the length of contact were two important predictors of smoking cessation success (Kottke 1988). Since relapse risk is greatest soon after quitting (Kottke 1989; Benowitz 1992), continued support for smoking abstinence by the physician could result in long-term benefits (Wilson 1988).

Two of the obstacles preventing many physicians from delivering smoking cessation advice are the perceived low success rate and inexperience in this type of counseling. While it is true that long-term smoking cessation rates are low with physician intervention, if physicians counsel all smokers to stop, approximately 2 million would become nonsmokers each year. Thus, improved physician counseling skills may have a large public health impact. Many physicians have expressed interest in more training to improve their preventive counseling skills (Ochene 1987). In response to the need for smoking intervention training, the National Cancer Institute has developed a manual and program for physician intervention training (Glynn 1990b). The recommended intervention is brief and focused, and it is designed to be delivered during a routine clinical visit (see Table 5.5). The training guide also reviews office systems

Table 5.5. Physician Counseling Guidelines for Smoking Cessation

---

Ask about smoking at every clinical visit.
Advise all smokers to stop.
Assist the patient by advising a quit date and providing self-help materials.
Arrange follow-up visits to assess smoking status and encourage continued abstinence.

Source: From Glynn (1990b).

and procedures which will enhance the physician intervention by improving both physician comfort and patient compliance with smoking intervention, yet allow individual counseling for each patient.

Pharmacologic Therapy

Cigarettes and other forms of tobacco are addicting and lead to patterns of regular and compulsive use (US DHSS 1988). Nicotine is the substance in tobacco that is responsible for its addictive qualities (US DHSS 1988). Abstinence from tobacco causes a withdrawal syndrome including symptoms of restlessness, irritability, anxiety, impaired concentration, and strong craving for cigarettes (Benowitz 1992). Relapse to smoking approaches 50% within a month of quitting and gradually declines thereafter (Kottke 1988; US DHSS 1988; Benowitz 1992). Relief of withdrawal symptoms can improve initial abstinence rates, reduce early relapse and thereby improve long-term abstinence rates. This rationale stands behind the major forms of drug therapy used for treatment of nicotine dependence.

Transdermal Nicotine Patch. Nicotine replacement therapy via application of a transdermal delivery system has been used extensively in clinical trials since 1989. Transdermal nicotine effectively reduces cigarette craving and withdrawal compared with placebo treatment (Daughton 1991; Tonneson 1991; Russell 1993; Hurt 1994). The differences in withdrawal symptoms between placebo and active treatment groups in these studies declined after two to three weeks of abstinence. Withdrawal symptom relief may depend on achieving adequate blood levels of nicotine and calls for individualizing patch dosage rather than following a fixed schedule for every smoker (Hurt 1994). The level of blood nicotine achieved with a fixed 22-mg patch dose is about half the level found when smokers are smoking their usual number of cigarettes (Hurt 1993).

Short-term efficacy of nicotine patch therapy has been demonstrated in multiple studies (Fiore 1992b). Although duration, dose, and adjuvant treatments vary, the mean smoking cessation rate at the end of active treatment is approximately 40%. Abstinence rates in placebo groups in these studies were about half those of active patch groups (Table 5.6). The type of adjuvant therapy used did not significantly affect outcome. These studies demonstrate reasonable long-term efficacy of patch therapy after six to 12 months of follow-up, with mean cessation rates of 20% to 25% compared with 5% to 10% in placebo groups. Unfortunately, there is also a uniform and sometimes dramatic fall in smoking cessation rates after active nicotine patch therapy is discontinued. Relapse after withdrawal of nicotine replacement points out the importance of ongoing support and relapse prevention. The end-of-treatment smoking cessation rates with nicotine patch therapy are impressive; thus, the challenge is to develop equally effective relapse-prevention techniques.

Fiore (1992b) has reviewed the reported frequency of several common systemic and local side effects. Skin reactions have been common, with mild reactions including itching and erythema at the patch sites occurring in up to 50% of patch users (Fiore 1992b). Severe skin reactions occur uncommonly, and generalized skin reactions, for example, urticaria, have been reported in only 2% to 3% of patients in clinical trials.

Table 5.6. Smoking Cessation Rates in Randomized Trials of Transdermal Nicotine (Percent)

Reference	End of Active Treatment		End of Study		N	Duration of Observation (months)
	Active	Placebo	Active	Placebo		
Westman 1993	29.5	8.8	20.5	2.5	159	6
Sachs 1993	45	26	25	9	220	12
Hurt 1990	77	39	29	26	70	13
TNSG 1991[a]	54.5	27	26	12	935	6
Daughton 1991	37	13.5	26	8	158	6
Tonnesen 1991	41	10	17	4	289	12
Russel 1993	17.5	7.5	9.3	5	600	12
Hurt 1994	46.7	20	27.5	14.2	240	12

Only studies with minimum 6 months follow-up are included.

[a]Transdermal Nicotine Study Group.

None of the clinical trials of transdermal nicotine have reported a significant number of any systemic adverse effects. The interpretation of reported side effects such as sleep disturbance and change in bowel habits, is confounded because of the overlap between symptoms of nicotine withdrawal and nicotine toxicity. Although there has been concern about serious cardiovascular effects from nicotine patch use, Orleans (1994) reported that an investigation by the Food and Drug Administration found only 33 reports of serious adverse cardiovascular events out of an estimated 2 million patch users. Concomittant smoking and nicotine patch use should be discouraged, but has not been associated with serious nicotine toxicity (Hurt 1994; Orleans 1994). Smokers who have decreased their smoking rate while on patch therapy and remain motivated to quit, may be continued on patch therapy while being monitored closely. For those who continue to smoke at baseline levels after two weeks of patch therapy, nicotine patches should be discontinued and a new quit date should be set (Fiore 1994).

Future directions for nicotine patch therapy investigations include higher doses and dose titration studies to determine optimum nicotine replacement strategies. Use of a 44-mg patch dose appears to be safe and tolerable (Fredrickson 1993) in heavy smokers consuming 25 or more cigarettes per day. It is not known whether higher patch doses will improve smoking cessation rates, or whether a tapering nicotine patch withdrawal schedule is better than abrupt withdrawal. Finally, the optimum length of therapy with nicotine patches has not been determined, although available information suggests that six to eight weeks is adequate.

Nicotine Gum. Nicotine-containing gum became available in 1984 and quickly became one of the fastest-selling prescription drugs (Schwartz 1992). However, results of trials with nicotine gum are far from uniform. Schwartz (1987) found a median smoking cessation rate of 11% after one year of follow-up in studies that provided no behavioral component. When behavioral therapy in specialized clinics was added, one-year cessation rates were improved at 29% for gum treatment versus 13.5% in placebo groups. When counseling intervention was provided by physicians, along with the use of nicotine gum, one-year cessation rates ranged from 6% to 10% (Schwartz 1987). In the physician intervention studies sponsored by the National Cancer Institute, nicotine gum provided small benefits in addition to counseling (Wilson 1988; Cohen 1989; Ockene 1991). Nicotine gum alone with minimal intervention yielded results similar to control group cessation rates (Wilson 1988; Cohen 1989). One study found significantly better cessation rates in smokers offered nicotine gum, but only 29% used gum for more than one month (Ockene 1991). In a similar multicenter trial of minimal physician intervention and nicotine gum, Gilbert (1989) reported no difference between gum and no-gum groups. Hughes (1989) also found no improvement in smoking cessation for nicotine versus placebo gum treatment when combined with physician advice. The Stanford Stop Smoking Project reported six-month cessation rates of 30% and 22% in nicotine gum versus no-gum users, respectively (Fortmann 1988), although these differences were not maintained at one year (Killen 1990).

Though no direct comparisons have been made, nicotine gum does not appear to be as efficacious as the nicotine transdermal patch in studies of physician counseling plus nicotine replacement therapy. The primary reason for these differences is poor patient compliance due to inadequate instruction in the proper technique of gum use (see Appendix B). Change in salivary pH caused by many beverages and foods may also interfere with nicotine absorption (Henningfield 1990). Nicotine gum may have an advantage over the nicotine patch for use in high-stress situations by allowing the user to titrate nicotine levels and alleviate acute urges to smoke. Fagerstrom (1993) found combined nicotine gum and patch therapy provided better withdrawal symptom relief than either one alone.

Clonidine. The rationale for the use of the antihypertensive clonidine in smoking cessation treatment is its demonstrated efficacy in alleviating opiate withdrawal symptoms (US DHSS 1988). Clonidine has not been used extensively for smoking cessation treatments, and published results have shown modest benefit at best. Glassman and coworkers (1988) demonstrated a significant effect favoring clonidine. At the end of four weeks of treatment, 17% of clonidine-treated subjects versus 8% of placebo controls had verified continuous abstinence. The difference in the two groups was entirely accounted for by a beneficial effect in women. The same gender effect was noted for clonidine in a later study (Glassman 1993), although these data did not show an overall significant long-term benefit, with cessation rates at 12 months of 15% and 11% in clonidine and placebo groups, respectively. In both these investigations, the presence of a history of depression had a significant negative impact on smoking cessation.

Using a minimal counseling intervention format, Franks (1989) and Prochazka (1992) demonstrated no difference in smoking cessation in clonidine versus placebo groups. Clonidine had minimal effect in reducing withdrawal symptoms in one study (Prochazka 1992), while significantly reducing craving, irritability, anxiety, and restlessness in another (Ornish 1988). A recent study also concluded that clonidine reduced craving after smoking cessation, but at the cost of significant adverse effects (Gourlay 1994).

If clonidine has any role in smoking cessation therapy, it appears to be in women who are highly nicotine-dependent (Glassman 1993). It may serve as a second tier treatment in the patient who cannot tolerate transdermal nicotine replacement. Like nicotine gum, in a typical office setting with minimal counseling intervention, no beneficial effect can be expected (Prochazka 1992).

Other Pharmacologic Treatments. Many other drug treatments have been tried in nicotine dependence but have shown no consistent efficacy (Schwartz 1987; US DHSS 1988). A recent study of the anxiolytic buspirone demonstrated significantly diminished withdrawal symptoms in the active drug versus placebo group (Hilleman 1992). Nicotine replacement in the form of a nicotine inhaler proved beneficial in an initial randomized, controlled trial (Tonneson 1993); no other trials of this novel treatment have been reported. Hjalmarson (1994) reported the first use of nicotine nasal spray for smoking cessation and demonstrated doubling of the one-year continuous abstinence rate in the active drug group over the placebo group. More randomized trials are planned for this promising treatment. Since prevalence of depression among smokers appears to be high (Glassman 1988, 1993; Breslau 1993), treatment of selected smokers with antidepressant medication may improve their ability to quit smoking. Doxepin has been shown to reduce withdrawal symptoms and craving for cigarettes in a double-blind study (Murphy 1990) and improved short-term smoking cessation in a pilot study (Edwards 1989). No studies have reported long-term follow-up of smoking cessation and antidepressant therapy.

Nicotine Dependence Treatment: A Comprehensive Model

The individual components of smoking cessation intervention such as self-help materials, advice and counseling regarding smoking cessation, and pharmacologic therapy do not operate independently. These components are blended by the care provider at the point of contact with the smoker, resulting in an individualized intervention and treatment plan. This model is applicable not only for large institutions with abundant resources, but also for small clinics and individual practitioners. In fact, the public health benefits will be greatest when this model is applied widely at the individual practitioner level.

The staff of the Mayo Nicotine Dependence Center has served over 8,000 smoking patients since its establishment in 1988. This program in a medical center setting has developed a clinically oriented approach to nicotine dependence treatment. The treatment philosophy is based on the principles of behavioral treatment, addictions treatment, pharmacologic therapy, and relapse prevention (Hurt 1992a). The intervention is initiated by a physician referral to see a nonphysician counselor. The counselors are masters degree-level professionals who provide a 45–60-minute consultation during which a comprehensive assessment is performed and a treatment plan formulated. The elements of this approach to nicotine dependence treatment can be outlined as follows (Hurt 1992a):

1. *Identification* of the smoker by the treating physician
2. *Advice to stop smoking* by the physician and referral for nicotine dependance consultation when indicated

3. *Comprehensive assessment* by the nicotine dependence counselor of medical and smoking history, previous stop attempts, degree of addiction, support systems, motivation to stop, and stage of readiness to change
4. *Preparation of a treatment plan* based on the individual's motivation level and stage of readiness to change, including a personalized message to quit, as well as counseling regarding the individual's addiction to nicotine and behavioral skills training
5. *Relapse prevention*, achieved through structured follow-up phone calls, letters, face-to-face counseling, and group support
6. *Intensive treatment* for more severe nicotine dependence or those smokers with life-threatening tobacco-related diseases. Treatment intensity is matched to individual patient needs and may include frequent individual counseling, group programs, or residential nicotine dependence treatment

This integrated effort of physicians, trained counselors, and experienced office personnel has produced quit rates of approximately 23% at one-year follow-up for patients receiving the consultation and structured relapse prevention program. Higher rates are achieved with group interventions and the residential treatment program (Hurt 1992b). Even though the resources of a specialized center for nicotine dependence treatment are not available to most physicians, the principles for smoking cessation intervention are directly transferable to most medical settings. There are many other health-care professionals besides physicians who can also be trained to provide smoking cessation intervention services. For example, nurses, respiratory therapists, physician assistants, and chemical dependency counselors have all provided this type of service in other medical centers.

Physicians play a vital role in smoking intervention because of their frequent contact with smoking patients (CDC 1993). As already pointed out, most physicians do not inquire about smoking status or intervene. Ockene (1987) summarized some of the barriers to physician intervention: perceived low success rate, lack of counseling skills and knowledge, lack of time and space, and concerns about reimbursement. A comprehensive, systematic approach will allow these barriers to be overcome:

1. Assess smoking status at each clinical encounter. Fiore (1990) has suggested this be done as part of routine vital signs. Chart reminders can facilitate smoking status assessment as well (Cohen 1987; Kottke 1989).
2. Obtain a brief smoking history as part of the medical database. This should include number of cigarettes consumed per day, an estimate of dependence on nicotine, and the number of previous quit attempts. The degree of dependence can be assessed by whether or not withdrawal symptoms are present during abstinence and how soon the first cigarette of the day is used. Orleans (1993) has suggested a simple smoking assessment form for office use.
3. Give a simple and direct message advising the patient to quit. The message should be personalized to the patient's specific needs (Glynn 1989). Reinforce the message with self-help literature about smoking cessation. This message should be delivered to each smoker regardless of their stage of readiness. This may move some who are precontemplative or contemplative to the action stage (Glynn 1990a). Encourage each patient to set a quit date. Counseling regarding

patient concerns and available support can be effectively performed by nurses (Hollis 1993; Orleans 1993; Hurt 1994).

4. Prescribe nicotine replacement therapy for patients who are motivated to stop. Transdermal nicotine has advantages over nicotine gum, but the latter may be effective when used properly.

5. See the patient for follow-up within two weeks of the quit date. This visit is to reinforce the smoking cessation message and discuss concerns about maintaining abstinence. Maintaining abstinence for the first two weeks is a critical step in achieving long-term success (Hurt 1994; Kenford 1994). Kottke (1988) noted the importance of repeated visits in maintaining abstinence. Nurses can effectively deliver follow-up and provide counseling regarding patient concerns (Hollis 1993; Hurt 1994).

6. Recycle and try again for those patients who fail to achieve abstinence and refer those patients with repeated relapse to specialized clinics or programs for more intensive treatment.

Successful office intervention need not be excessively time-consuming or use up valuable resources. It does require obtaining a few new skills and systematically implementing the comprehensive model outlined. Patient education and counselling materials are provided in an appendix at the end of this chapter. Referring highly addicted and recidivist patients to specialized centers for more intensive treatment will help match smokers to the appropriate treatment and enhance their chances of achieving abstinence.

Effectiveness of Intervention Strategies

Randomized trials of physician advice yield long-term smoking cessation rates of about 6% in the intervention groups. The addition of nicotine gum to physician advice marginally improves cessation rates. Nicotine patch therapy as an adjunct to minimal counseling has been associated with significantly improved cessation rates of over 20% in controlled studies. The strength of this data is good since the results have come from randomized trials in multiple settings with varying populations. Brief physician interventions as described in the National Cancer Institute manual (Glynn 1990b) and outlined in Table 5.4, combined with nicotine patch therapy and nurse follow-up can provide a clinically significant one-year smoking cessation rate of nearly 30% (Hurt 1994). Matching nicotine replacement dose to patients' needs and providing more effective relapse prevention will boost this rate higher in the future.

Strength of Evidence Supporting Benefit of Smoking Cessation

The evidence for a causal link between cigarette smoking and increased risk for fatal and nonfatal CHD is based on a large body of observational studies. Likewise, the evidence for beneficial effects of smoking cessation is not supported by any randomized trials but by cohort and case-control studies. For obvious reasons, a randomized study of smoking effects in previously unexposed subjects will never be performed. Intervention trials which deal with multiple risk factors (e.g., MRFIT) give us indirect evidence of the benefits of smoking cessation. Because of the large volume of data from observational studies, the overall strength of the evidence must be judged as excellent, even though there is a paucity of information from randomized trials. Two conclusions are indisputable:

1. Cigarette smoking is the most important modifiable risk factor for the development of CHD.
2. Smoking cessation significantly lowers the risk for both fatal and nonfatal CHD events regardless of sex, age, or presence of established CHD.

Cost-Effectiveness of Smoking Cessation Intervention

It is ironic that tobacco is the leading cause of death among Americans each year, yet the national investment in prevention is estimated to be less than 5% of the total annual health care cost (McGinnis 1993). The great public health burden of smoking-attributable mortality has already been discussed. With such a heavy death and disease load attributable to tobacco, it is surprising the paucity of information there is about the cost-effectiveness of smoking cessation. In a study by Oster (1986), it was estimated that smoking cessation using nicotine gum as an adjuvant could cost the smoker $4,113–$9,473 per year of life gained. In this study, the population base was hypothetical and assumed a 0% chance of relapse. The focus of the study was to evaluate the cost-effectiveness of using nicotine gum as an adjuvant to physician' advice. Cummings (1989b) found smoking cessation advice by physicians to cost a smoking individual $705–$2,058 per year of life gained. In contrast, the cost of smoking one pack of cigarettes daily is approximately $700 per year (based on the 1993 average retail price).

Compared with the cost-effectiveness of other medical services, nicotine dependence treatment is relatively inexpensive. For example, it is estimated that it costs $24,408 per year of life gained for treating mild hypertension (Edelson 1990) and $56,100 per year of life gained for the treatment of hypercholesterolemia with cholestyramine (Oster 1987). Such cost-outcome data should be considered by policy makers as they determine how best to allocate limited health care resources.

Summary

Quality of available data: A large body of well-designed observational (both case-control and cohort) studies comparing risks of MI in current and former smokers compared with nonsmokers.

Estimated risk reduction: 50–70% within 5 years of smoking cessation.

Comparability of effect in men and women: The benefits of smoking cessation apply equally to men and women.

Appendix A

Patient Education and Counseling Materials

Source	*Publication*
National Cancer Institute Office of Cancer Communications Building 31, Room 10A24 Bethesda, MD 20892 (800) 4-CANCER	• *Clearing the Air* (NIH publication no. 92-1647) The best succinct self-help smoking cessation pamphlet available • *How to Help Your Patients Stop Smoking* (NIH publication no. 90-3064) An excellent training manual for physicians in smoking cessation intervention and counseling • *Why Do You Smoke?* (NIH publication no. 83-1822) A simple self-administered questionnaire that may provide insight into many of the behavioral aspects of a smoker's addiction and cues to smoking.
Centers for Disease Control and Prevention Center for Chronic Disease Prevention and Health Promotion Office on Smoking and Health Rockville, MD 20857	• *The Health Benefits of Smoking Cessation.* *A Report of the Surgeon General, 1990, at* *a Glance.* (DHSS publication no. (CDC) 90-8419). A patient-oriented, brief summary of the 1990 Surgeon General's Report
American Heart Association 7272 Greenville Avenue Dallas, TX 75231-4596	• *Children and Smoking: A Message to* *Parents.* A pamphlet instructing parents in primary prevention of smoking in their children.

- *How to Avoid Weight Gain When Quitting Smoking.*

  A common-sense guide for this frequent problem.

American Cancer Society
(Local Office)
(800) ACS-2345

- *The Most Often Asked Questions About Tobacco and Health and . . . The Answers.*

  This booklet gives brief explanations about health effects of smoking and nicotine addiction.

- *Tobacco Free Young America Q & A. Questions and Answers for the Busy Practitioner.*

  This pamphlet contains a brief smoking intervention guide for physicians and offers suggestions for counseling smokers.

American Medical Association
Division of Health Science
515 North State Street
Chicago, IL 60610

- *How to Help Patients Stop Smoking. Guidelines for Diagnosis and Treatment of Nicotine Dependence* (Publication date 1/94)

  A brief state-of-the-art guide for physicians in smoking cessation intervention.

American Lung Association
(Local office)

- *Freedom from Smoking for You and Your Family.*

  This booklet is a self-help guide to smoking cessation for all adults.
  - *Freedom from Smoking for You and Your Baby.* (kit)

  A self-help, 10-day smoking cessation program aimed specifically at pregnant smokers.

- *Nicotine Addition and Cigarettes.*

  A brief pamphlet that discusses nicotine addition and specific ways family and friends can support and encourage smokers to quit.

W. R. Spence, M.D.
HEALTH EDCO
Waco, TX 76702-1207

- *The ABC's of Smoking.*

  This booklet contains graphic photographs of tobacco-related diseases. It is helpful for ''shock value'' in the carefully selected smoker.

• *Smokeless Tobacco. A Chemical Time Bomb.*

Similar to the publication noted above, this booklet shows graphic photographs of complications from smokeless tobacco use.

March of Dimes Birth Defects Foundation
1275 Mamaroneck Avenue
White Plains, NY 10605

• *Give Your Baby a Healthy Start: Stop Smoking.*

A very simply-written pamphlet about harmful effects of smoking on the fetus and a self-help guide for quitting.

Appendix B

Patient Instructions for Using Nicotine Polacrilex, Nicotine Patches, and Clonidine Hydrochloride for Smoking Cessation.

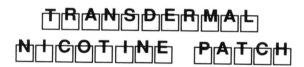

The Food and Drug Administration has approved four nicotine skin-patch systems to help you stop smoking. They include:

	mg	mg	mg
Habitrol™	21	14	7
Nicoderm™	21	14	7
Nicotrol™	15	10	5
Prostep™	22	11	

(mg = milligram)

Although these patches have different manufacturers, they all are used in the same way. The skin patch delivers a steady dose of nicotine through your skin. This reduces your craving for nicotine and lets you focus on changing the behaviors which accompany tobacco use. The amount of nicotine is gradually reduced over a period of several weeks.

Do not smoke while using this medication.

Reproduced with permission by Mayo Foundation for Medication Education and Research, Rochester, MN.

Dosing plan

Apply the patch on the first day you stop smoking. After that, apply a new patch each day — mornings or after bathing usually work best. The patch should remain attached **at all times**. If it comes off, apply a new patch. Do not remove the patch at night unless you are told to do so by your physician.

The following is a suggested treatment plan that gives some broad guidelines:

Step One: 15 mg, 21 mg or 22 mg patch per day for four to eight weeks

Step Two: 10 mg, 14 mg or 11 mg patch per day for two to four weeks

Step Three: 5 mg, 7 mg patch per day for two to four weeks (**Habitrol**™, **Nicotrol**™, **Nicoderm**™)

Each patient is different so your physician may give you an individualized treatment plan. Your physician may schedule you for treatment appointments at regular intervals. Or, you may get the entire treatment plan at your first appointment.

If you have heart disease, weigh less than 100 pounds, or smoke less than one-half pack per day, your physician may begin with a smaller dose. Other instructions are included with the medication and you should read them carefully. If you have any questions, ask your physician or pharmacist.

Application site

The patch may be placed anywhere on your upper body — including your arms and back. Non-hairy sites which are not rubbed by clothing are best. **Rotate the patch site.** On the next page is a rotation plan which you may use. Do **not** apply the patch to an area that has been shaved.

In each two-week cycle, place patches approximately as shown day by day (first day at location 1). Ideally, while the general location during each two-week cycle would follow this pattern, the exact location would be varied slightly so that no one body site is used more than once during the weeks of patch therapy.

Disposal

Before disposing a patch, fold it in half with the sticky sides together. Dispose patches out of the reach of children and pets.

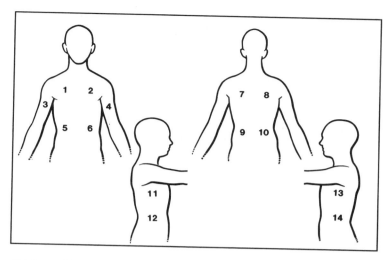

Side effects

Problems with the patches usually relate to skin irritation. These usually do not occur until after several weeks of use. After you remove a patch, you may want to use hydrocortisone cream to relieve any irritation. This cream can be bought in any drugstore or discount store. If you are troubled by irritation or other problems you think may be related to the nicotine patch, contact your physician or pharmacist.

Expectations

The nicotine patch is not magic. It will reduce your craving and your physical withdrawal symptoms, but it is not expected to give you the same levels of nicotine as smoking. You will probably have the urge to smoke at times. Having a plan for coping with situations where you may be tempted to smoke is important. The patch is only one part of a successful treatment program. It works best when combined with an individual or group counseling program.

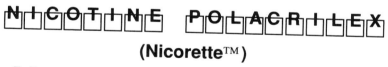

(Nicorette™)

Nicotine polacrilex (Nicorette™) is a gum-like product to help you stop smoking. There are two forms available: Nicorette™ which contains two milligrams of nicotine, and Nicorette DS™ (double strength) which contains four milligrams of nicotine. The double strength product is recommended for patients who have a more severe nicotine addiction.

The amount of nicotine acquired from one piece of the two milligram dose is about the equivalent of **one** inhaled cigarette. The nicotine is absorbed **only** through the lining of your cheeks. For this reason, using Nicorette™ like chewing gum is not effective. Avoid coffee, colas, orange juice, etc., while using Nicorette™ since they can slow or prevent the absorption of nicotine.

Nicotine polacrilex is available only with a physician's prescription. Your physician will decide which strength to prescribe based on the severity of your addiction. Nicotine polacrilex is sold in boxes of 96 pieces. Most patients initially use 10 to 12 pieces per day (some patients will need more) with a box lasting approximately one week. Nicotine replacement reduces physical withdrawal symptoms and lets you concentrate on the other changes you need to make as you quit smoking.

Do not smoke while using this medication.

Nicotine replacement therapy is a temporary aid used as part of a smoking cessation program. It usually is used for several weeks and almost always less than six months. For those who are still using it at the end of three months, a reduction plan should be initiated. The tapering schedule will vary for each user. When only one or two pieces are being used per day, usage should be discontinued altogether.

Instructions for use of Nicotine Polacrilex
(Nicorette™) • (Nicorette DS™)

You **must** stop smoking completely before beginning to use the gum.

1. Plan to use the gum on a regular schedule, such as one piece per hour.

2. Bite the gum a few times until a tingling sensation is felt or you taste the nicotine. **Do not chew it like gum.**

3. Stop biting and hold the gum next to your cheek toward the front of your mouth.

4. When you no longer notice a tingling sensation, repeat steps two and three, moving the gum to a different part of your mouth.

5. Continue the process of biting and holding the gum until only a mint flavor remains. This takes about 30 minutes.

6. Do not eat or drink anything while using the gum. Any nicotine that is swallowed with saliva or washed down with liquids will **not** be effective and may cause side effects such as heartburn or nausea.

7. Avoid acidic beverages before using the gum. If you have drunk coffee, colas, orange juice or other acidic liquids, rinse your mouth with water before using the gum.

8. Do not swallow the gum.

9. Keep the product out of reach of children at all times.

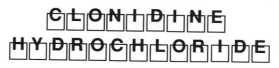

(Catapres™)

Your doctor has prescribed clonidine to help you quit smoking. It has been shown to be helpful in reducing nicotine withdrawal symptoms such as craving, irritability, anxiety and restlessness. This medication is usually prescribed for the treatment of high blood pressure. While the use of clonidine for smoking cessation has not been approved by the Food and Drug Administration, your physician may recommend it under special circumstances for nicotine withdrawal.

Use

This medication does not contain nicotine and it is not addicting. It comes in two forms: a pill that usually is taken twice a day, or a patch that is applied once a week. As with any medication, it is important to take it as prescribed. If you forget a dose, do not try to make up by taking two doses the next time.

Patch application

Apply the patch to a clean, dry area of skin on your upper arm or chest. Select an area with little or no hair. Each dose is best applied to a different area of skin to prevent skin irritation. Patches normally will stay in place during bathing or swimming. If the patch becomes loose, cover it with the extra adhesive provided with the patch.

Local irritation may form under the adhesive holding the patch. Change the location of the patch each week to avoid this irritation. If you develop a generalized body rash, contact your physician.

Disposal

Before disposing a patch, fold it in half with the sticky sides together. Dispose patches out of the reach of children and pets.

Side effects

The most common **side effects** of clonidine are
• lightheadedness
• drowsiness
• dry mouth
• decreased sexual ability which is a less common side effect

If any of these side effects occur, talk with your physician before you decide to stop the medication. The side effects usually subside with continued use of the medication.

The lightheadedness may be caused by a drop in your blood pressure, usually within the first few weeks of using clonidine. It is best to deal with this by rising slowly from a chair or bed, allowing enough time for your blood pressure to adjust. If lightheadedness persists, have your blood pressure checked, sitting and standing.

Clonidine will add to the effects of alcohol and other medicines that may make you drowsy. Examples of medicines that may cause drowsiness are antihistamines, medicines for depression or anxiety, sleeping medicine, prescription medicines for pain, medicines for seizures, and muscle relaxants. Be sure to tell your doctor about all the medicines you are taking, including those that you buy without a prescription. Limit your alcohol intake while taking clonidine.

Make sure you know how you react to clonidine before you drive, use machines, or do anything else that could be dangerous if you are not alert.

The safety of clonidine use during pregnancy is unproven. You should not smoke during pregnancy. In addition, you should not use any medications during pregnancy unless they are prescribed or approved by your physician.

References

Allen, DR, Browse NL, Rutt DL. Effects of cigarette smoke, carbon monoxide and nicotine on the uptake of fibrinogen by the canine arterial wall. Atherosclerosis 1989;77:83–8.

Asmussen I. Mitochondrial proliferation in endothelium: observations on umbilical arteries from newborn children of smoking mothers. Atherosclerosis 1984;50:203–8.

Auerback O, Carter HW, Garfinkel L, Hammond EC. Cigarette smoking and coronary artery disease: a macroscopic and microscopic study. Chest 1976;70:697–705.

Beard CM, Kottke TE, Annegers JF, Ballard DJ. The Rochester Coronary Heart Disease Project: effect of cigarette smoking, hypertension, diabetes and steroidal estrogen use on coronary heart disease among 40- to 59-year-old women, 1960 through 1982. Mayo Clinic Proc 1989;64:1471–80.

Benfante R, Reed D, Frank J. Does cigarette smoking have an independent effect on coronary heart disease incidence in the elderly? Am J Public Health 1991;81:897–9.

Benowitz NL. Cigarette smoking and nicotine addiction. Med Clin North Am 1992;76:415–37.

Breslasu N, Kilbey MM, Andreski P. Nicotine dependence and major depression: new evidence from a prospective investigation. Arch Gen Psychiatry 1993;50:31–5.

Caro CG. Cigarette smoking causes acute changes in arterial wall mechanics and the pattern of arterial blood flow in healthy subjects: possible mechanism into atherogenesis. Adv Exp Med Biol 1990;273:273–80.

Cavender, JB, Rogers WJ, Fisher LD, et al. Effects of smoking on survival and morbidity in patients randomized to medical or surgical therapy in the Coronary Artery Surgery Study (CASS): 10 year follow-up. J Am Coll Cardiol 1992;20:287–94.

Centers for Disease Control and Prevention. Cigarette smoking among adults: United States, 1991. MMWR 1993a; 42:230–3.

Centers for Disease Control and Prevention. Cigarette smoking-attributable mortality and years of potential life lost: United States, 1990. MMWR 1993b;42:645-9.

Centers for Disease Control and Prevention. Physician and other health-care professional counseling of smokers to quit: United States, 1991. MMWR 1993c;42:854–7.

Cohen SJ, Christen AD, Katz BP, et al. Encouraging primary care physicians to help smokers quit: a randomized, controlled trial. Ann Intern Med 1989;110:648–52.

Cohen SJ, Stookey GK, Katz BP, et al. Encouraging primary care physicians to help smokers quit: a randomized, controlled trial. Ann Intern Med 1989;110:648–52.

Cummings SR, Coates TJ, Richard RJ, et al. Training physicians in counseling about smoking cessation: a randomized trial of the "Quit for Life" program. Ann Intern Med 1989a; 110:640–7.

Cummings SR, Oster G. The cost-effectiveness of counseling smokers to quit. JAMA 1989b; 261:75–79.

Daughton DM, Heatley SA, Prendergast JJ, et al. Effect of transdermal nicotine delivery as an adjunct to low-intervention smoking cessation therapy: a randomized, placebo-controlled, double-blind study. Arch Intern Med 1991;151:749–52.

Deanfield JE, Shea MJ, Wilson RA, et al. Direct effects of smoking on the heart: silent ischemic disturbances of coronary flow. Am J Cardiol 1986;57:1005–9.

DiClemente CC, Prochaska JO, Fairhurst SK, et al. The process of smoking cessation: an analysis of precontemplation, contemplation and preparation stages of change. J Consult Clin Psychol 1991;59:295–304.

Doll R, Hill, AB. Lung cancer and other causes of death in relation to smoking: a second report on the mortality of British doctors. Br Med J 1956;2:1071–81.

Doll R, Peto R. Mortality in relation to smoking: 20 years' observation on male British doctors. Br Med J 1976;2:1525–36.

Edelson JT, Weinstein MC, Tosteson ANA. Long-term cost-effectiveness of various initial monotherapies for mild to moderate hypertension. JAMA 1990;263:408–13.

Edward NB, Murphy JK, Downs AD, et al. Doxepin as an adjunct to smoking cessation: a double-blind pilot study. Am J Psychiatry 1989;146:373–6.

Ernst E, Koenig W. Smoking and blood rheology. Adv Exp Med Biol 1990;273:295–300.

FAgerstrom KO, Schneider NG, Lunell E. Effectiveness of nicotine patch and nicotine gum as individual versus combined treatments for tobacco withdrawal symptoms. Psychopharmacology 1993:111:271–7.

Feher MD, Rampling MW, Brown J, et al. Acute changes in atherogenic and thrombogenic factors with cessation of smoking. J R Soc Med 1990;83:146–8.

Fiore MC. The new vital sign: assessing and documenting smoking status. JAMA 1991;266:3193-4.

Fiore MC. Trends in cigarette smoking in the United States: the epidemiology of tobacco use. Med Clin North Am 1992a;76:289–303.

Fiore MC, Jorenby DE, Baker TB, Klinford SL. Tobacco dependence and the nicotine patch: clinical guidelines for effective use. JAMA 1992b;268:2687–94.

FitzGerald GA, Oates JA, Nowak J. Cigarette smoking and hemostatic function. Am Heart J 1988;115:267–71.

Fortmann SP, Killen JD, Telch MJ, Newman B. Minimal contact treatment for smoking cessation. A placebo controlled trial of nicotine polacrilex and self-directed relapse prevention: initial results of the Stanford Stop Smoking Project. JAMA 1988;260:1575–80.

Frank E, Winkleby MA, Altman DG, et al. Predictors of physicians' smoking cessation advice. JAMA 1991;266:3139–44.

Franks P, Harp J, Bell B. Randomized, controlled trial of clonidine for smoking cessation in a primary care setting. JAMA 1989;262:3011–13.

Fredrickson PA, Lee GM, Wingender LA, et al. Safety and tolerance of high-dose transdermal nicotine therapy in light and heavy smokers [Abstract]. J Addict Dis 1993;12:177.

Fuster V, Badimon L, Badimon JJ, Chesebro JH. The pathogenesis of coronary artery disease and the acute coronary syndromes. N Engl J Med 1992;326:242–50, 310–18.

Gilbert JR, Wilson DCM, Best JA, et al. Smoking cessation in primary care: a randomized controlled trial of nicotine-bearing chewing gum. J Fam Prac 1989;28:49–55.

Gilbert JR, Wilson DMC, Singer J., et al. A family physician smoking cessation program: an evaluation of the role of follow-up visits. Am J Prev Med 1992;8:91–5.

Glassman AH, Stetner F, Walsh T, et al. Heavy smokers, smoking cessation, and clonidine: results of a double-blind, randomized trial. JAMA 1988;259:2863–6.

Glassman AH, Covey LS, Dallack GW, et al. Smoking cessation, clonidine, and vulnerability to nicotine among dependent smokers. Clin Pharmacol Ther 1993;54:670–9.

Glynn TJ, Boyd GM, Gruman JC. Essential elements of self-help/minimal intervention strategies for smoking cessation. Health Educ Q 1990a;17:329–45.

Glynn TJ, Manley MW. How to help your patients stop smoking: a National Cancer Institute manual for physicians. Washington, DC: Government Printing Office, 1990b. (NIH publication no. 90-3064).

Goldman L, Cook EF. The decline in ischemic heart disease mortality rates: an analysis of the comparative effects of medical interventions and changes in lifestyle. Ann Intern Med 1984;101:825–36.

Gordon T, Kannel WB, McGee D. Death and coronary attacks in men after giving up cigarette smoking: a report from the Framingham Study. Lancet 1974;2:1345–8.

Hammond EC, Horn D. Smoking and death rates: report on forty-four months of follow-up of 187,783 men. II. Death rates by cause. JAMA 1958;166:1294–308.

Henningfield JE, Radyius A, Coger RM, Clayton RR. Drinking coffee and carbonated beverages blocks absorption of nicotine from nicotine polacrilex gum. JAMA 1990;264:1560–4.

Hermanson B, Omenn GS, Kronmal RA, Gersh, BJ. Beneficial six-year outcome of smoking cessation in older men and women with coronary artery disease: results from the CASS registry. N Engl J Med 1988;319:1365–9.

Hilleman DE, Mohiuddin SM, Del Core MG, Sketch MH. Effect of buspirone on withdrawal symptoms associated with smoking cessation. Arch Intern Med 1992;152:350-2.

Hjalmarson A, Franzon M, Westin A, Wiklund O. Effect of nicotine nasal spray on smoking cessation. A randomized, placebo-controlled, double-blind study. Arch Int Med 1994;154:2567–72.

Hollis JF, Lichtenstein E, Vogt TM, et al. Nurse-assisted counseling for smokers in primary care. Ann Intern Med 1993;118:521–5.

Hughes JR, Gust SW, Keenan RM, et al. Nicotine vs placebo gum in general practice. JAMA 1989;261:1300–5.

Hurt RD, Lauger GG, Offord KP, et al. Nicotine-replacement therapy with use of a transdermal nicotine patch: a randomized, double-blind placebo-controlled trial. Mayo Clin Proc 1990;65:1529–37.

Hurt RD, Dale LC, McClain FL, et al. A comprehensive model for the treatment of nicotine dependence in a medical setting. Med Clin North Am 1992a:76:495–514.

Hurt, RD, Dale LC, Offord KP, et al. Inpatient treatment of severe nicotine dependence. Mayo Clin Proc 1992b;67:823–8.

Hurt, RD, Dale LC, Offord KP, et al. Serum nicotine and continue levels during nicotine-patch therapy. Clin Pharmacol Ther 1993;54:98–106.

Hurt RD, Dale LC, Fredrickson PA, et al. Nicotine patch therapy for smoking cessation combined with physician advice and nurse follow-up: one-year outcome and percentage of nicotine replacement. JAMA 1994;271:595–600.

Jeremy JY, Mikhailidis DP. Vascular and platelet eicosanoids, smoking and atherosclerosis. Adv Exp Med Biol 1990;273:135–46.

Kawachi I, Colditz GA, Stampfer MJ, et al. Smoking cessation and time course of decreased risks of coronary heart disease in middle-aged women. Arch Intern Med 1994;154:169–75.

Kenford SL, Fiore MC, Jorenby DE, et al. Predicting smoking cessation: who will quit with and without the nicotine patch. JAMA 1994;271:589–94.

Killen JD, Fortmann SP, Newman B, Varady A. Evaluation of a treatment approach combining nicotine gum with self-guided behavioral treatment for smoking relapse prevention. J Consult Clin Psychol 1990;58:85–92.

Klein LW, Volgman AS. Effects of cigarette smoking on coronary vascular dynamics: relationship to coronary atherosclerosis. Adv Exp Med Biol 1990;273:301–10.

Kottke TE, Battista RN, DeFriese GH, Brekke ML. Attributes of successful smoking cessation interventions in medical practice: a meta-analysis of 39 controlled trials. JAMA 1988;259:2882–9.

Kottke TE, Brekke ML, Solberg LI, Hughes JR. A randomized trial to increase smoking intervention by physicians: doctors helping smokers, round 1. JAMA 1989;261:1201–6.

Kuller LH, Ockene JK, Meilahn E, et al. Cigarette smoking and mortality. Prev Med 1991;20:638–54.

LaCroix AZ, Lang J, Scherr P, et al. Smoking and mortality among older men and women in three communities. N Engl J Med 1991;324:1619–25.

McGinnis JM, Foege WH. Actual causes of death in the United States. JAMA 1993;270:2207–12.

Mjos OD. Lipid effects of smoking. Am Heart J 1988;115:272–5.

Moreyra AE, Lacy CR, Wilson AC, et al. Arterial blood nicotine concentration and coronary vasoconstrictive effect of low-nicotine cigarette smoking. Am Heart J 1992;124:392–7.

Multiple Risk Factor Intervention Trial Research Group. Mortality rates after 10.5 years for participants in the Multiple Risk Factor Intervention Trial: findings related to a priori hypotheses of the trial. JAMA 1990;263:1795–1801.

Murphy JK, Edward NB, Downs AD, et al. Effects of doxepin on withdrawal symptoms in smoking cessation. Am J Psychiatry 1990;147:1353–7.

Murray JJ, Nowak J, Oates JA, FitgGerald GA. Platelet-vessel wall interactions in individuals who smoke cigarettes. Adv Exp Med Biol 1990;273:189–98.

Neaton JD, Wentworth D. Serum cholesterol, blood pressure, cigarette smoking and death from coronary heart disease: overall findings and differences by age for 316,099 white men. Arch Intern Med 1992;152:56–64.

Ockene JK. Physician-delivered intervention for smoking cessation: strategies for increasing effectiveness. Prev Med 1987;16:723–37.

Ockene JK, Kristeller J, Goldberg R, et al. Increasing the efficacy of physician-delivered smoking interventions: a randomized clinical trial. J Gen Intern Med 1991;6:1–8.

O'Connor NTJ, Cederholm-Williams S, Copper S, Cotter L. Hypercoagulability and coronary artery disease. Br Heart J 1984;52:614–6.

Omenn GS, Anderson KW, Krommal RA, Vliestra RE. The temporal pattern of reduction of mortality risk after smoking cessation. J Prev Med 1990;6:251–7.

Orleans CT, Glynn TJ, Manley MW, Slade J. Minimal-contact quit smoking strategies for medical settings. In: Nicotine addiction: principles and management. New York: Oxford University Press, 1993:181–220.

Orleans CT, Resch N, Noll E, et al. Use of transdermal nicotine in a state-level prescription plan for the elderly: a first look at "real-world" patch users. JAMA 1994;271:601–7.

Ornish SA, Zisook S, McAdams LA. Effects of transdermal clonidine treatment on withdrawal symptoms associatged with smoking cessation: a randomized controlled trial. Arch Intern Med 1988;148:2027–31.

Oster G, Huse DM, Delea TE, Colditz GA. Cost-effectiveness of nicotine gum as an adjunct to physician's advice against cigarette smoking. JAMA 1986;256:1315–1318.

Oster G, Epstein AM. Cost-effectiveness of antihyperlipemic therapy in the prevention of coronary heart disease. JAMA 1987;258:2381–7.

Pittilo RM. Cigarette smoking and endothelial injury: a review. Adv Exp Med Biol 1990;273:61–78.

Pooling Project Research Group. Relationship of blood pressure, serum cholesterol, smoking habit, relative weight and ECG abnormalities to incidence of major coronary events: final report of the pooling project. J Chron Dis 1978;31:201–306.

Prochaska JO, Goldstein MG. Process of smoking cessation: implications for clinicians. Clin Chest Med 1991;12:727–35.

Prochazka AV, Petty TL, Nett L, et al. Transdermal clonidine reduced some withdrawal symptoms but did not increase smoking cessation. Arch Intern Med 1992;152:2065–9.

Reed D, Marcus E, Hayashi T. Smoking as a predictor of atherosclerosis in the Honolulu Heart Study Program. Adv Exp Med Biol 1990;273:17–25.

Robertson D, Tseng CJ, Appalsamy M. Smoking and mechanisms of cardiovascular control. Am Heart J 1988;115:258–63.

Rogot E, Murray JL. Smoking and causes of death among U.S. veterans: 16 years of observation. Public Health Rep 1980;95:213–22.

Rose G, Hamilton PJS, Colwell L, Shipley MJ. A randomized controlled trial of anti-smoking advice: 10-year results. J Epidemiol Comm Health 1982; 36:102–8.

Rosenberg L, Kaufman DW, Helmrich SP, Shapiro S. The risk of myocardial infarction after quitting smoking in men under 55 years of age. N Engl J Med 1985;313:1511–4.

Rosenberg L, Palmer JR, Shaprio S. Decline in the risk of myocardial infarction among women who stop smoking. N Engl J Med 1990;322:213–7.

Russell MAH, Stapleton JA, Feyerabend C, et al. Targeting heavy smokers in general practice: randomized controlled trial of transdermal nicotine patches. Br Med J 1993;306:1308–12.

Sacks DPL, Sawe U, Leischow SJ. Effectiveness of a 16-hour transdermal nicotine patch in a medical practice setting, without intensive group counseling. Arch Intern Med 1993; 153:1881–90.

Schwartz JL. Review and evaluation of smoking cessation methods: the United States and Canada 1978-1985. Washington, DC: Government Printing Office, 1987. (NIH publication no. 87-2940).

Schwartz JL. Methods of smoking cessation. Med Clin North Am 1992;76:451–76.

Sytkowski PA, Kannel WB, D'Agostino RB. Changes in the risk factors and the decline in mortality from cardiovascular disease: the Framingham Heart Study. N Engl J Med 1990; 322:1635–41.

Tonneson P, Norregaard J, Simonsen K, Sawe U. A double-blind trial of a 16-hour transdermal nicotine patch in smoking cessation. N Engl J Med 1991;325:311–5.

Tonnesen P, Norregaard J, Mikkelsen K, et al. A double-blind trial of a nicotine inhaler for smoking cessation. JAMA 1993;269:1268–71.

Transdermal Nicotine Study Group: transdermal nicotine for smoking cessation: six-month results from two multicenter controlled clinical trials. JAMA 1991;266:3133–8.

U.S. Department of Health and Human Services. The health consequences of smoking: cardio-vascular disease: a report of the Surgeon General. Washington, DC: Government Printing Office, 1983. (DHHS publication no. (PHS) 84-50204.

U.S. Department of Health and Human Services. The health consequences of smoking: nicotine addiction: a report of the Surgeon General. Washington, DC: Government Printing Office, 1988. (DHSS publication no. (CDC) 88-8406).

U.S. Department of Health and Human Services. Reducing the health consequences of smoking: 25 years of progress: a report of the Surgeon General. Washington DC: Government Printing Office, 1989. (DHSS publication no. (CDC) 89-8411).

U.S. Department of Health and Human Services. The health benefits of smoking cessation: a report of the Surgeon General. Washington, DC: Government Printing Office, 1990. (DHHS publication no. (CDC)90-8416).

U.S. Department of Health and Human Services. Smoking and health in the Americas: a 1992 report of the Surgeon General in collaboration with the Pan American Health Organization. Washington, DC: Government Printing Office, 1992. (DHSS publication no. (CDC)92-8419).

U.S. Public Health Service. Smoking and health: report of the advisory committee to the Surgeon General of the Public Health Service. Washington, DC: Government Printing Office, 1964. (PHS publication no. 1103).

Weintraub WS. Cigarette smoking as a risk factor for coronary artery disease. Adv Exp Med Biol 1990;273:27–37.

Westman EC, Levin ED, Rose JE. The nicotine patch in smoking cessation: a randomized trial with telephone counseling. Arch Intern Med 1993;153:1917–23.

Willett WC, Green A, Stampfer MJ, et al. Relative and absolute excess risks of coronary heart disease among women who smoke cigarettes. N Engl J Med 1987;317:1303–9.

Wilson DM, Taylor W, Gilbert JR, et al. A randomized trial of a family physician intervention for smoking cessation. JAMA 1988;260:1570–4.

Zimmerman M, McGeachie J. The effect of nicotine on aortic endothelium: a quantitative ultrastructural study. Atherosclerosis 1987;63:33–41.

6

Cholesterol Reduction

Lee Goldman

The importance of cholesterol as a risk factor for atherosclerosis and myocardial infarction (MI) has been well established in both animal studies and human investigations. Cholesterol reduction by diet or medication will lower the risk of MI when used for either primary or secondary prevention. Because it remains unclear whether or not cholesterol reduction, especially with medications, has adverse effects on noncardiovascular mortality, recommendations regarding cholesterol reduction at both the population and the individual level must include a balanced assessment of the risks and benefits. The cost effectiveness of cholesterol reduction depends on both the cost of the intervention and the benefits to be realized by the individual, which are largely determined by the individual's underlying risk for coronary and noncoronary diseases.

Mechanisms

Cholesterol is transported in the plasma by lipoproteins. Most cholesterol is transported by low density lipoproteins (LDL), which are about 45% cholesterol by weight. Intermediate density lipoproteins are an intermediary between very low density lipoproteins, which themselves are derived from chylomicrons, and LDL. In most individuals, intermediate density lipoproteins are present in small amounts. High density lipoproteins (HDL) are produced both by the liver and the gastrointestinal tract and by the breakdown of chylomicrons and very low density lipoproteins in peripheral tissues (Ross 1992).

Cholesterol is an intrinsic component of the atherosclerotic process. The oxidation of LDL cholesterol allows it to be incorporated by scavenger macrophages into foam cells and to start the formation of the fatty streak, the earliest endothelial manifestation of atherosclerosis. Fatty streaks expand the endothelial surface, especially at areas of bifurcation or turbulence, and endothelial cells retract. Lipid-laden macrophages, which are now exposed to the circulating blood, attract platelets and continue the process of forming fibrous plaques. These plaques commonly begin in an area of endothelial injury with the accumulation of lipids and macrophages, followed by pro-liferation of smooth muscle (Fuster 1992; Ross 1992). HDL particles, which help remove free cholesterol from the endothelium by a process termed reverse transport, are protective against the development of atherosclerosis. Although some subfractions of HDL have been suspected of conveying greater protection, epidemiologic studies have generally indicated that all subfractions are protective. Reduction of LDL cho-lesterol appears to limit the substrate available for the atherosclerotic process, while HDL appears to serve as a scavenger that removes potential substrate.

Observational Studies

The most convincing epidemiologic data on the relationship between cholesterol levels and coronary heart disease (CHD) are derived from observational studies of middle-aged men. Such investigations have shown a consistent relationship of total cholesterol and LDL cholesterol levels with an increased risk of CHD, and an inverse relationship between HDL cholesterol levels and CHD. This relationship holds among populations (Figure 6.1) as well as individuals within a population. These relationships are con-tinuous and graded, so that a 1% change in serum cholesterol level corresponds to about a 2% change in the incidence of CHD (Lipid Research I 1984a; Lipid Research II 1984b; Martin 1986; Frick 1987; Tryoler 1987; Brown 1990; Buchwald 1990; Cashin-Hemphill 1990; Davis 1990; Kane 1990; MacMahon 1990; Rossouw 1990). Because many of the epidemiologic analyses have been based on a single cholesterol measurement, it has been postulated that regression-dilution bias may lead to a sub-stantial underestimate of the true relationship: a 1% change in cholesterol may actually correspond to a 3% change in coronary risk (Davis 1990; MacMahon 1990). As the serum cholesterol level increases from 160 mg/dl to the highest cholesterol values, the increase in risk is between four- and sixfold (Martin 1986; Davis 1990; MacMahon 1990).

Levels of HDL cholesterol have shown a consistent inverse relationship with CHD. In men, each 1 mg/dl increase in HDL cholesterol is associated with about 2–3% decrease in CHD, and the association may be even stronger in women (Gordon 1989).

Data suggest that the ratio of total:HDL cholesterol or LDL:HDL cholesterol is even more important than any of these levels alone. Each one unit change in the ratio of total:HDL cholesterol has been associated with about a 50% change in the risk of CHD (Stampfer 1991). The protective effect of HDL cholesterol may be even greater in individuals with lower levels of total cholesterol.

Data are less plentiful to substantiate the relationship between the cholesterol level and the risk of CHD in women, children, and the elderly, since studies have tended to concentrate on middle-aged men. Epidemiologic evidence indicates that elevated cholesterol levels are associated with higher risks of coronary mortality when choles-terol levels are measured in early adulthood (Klag 1993). The relationship between total cholesterol and CHD is also strong and consistent for women under age 65 but is less clear for older women (Manolio 1992). However, because CHD is not a major cause of death in middle-aged women, the relationship betwen total cholesterol and mortality is less strong in middle-aged women than in middle-aged men (Jacobs 1992).

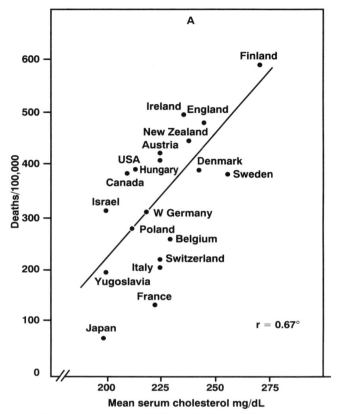

Fig. 6.1. Relationship of mean serum cholesterol level with the coronary heart disease mortality rate. [Reproduced from Simons et al. (1986), with permission.]

Elevated total cholesterol levels are predictive of CHD in elderly men, but the relative risk associated with hypercholesterolemia is only about half as strong in elderly men as in middle-aged men (Manolio 1992). Data for racial minority groups in North America and for populations from other continents are generally similar to what has been found for white Americans.

Substantial data indicate that individuals with low total cholesterol levels have higher noncardiovascular mortality rates, even after eliminating deaths in the first 5 years after study entry as a method of controlling for the possibility that low cholesterol levels may be a manifestation of severe, preexisting noncardiovascular conditions (Table 6.1) (Jacobs 1992). These trends generally appear to be consistent in smokers and nonsmokers and unaffected by alcohol intake, but debate continues as to whether low cholesterol is a cause or a marker of higher noncardiovascular risk (Stamler 1993). In a recent review by Law et al. (1994), the association of increased non-CHD mortality from prospective cohort studies varied depending on whether the populations studied were employment- or community-based. In employment-based cohorts, there was no evidence of increased non-CHD mortality among those with low cholesterol,

Table 6.1. Rate Ratios[a] for Deaths Occurring ≥5 Years After Cholesterol Measurement

Blood Cholesterol (mg/dl)	Coronary Heart Disease	Total Cardiovascular	Total Cancer	Noncardiovascular Noncancer	All Causes
Pooled, except					
MRFIT, men (*N* = 172,760)					
<160	0.92	1.04	1.18*	1.32**	1.17**
160–199	1.00	1.00	1.00	1.00	1.00
200–239	1.23**	1.16**	0.95***	0.89*	1.02
≥240	1.69**	1.48**	0.95	0.87**	1.14**
MRFIT men (*N* = 350,977)					
<160	0.78*	0.89***	1.23**	1.48**	1.17**
160–199	1.00	1.00	1.00	1.00	1.00
200–239	148**	1.31**	0.95***	0.87**	1.05*
≥240	2.20**	1.86**	0.91*	0.84**	1.22**
Pooled women (*N* = 124,814)					
<160	1.02	0.96	1.05	1.41*	1.10
160–199	1.00	1.00	1.00	1.00	1.00
200–239	1.12	0.95	1.01	0.92	0.94
≥240	1.56**	1.09	0.97.	0.82*	0.97

Source: Adapted from Jacobs et al. (1992), with permission.
[a]Rate in treated group ÷ rate in control group.
*$p < .05$.
**$p < .01$
***$p < .10$.

which was defined as less than 5 mmol/l (193 mg/dl) (RR = 1.00; 95% CI: 0.94–1.06). In addition to the point estimate indicating a null result, the upper bound of the confidence interval (1.06) excludes any substantial risk. In contrast, there was an apparent increased risk of non-CHD deaths among those in community-based cohorts (RR = 1:20; 95% CI: 1.15–1.24). If we assume a causal link between low cholesterol and non-CHD mortality, these discrepant results are difficult to explain. An alternative explanation for the inverse relationship in the less healthy community-based populations may be the higher prevalence of premorbid disease, such as cancer, liver disease, and depression, all of which are associated with low cholesterol.

Randomized Trials

Overwhelming evidence indicates that the likelihood of developing CHD will be reduced when cholesterol levels are lowered (Expert Panel 1988; Preventive Services 1989; Toronto 1990). Randomized interventional trials have conclusively demonstrated that cholesterol reduction is beneficial for reducing atherosclerosis and clinical coronary events. The aggressive treatment of high cholesterol levels slows the progression of atherosclerosis and increases the likelihood of regression (Brown 1990; Buchwald 1990; Cashin-Hemphill 1990; Kane 1990; Watts 1992). Large-scale clinical trials, primarily in middle-aged hypercholesterolemic men, have demonstrated that cholesterol reduction achieves the predicted epidemiologic benefit of reducing coronary events when used as primary prevention in persons without preexisting CHD, or when used as secondary prevention in persons with known CHD (Lipid I 1984a; Lipid II 1984b; Frick 1987; Rossouw 1990). Metanalyses of the primary prevention data demonstrate no reduction in overall deaths (Canadian 1993) because of a small but consistent increase in noncardiovascular mortality (Table 6.2). This increase in noncardiovascular mortality in the primary prevention trials is also consistent with the higher levels of noncardiovascular mortality seen with lower cholesterol levels in observational studies (Jacobs 1992). Conversely, analysis of the secondary prevention trials (Rossouw 1990; Scandinavian Simvastatin Study Group (1994)) indicates that the reduction in coronary deaths in these higher risk patients with preexisting CHD appears to more than offset any small increase in noncardiovascular deaths (Table 6.3).

Diet

Despite the manifest benefit of dietary interventions in short-term controlled experiments, the impact of dietary interventions in long-term trials of free-living subjects has been much less impressive. In one of the earliest studies, the MRFIT intervention, only a 2% net reduction in total cholesterol levels was achieved, apparently because of poor compliance (MRFIT 1982). Similarly disappointing results have been achieved in a variety of other studies in the workplace (Rose 1980), in the community (Orchard 1983), and in men with hypertension (Burr 1989) or previous MI (Curzio 1989).

Intensive community-based educational programs in Finland and in the United States have generally resulted in only 1–3% net reductions in cholesterol levels superimposed on modest secular changes (Fortmann 1981; Taskanen 1983; Farquhar 1990). Interventions in school-aged children have also shown similarly modest results (Puska 1982; Tell 1987; Walter 1988; Newman 1990). Thus, the impressive dietary results that were found in early, very intensive interventional trials of adults who were consuming very high fat diets (Leren 1970; Hjermann 1981; Choudhury 1984) have generally not been duplicated in subsequent interventional trials of diet. The effect of diet in lowering cholesterol levels is enhanced in individuals who increase their exercise levels (Tran 1983) and in those who also have substantial weight loss (Cagguilu 1981).

The two major randomized trials of the primary prevention of CHD in large numbers of free-living individuals, the Los Angeles Veterans Study (Dayton 1969) and the Minnesota Coronary Survey (Frantz 1989), mainly intervened on the polyunsaturated:saturated fat ratio. The former included a small proportion of patients with previous CHD, while the latter was purely a primary prevention trial. Total cholesterol levels were reduced by 13% and 14%, respectively, in the two trials, and nonfatal CHD events were reduced by 40% and 17%, respectively, with an overall odds ratio in the two combined of 0.77 (95% CI: 0.55–1.09) (Table 6.2) (Canadian 1993). The change in fatal coronary events was less impressive, with an odds ratio of 0.93 (0.63–1.37). The overall death rate was unchanged (odds ratio: 1.00) because of a small, insignificant increase in noncardiac mortality (odds ratio: 1.02; 0.85–1.24) (Canadian 1993).

Table 6.2. Primary Prevention Trials: Effects of Lowering the Cholesterol Level on Cause-Specific and Overall Death Rates

Trial	Cause; OR (and 95% CI)				
	Cardiac	All Noncardiac	Cancer	Violence	Total
Dietary therapy					
Dayton, 1969 (N = 846)	0.80 (0.50–1.26)	1.06 (0.78–1.44)	1.70 (0.93–3.12)	9.04[a] (0.65–>99)	0.96 (0.73–1.28)
Frantz, 1989 (N = 4,393)	1.39 (0.65–3.00)	1.00 (0.78–1.28)	1.34 (0.60–3.01)	1.50 (0.73–3.12)	1.03 (0.82–1.31)
Total (N = 5,239)	0.93 (0.63–1.37)	1.02 (0.85–1.24)	1.55 (0.96–2.51)	1.79 (0.89–3.63)	1.00 (0.84–1.20)
Drug therapy					
Lipid I, 1984 (N = 3,806)	0.78 (0.47–1.30)	1.34 (0.79–2.27)	1.06 (0.50–2.27)	2.75 (0.81–10.2)	0.96 (0.67–1.36)
Frick, 1987 (N = 4,081)	0.84 (0.35–1.99)	1.30 (0.73–2.32)	0.99 (0.40–2.45)	2.48 (0.72–9.39)	1.13 (0.70–1.82)
Report, 1978 (N = 10,627)	1.05 (0.64–1.72)	1.74 (1.22–2.48)	1.66 (0.97–2.84)	1.19 (0.57–2.49)	1.47 (1.11–1.96)
Dorr, 1968 (N = 1,094)	0.59 (0.14–2.25)	1.60 (0.47–5.66)	1.00 (0.18–9.90)	5.00[c] (0.25–>99)	0.62 (0.32–1.19)
Total (N = 19,608)	0.88 (0.64–1.20)	1.54 (1.20–1.98)	1.32 (0.91–1.93)	1.77 (1.04–3.05)	1.14 (0.95–1.38)
Overall total (N = 24,847)	0.90 (0.71–1.14)	1.19 (1.03–1.39)	1.41 (1.05–1.89)	1.78 (1.17–2.72)	1.07 (0.94–1.22)

Source: Adapted from Canadian Task Force on the Periodic Health Examination (1993), with permission.
OR, odds ratio (odds in treated group divided by odds in control group); CI, confidence interval.
[a]Because there were no violent deaths in the control groups in the UCS and Dayton, 1969, the odds ratios and confidence intervals were calculated by first adding 0.5 to each cell of the @ × @ table.

Table 6.3. Secondary Prevention: Metanalysis of Rates of Events in Trials of Cholesterol Lowering Through 1988

Trial	No. of Patients Randomized		Myocardial Infarctions		Cardiovascular Deaths		Deaths from Cancer		All Noncardiovascular Deaths		All Deaths	
	Treated	Control	Treated	Control	Treated	Control	Treated	Control	Treated	Control	Treated	Control
Coronary Drug Project Research Group 1975												
Clofibrate	1,103	2,789	28.0	30.1	21.8	22.7	0.9	0.9	2.6	1.9	25.5	25.4
Niacin	1,119	2,789	25.6	30.1	21.3	22.7	0.8	0.9	2.7	1.9	24.4	25.4
Newcastle Physicians 1971 (Clofibrate)	244	253	21.3	32.0	NA		NA		NA		NA	
Scottish Society of Physicians 1971 (Clofibrate)	350	367	15.4	19.6	NA		NA		NA		12.3	11.7
Carlson 1988 (Clofibrate + niacin)	279	276	25.8	36.2	19.4	27.2	1.4	2.1	2.5	2.5	21.9	29.7
Leren 1966	206	206	29.6	39.3	18.4	25.2	0.5	1.5	1.5	1.5	19.9	26.7
Medical Research Council												
1965 Low-fat diet	123	129	24.4	24.0	NA		NA		NA		16.3	18.6
1968 Soybean oil	199	194	22.6	26.3	13.6	12.9	0.5	3.1	0.5	3.1	14.1	16.0
Odds ratio[a] (95% confidence interval)			0.78 (0.70–0.86)*		0.88 (0.77–0.99)**		0.75 (0.46–1.23)		1.30 (0.93–1.83)		0.91 (0.82–1.02)	

Source: Adapted from Rossouw et al. (1990), with permission.

[a] Odds of events in treatment group ÷ odds of events in control group.

**p < .01.

*p < .05.

Medications

The primary prevention trials (Table 6.2) present clear evidence that medications to reduce cholesterol will result in a significant reduction in nonfatal cardiac events, a result consistent with the predicted benefit based on the observed changes in lipid levels in the treated groups. For the duration of these studies, all 7.5 years or less, this significant and substantial reduction in nonfatal cardiac events was associated with a smaller and nonsignificant reduction in fatal cardiac events (odds ratio: 0.88; 0.64–1.20) (Smith 1993). This reduction in cardiac events, however, was associated with a significant increase in noncardiac deaths, primarily from cancer and violence. The overall odds for death were 1.14 in the treated group, a nonsignificant *increase* in deaths. Recent results from the West of Scotland Coronary Prevention Study, a primary prevention trial of an HMG-CoA reductase inhibitor, indicate clear reductions in fatal and nonfatal CHD and a 22% reduction ($p = 0.051$) in total mortality (Shepard 1995).

In secondary prevention trials (Table 6.3), the proportional benefits from cholesterol reduction were similar to those found in the primary prevention trials and to those that would be predicted based on epidemiologic evidence. In the secondary prevention setting, however, the cause-specific distribution of death tends to be more heavily weighted toward coronary deaths, so that the significant reduction in coronary deaths outweighs any increase in noncardiovascular deaths, and cholesterol reduction is associated with a net benefit in mortality (Figure 6.2) (Scandinavian Simvastatin Survival Study Group 1994). These findings underscore the critical importance of considering cause-specific risks in making recommendations about cholesterol reduction (Smith 1993).

The benefits of cholesterol reduction in populations other than middle-aged men can only be estimated from the relationship of cholesterol to CHD and total mortality in these other groups and the assumption, perhaps fallacious, that cholesterol reduction will have the same proportional impact on relative risk. To the extent that all other age-sex groups have either a lower risk of coronary disease than middle-aged men or rates that are less dependent on cholesterol levels, the risk:benefit ratios for cholesterol reduction may be less favorable.

In assessing the potential benefit of cholesterol reduction, it is critical to consider the overall risk of CHD, which will be reduced by cholesterol lowering. The higher the former and the lower the latter, the more benefit will be realized from cholesterol reduction. Conversely, when the CHD risk is low compared with the risks of death from other causes, cholesterol reduction may be detrimental (Figure 6.2) (Smith 1993). When analyzed in such a way, the data demonstrate that diet therapies tend to have approximately the same benefit for reducing death from CHD as does drug therapy, but diet does not appear to have as strong an effect on increasing noncoronary deaths (Table 6.4).

Strength of Evidence Supporting Benefit of Cholesterol Lowering

The data to support the benefit of lowering LDL cholesterol to reduce CHD are clear and convincing. However, two issues remain unresolved. First, it is uncertain whether there is benefit from a reduction in total cholesterol levels if it is accomplished by a

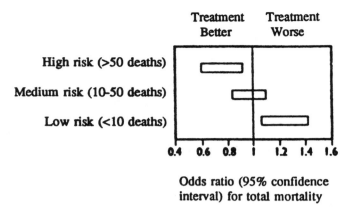

Fig. 6.2. Effect of cholesterol lowering treatment on total mortality stratified by number of deaths from coronary heart disease per 1,000 person years in control subjects. [Adapted from Smith et al. (1993), with permission.]

symmetric, proportional reduction in both LDL and HDL cholesterol levels. Data suggest that the ratio of LDL to HDL cholesterol may be more important than the values of either one alone (Stampfer 1991). If this relationship is true, then dietary interventions that cause symmetric reductions in both LDL and HDL cholesterol levels, and hence no change in their ratios, would be expected to have no benefit. For example, diets that emphasize an increase in polyunsaturated fats appear to reduce LDL cholesterol levels but also to reduce HDL cholesterol levels by nearly the same proportion (Mattson 1985). Similarly, the American Heart Association Step Three Diet, which emphasizes reduction of total fat intake to 20% of the total energy intake by substituting carbohydrates for saturated fats, reduces not only LDL cholesterol but also HDL cholesterol (Nutrition 1986; Grundy 1986, 1988). The most favorable changes in LDL and HDL cholesterol, with a lowering of the former and little change in the latter, appear to be induced by diets that are rich in *cis*-monounsaturated fatty acids, which are found especially in olive and canola oils. By comparison, the *trans*-monounsaturated fatty acids that are produced by the hydrogenation or hardening of monounsaturated fats tend to increase LDL cholesterol and reduce HDL cholesterol levels.

The second issue is the debate over the relationship of cholesterol levels with noncardiovascular mortality. As noted above, the increase in noncardiovascular deaths as the total cholesterol level is lowered appears in meta-analyses of both observational and interventional studies. However, additional data from ongoing trials of the newer and more powerful HMG-CoA reductase inhibitors will be required to better evaluate this issue. Nevertheless, in the highest risk individuals with very elevated cholesterol levels or with preexisting CHD, the CHD-related benefits of cholesterol reduction clearly seem to outweigh any noncardiovascular hazards (Smith 1993). Furthermore, the benefit of cholesterol reduction for prevention of coronary morbidity must be considered. Thus, the benefits demonstrated by the recent simvastatin study were perfectly predictable based on prior studies (Scandanavian Simvastatin Survival Study Group 1994).

Table 6.4. Effects of Cholesterol Lowering in Trials Using Drug and Nondrug Interventions

Trials Stratified by Risk of Death from CHD	No. of Trials	No. of Subjects	Odds Ratio (95% Confidence Interval)		
			Death from CHD	Death from Other Causes	Total Deaths
Drug trials					
Higher risk group[a]	11	11,106	0.78 (0.60–1.02)	1.14 (0.92–1.41)	0.81 (0.64–1.04)
Lower risk group[b]	13	31,165	0.97 (0.75–1.27)	1.27 (1.05–1.53)	1.08 (0.90–1.28)
All drug trials	24	42,271	0.87 (0.73, 1.03)	1.21 (1.05–1.39)	0.94 (0.81, 1.08)
Nondrug trials					
Higher risk group[a]	6	4,009	0.79 (0.63–0.98)	0.98 (0.76–1.26)	0.80 (0.63–1.01)
Lower risk group[b]	6	10,874	1.09 (0.80–1.49)	1.05 (0.87–1.27)	1.07 (0.82–1.40)
All nondrug trials	12	14,883	0.90 (0.74, 1.10)	1.02 (0.88–1.19)	0.90 (0.76, 1.09)

Source: Adapted from Smith et al. (1993), with permission. Not including Scandinavian Simvastatin Survival Group, 1994. CHD, coronary heart disease.

One study (Watts 1992) had a drug and a diet arm and is reported here as two separate trials.

[a] ≥ 30 deaths from CHD per 1,000 person years.

[b] < 30 deaths from CHD per 1,000 person years.

139

Intervention Strategies

Although cholesterol levels have been declining in American adults over the past three decades (Johnson 1993), the prevalence of hypercholesterolemia is so substantial that any widespread intervention or recommendations could have major national implications. Even in 1991, 20% of American adults aged 20 through 74 had cholesterol levels of 240 mg/dl or higher, and another 31% had levels of 200–239 mg/dl (Sempos 1993). If the recommendations of the Adult Treatment Panel II of the National Cholesterol Education Program were to be followed, about 52 million Americans, or nearly 30% of the adult population, would be candidates for dietary treatment, and a projected 7% of American adults, representing nearly 13 million individuals, are projected to be candidates for medications to lower cholesterol levels (Sempos 1993; Expert Panel 1993). In this context, it is critical that potential intervention strategies be carefully evaluated and that their costs and effectiveness be understood.

The 1993 Canadian Task Force on the Periodic Health Examination (Canadian 1993) concluded that no evidence from even one high-quality randomized trial documented that the dietary recommendations of the American Heart Association (Nutrition 1986), the Canadian Consensus Conference on Cholesterol (Canadian 1988), or the National Cholesterol Education Program's Expert Panel (Expert Panel 1993) will reduce CHD risks, either in the overall population or even in any identifiable high-risk subgroup. However, previous dietary trials did show a benefit when cholesterol reduction was combined with smoking cessation and when cholesterol reduction was achieved by using diets that substituted polyunsaturated fats for saturated fats. Since current recommendations emphasize a reduction in total fat intake and tend to advocate an increase in monounsaturated rather than polyunsaturated fats, it would be predicted from experimental evidence that the current dietary recommendations would be *even more beneficial* than the diets that have previously been shown to reduce CHD. It is therefore unlikely that future randomized trials will be conducted, at least in higher risk populations, and hence unlikely that the strength of evidence will be increased. More likely, future dietary interventions will be targeted to lower risk groups, such as women in the Women's Health Initiative sponsored by the National Institutes of Health, in whom a "control" diet can be proposed as a reasonable alternative because of uncertainties regarding the benefit of cholesterol-reduction in American women of average risk.

As emphasized by the Canadian Task Force on the Periodic Health Examination (Canadian 1993), the relationships among diet, dietary modifications, CHD, and overall mortality are controversial. Although the relationship between cholesterol level and coronary risk appears to be clear in women, the effects of dietary modification on cholesterol levels are less clear, and dietary interventions in women have not shown consistent reductions in cholesterol levels or in coronary deaths (Miettinen 1972; Frantz 1989). Much of the uncertainty may arise because elevated total cholesterol levels in women may more commonly be associated with favorable LDL:HDL ratios, especially in premenopausal women or women who are taking postmenopausal hormone replacement therapy. At the current time, perhaps the most convincing argument in favor of dietary interventions in women would be that there is no compelling evidence to suggest any deleterious effects, especially from the diets that are currently recommended in men, and that most studies of women have not focused on those in their 60s to 80s, among whom the risk of CHD is highest.

In children and young adults, cholesterol levels are variable and are a less reliable predictor of future events than in middle-aged adults. Nevertheless, higher cholesterol levels in young adults correlate with higher risks of CHD in later life, and childhood is the ideal time to diagnose familial hypercholesterolemic disorders. However, there is substantial debate regarding the wisdom of routine screening and the age at which it should be started. Some experts argue against the need for very early detection because treatment will yield benefits within about 2 years so that most of the benefit of cholesterol reduction may be achieved even when interventions are begun much later in life (Hulley 1992). The alternative argument is that atherosclerosis is a gradual and progressive disorder, so earlier interventions will be far preferable to those that are begun after the pathologic process is more advanced. The National Cholesterol Education Program's Expert Panel recommends that screening should begin with a total serum cholesterol level in all adults at the age of 20 years and be repeated at least every five years (Expert Panel 1993). Conversely, the Canadian Task Force found that evidence is insufficient to recommend for or against universal screening but did recommend that total cholesterol screening be considered in men between the ages of 30 and 59 (Canadian 1993). The striking discrepancy between these two recommendations underscores uncertainties in the available evidence regarding the importance of cholesterol as a risk factor in some subgroups, the risk-benefit ratio of interventions, and the cost-effectiveness of potential therapies.

In the opinion of the Canadian Task Force (Canadian 1993), the strength of evidence supporting a reduction in the intake of total fat, saturated fat, and cholesterol and a modest increase in unsaturated fat in middle-aged men was only fair, while the evidence for similar interventions in women, the elderly, and children was poor. Although the National Cholesterol Education Program's Expert Panel did not provide a similar rating scale, their overall recommendations imply substantially more enthusiasm for cholesterol reduction in all segments of the population (Expert Panel 1993).

Based on the available evidence, there appears to be good data for recommending medications to reduce cholesterol in individuals with known CHD. In these individuals, the benefits of medications to lower cholesterol levels clearly seem to outweigh the risks.

For primary prevention, recommendations regarding medications must be considered at lower levels of evidence. The key determinant appears to be the individual's comparative risks of CHD (Smith 1993). In individuals with very marked hyperlipidemia, and especially individuals with familial homozygous or heterozygous hyperlipidemia, the risks of CHD appear to be sufficiently high to warrant aggressive medications (Goldman 1993). But for individuals with more modest hypercholesterolemia and hence more modest risks, the risk-benefit ratio is clearly different. In assessing the risk attributable to an elevated cholesterol level, it is important that the individual's overall risk profile be considered (Expert Panel 1993). In individuals who are male or who have other cardiac risk factors, the same elevation in serum cholesterol carries more attributable risk than among individuals with similar cholesterol levels who are without these other risk factors.

If the primary prevention pooled analyses are correct, then the proportional increase in noncardiac death rates is perhaps twice as great as the proportional decrease in coronary deaths during the first five or seven years of follow-up. Thus, during this time interval, one could argue that an individual's risk of dying from cardiac causes should be at least twofold higher than his or her risk of dying from other causes, especially cancer and accidents or violence, if cholesterol reduction from medications is to be recommended. Such risk profiles are found only at substantially increased levels of serum cholesterol.

Appendices concerning nutritional guidelines for reducing cholesterol and cholesterol-lowering medications (dosages, benefits, risks, and relative costs) are provided at the end of this textbook.

Cost Effectiveness

At the population level, educational interventions to encourage individuals to change their lifestyle to lower cholesterol levels are of marginal benefit, but their cost is low. No data are available to assess the costs to an individual or to the population of making the types of dietary changes that are currently recommended by various organizations and expert panels (Canadian 1993; Expert Panel 1993). It is currently estimated that the production of excess fat on live cattle generates substantial costs that might be reduced by changes in the feeding and production approach (National Cattlemen's 1990), so it is possible that some changes in diet may lower costs as well as increase costs.

Using estimates ranging from $4 to $5 per person per year in the Stanford Five Community Study (Farquhar 1990) to about $15 per year in the North Karelia study (Keeler 1985), even adjusting for inflation rates since the conclusion of the studies, nationwide programs would have reasonable costs and might still be cost effective even if they yielded relatively small changes in cholesterol. However, the true cost effectiveness of such programs may be more dependent on their ability to alter smoking rates, salt intake, and the rates of detection, treatment, and control of hypertension. If all the risk factor changes that were noted in the Stanford studies could be achieved at the same price per person as found in those studies, then the cost effectiveness of the multifactorial intervention is favorable (Tosteson 1991).

Medications to reduce cholesterol levels appear to have very favorable cost effectiveness ratios when used for secondary prevention of recurrent events in individuals who have already had evidence for preexisting CHD (Goldman 1991, 1992). These recommendations appear to be sound even if the cholesterol level is relatively normal (Goldman 1991, 1992, 1993).

Medications for primary prevention also appear to be worthwhile from a cost effectiveness standpoint in individuals with familial heterozygous hypercholesterolemia (Goldman, 1993). This favorable cost effectiveness ratio for primary prevention is based on the extremely high risk of coronary events by age 50 in these individuals.

Cost effectiveness estimates are not nearly so favorable when medications are used for primary prevention in other types of individuals. In several different analyses, cholestyramine, lovastatin, and other medications have been estimated to have reasonable cost effectiveness ratios when used in middle-aged men with hypercholesterolemia and additional risk factors, but usually to be very costly when used for primary prevention in women, young men, and men without other risk factors (Oster 1987; Schulman 1990; Goldman 1991). Even if the potentially deleterious noncardiovascular effects of cholesterol lowering are not considered, only the highest risk individuals would be projected to have benefits from cholesterol reduction at a reasonable cost (Tables 6.5 and 6.6). Although niacin is less costly than other medications, its effectiveness in lowering cholesterol per dollar of cost is only slightly better. Medications that raise the HDL cholesterol level as well as lower the LDL cholesterol level are more beneficial and cost effective than medications that alter only the LDL level. The cost effectiveness of medications is also influenced by the potential for deleterious effects of cholesterol lowering. Essentially none of the cost effectiveness analyses to date have incorporated the deleterious noncardiovascular effects of cholesterol lowering into their estimates. Future reductions in the costs of medications, because of either the expiration of patents or pressure from managed care, as well as increased potency of the newer statins, could improve these cost effectiveness ratios.

Recommendations of Expert Groups in North America

The debate over the appropriate role for screening and treating hypercholesterolemia is best exemplified by the recommendations of the Canadian Task Force on the Periodic Health Examination as compared with the United States' National Cholesterol Education Programs Expert Panel on detection, evaluation and treatment of high cholesterol in adults. The Canadian approach is to screen only in men aged 30–59 (Table 6.7), and to reserve dietary and drug therapy to this group (Figure 6.3). By comparison, the US Panel recommends routine screening with a substantially more aggressive treatment approach (Figures 6.4–6.6; Table 6.8).

These two expert groups have provided what might be considered two extremes of approach to screening and treating hypercholesterolemia. The Canadian approach required clear evidence of benefit, while the United States' approach was based on lower levels of proof. The difference between these two approaches is likely to be critically dependent on the true deleterious effects of cholesterol reduction on noncoronary mortality and the extent to which individuals perceive a change in their quality of life from diet changes or medications (Krahn 1991).

At the current time, the benefits and favorable cost effectiveness implications of cholesterol reduction for secondary prevention must be emphasized, especially if the cholesterol level is elevated. Ongoing trials will determine whether these conclusions hold even for individuals with cholesterol levels of about 200 mg/dl or lower.

For primary prevention, population recommendations for dietary changes should be encouraged because they have potential benefits at low risk. More aggressive dietary recommendations, especially to increase monounsaturated fat and reduce saturated fats further, appear to be appropriate for primary prevention in higher risk patients. Medications should be reserved for the higher-risk primary prevention situations, in which the benefits of such medications clearly outweigh the risks. Since the pooled analysis of drug therapy trials for primary prevention reveal a 54% increase

Table 6.5. Estimated Cost (US Dollars) per Year of Life Saved for Lovastatin as Secondary Prevention in Patients with Preexisting Coronary Heart Disease

Lovastatin dose	Age				
	35–44	45–54	55–64	65–74	75–84
Pretreatment Cholesterol Level ≥250 mg/dl (6.47 mmol/l)					
20 mg/day					
Men	—[a]	—[a]	1,600	10,000	19,000
Women	4,500	3,500	8,100	12,000	15,000
40 mg/day[b]					
Men	14,000	8,600	17,000	27,000	38,000
Women	49,000	30,000	29,000	30,000	29,000
80 mg/day[b]					
Men	120,000	72,000	73,000	84,000	130,000
Women	210,000	130,000	100,000	93,000	83,000
Pretreatment Cholesterol Level <250 mg/dl (6.47 mmol/l)					
20 mg/day					
Men	38,000	16,000	17,000	25,000	30,000
Women	210,000	73,000	36,000	30,000	23,000
40 mg/day[b]					
Men	120,000	57,000	48,000	53,000	58,000
Women	310,000	150,000	81,000	62,000	45,000

Source: From Goldman et al. (1991), with permission.
[a] The savings from future coronary heart disease that is averted outweigh the costs of treatment; thus, therapy saves lives and money.
[b] Each dose is compared with the next lower dose to calculate the incremental cost-effectiveness ratio.

Table 6.6. Estimated Cost-Effectiveness[a] (in US Dollars Per Year of Life Saved) of 20 mg Lovastatin for Primary Prevention in Adults, Aged 34–44 Years

Other Risk Factors	Pretreatment Cholesterol Level (mg/dl)					
	275		330		400	
	Men	Women	Men	Women	Men	Women
None	840,000	2,500,000	400,000	1,000,000	160,000	360,000
Smoking	460,000	1,500,000	220,000	670,000	80,000	220,000
Smoking and overweight[b]	320,000	1,000,000	150,000	450,000	50,000	150,000
Smoking, overweight, and mild hypertension[c]	190,000	500,000	80,000	200,000	21,000	55,000

[a] Incremental cost-effectiveness when added to secondary prevention.
[b] 110–130% if ideal body weight.
[c] Diastolic blood pressure 95–104 mmHg.

Table 6.7. Summary of Interventions, Effectiveness, Level of Evidence and Recommendations for Lowering of Blood Total Cholesterol Level to Prevent CHD as Reported by the Canadian Task Force

Maneuver	Effectiveness	Level of Evidence[a]	Recommendation[a]
Measurement of blood total cholesterol level	Average of three or more readings accurately reflects "true" level if measured in standardized laboratory. Although not evaluated for its effectiveness, screening should be considered in all men aged 30 to 59 years; individual clinical judgment should be exercised in all other cases	Expert opinion	Insufficient evidence to include in or exclude from PHE
Stepped fat-modified diet to which a cholesterol-lowering drug is added if response is inadequate (mean total cholesterol level of more than 265 mg/dl (6.85 mmol/l) or LDL-C level of more than 175 mg/dl (4.50 mmol/l)	For men 30 to 59 years old with a mean total cholesterol level of more than 265 mg/dl (6.85 mmol/l) or an LDL-C level of more than 175 mg/dl (4.90 mmol/l) treatment is efficacious in reducing incidence of CHD	Randomized contolled trials	Fair evidence to include in PHE
	For all others the value of treatment has not been demonstrated	Expert opinion	Insufficient evidence to include in or exclude from PHE
General dietary advice	For men 30 to 69 years decreased intake of total fat, saturated fat and cholesterol is associated with decreased incidence of CHD	Prospective cohort studies	Fair evidence to include in PHE
	For all others value of such advice has not been demonstrated	Expert opinion	Insufficient evidence to include in or exclude from PHE

Source: Canadian Task Force on the Periodic Health Examination (1993), with permission.
PHE, periodic health examination; LDL-C, low density lipoprotein cholesterol; CHD, coronary heart disease.
[a]For descriptions of the other levels of evidence and classification of recommendations see Appendix 1 in part 1 of the 1992 update (Can Med Assoc J 1992;147:443).

145

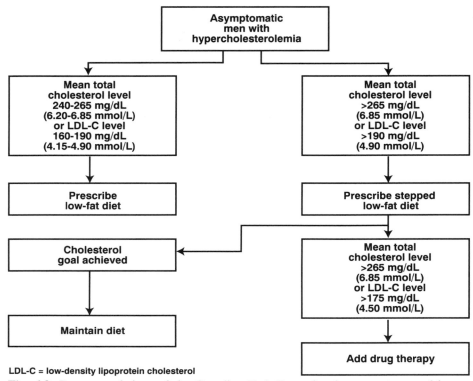

LDL-C = low-density lipoprotein cholesterol

Fig. 6.3. Recommendations of the Canadian Task Force for the management of hyper-cholesterolemia in asymptomatic men aged 30 to 59 years. [From Can Med Assoc J (1993) with permission.]

in noncardiac death, the cardiac benefit from cholesterol reduction with medications must be substantial to outweigh these risks. Assuming that medications may lower the cholesterol level by up to 25% and hence yield perhaps a 50% reduction in coronary events and mortality, the risk of death from cardiac causes must at least exceed the risk of death from noncardiac causes if such medical therapy is to be effective. For such therapy to be cost effective, the relative proportion of deaths from cardiac causes must be even higher. Further investigations will be required to determine conclusively the types of situations in which primary prevention will be both effective and cost effective, but at the present time it is clear that such recommendations must be limited to the high risk primary prevention situations.

Summary

Quality of available data: A large number of randomized trials testing the effects of cholesterol-lowering interventions.

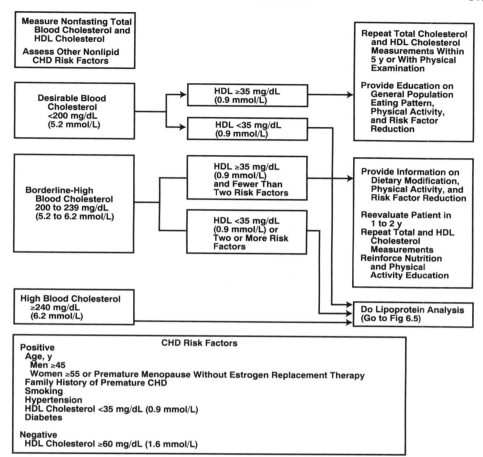

Fig. 6.4. Recommendation of the U.S. NCEP-ATP for primary prevention in adults without evidence of coronary heart disease (CHD). Initial classification is based on total cholesterol and high-density lipoprotein (HDL) cholesterol levels. [From JAMA (1993) with permission.]

Estimated risk reduction: A 2–3% reduction in risk of MI for each 1% reduction in serum cholesterol level. On average, dietary interventions result in about 10% reductions in cholesterol, while reductions with pharmacologic therapy often exceed 20%.

Comparability of effect in men and women: The relationship between total cholesterol and MI is less well studied in women than in men. Available evidence suggests efficacy of cholesterol reduction for both sexes but is stronger and more consistent in men than in women.

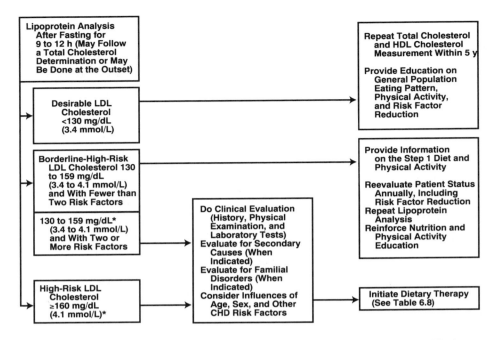

* On the basis of the average of two determinations. If the first two LDL-cholesterol test results differ by more than 30 mg/dL (0.7 mmol/L), a third test result should be obtained within 1 to 8 weeks and the average value of the three tests used.

Fig. 6.5. Recommendations of the U.S. NCEP-ATP for primary prevention in adults without evidence of coronary heart disease (CHD). Subsequent classification is based on low-density lipoprotein (LDL) cholesterol level. [From JAMA (1993) with permission.]

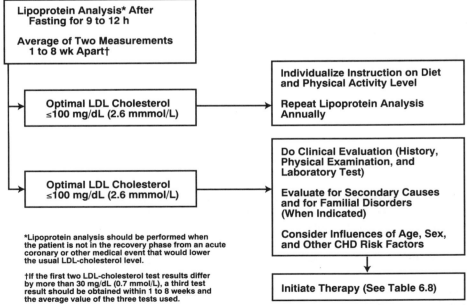

Fig. 6.6. Recommendations of the U.S. NCEP-ATP for secondary prevention in adults with evidence of coronary heart disease (CHD). Classification is based on low-density lipoprotein (LDL) cholesterol level. [From JAMA (1993) with permission.]

Table 6.8. Recommended Treatments of US NCEP-ATP Based on LDL Cholesterol Level

Patient Category	Initiation Level, mg/dl (mmol/l)	LDL Goal, mg/dl (mmol/l)
Dietary Therapy		
Without CHD and with fewer than two risk factors	≥160 (4.1)	<160 (4.1)
Without CHD and with two or more risk factors	≥130 (3.4)	<130 (3.4)
With CHD	>100 (2.6)	≤100 (2.6)
Drug Treatment		
Without CHD and with fewer than two risk factors	≥190 (4.9)	<160 (4.1)
Without CHD and with two or more risk factors	≥160 (4.1)	<130 (3.4)
With CHD	>130 (3.4)	≤100 (2.6)

Source: From Johnson et al. (1993), with permission.
NCEP-ATP, National Cholesterol Education Programs.
LDL, low-density lipoprotein; CHD, coronary heart disease.

References

A Research Committee. Low-fat diet in myocardial infarction: a controlled trial. Lancet 1965; 2:501–4.

Brown G, Albers JJ, Fisher LD, et al. Regression of coronary artery disease as a result of intensive lipid-lowering therapy in men with high levels of apolipoprotein B. N Engl J Med 1990;323:1289–98.

Buchwald H, Varco RL, Matts JP, et al. Effect of partial ileal bypass surgery on mortality and morbidity from coronary heart disease in patients with hypercholesterolemia. N Engl J Med 1990;323:946–55.

Burr ML, Fehily AM, Gilbert JF, et al. Effects of changes in fat, fish, and fibre intakes on death and myocardial reinfarction: diet and reinfarction trial (DART). Lancet 1989;2: 757–61.

Cagguilu AW, Christakis G, Farrand M, et al. The Multiple Risk Factor Intervention Trial (MRFIT): IV. Intervention on blood lipids. Prev Med 1981;10:443–75.

Canadian Consensus Conference on Cholesterol. Final Report, Canadian Consensus Conference on the Prevention of Heart and Vascular Disease by Altering Serum Cholesterol and Lipoprotein Risk Factors. Can Med Assoc J 1988;139:Suppl II:II1–II8.

Canadian Task Force on the Periodic Health Examination. Periodic health examination, 1993 update. 2. Lowering the blood total cholesterol level to prevent coronary heart disease. Can Med Assoc J 1993;148:521–38.

Carlson LA, Rosenbaumer G. Reduction of mortality in the Stockholm Ischaemic Heart Disease Secondary Prevention Study by combined treatment with clofibrate and nicotinic acid. Acta Med Scand 1988;223:405–18.

Cashin-Hemphill L, Mack WJ, Pogoda JM, et al. Beneficial effects of colestipol-niacin on coronary atherosclerosis. JAMA 1990;264:3013–17.

Choudhury S, Jackson P, Katan MB, et al. A multifactorial diet in the management of hyper-lipidemia. Atherosclerosis 1984;50:93–103.

Controlled trial of soya-bean oil in myocardial infarction: report of Research Committee to the Medical Research Council. Lancet 1968;2:693–700.

Coronary Drug Project Research Group. Clofibrate and niacin in coronary heart disease. JAMA 1975;23:1360–81.

Curzio JL, Kennedy SS, Elliott HL, et al. Hypercholesterolemia in treated hypertensives: a controlled trial of intensive dietary advice. J Hypertension 1989;7:Suppl 6:S254–S255.

Davis CE, Rifkind BM, Brenner H, Gordon DJ. A single cholesterol measurement underesti-mates the risk of coronary heart disease. JAMA 1990;264:3044–46.

Dayton S, Pearce ML, Hashimoto S, et al. A controlled clinical trial of a diet high in unsaturated fat in preventing complications of altherosclerosis. Circulation 1969;40:Suppl II:II1–II63.

Dorr AE, Gundersen K, Schneider JC Jr, et al. Colestipol hydrochloride in hypercholesterolemic patients—effect on serum cholesterol and mortality. J Chronic Dis 1978;31:5–14.

Expert Panel. Report of the National Cholesterol Education Program Expert Panel on Detection, Evaluation, and Treatment of High Blood Cholesterol in Adults. Arch Intern Med 1988; 148:36–69.

Expert Panel on Detection, Evaluation, and Treatment of High Blood Cholesterol in Adults. Summary of the Second Report of the National Cholesterol Education Program (NCEP) Expert Panel on Detection, Evaluation, and Treatment of High Blood Cholesterol in Adults (Adult Treatment Panel II). JAMA 1993;269:3015–23.

Farquhar JW, Fortmann SP, Flora JA, et al. Effects of community-wide education on cardio-vascular disease risk factors. JAMA 1990;264:359–65.

Fortmann SP, Williams PT, Hulley SB, et al. Effect of health education on dietary behavior: the Stanford Three-Community Study. J Clin Nutr 1981;34:2030–8.

Frantz ID, Dawson EA, Ashman PL, et al. Test of effect of lipid lowering by diet on cardiovascular risk: the Minnesota Coronary Survey. Atherosclerosis 1989;9:129–35.

Frick MH, Elo O, Haapa K, et al.: Helsinki Heart Study: Primary prevention trial with gemfibrozil in middle-aged men with dyslipidemia. N Engl J Med 1987;317:1237–45.

Fuster V, Badimon L, Badimon JJ, Chesebro JH. The pathogenesis of coronary artery disease and the acute coronary syndromes. N Engl J Med 1992;326:242–50.

Goldman L, Weinstein MC, Goldman PA, Williams LW. Cost-effectiveness of HMG-CoA reductase inhibition for primary and secondary prevention of coronary heart disease. JAMA 1991;265:1145–51.

Goldman L, Gordon DJ, Rifkind BM, et al. Cost and health implications of cholesterol lowering. Circulation 1992;85:1960–8.

Goldman L, Goldman P, Williams L, Weinstein MC. Cost-effectiveness considerations in the treatment of heterozygous familial hypercholesterolemia with medications. In: Proceedings of the National Heart, Lung, and Blood Institute Workshop on Identification and Management of Heterozygous Familial Hypercholesterolemia. Am J Cardiol 1993;72: 75D–9D.

Gordon DJ, Probstfield JL, Garrosons RJ, et al. High-density lipoprotein cholesterol and cardiovascular disease: four prospective American studies. Circulation 1989;79:8–15.

Grundy SM, Nix D, Whelan MF, et al. Comparison of three cholesterol-lowering diets in normolipidemic men. JAMA 1986;256:2351–5.

Grundy SM, Barrett-Connor E, Rudel LL, et al. Workshop on the impact of dietary cholesterol on plasma lipoproteins and atherogenesis. Arteriosclerosis 1988;8:95–101.

Hjermann I, Velve BK, Holme I, et al. Effect of diet and smoking intervention on the incidence of coronary heart disease: report from the Oslo Study Group of a randomised trial in healthy men. Lancet 1981;2:1303–10.

Hulley SB, Newman TB, Grady D, et al. Should we be measuring blood cholesterol levels in young adults? JAMA 1992;269:1416–19.

Jacobs D, Blackburn H, Higgins M, et al. Report of the Conference on Low Blood Cholesterol: Mortality Associations. Circulation 1992;86:1046–60.

Johnson CL, Rifkind BM, Sempos CT, et al. Declining serum total cholesterol levels among US adults. JAMA 1993;269:3002–8.

Kane JP, Malloy MJ, Ports T, et al. Regression of coronary atherosclerosis during treatment of familial hypercholesterolemia with combined drug regimens. JAMA 1990;264:3007–12.

Keeler EB, Operskalsi BH, Sloss EM. Cost-effectiveness of health promotion programs. Report to the Henry J. Kaiser Family Foundation. Santa Monica, California, RAND, 1985.

Klag MJ, Ford DE, Mead LA, et al. Serum cholesterol in young men and subsequent cardiovascular disease. N Engl J Med 1993;328:313–18.

Krahn M, Naylor D, Basinski AS, Detsky AS. Comparison of an aggressive (U.S.) and a less aggressive (Canadian) policy for cholesterol screening and treatment. Ann Intern Med 1991;115:248–55.

Law MR, Thompson SG, Wald NJ. Assessing possible hazards of reducing serum cholesterol. Br Med J 1994;308:373–9.

Leren P. The effect of plasma cholesterol lowering diet in male survivors of myocardial infarction: a controlled clinical trial. Acta Med Scand Suppl 1966;466:1–92.

Leren P. The Oslo diet heart study: 11-year report. Circulation 1970;40:935–42.

Lipid Research Clinics Program. The Lipid Research Clinics Coronary Primary Prevention Trial results: I. Reduction in incidence of coronary heart disease. JAMA 1984a;251:351–64.

Lipid Research Clinics Program. The Lipid Research Clinics Coronary Primary Prevention Trial results. II. The relationship of reduction in incidence of CHD to cholesterol lowering. JAMA 1984b;251:365–74.

MacMahon S, Peto R, Cutler J, et al. Blood pressure, stroke, and coronary heart disease: Part I. Prolonged differences in blood pressure: prospective observational studies corrected for the regression dilution bias. Lancet 1990;335:765–74.

Manolio TA, Pearson TA, Wenger NK, et al. Cholesterol and heart disease in older persons and women. Review of an NHLBI Workshop. Ann Epidemiol 1992;2:161–76.

Martin M, Hulley S, Browner W, Kuller L, Wentworth D. Serum cholesterol, blood pressure, and mortality: implications from a cohort of 361,662 men. Lancet 1986;2:933–6.

Mattson FH, Grundy SM. Comparison of effects of dietary saturated, monounsaturated and polyunsaturated fatty acids on plasma lipids and lipoproteins in man. J Lipid Res 1985; 26:194–202.

Miettinen M, Turpeinen O, Karvonen MJ, et al. Effect of cholesterol-lowering diet on mortality from coronary heart disease and other causes: a twelve-year clinical trial in men and women. Lancet 1972;2:835–8.

Multiple Risk Factor Intervention Trial Research Group. Multiple Risk Factor Intervention Trial: Risk factor changes and mortality results. JAMA 1982;248:1465–77.

National Cattlemen's Association. War on fat: A report of the value-based marketing task force. Summer Meeting of the National Cattlemen's Association. Denver, Colorado, 1990.

Newman TN, Browner WS, Hulley SB. The case against childhood cholesterol screening. JAMA 1990;264:3039–43.

Nutrition Committee, American Heart Association. Dietary guidelines for healthy American adults. Circulation 1986;74:1465A–8A.

Orchard TJ, Donahue RP, Kuller LH, et al. Cholesterol screening in childhood: Does it predict adult hypercholesterolemia? The Beaver County experience. J Pediatr 1983;103:687–91.

Oster G, Epstein AM. Cost-effectiveness of antihyperlipidemic therapy in the prevention of coronary heart disease: the case of cholestyramine. JAMA 1987;285:2381–7.

Preventive Services Task Force. Guide to Clinical Preventive Services. Baltimore, Williams & Wilkins, 1989;11–21.

Puska P, Variainen E, Pallonen U, et al. The North Karelia Youth Project: evaluation of two years of intervention on health behavior and CVD risk factors among 13- to 15-year-old children. Prev Med 1982;11:550–70.

Report from the Committee of Principal Investigators. A cooperative trial in the primary prevention of ischaemic heart disease using clofibrate. Br Heart J 1978;40:1069–118.

Report by a Research Committee of the Scottish Society of Physicians. Ischaemic heart disease: a secondary prevention trial using clofibrate. Br Med J 1971;4:775–84.

Rose G, Heller RF, Pedoe HT, et al. Heart disease prevention project: a randomized controlled clinical trial in industry. Br Med J 1980;280:747–51.

Ross R. The pathogenesis of atherosclerosis. In: Braunwald E (ed), Heart Disease, 4th edition. Philadelphia: WB Saunders, 1992:1106–24.

Rossouw FE, Lewis B, Rifkind BM. The value of lowering cholesterol after myocardial infarction. N Engl J Med 1990;323:1112–19.

Scandinavian Simvastatin Survival Study Group. Randomized trial of cholesterol lowering in 4444 patients with coronary heart disease: the Scandinavian Simvastatin Survival Study (4S) Lancet 1994;344:1383–9.

Schulman K, Kinosian B, Jacobson T, et al. Reducing high blood cholesterol with drugs: Cost-effectiveness of pharmacologic management. JAMA 1990;264:3025–33.

Sempos CT, Cleeman JI, Carroll MD, et al. Prevalence of high blood cholesterol among US adults: an update based on guidelines from the Second Report of the National Cholesterol Education Program Adult Treatment Panel. JAMA 1993;269:3009–14.

Shepard J, Cobbe SM, Ford I. Prevention of coronary heart disease with Pravastatin in men with hypercholesterolemia. N Engl J Med 1995;333:1301–7.

Smith GD, Song F, Sheldon TA. Cholesterol lowering and mortality: the importance of considering initial level of risk. Br Med J 1993;306:367–73.

Stamler J, Stamler R, Brown WV, et al. Serum cholesterol: doing the right thing. Circulation 1993;88:1954–60.

Stampfer MJ, Sacks FM, Salvini S, et al. A prospective study of cholesterol, apolipoproteins, and the risk of myocardial infarction. N Engl J Med 1991;325:373–81.

Taskanen A, Ronnqvist P, Koskela K, Huttunen J. Change in risk factors for coronary heart disease during 10 years of a community intervention program (North Karelia Project). Br Med J 1983;287:1840–4.

Tell GS, Vellar OD. Noncummunicable disease risk factor intervention in Norwegian adolescents: the Oslo Youth Study. In: Hetzel BX, Berenson GS (eds), Cardiovascular Risk Factors in Childhood: Epidemiology and Prevention. Amsterdam: Elsevier, 1987:203–17.

Toronto Working Group on Cholesterol Policy. Asymptomatic hypercholesterolemia: A clinical policy review. J Clin Epidemiol 1990;43:1021–112.

Tosteson ANA, Weinstein MC, Williams L, Goldman L. Cost-effectiveness of population-wide approaches to reduce serum cholesterol levels. Clin Res 1991;39:298A.

Tran ZV, Weltman A. Differential effects of exercise on serum lipids and lipoprotein levels seen with changes in body weight. JAMA 1983;254:919–24.

Trial of clofibrate in the treatment of ischaemic heart disease: Five-year study by a group of physicians of the Newcastle upon Tyne region. Br Med J 1971;14:767–75.

Tyroler HA. Review of lipid-lowering clinical trials in relation to observational epidemiologic studies. Circulation 1987;76:515–22.

Walter HJ, Hofman A, Vaughan RD, Wynder EL. Modification of risk factors for coronary heart disease: five-year results of a school-based intervention trial. N Engl J Med 1988;318:1093–100.

Watts GF, Lewis B, Brunt JNH, et al. Effects on coronary artery disease of lipid-lowering diet, or diet plus cholestyramine, in the St. Thomas' Atherosclerosis Regression Study (STARS). Lancet 1992;339:563–9.

7

Treatment and Prevention of Hypertension

PAUL K. WHELTON, JIANG HE, AND LAWRENCE J. APPEL

Age-Blood Pressure Relationship and Prevalence of Hypertension

Average blood pressure (BP) and the prevalence of hypertension (high BP or treatment with antihypertensive medications) both tend to rise progressively with increasing age. With the exception of relatively isolated societies, this is true in almost every population (Whelton 1985, 1994a). The pattern of age-related changes in systolic and diastolic BP in residents of six economically developed countries is illustrated in Figure 7.1 (Italian National Research Council 1981; MacMahon 1984; National Center for Health Statistics 1986; Ueshima 1987; Appleyard 1989; Joffres 1992). Systolic BP tends to rise progressively until the eighth or ninth decade, while diastolic BP remains constant or declines after the fifth decade.

Hypertension prevalence estimates from the recent National Health and Nutrition Examination Survey (NHANES III) indicate that approximately one in every four adult residents of the United States has hypertension, based on current treatment with antihypertensive medications or an average of three systolic or diastolic BP readings ≥140 or 90 mmHg, respectively, at a single visit (Working Group on Primary Prevention of Hypertension 1993). As indicated in Table 7.1, there was a marked age-related rise in the prevalence of hypertension. Thus, the prevalence of hypertension ranged from 4% in young adults, aged 18–29, to 65% for those ≥80 years. In youth and middle-age, hypertension tends to be more common in men than in women (Whelton 1994a); the reverse is true in later life. Throughout the adult years, the prevalence of hypertension is higher in African-Americans and in those of lower socioeconomic status. Overall, approximately half of the hypertensives identified in the NHANES III were being treated with BP-lowering medications. About half of them or 20% of all hypertensives were well controlled (systolic and diastolic BPs less than 140/90 mmHg, respectively).

Although BP tends to rise with age in most countries, this is not a uniform finding. Populations with a low average BP and little evidence of age-related change in their BP have been described in several parts of the world (Poulter 1984; Whelton 1985; Carvalho 1989; He 1991). Typically, these ''normotensive'' populations tend to be found in relatively isolated societies who have a high level of physical activity and consume a natural diet which is low in sodium and high in potassium (Carvalho 1989; Stamler 1991). The infrequency of hypertension in such populations is extremely interesting since it indicates that age-related increases in BP are not a biologic necessity. When these populations have adopted a Western lifestyle, their BPs have begun to rise with age, and they have lost their immunity to hypertension (Poulter 1984; He 1991). The explanation for this change in BP pattern must lie in an alteration of environmental rather than genetic influences. Dietary changes, including consumption of processed foods with relatively high sodium/potassium ratios and more calories, as well as an increase in emotional stress have frequently been suggested as etiological factors of greatest importance in this change (Whelton 1994b).

Classification of High Blood Pressure

The recently published Fifth Report of The Joint National Committee for Detection, Evaluation, and Treatment of High BP (JNC-V) recommended use of the schema presented in Figure 7.2 to categorize adults according to their BP level (The Joint National Committee 1993). In this classification system, optimal BP is defined as a systolic BP less than 120 mmHg and a diastolic BP below 80 mmHg. Those with a systolic BP between 130 and 139 mmHg or a diastolic BP between 85 and 89 mmHg are designated as having a high normal BP. Hypertention is characterized by a confirmed elevation of systolic ($\geq$140 mmHg) or diastolic ($\geq$90 mmHg) BP. Hypertension is further characterized into four stages according to the patients' level of systolic and diastolic BP. Stage 1 is the mildest and most common (80%) form of hypertension, while stage 4 is the most severe and least common (less than 3%) category of hypertension (Stamler 1993).

Blood Pressure-Related Risk of Myocardial Infarction

Prospective studies have repeatedly identified an increasing risk of myocardial infarction (MI) as well as stroke, congestive heart failure, and renal insufficiency, with progressively higher levels of both systolic and diastolic BP (Shaper 1981; Keil 1987; Fiebach 1989; Reed 1989; Stokes 1989; Collins 1990; MacMahon 1990; Wilson 1991; Whelton 1992; Stamler 1993). Pooling of the experience in different studies provides the most stable estimates of risk. The results presented in Figure 7.3 are based on pooling of information from 418,343 participants in nine prospective observational studies (Collins 1990; MacMahon 1990). None had a history of MI at baseline and the average period of follow-up was 10 years. Analyses, which were corrected for the regression dilution bias resulting from attempts to estimate average BP with a single measurement, identified a striking positive relationship between diastolic BP and the risk of a subsequent coronary heart disease (CHD) event. There was no evidence of a J-shaped relationship between diastolic BP and incidence of CHD, a phenomenon which has been noted in secondary analyses of smaller data sets (Cruickshank 1987; Alderman 1989; Hansson 1990; Farnett 1991). Indeed, there was no threshold for risk

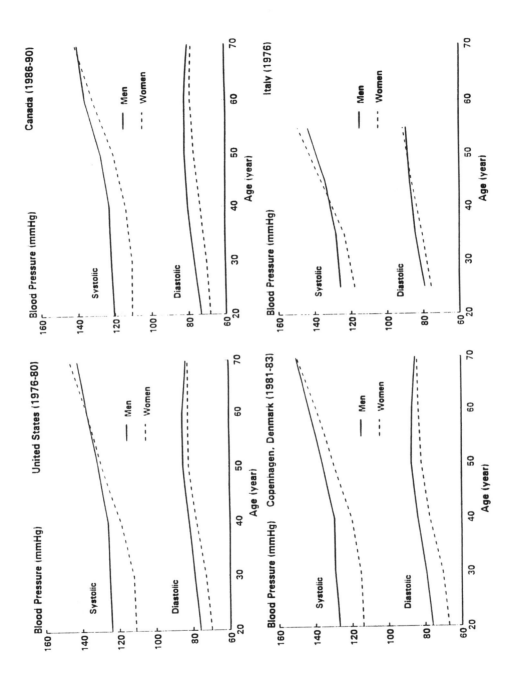

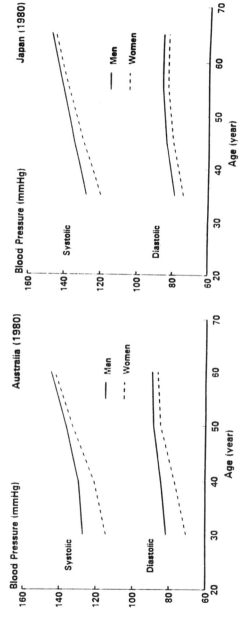

Fig. 7.1. Association between age and average levels of systolic and diastolic blood pressure in six economically developed countries. Diastolic blood pressure reflects the use of Phase 5 Korotkoff sounds. [From Whelton et al. (1990), with permission.]

Table 7.1. Prevalence of Hypertension in the Civilian Noninstitutionalized Adult Population of the United States during 1988–1991

Age	% Hypertension[a]
18–29	4
30–39	11
40–49	21
50–59	44
60–69	54
70–79	64
≥80	65

Source: From Working Group on Primary Prevention of Hypertension (1993), with permission.

[a]Average of three blood pressure measurements ≥140/90 mmHg on one occasion or taking antihypertensive medications

reduction even at the lowest end of the BP distribution. The relationship between diastolic BP and fatal and nonfatal CHD was equally impressive. The data suggest that a 5–6 mmHg lower level of diastolic BP is likely to be associated with a 20–25% reduction in the incidence of CHD.

Most (84%) of the participants and the vast majority of the 4,856 CHD events in the previously mentioned metanalysis reflect follow-up of the 350,977 men who were free from CHD when they were screened for possible participation in the Multiple Risk Factor Intervention Trial (MRFIT). In the more recent report from this prospective study, 7,150 CHD deaths were noted during an average of 11.6 years of follow-

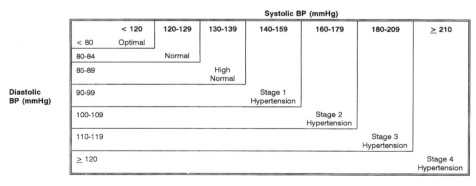

Fig. 7.2. National High Blood Pressure Education Program criteria for classification of adults by average level of blood pressure. Average blood pressure represents mean of two or more readings on two or more occasions in an individual who is not acutely ill and is not taking antihypertensive medications. When the average of the systolic and diastolic measurements fall into different categories, the higher reading should be selected for classification of blood pressure status. [Adapted from The Joint National Committee on Detection, Evaluation, and Treatment of High Blood Pressure (1993), with permission.]

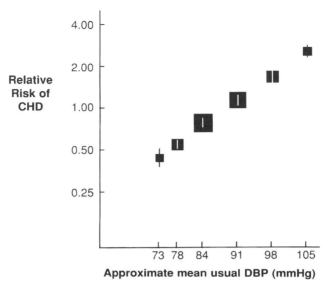

Fig. 7.3. Pooled estimates of the relationship between diastolic blood pressure and subsequent coronary heart disease (CHD) during an average of 10 years of follow-up in nine prospective observational studies of 418,343 persons who were initially free of CHD (Multiple Risk Factor Intervention Trial Screenee Cohort Study, Chicago Heart Association Study, Framingham Heart Study, Honolulu Heart Study, Lipid Research Clinics Screenee Study, Peoples Gas Study, Chicago Electric Study, Puerto Rico Heart Study, and Whitehall Study) CHD (N = 4,856) includes fatal events which were monitored in all nine studies (N = 4,260) and nonfatal myocardial infarction which were measured in only three of the studies (N = 596). The size of the squares are proportional to the number of events which occurred in each category of blood pressure and the vertical lines within the boxes reflect 95% confidence intervals for each estimate of relative risk. [Adapted from MacMahon et al. (1990), with permission.]

up of the overall cohort of 347,978 MRFIT screenees (Stamler 1993). For both systolic and diastolic BP, the absolute and relative risk of CHD mortality increased with progressively higher levels of BP, independent of age, race, serum cholesterol, cigarette smoking, diabetes mellitus, and income (Table 7.2). Compared with those having a systolic BP less than 110 mmHg, the risk of CHD mortality rose steadily with progressively higher levels of BP. The screenees in the highest BP category ($\geq$180 mmHg) had a relative risk of 5.65, but even those whose pressures were within the normotensive range experienced a higher relative risk of CHD mortality with each succeeding level of systolic BP. Given the fact that approximately 75% of the MRFIT screenees with a BP in excess of 110 mmHg were within the normotensive range (110–139 mmHg), this group accounted for roughly 32% of the systolic BP-related excess of CHD mortality. Those with a systolic BP between 140–159 mmHg represented only 20% of the population at risk. However, since their average relative risk of CHD mortality was increased about twofold, this group accounted for almost 43% of the excess risk of systolic BP-related CHD mortality. Those with a systolic BP

Table 7.2. Baseline Systolic Blood Pressure and Adjusted Coronary Heart Disease (CHD) Death Rates for Men Screened for the Multiple Risk Factor Intervention Trial

Systolic Blood Pressure, mmHg	Number (%)	Number of CHD Deaths	Rate[a]	Relative Risk[b]	Excess Deaths[c]	% of All Excess Deaths	
<110	21,379 (6.1)	197	9.8	1.00	0	00	
110–119	66,080 (19.0)	712	11.1	1.12	77	1.3	
120–129	98,834 (28.4)	1,349	12.9	1.32*	319	9.9	31.9
130–139	79,308 (22.8)	1,587	17.0	1.76*	669	20.7	
140–149	44,388 (12.8)	1,328	22.8	2.35*	755	23.4	
150–159	21,477 (6.2)	938	30.5	3.14*	631	19.5	42.9
160–169	9,308 (2.7)	470	34.0	3.41*	328	10.1	
170–179	4,013 (1.2)	286	47.6	4.30*	221	6.8	24.1
≥180	3,191 (0.9)	283	57.2	5.65*	232	7.2	

Source: From Stamler et al. (1993), with permission.

Excess deaths were derived by first calculating expected number of deaths within deciles of a risk score based on age, race, serum cholesterol, cigarettes per day, use of medication for diabetes, and income, then summing these estimates across risk score deciles within each blood pressure category and subtracting this number from the observed number of deaths.

[a]Rate per 10,000 person-years adjusted by direct method of age, race, serum cholesterol, cigarettes per day, use of medication for diabetes, and income; average follow-up was 11.6 years.

[b]Adjusted by proportional hazards regression for age, race, serum cholesterol, cigarettes per day, use of medication for diabetes, and income.

[c]Estimated number of excess deaths compared with the baseline systolic blood pressure category of less than 110 mmHg during 11.6 years of follow-up.

*p < .001.

above 160 mmHg had at least a threefold increase in their relative risk of CHD mortality. Fortunately, only 5% of the MRFIT screenees with a BP greater than 110 mmHg were in this category. This group was responsible for about 24% of the overall excess of systolic BP-related CHD mortality.

These data and similar findings from other studies have important implications for prevention of BP-related CHD. First, they indicate that there is a strong epidemiologic basis for efforts aimed at the detection, treatment, and control of hypertension. Successful treatment provides the potential for a meaningful reduction in the population burden of CHD in addition to providing the potential for a clinically relevant reduction in risk for the individual patient. Second, they underscore the importance of treating mild hypertension, since approximately two-thirds of all the hypertension-related CHD mortality occurs within this range of BP. Finally, the data indicate that treatment of hypertension represents an incomplete response to the overall burden of BP-related CHD in the community. Even with completely effective treatment and control of hypertension, only 60–70% of the BP-related CHD events could be eliminated. To maximize the benefit for the community, treatment must be accompanied by equally vigorous attempts to prevent the development of hypertension.

The relationship between BP and risk of CHD has been similar in study participants with varying sociodemographic characteristics and in the presence or absence of other cardiovascular disease risk factors. In the MRFIT screenee cohort, the adjusted relative risk for those with a 20-mmHg higher systolic BP at baseline was 1.56 for whites, 1.53 for African Americans, 1.62 for Hispanics, and 1.39 for Asians (Stamler 1993). In the Nurses Health Study, 308 incident cases of CHD were noted during a 6-year follow-up of 119,963 women aged 30–54 at baseline (Fiebach 1989). After adjustment for age, serum cholesterol, cigarette smoking, body mass index, parental history of MI, menopausal status, current and past postmenopausal hormone use, and time period, self-reported hypertension was associated with a 3.5-fold increase in the risk of subsequent CHD mortality (95% CI: 1.8–3.5). Elevation of systolic and diastolic BP have also been identified as independent predictors of CHD risk in men and women followed in the Framingham Heart Study (Stokes 1989) and in the Framingham Offspring Study (Wilson 1991). The relationship between BP and CHD risk has proven to be quite similar in studies conducted in different cultures and in different geographic locations (Shaper 1981; Keil 1987; Reed 1989). Likewise, the association has been apparent both in the presence and absence of other cardiovascular disease risk factors. The absolute risk is, however, always considerably higher when high BP is accompanied by cigarette smoking, hypercholesterolemia, or one of the other cardiovascular disease risk predictors (Stamler 1993).

Overall Goals and Strategies for Treatment of Hypertension

The overal goals of treating patients with hypertension are to prevent BP-associated morbidity and mortality and to lower BP using the least invasive means possible. BP can be lowered by application of either pharmacologic or nonpharmacologic lifestyle modification interventions. In either case, the therapist should strive to achieve and maintain a systolic BP $\leq$ 140 mmHg and a diastolic BP $\leq$ 90 mmHg, while concurrently optimizing the profile of other cardiovascular disease risk factors. The extent to which BP should be lowered below 130 mmHg systolic and 85 mmHg diastolic is unclear (Fletcher 1992). Lifestyle modifications constitute the initial approach to treatment. The decision to add a pharmacologic intervention should be dependent on the extent to which lifestyle modifications result in a lowering of BP and the presence or absence of target organ disease, other medical conditions, and other cardiovascular disease risk factors.

The frequency of follow-up visits should be based on the patient's average BP level as well as on the complexity of his or her treatment regimen and other health needs. Recommendations based on a patient's initial average systolic and diastolic BP are provided in Table 7.3.

Achievement and maintenance of the desired level of BP control necessitates ongoing monitoring of the patient and may include adjustment of the treatment regimen. In general, patients with stage 1 hypertension and no target organ disease should be reevaluated within one to two months following initiation of therapy. Those with more severe hypertension, target organ disease, or treatment-related adverse effects may need to be seen at an earlier stage. Once the goal BP has been achieved, follow-up visits can be reduced to a 3- to 6-month frequency.

Maximizing adherence to the prescribed therapy should be an important component of the treatment plan. A series of approaches that can be used to improve compliance are outlined in Table 7.4. Simplification of the regimen, inclusion of the patient

Table 7.3. Recommendations for Follow-Up of Adults Based on Their Initial Average Levels of Blood Pressure

Systolic	Diastolic	Follow-Up Recommendations[a]
<130	<85	Recheck in 2 years
130–139	85–89	Recheck in ±1 years.
140–159	90–99	Confirm within 2 months.
160–179	100–109	Evaluate or refer to source of care within 1 month.
180–209	110–119	Evaluate or refer to source of care within 1 week.
≥210	≥210	Evaluate or refer to source of care immediately.

[a]If the systolic and diastolic categories are different, follow recommendation for the shorter-time follow-up (e.g., 160/85 mmHg should be evaluated or referred to source of care within 1 month). The scheduling of follow-up visits should be modified by reliable information about past blood pressure measurements, target-organ disease, and other cardiovascular risk factors and medical conditions.

in decision-making, active discussion of compliance issues, and strengthening of the social environment are fundamental to improving adherence to the prescribed regimen. Over time, the patient's needs and social environment may change, necessitating a shift in emphasis for implementation of these strategies.

Intervention Strategies

Lifestyle Modification

Lifestyle alterations leading to weight loss, a decreased intake of dietary sodium, moderation of alcohol intake, and increased physical activity provide effective means to treat hypertension and to modify favorably other risk factors for cardiovascular disease (Joint National Committee 1993). Other measures such as supplementation with potassium, calcium, magnesium, fiber, or fish oils and a reduction in stress or

Table 7.4. Strategies for Enhancement of Adherence to the Treatment Plan

- Improve the patients' knowledge of hypertension and goals of therapy.
- Involve patient as a partner in decision-making. Provide feedback on blood pressure levels and laboratory findings. Encourage self-monitoring.
- Simplify and individualize the treatment plan. Where possible, incorporate treatment plan into the patient's lifestyle. Provide patient with written details of the treatment plan and confirm patients understanding of the plan prior to end of visit. Minimize the cost of treatment.
- Set realistic goals and time-lines for completion of tasks. At each visit, discuss achievement of goals and methods for maximizing adherence with therapy. Consider use of physician-patient contracts to achieve goals.
- Schedule next appointment before end of visit. Between visits, use phone, mail, or home visit contacts as opportunities to discuss progress, problem solve, and confirm time and date of next appointment.
- Strengthen social support by involvement of family and friends in implementation of treatment plan. Consider participation of patient in small group meetings to enhance motivation and provide peer support.
- Draw on complementary skills of other health professionals and refer patient for more intensive counseling as necessary.

dietary fat may also be helpful but are less well proven. Lifestyle modifications can be effective as a definitive form of therapy in patients with stage 1 hypertension but are better considered as adjunctive therapy in stages 2–4 hypertension. Typical goals for weight loss and sodium restriction are to achieve and maintain a 10-lb weight loss and to reduce urinary excretion of sodium to ≤80 mmol/24 h. Even partial success in meeting these goals can lead to a meaningful reduction in BP, an improvement in the patient's response to antihypertensive drug therapy, an improvement in the patient's lipid profile and carbohydrate metabolism (weight loss), and a reduction in the prevalence of hypokalemia and symptomatic congestive heart failure (sodium restriction). In addition, weight loss may yield general health benefits such as a reduction in the incidence of gout, osteoarthritis, and neoplasms such as breast cancer. The goal of physical activity should be incorporation of regular low-intensity exercises, such as walking, swimming, dancing, cycling, or gardening into the patient's day-to-day routine. A reasonable goal for alcohol consumption would be moderation of alcohol intake to fewer than three drinks per day.

Achievement and maintenance of a lifestyle modification requires a greater committment of time and effort on the part of the patient and the therapist than is the case for pharmacologic interventions. Long-term success revolves around the achievement and maintenance of behavioral changes which impact on nutrition, physical activity, and consumption of alcohol. Some of the elements which facilitate achievement of a successful lifestyle change are outlined in Table 7.5. Most of these revolve around understanding how to influence antecedents of the desired behavior change and how to structure positive or negative consequences which promote the desired change in behavior. In practice, interventions involving nutritional changes can be greatly facilitated by having the patient keep a food diary and by calculating the contribution of specific dietary elements to the consumption of calories, salt, or other nutrients of interest (Figure 7.4). Such calculations can be made with the help of quite simple food composition books that can be purchased in most book stores and many supermarkets. Even relatively crude food diaries maintained over short periods of time can highlight dietary practices that can be easily changed. Instructing the patient and fam-

Table 7.5. Elements Necessary for Successful Implementation of a Behaviorally Oriented Change in Nutrition Practices

Patient	Therapist
• Value proposed change	• Specify nutrition goals
• Feel capable of making change	• Translate nutrition goals into behavior change goals
• Learn basic skills for achieving behavior change	• Provide patients the instruments necessary to achieve their lifestyle change goals
• Set explicit, achievable, incremental short-term behavior change goals	• Understand antecedents and consequences of behavior to be changed
• Obtain rapid, ongoing feedback on achievement of goals	• Negotiate small, incremental and progressive changes in behavior to be achieved over defined interval
• Engage family and friends in process	• Develop problem-solving partnership with patient

NAME: DATE:

TIME	AMOUNT	FOOD ITEM	CAL	FAT(G)	Na(mg)
7:00 am	8 oz	Coffee, regular	5	0	5
	1 tbsp	Half & Half	20	2	5
	1	Croissant	235	16	280
	2 tsp	Butter	70	8	80
12:00 Noon	2 sl	Pepperoni Pizza	460	18	825
	12 oz	Cola	150	0	25
	2"x2"	Brownie	140	6	90

Fig. 7.4. Example of food record indicating the calorie, fat and sodium content of two sample meals.

ily members to read nutrition information labels before purchasing food products can also be very helpful. Optimally, the patient's primary health care provider should play a lead role in implementing the behavior change. If this is not feasible, he or she should at least be supportive and willing to refer the patient to a professional who is more experienced in behavior counseling. A more detailed discussion of the theory and practice of behavior changes is beyond the scope of this chapter but can be found elsewhere (Ewart 1991).

Pharmacologic Treatment

Over the past three decades, numerous drug treatment trials have been conducted to determine whether BP reduction in middle age decreases the risk of cardiovascular disease. For accelerated and malignant hypertension, the effect on all-cause mortality was so impressive that nonrandomized, historically controlled trials with some of the earliest and least well tolerated antihypertensive medications provided enough evidence to convince practitioners of the wisdom of treatment (Harrington 1959; Bjork 1961). During the 1960s, results from three trials provided persuasive evidence of the value of antihypertensive drug therapy in patients with severe (Stages 3–4) hypertension. The treatment benefits, which were apparent within months of initiating therapy, resulted primarily from an impressive reduction in the frequency of hypertensive complications such as hemorrhagic stroke, congestive heart failure, and uremia. Atherosclerotic complications such as CHD and atherothrombotic stroke were rare, presumably reflecting the relatively short duration of follow-up in these trials.

Evidence of a beneficial effect of antihypertensive drug therapy on CHD and other atherosclerotic complications of hypertension has largely been based on experience in trials conducted in patients with mild to moderate (stages 1–2) hypertension. Results from almost 20 such trials have been reported (Cutler 1985; Whelton 1988; Collins 1990; Hebert 1993). Most have demonstrated a statistically significant and impressive reduction in stroke event rate. The impact on CHD event rate has been less striking and, with two exceptions (Hypertension Detection and Follow-up Program Cooperative Group 1988; SHEP Cooperative Research Group 1991), reductions have not been statistically significant. Some authors have attributed this to a lack of effect of anti-hypertensive drug therapy, as prescribed in these studies, on CHD (Giles 1991; Hansson 1991; Pool 1991). In large part, however, the failure to achieve a statistically significant reduction in CHD event rates in individual trials results from a lack of sufficient power to provide a definitive answer. To overcome this problem, data from individual trials have been pooled in order to obtain more precise estimates of the effect of treatment. In one of the most recent such analyses, results from 17 trials with a combined sample size of 47,653 were pooled (Hebert 1993). The average weighted difference in diastolic BP between active and control therapy in this analysis was 5–6 mmHg. As indicated in Table 7.6, the corresponding reduction in total and fatal CHD events was important (16% reduction for both endpoints) and highly statistically significant ($p = .0001$ and .006, respectively). Although the relative reduction in fatal (40%) and nonfatal (38%) stroke event rates was far greater, the overall reduction in number of coronary ($N = 90$) and stroke ($N = 94$) deaths was about the same given the much higher prevalence of CHD in the community.

Based on the experience in observational studies, the expected pooled reduction in CHD in the 17 trials was approximately 20% to 25%. The difference between the observed and expected reduction in CHD mortality may reflect the fact that the period of follow-up in the observational studies was much longer than was the case for the experimental trials. In most experimental studies, the beneficial effect of interventions on atherosclerosis is not seen for at least 2 to 3 years, and the maximal impact may not become apparent for several more years (Lipid Research Clinics Program 1984; Frick 1987; Multiple Risk Factor Intervention Trial Research Group 1990). Alternatively, the discrepancy may simply reflect the effect of random variation. The 95% confidence interval for a beneficial antihypertensive drug treatment effect on total and fatal CHD in the pooled analysis was 4% to 22% and 4% to 24%, respectively. A third possible explanation for the difference in observed and expected rates is that the primary drugs used in the 17 trials conducted to date may have provided less cardiac protection than would have been the case for an optimal agent that produced a similar degree of BP reduction. Diuretics, often administered in relatively high doses, were the principal form of drug therapy prescribed in most of the trials. Beta-blockers were included as first-line therapy in four trials (Medical Research Council Working Party 1985; Coope 1986; Dahlof 1991; MRC 1992). In the two Medical Research Council trials, hypertensives were assigned at random to either a diuretic or a beta-blocker

Table 7.6. Pooled Effect of Antihypertensive Drug Therapy on Stroke and Coronary Heart Disease in 47,653 Hypertensives Studied in 17 Clinical Trials

	% Risk Reduction (95% CI)	
	Total	Fatal
Stroke	38 (31–45)	40 (26–51)
CHD	16 (8–23)	16 (5–26)

Source: From Hebert et al. (1993), with permission.

(Medical Research Council Working Party 1985; MRC 1992). Both drugs reduced BP, but diuretic therapy was accompanied by a greater reduction in event rates. Newer classes of antihypertensive drugs such as the angiotensin-converting enzyme inhibitors, calcium channel blockers, and α-receptor blockers have theoretic advantages compared to treatment with diuretics or beta-blockers. The newer agents are, however, considerably more expensive (Manolio 1995). Whether these newer agents are more effective than diuretics in reducing CHD event rates is the primary question being addressed in the Antihypertensive and Lipid-Lowering Treatment To Prevent Heart Attack Trial (ALLHAT). The results of this large, community-based trial will not be available until the latter part of this decade. Based on the available evidence, JNC-V has recommended diuretics and beta-blockers as the preferred form of initial therapy, unless there are specific indications that would warrant use of an alternative agent (The Joint National Committee 1993).

An appendix concerning antihypertensive agents (dosages, benefits, risks, and relative costs) is provided at the end of this textbook.

Cost of Care

Treatment of hypertension is one of the most cost-effective means available for prevention of CHD and other cardiovascular risk factors (Goldman 1992). This is especially the case for high-risk hypertensives who comply fully with their assigned treatment regimen and who can be managed satisfactorily with cheaper forms of therapy. In contrast, the cost-benefit relationship is most tenuous for patients with the mildest forms of hypertension and for those who are noncompliant or require expensive forms of evaluation, treatment or monitoring.

Given that antihypertensive therapy usually requires a lifelong commitment and that approximately 50 million Americans have hypertension, maximizing the cost effectiveness of treatment is an important goal not only for the individual patient but also for society. Avoiding misclassification of hypertensives with a consequent reduction in the number of individuals who are candidates for treatment is one approach to improving the cost effectiveness of antihypertensive therapy. Self-monitoring of BP by the patient and ambulatory monitoring of BP by means of automated devices have both been advocated as means to achieve this goal. The latter approach, however, should be used with caution as the risk and treatment implications of ambulatory BP measurements are likely to be quite different from those which have been accrued in studies using standard methods of BP measurement. Cost effectiveness can also be improved by minimizing the intensity of the initial evaluation and minimizing the frequency and complexity of follow-up visits.

Drug costs account for approximately 70% to 80% of the total expenditure for treatment of hypertension (Joint National Committee 1993). As such, choice of drug therapy has the potential to play a major role in contributing to the cost-effectiveness of the treatment. In recent years, there has been a progressive shift from prescription of diuretics and beta-blockers to prescription of newer and more expensive drugs, such as calcium channel blockers and angiotensin-converting enzyme inhibitors. This shift has led to an almost twofold increase in the cost of providing drug therapy for hypertensives in the United States (Manolio 1995). In the individual patient, drug costs can vary by more than 30-fold, depending on the choice of medications used for treatment. Regardless of the specific choice of pharmaceutical agents, drug doses and associated costs can be decreased by maximizing compliance with the assigned therapy and by encouraging adoption of a healthy lifestyle aimed at reducing the need for drug therapy. In addition, drug costs can often be diminished by prescribing scored tables containing twice the required dosage and instructing the patient to halve the tablet in order to achieve the desired dose.

Prevention of Hypertension

Despite its obvious benefits, treatment of hypertension does not provide a complete solution to the current epidemic of BP-related cardiovascular disease (Working Group on Primary Prevention of Hypertension 1993). First, treatment of hypertension reduces but does not eliminate risk. Second, it is extremely hard to detect, treat, and control all hypertensives. Furthermore, a variety of factors including cost, medication side effects, and miscommunication may result in discontinuation of therapy. Finally, treatment of hypertension has no impact on the substantial burden of BP-related CHD that results from an elevation of BP within the normotensive range. For all of these reasons, treatment of hypertension represents only one component of a comprehensive response to the problem of BP-related cardiovascular disease.

Hypertension treatment should be complemented by an equally vigorous attempt to prevent the development of hypertension. Primary prevention of hypertension is a natural extension of hypertension treatment. More than this, the two approaches are mutually reinforcing and complementary. Primary prevention of hypertension can be accomplished by means of lifestyle modification interventions, which result in a slight downward shift in the entire distribution of BP (general population strategy), and by more intensive modification of lifestyles in those who are at special risk of development of hypertension (individual-targeted strategy). The latter group includes persons with a high normal BP, African-Americans, and those who are overweight, inactive, or comsuming excess amounts of salt or alcohol. For both strategies, a small reduction in BP can yield substantial health benefits. For instance, a downward shift in the general population's distribution of BP by 2, 3, or 4 mmHg is likely to result in an annual reduction in CHD mortality of 4%, 5%, and 9%, respectively (Stamler 1991). Likewise, targeted interventions that have resulted in as little as a 2- to 3-mmHg decrement in BP have yielded a 25% to 50% reduction in the subsequent incidence of hypertension (Stamler 1989; Hypertension Prevention Trial 1990; the Trials of Hypertension Prevention Collaborative Research Group 1992; Working Group on Primary Prevention of Hypertension 1993). The lifestyle changes that are most effective in prevention of hypertension are identical to those previously recommended for treatment of hypertension, namely, weight loss, a decreased intake of dietary sodium, moderation in consumption of alcoholic beverages, and an increase in physical activity.

The population strategy is best implemented by:

1. delivering simple, action-oriented messages that enhance and complement the existing base of health advice being directed at the general public;
2. favorably influencing the manufacture and preparation of foods;
3. improving product and shelf labeling of raw and processed foods; and
4. increasing the opportunities for physical activity in schools, the work place, and the community.

The targeted strategy is best achieved by enhancing education and support of health care providers in order to facilitate their active participation in hypertension prevention counseling. Although challenging, primary prevention provides the best hope for interruption of the continuing, costly cycle of managing hypertension and its complications. Through achievement of healthier lifestyles, much of the current epidemic of BP-related atherosclerotic CHD can potentially be eliminated.

Summary

Quality of available data: A large number of randomized trials testing the effects of both pharmacologic and lifestyle interventions on hypertension.
Estimated risk reduction: A 2–3% decline in risk for each 1-mmHg reduction in diastolic BP, which average 5–6 mmHg with a combination of dietary and pharmacologic therapies. In clinical practice, decreases of 20 mmHg or more are often achieved. Comparable reductions in MI risk can be achieved by treating patients with isolated systolic hypertension.
Comparability of effect in men and women: There is strong and consistent evidence of a relationship between elevated BP and increased MI risk among both men and women. Treatment of diastolic and/or systolic hypertension is indicated in both men and women.

References

Alderman MH, Ooi WL, Madhaven S, Cohen H. Treatment-induced blood pressure reduction and risk of myocardial infarction. JAMA 1989;262:920–4.
Appleyard M. The Copenhagen City Heart Study. Osterbroundersogelsen. A book of tables with data from the first examination (1976–78) and a five-year follow-up (1981–83). Scand J Soc Med 1989;17(Suppl 41):106–11.
Bjork S, Sannerstedt R, Falkheden T, Hood B. The effect of active drug treatment in severe antihypertensive disease. Acta Med Scand 1961;169:673–89.
Carvalho JJM, Baruzzi RG, Howard PF, et al. Blood pressure in four remote populations in the INTERSALT Study. Hypertension 1989;14:238–46.
Collins R, Peto, Goodwin J, MacMahon S. Blood pressure and coronary heart disease [Letter]. Lancet 1990a;335:370–1.
Collins R, Peto R, MacMahon S, et al. Blood pressure, stroke, and coronary heart disease, II: short-term reductions in blood pressure: overview of randomized drug trials in their epidemiological context. Lancet 1990b;335:827–38.

Coope J and Warrender T. Randomized trial of treatment of hypertension in the elderly patients in primary health care. Br Med J 1986;293:1145–51.

Cruickshank JM, Thorp JM, Zacharias FJ. Benefits and potential harm of lowering blood pressure. Lancet 1987;1:581–4.

Cutler JA, Furberg CD. Drug treatment trials in hypertension: a review. Prev Med 1985;14: 499–518.

Dahlof B, Lindholm LH, Hansson L, et al. Morbidity and mortality in the Swedish Trial in Old Patients with Hypertension. Lancent 1991;338:1281–5.

Ewart CK. Social action theory for a public health psychology. Am Psychologist 1991;46: 931–46.

Farnett L, Mulrow CD, Linn WD, et al. The J-curve phenomenon and treatment of hypertension: is there a point beyond which pressure reduction is dangerous? JAMA 1991;265:489–95.

Fiebach NH, Hebert PR, Stampfer MJ, et al. A prospective study of high blood pressure and cardiovascular disease in women. Am J Epidemiol 1989;130:646–54.

Fletcher AE, Bulpitt CJ. How far should blood pressure be lowered? N Engl J Med 1992;326: 251–4.

Frick MH, Elo O, Haapa K, et al. Helsinki Heart Study: primary-prevention trial with gemfibrozil in middle-aged men with dyslipidemia: safety of treatment, changes in risk factors, and incidence of coronary heart disease. N Engl J Med 1987;317:1237–45.

Giles TD. Antihypertensive therapy and cardiovascular risk: are all antihypertensives equal? Hypertension 1991;19(Suppl 1);I-124–I-129.

Goldman L. Gordon DJ, Rifkind BM, et al. Cost and health implications of cholesterol lowering. Circulation 1992;85:1960–8.

Hansson L. How far should blood pressure be lowered? What is the role of the so-called J-curve? Am J Hypertens 1990;3:726–9.

Hansson L. Shortcomings of current antihypertensive therapy. Am J Hypertens 1991;4:84S–7S.

Harrington M, Kincaid-Smith P, McMichael J. Results of treatment of malignant hypertension. Br Med J 1959;ii:969–989.

He J, Klag MJ, Whelton PK, et al. Migration, blood pressure pattern, and hypertension: the Yi Migrant Study. Am J Epidemiol 1991;134:1085–101.

Hebert P, Moser M, Mayer J, et al. Recent evidence on drug therapy of mild to moderate hypertension and decreased risk of coronary heart disease. Arch Intern Med 1993;153: 578–81.

Houston MC. New insights and new approaches for the treatment of essential hypertension: selection of therapy based on coronary heart disease risk factor analysis, hemodynamic profiles, quality of life, and subsets of hypertension. Am Heart J 1989;117:911–51.

Hypertension Detection and Follow-up Program Cooperative Group. Persistence of reduction in blood pressure and mortality of participants in the Hypertension Detection and Follow-up Program. JAMA 1988;259:2113–22.

Hypertension Prevention Trial Research Group. The Hypertension Prevention Trial: three-year effects of dietary changes on blood pressure. Arch Intern Med 1990;150:153–62.

Joffres MR, Hamet P, Rabkin SW, et al., and Canadian Heart Health Surveys Research Group. Prevalence, control and awareness of high blood pressure among Canadian adults. Can Med Assoc J 1992;146:1997–2005.

Joint National Committee on Detection, Evaluation and Treatment of High Blood Pressure: the Fifth Report of The Joint National Committee on the Detection, Evaluation, and Treatment of High Blood Presure (JNC V). Arch Intern Med 1993;153:154–83.

Keil JG, Gazes PC, Loadholt CB, et al. Coronary heart disease mortality and its predictors among women in Charleston, South Carolina. In: Eaker ED, Packard B, Wenger NK,

Clarkson TB, Tyroler HA, eds. Coronary heart disease in women: Proceedings of an NIH workshop. New York: Haymarket Doyma, 1987:90–8.

Lipid Research Clinics Program. The Lipid Research Clinics Coronary Primary Prevention Trial results. I. Reduction in incidence of coronary heart disease. JAMA 1984;251:351–64.

MacMahon SW, Blacket RB, Macdonald GJ, Hall W. Obesity, alcohol consumption and blood pressure in Australian men and women: the National Heart Foundation of Australia Risk Factor Prevalence Study. J Hypertens 1984;2:85–91.

MacMahon S, Peto R, Cutler J, et al. Blood pressure, stroke, and coronary heart disease. Part 1: Prolonged differences in blood pressure: prospective observational studies corrected for the regression dilution bias. Lancet 1990;335:765–74.

Manolio TA, Cutler JA, Furberg CD, et al. Trends in pharmacologic management of hypertension in the United States. Arch Intern Med 1995;155:829–37.

Medical Research Council Working Party: MRC trial of treatment of mild hypertension: principal results. Br Med J 1985;291:97–104.

MRC Working Party. Medical Research Council trial of treatment of hypertension in older adults: principal results. Br Med J 1992;304:405–12.

Multiple Risk Factor Intervention Trial Research Group. Mortality rates after 10.5 years for participants in the Multiple Risk Factors Intervention Trial: findings related to a priori hypotheses of the trial. JAMA 1990;263:1795–801.

National Center for Health Statistics: Drizd T, Dannenberg AL, Engel A. Blood pressure levels in persons 18–74 years of age in 1976-80, and trends in blood presure from 1960 to 1980 in the United States. Vital and Health Statistics. Series 11, N. 234., DHHS Pub. No. (PHS) 86-1684. Public Health Service. Washington, DC: U.S. Government Printing Office, July 1986.

Pool PE, Seagren SC, Salel AF. Metabolic consequences of treating hypertension. Am J Hypertens 1991;4:494S–502S.

Poulter N, Khaw KT, Hopwood BEC, et al. Blood pressure and associated factors in a rural Kenyan community. Hypertension 1984;6:810–13.

Reed D, MacLean C. The nineteen-year treand in CHD in the Honolulu Heart Program. Int J Epidemiol 1989;18:S82–7.

The Research Group ATS-RF2 of the Italian National Research Council. Distribution of some risk factors for atherosclerosis in nine Italian population samples. Am J Epidemiol 1981; 113:338–46.

Shaper AG, Pocock SJ, Walker M, et al. British Regional Heart Study: cardiovascular risk factors in middle-aged men in 24 towns. Br Med J 1981;283:179–86.

SHEP Cooperative Research Group. Prevention of stroke by antihypertensive drug treatment in older persons with isolated systolic hypertension: final results of the Systolic Hypertension in the Elderly Program (SHEP). JAMA 1991;265:3255–64.

Stamler R, Stamler J, Gosch FC, et al. Primary prevention of hypertension by nutritional-hygienic means: final report of a randomized, controlled trial. JAMA 1989;262:1801–7.

Stamler R. Implications of the INTERSALT Study. Hypertension 1991;17(Suppl. 1):I-16–20.

Stamler J, Stamler R, Neaton JD. Blood pressure, systolic and diastolic, and cardiovascular risks: U.S. population data. Arch Intern Med 1993;153:598–615.

Stokes J III, Kannel WB, Wolfe PA, et al. Blood pressure as a risk factor for cardiovascular disease: the framingham study: 30 years of follow-up. Hypertension 1989;13(Suppl I): I-13–18.

The Trials of Hypertension Prevention Collaborative Research Group. The effects of non-pharmacologic interventions on blood pressure of persons with high normal levels: results of the Trials of Hypertension Prevention, Phase I. JAMA 1992:267:1213–20.

Ueshima H, Tatara K, Asakura, Okamoto M. Declining trends in blood pressure level and the prevalence of hypertension, and changes in related factors in Japan, 1956–1980. J Chron Dis 1987;40:137–47.

Whelton PK. Blood pressure in adults and the elderly. In: Bulpitt CJ, ed. Epidemiology of hypertension. Amsterdam: Elsevier, 1985:51–69.

Whelton PK, Russell RP. Systemic hypertension. In: Harvey AM, Johns RJ, McKusick VA, Owens AM, Ross RS, eds. The principles and practice of medicine, 22nd ed. Norwalk CT: Appleton & Lange, 1988:127–44.

Whelton PK, Pernerger TV, Klag MJ, Brancati FL. Epidemiology and prevention of blood pressure-related renal disease. J Hypertens 1992;10(Suppl 7):S77–S84.

Whelton PK, He J, Klag MJ. Blood pressure in westernized populations. In: Swales JD, ed. Textbook of hypertension. Oxford: Blackwell Scientific Publications 1994:11–21.

Whelton PK. Epidemiology of Hypertension. Lancet 1994;344:101–106.

Wilson PW, Anderson KM, Castelli WP. Twelve-year incidence of coronary heart disease in middle-aged adults during the era of hypertensive therapy: the Framingham Offspring Study. Am J Med 1991;90:11–16.

Working Group on Primary Prevention of Hypertension. Report of the National High Blood Pressure Education Program Working Group on Primary Prevention of Hypertension. Arch Intern Med 1993;153:186–208.

8

Exercise and Fitness

RALPH S. PAFFENBARGER, JR. AND I-MIN LEE

Most of the evidence relating increasing levels of exercise and fitness to decreasing incidence of myocardial infarction (MI) is based on epidemiologic study of total coronary heart disease (CHD) or cardiovascular disease (CVD), rather than MI specifically. Nonetheless, MI accounts for the bulk of CHD, and most epidemiologic studies that have treated MI as a distinct entity (Paffenbarger 1978; Salonen 1982; 1988; Leon 1987) have shown associations between exercise and reduced risk of MI that are equally as strong as associations between exercise and reduced risks of sudden death, angina pectoris, coronary insufficiency, total CHD, and total CVD. Thus analysis of the larger numbers provided by study of total CHD or CVD seems appropriate, and we can be reasonably confident that observations linking exercise and CHD or CVD reflect those between exercise and MI. Accordingly, this chapter is concerned more with the primary prevention of CHD or CVD, rather than MI per se, by exercise and fitness.

Level of physical activity is related inversely to incidence of nonfatal and fatal CHD in observational epidemiologic studies, and this association appears to be at least partly independent of other influences. The benefits of physical activity can be appreciated in the hypothesis that where exercise is adequate, physiologic fitness is maintained or improved, systemic disease such as CHD is prevented or delayed, and longer life may be attained. Since physical activity is an optional behavior and physiologic fitness an achieved condition, each may act independently to favor health and longevity. However, activity and fitness are interrelated because activity modifies fitness over time, and fitness establishes benchmarks and limitations for activity.

Proposed Mechanisms of Benefit

A reduced risk of CHD from a physically active lifestyle may be mediated by direct action on the heart: increasing myocardial oxygen supply, decreasing oxygen demand, and improving myocardial contraction or its electrical stability (Clausen 1977; Blomqvist 1983; Saltin 1990). That endurance exercise reduces oxygen demand and myocardial work is reflected in lowered heart rate and blood pressure at rest and a general reduction in sympathetic tone (Péronnet 1981; Palatini 1988). Notably, physical activity increases blood levels of high density lipoproteins, reduces blood levels of low density lipoproteins and fibrinogen, promotes the blood clearance of triglycerides, increases insulin sensitivity, and helps maintain normal glucose tolerance (Haskell 1984; Rauramaa 1984; Gordon 1989; Ernst 1991). Other likely acute and chronic mechanisms include a reduced tendency for platelet aggregation and increased fibrinolytic activity, increased diameter and dilating capacity of coronary arteries, increased collateral artery formation, reduced rates of progression of coronary artery atherosclerosis, and modification of deleterious effects of other personal characteristics and lifestyle habits (Richardson 1989; Blair 1990; Fuster 1992; Hambrecht 1993; Kestin 1993). All of these potential mechanisms, singly or in combination, can reduce the risk of CHD events.

Evidence from Animal Studies

Animal studies have demonstrated that moderate conditioning (endurance) exercise retards the development of coronary atherosclerosis. Kramsch and his associates (1981) compared treadmill-exercised and sedentary adult male *Macaca fascicularis* on an atherogenic diet for ischemic electrocardiographic (EKG) changes, angiographic signs of coronary narrowing, and for gross and microscopic myocardial changes. Moderate, sustained physical activity in these primates was accompanied by

1. Lowered heart rates at rest and after exercise
2. Increased heart size
3. A loss and regain of body weight (presumably, a sequential loss of body fat followed by a gain of body muscle)
4. Small increases in serum HDL cholesterol, and large decreases in both LDL and VLDL cholesterol
5. Little change in blood pressure levels

More importantly, with respect to coronary artery disease, moderate exercise led to reduced coronary intimal involvement, smaller lesion size (surface thickening), less collagen accumulation, and widened lumina, in contrast to findings in sedentary animals. Also, delayed lesion growth in coronary vessels was accompanied by similarly inhibited atherosclerotic changes in the aorta and other arteries of the exercised monkeys.

Exercise training of rats in which an experimental MI had been induced lowered heart rate and protected against ventricular dysrhythmias (Williams 1984). Noakes (1983), observing the effect of a period of treadmill exercise on the ventricular fibrillation threshold of the isolated myocardial fibers of rats, demonstrated that resistance of the heart to fibrillation was increased in these exercised rats as contrasted with such resistance in sedentary rats. Perhaps reductions in the number of myocardial alpha-receptors and muscarinic cholinergic receptors in exercise-trained rats contributes to the protection against arrhythmias (Williams 1984). Such findings are compatible with human data that physical activity protects against sudden unexpected cardiac death (Paffenbarger 1975; Siscovick 1984; Kohl 1992).

Physical Activity: Evidence from Human Studies

The evidence for a role of physical activity in the primary prevention of CHD in humans derives exclusively from observational studies. Although randomized, controlled clinical trials would allow for a more rigorous assessment of cause and effect, such studies have not been conducted because of feasibility issues related to compliance and cost.

The modern story of exercise and CHD began in 1949 when Morris and his colleagues in London first began to understand how both vocational and leisure-time physical activity relate to cardiovascular fitness and risk of CHD (Morris 1953). Initially they found that highly active conductors on London's double-decker buses were at lower risk for CHD than the bus drivers who worked sitting at the wheel; what disease the conductors did develop was less severe, and they were more likely to withstand an attack. Morris et al. (1953) also found that postmen delivering mail on foot had lower rates of CHD then sedentary supervisors and telephonists, and a gradient appeared for positions of intermediate physical activity.

Since the early research by Morris and coworkers, further studies of occupational or leisure physical activity and CHD rates have concerned farmers and nonfarmers (Zukel 1959; Pomrehn 1982); American letter carriers and mail clerks (Kahn 1963); American and Italian railroad trackmen and clerks (Taylor 1970; Menotti 1979); Israeli kibbutzim workers in various occupations (Brunner 1974); San Francisco cargo handlers and warehousemen (Paffenbarger 1975); those insured by the Health Insurance Plan of New York (Shapiro 1965); college students and alumni in various activities (Paffenbarger 1978); residents of Framingham, Massachusetts (Kannel 1986); American Cancer Society volunteers (Garfinkel 1988); Japanese-American men in Hawaii (Donahue 1988; Rodriquez 1994); and those from various regions of Denmark (Hein 1992), Finland (Punsar 1976; Salonen 1982; 1988; Lakka 1994), Holland (Magnus 1979), and Puerto Rico (Garcia-Palmieri 1982). While these studies showed lower CHD risk with higher exercise level, they often did not address potential confounding by cigarette smoking, diet, heredity, stress, or other factors (Curfman 1993). Many of these studies have been summarized by Powell et al. (1987) and Berlin and Colditz (1990).

Some studies have failed to show differences in CHD risks, such as those among groups of civil service workers in Los Angeles (Chapman 1957) and among industrial workers in Chicago (Stamler 1960). This result may have occurred because differences in physical activity on the job were insufficient, or because other influences such as leisure-time exercise were not taken into account (Berlin 1990). A 1-year follow-up of men comprising 16 culturally varied cohorts in seven countries produced mixed results (Keys 1980). Difficulties arise in defining or assessing physical activity levels in diverse international settings that complicate comparison within or among groups (Berlin 1990). On a global scale the relation between CHD and its predisposing characteristics is complex and may appear contradictory. Various lifestyles must be carefully characterized and closely studied if valid conclusions are to be drawn concerning them (Curfman 1993), but research in all countries and societies can provide valuable input toward a better understanding of CHD and its determinants.

Since many of the above cited observational studies were qualitative rather than quantitative in nature, the next series of paragraphs elaborate on findings from some of the more important and representative studies of exercise and CHD or CVD (Table 8.1).

British Civil Servants

In later study of leisure-time exercise levels of sedentary civil servants, Morris et al. (1973, 1980) devised a two-day diary-style report form, which, without advance notice, the civil servants were asked to fill out on a Monday morning with reference to their activities of the preceding Friday and Saturday. These seven-page, handwritten, 5-minute-by-5-minute diaries were submitted by 17,944 middle-aged men during the years 1968–1970 and carefully coded by researchers having no knowledge of the medical histories of the study subjects. Findings were based on analysis of 3,590 (a 20% sample) of the activity diaries. Health and mortality records were obtained from official sources and assessed by cross-tabulation with leisure-time physical activity levels coded from the personal diaries.

Between 1968 and 1978 there were 1,138 first clinical episodes of CHD, of which 475 were fatal, among men aged 40 to 65 years at time of activity survey. Among those who reported engaging in vigorous exercise (VE) sports, there were 66 first attacks, a rate of 3.1%, in contrast to 981 cases and a rate of 6.9% among men who reported no vigorous exercise. Fatal first attacks were less than half as likely for VE sports men as for sedentary men, the rates being 1.1% and 2.9% respectively ($p<.001$), and 0.65% and 1.6% for sudden deaths ($p<.01$). Similar trends were found in available data on civil servants who had retired. Of particular interest, the rise in mortality with age was markedly less among men who reported VE sports, and a similar divergence was even more pronounced for overall CHD incidence. Such evidence of a long-term effect and continuing habits of VE sports activity tend to refute the likelihood that observed differences were due to a selection process where men already ill chose not to engage in VE sports. A sample tally showed that 13% of men aged 40 to 54 and 10% aged 55–65 reported VE sports activity; seven years later 40% of these were still this active at least twice a week. Since the CHD rates for sedentary men continued to climb at a geometrically increasing pace while the rates for VE sports active men remained nearly level at all ages, the figures suggest a protective effect of maintained habitual vigorous exercise, not merely an initial selection of unhealthy and healthy individuals. Rather, the likelihood is that many of the men who did not engage in vigorous exercise chose to be sedentary not because of ill health, but because of indolence or conflicts in lifestyle.

It is undoubtedly true that the VE sports men may have had other protective advantages. They may have been less likely to smoke cigarettes, and diet, stress, and other risk patterns may have been more favorable than those of less active individuals. Nevertheless, the principal ''selection process'' that singled out the men with low risk of CHD in this study was simply their report of habitual engagement in vigorous exercise. The validity of this basis was demonstrated by their subsequent lower incidence of first clinical attacks of CHD within strata defined by presence as well as absence of other characteristics affecting risk (e.g., among smokers, as well as non-

Table 8.1. Relative Risks of Coronary Heart Disease (CHD) or Cardiovascular Disease (CVD), by Gradients of Physical Activity

A. Rates and relative risks of CHD[a] among 9,376 British civil servants aged 45–64 years at entry, in a ≥9-year follow-up, 1976–1986 (87,563 man-years), by patterns of sports play

Episodes of Sports Play in Past 4 Weeks	Vigorous Sports Play				Nonvigorous Sports Play			
	Man-years (%)	No. CHD Cases	Cases per 1000 Man-years	Relative Risk of CHD*	Man-years (%)	No. CHD Cases	Cases per 1000 Man-years	Relative Risk of CHD**
None	82	413	5.8	1.00	67	310	5.4	1.00
1–3	9	37	4.5	0.78	16	85	5.9	1.09
4–7	5	17	4.1	0.71	10	52	5.9	1.09
8–11	4	7	2.1	0.36	6	19	3.5	0.65
12+					1	8	6.8	1.26

B. Rates and relative risks of CHD[b],*** among 16,936 Harvard alumni aged 35–74 years at entry, in a 10-year follow-up, 1962–1972, by physical activity in kilocalories per week

Physical Activity Index in kcal/wk	Man-years of Observation	No. CHD Cases	CHD Rate per 10,000 Man-years	Relative Risk of CHD
<2,000	56,459	307	57.9	1.00
2,000+	38,027	122	35.3	0.61
Undetermined	23,184	143	47.6	0.82

176

C. Rates and relative risks of CVD death[c] among 14,623 Harvard alumni aged 45–84 years at entry, in a 12-year follow-up, 1977–1988, by physical activity in kilocalories per week and patterns of sports play

Physical Activity Index in kcal/wk	Man-years (M-Y) %	No. CVD Deaths	CVD Deaths per 10,000 M-Y	Relative Risk of CVD Death	p-value
<1,000	31	512	78.8	1.00	—
1,000–2,499	39	317	56.3	.71	<0.001
2,500+	30	170	43.0	.54	<0.001
Sports play					
None	12	264	83.0	1.00	—
Light only	11	187	66.0	.79	0.017
Moderately vigorous	77	506	52.4	.63	<0.001

D. Relative risks of nonfatal myocardial infarction and sudden death[a] among New Zealand men and women aged 35–64 years in a case-control study, 1981–1982, by duration of regular exercise

Study Subjects	No. Subjects	Relative Risk of CHD by Duration of Regular Exercise in Years				
		None	<5	5–10	11+	Any
Men						
Control subjects	653					
MI patients	363	1.0	1.2	0.5****	0.2****	0.4****
Sudden deaths	130	1.0	1.9	0.5	0.1****	0.4****
Women						
Control subjects	390					
MI patients	100	1.0	0.9	0.7	0.2****	0.1****
Sudden deaths	32	1.0	—	—	0.2	0.1****

E. Rates and relative risks of CHD***** among 12,138 men aged 35–57 years at entry in the Multiple Risk Factor Intervention Trial, in an 8-year follow-up, 1973–1981, by thirds of leisure-time physical activity in kilocalories per day

Thirds of Leisure-Time Physical Activity in kcal/day	No. of CHD Cases	CHD Rate per 1,000 Men	Relative Risk
Low	286	71.8	1.00
Moderate	260	63.5	0.88
High	235	58.0	0.81

(continued on following page)

Table 8.1. Continued

F. Relative risks of CHD[a] among 2,548 U.S. railroad workers in a 17- to 20-year follow-up, 1957–1977, by levels of leisure-time physical activity in kilocalories per week

Leisure-Time Physical Activity, kcal/week	Relative Risk of CHD Mortality (95% CI)
3,632	1.0
1,372	1.05 (1.00–1.11)
554	1.11 (1.00–1.23)
40	1.28 (0.99–1.63)

G. Relative risks of CHD mortality among 7,630 men aged 40–59 years at entry in the British Regional Heart Study, in an 8-year follow-up, by levels of physical activity

Physical Activity	Number of Men (%)	Relative Risk of CHD	
		Adjusted[e] (95% CI)	Further Adjusted[f] (95% CI)
Inactive	686 (9.0)	1.0	1.0
Occasional	2345 (30.7)	0.8 (0.5–1.2)	0.9 (0.5–1.3)
Light	1761 (23.1)	0.8 (0.5–1.2)	0.9 (0.6–1.4)
Moderate	1205 (15.8)	0.4 (0.2–0.8)	0.5 (0.2–0.8)
Moderately vigorous	1120 (14.7)	0.4 (0.2–0.8)	0.5 (0.3–0.9)
Vigorous	513 (6.7)	0.8 (0.4–1.4)	0.9 (0.5–1.8)

[a]Adjusted for age differences.

[b]Adjusted for differences in age, cigarette habit, and blood pressure status.

[c]Adjusted for differences in age, cigarette habit, hypertension, obesity, alcohol consumption, early parental mortality, and selected chronic diseases (CHD, stroke, non-skin cancer, chronic lung disease, diabetes, and cancer).

[d]Adjusted for differences in age, cigarette habit, blood pressure, and serum cholesterol.

[e]Adjusted for differences in age, cigarette habit, body mass index, and social class.

[f]Also adjusted for systolic blood pressure, total cholesterol, HDL cholesterol, FEV1, breathlessness, and heart rate.

*p of trend <.005.

**p of trend >.05.

***p < .001.

****p < .05.

*****p of trend < .01.

178

smokers). It would be remarkable if vigorous exercise per se had nothing to do with this result, even though acting through its effects on various physiologic systems. The absence of such findings in some other studies must invite questions as to the adequacy of their modes of assessing exercise or even defining it, in contrast to the techniques that were used in this investigation. There was advantage in having a "captive" population of civil servants who could be "invited" to fill out "on official time" a surprise Monday-morning report of their recent exercise activities, and their subsequent health records also were quite firmly available for study. The exercise diaries may have been a tedious task to review, but their reliability as a sampling instrument in this study population was probably good. However, one potential limitation of this study was the inability of investigators to examine dietary differences among those active and inactive.

Morris and colleagues (1990) have extended their studies further to include men who worked at sedentary jobs and obtained most of their physical exercise during their leisure time as determined from mail questionnaires in 1976 (Table 8.1A). Their observations on lifestyles and health records of British civil servants concerned men in the executive grade who often were habitual gardeners, do-it-yourself handymen, and, less often, those involved in recreational sports after work or on holidays. No evidence was found in prospective data to support the idea that these men with high levels of physical activity would experience less CHD than otherwise similar men with low activity levels. Instead, only men engaging in VE sports showed a reduced incidence of the disease. Table 8.1A gives their rates and relative risks of CHD by patterns of sports play characterized by frequency and intensity. Sports defined as vigorous demanded 7.5 kcal/min or 6 metabolic equivalents (METs) or greater, while less intense recreational activities were considered nonvigorous. Frequency was ranked by the number of episodes of play during the four weeks prior to study entry. Only 33% of the total man-years represented any sports play, and 18% VE sports play. Increasing frequency of the latter was associated with a gradient reduction in risk of CHD. Not shown here, men aged 45 to 54 years required more energy expenditure to achieve beneficial effects than their elders, 55 to 64 years. Nonvigorous sports play in any quantity showed no benefit over no sports play at all. It is unclear whether quantity of activity, or intensity of activity is important for CHD risk. Findings from different studies have been inconsistent; this may result largely from the difficulty with which physical activity assessment can be precisely measured in epidemiologic studies.

Other observations by Morris and coworkers (1990) indicated clearly that to be "beneficial," the exercise had to be current, not historical in nature. Rates of CHD were similarly high among men who played no vigorous sports previously and those who stopped play from 20 to more than 40 years before. More interestingly, men who reported being vigorously active at study entry had the same low incidence over the 8-year follow-up, whether or not they had been physically active previously. The rates of CHD in men reporting vigorous sports play at least once a week at study entry were 3.2 and 3.0 per 1,000 man-years in those with and without such a history, respectively, as compared with 5.8 per 1,000 among men who were not vigorous sports players at study entry. As in previous investigations, these differences persisted after accounting for smoking habit, body mass index, and personal and family medical history. Dietary data were unavailable.

U.S. College Alumni

Table 8.1B gives results from a U.S. study (somewhat comparable to that among British civil servants) of chronic disease risks among college alumni who had been undergraduate students at Harvard University in the years 1916–1950 (Paffenbarger 1978). Baseline data were obtainable from archives of student health examinations and other university records, and follow-up information through the help of the university alumni office, leading to mortality data from official death certificates. Eventually, beginning in the 1960s, a series of self-administered mail questionnaires were issued to obtain information from alumni about their adult lifestyles and health histories, including exercise habits and occurrence of physician-diagnosed nonfatal CHD, among other data. Like the British civil servant diaries, these questionnaires asked study subjects to volunteer information as to their habitual sports or recreational activities and certain other exercise such as stair-climbing and walking (Lee 1992). The alumni were a more geographically dispersed population than the British civil servants, and hence the American data-gathering systems (such as mail questionnaires) were somewhat less neat. However, the large, highly educated population with quite detailed baseline information and a long span of subsequent time for follow-up analyses have provided opportunities for epidemiologic studies of considerable interest, especially with reference to lifestyle and CHD risk. For example, cross-tabular evaluations of student athleticism and alumnus exercise pattern versus CHD incidence have shown that the benefits of sports activity in youth tend to fade in adult years unless adequate exercise habits are continued during middle and later life (Paffenbarger 1978). This finding supports the British view that vigorous exercise, and not mere constitutional selection, is responsible for the observed reduced risk of CHD among physically active individuals.

The college alumni health studies used an index to evaluate weekly exercise effort. This composite index was established from questionnaire responses concerning stair climbing, walking, and leisure-time sports and recreational activities. Each activity, such as the various types of sports play, was rated in energy-output kilocalories per minute, and individual index totals were expressed in kilocalories per week. A physical activity index of 2,000 kcal/week, which left about two-thirds of the alumni on the low side of that figure, was chosen as the breakpoint between low and high exercise rating. The latter definition of adequate exercise was subsequently refined by noting whether vigorous ("strenuous") sports rated at 10 kcal/min were included or absent. On the average (Table 8.1B), rate of CHD was 39% lower among vigorously active alumni than among those indexed by fewer than 2,000 kcal of energy output per week, whether or not other adverse characteristics were present during their study days.

When alumni were cross-classified by vigorous sports play and total of other reported exercise expressed in kilocalories per week, there was a steady increase in CHD rate from 30 per 10,000 man-years for the most active alumni (>2,000 kcal/week) to 72 per 10,000 for the least active (<500 kcal/week), with an increment of added benefit associated with the presence of vigorous sports play versus its absence (Paffenbarger 1994). Results were similar in each 10-year age bracket included.

A multiple logistic regression analysis of the percent reduction in risk of first CHD attack associated with the weekly total of kilocalories expended in stair climbing, walking, light sports play, or vigorous sports activity controlled for age, cigarette habit, blood pressure status, body mass index, stature, and parental history of MI. There was a reduction in CHD risk as energy output from each type of exercise was increased, adjusting for the other three kinds of activity (Paffenbarger 1994). This analysis also revealed an extra benefit attached to vigorous sports as compared with less demanding types of exercise, at any given level of kilocalorie expenditure.

In 1977 these Harvard alumni were queried again as to their physical activity, personal characteristics, and other social habits. Classified by a variety of personal characteristics and lifestyle patterns, roughly 15,000 men were observed with relation to fatal CVD, determined from death certificates, in the ensuing 12 years (Paffenbarger 1993, 1994). Walking, stair-climbing, and sports play or recreational activity were combined as before into an index of energy expenditure. Sports and recreational activities were dichotomized into light and moderately vigorous recreation, at an intensity level of 4.5 METs. As seen in Table 8.1C, there was an inverse gradient relation between physical activity index and CVD risk, with the most active men (expending >2,500 kcal/week) at 46% lower risk of mortality than the least active (<1,000 kcal/week). Also, light sports play (including recreational activity) was accompanied by a 21% lower risk, and moderately vigorous (also including recreational activity) by a 37% lower risk, than the risk for not playing sports at all.

Uncertainty remains as to whether quantity alone or intensity of physical activity is of primary importance. Separating alumni into those whose activities require less than 4.5 METs, and those who include some activities requiring 4.5 METs or more, Figure 8.1 shows that with increasing levels of energy expenditure, both light and moderately vigorous activities are associated with a reduced risk of CVD mortality. But at any given level of energy expenditure, at least up to, say, 4,000 kcal/week, the risk tends to be lower with moderately vigorous than with more casual activities.

One potential limitation of those observations among alumni is the inability to take into account any differences in dietary habits between active and inactive alumni.

New Zealand Men and Women

As seen in Table 8.1D, Scragg et al. (1987) found that the risks of MI and sudden death were progressively reduced among New Zealand men and women, aged 45–64, who habitually had engaged in vigorous sports play or recreational exercise (such as running) for at least 5 years, after which their relative risk dropped to half that of nonexercisers as the 10-year mark passed. After additional time, the risks were 0.20 or less for both men and women. The longer intervals seem to imply that the exercise had become a well-established habit and had been sufficient to maintain cardiovascular fitness at a protective level. These observations were adjusted for age differences; further consideration of smoking, hypertension, and serum cholesterol did not materially change findings.

The Multiple Risk Factor Intervention Trial (MRFIT)

Table 8.1E presents data from MRFIT, as described by Leon and his associates (1987). Those high-risk (for CVD), predominantly sedentary men, were categorized into thirds

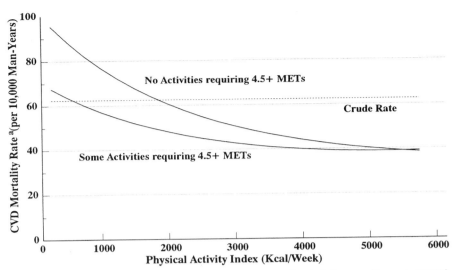

^aAdjusted for differences in age, cigarette habit, hypertension, obesity, alcohol consumption, early parental mortality, and selected chronic diseases (CHD,stroke,non-skin cancer,chronic lung disease,diabetes).

Fig. 8.1. Mortality rates from cardiovascular disease (CVD) per 10,000 man-years of observation among 14,623 Harvard alumni aged 45–84 at entry and followed from 1977 through 1988, by a continuous physical activity index in two levels of physical activity intensity. The data are adjusted for differences in age, cigarette habit, hypertension, obesity, alcohol consumption, early parental mortality, and selected chronic diseases (CHD, stroke, diabetes, chronic lung disease, and cancers other than skin cancer).

by levels of energy expenditure in kilocalories per day from a leisure-time physical activity questionnaire. In a 7-year follow-up period, the middle group of men was found to be more than twice as active as was the low group, and the high group was more than twice as active as the middle group. A consistent gradient of reduction in risk of CHD was seen across the three physical activity thirds of the MRFIT population. Investigators did not take dietary differences into consideration, although differences in serum cholesterol levels were adjusted for. No added benefit was recognized from what was described as vigorous effort over more moderate activities, in contrast to results from the studies of British civil servants. These results may have been due to less precise assessment of the intensity or frequency of activity in the MRFIT men.

U.S. Railroad Workers

Slattery and colleagues (1989) studied leisure-time physical activity among male U.S. railroad workers for relation to death from CHD in a 17- to 20-year follow-up period (Table 8.1F). Some 2,500 men who had been queried as to activity patterns and examined for other characteristics between 1957 and 1960 were reexamined from 1962 to 1964, and followed until 1977. The relative risk of death was 1.28 for men who were essentially sedentary (expending <40 kcal/week) as compared with very active men. These analyses were adjusted for age, cigarette habit, blood pressure, and serum cholesterol.

British Regional Heart Study

Table 8.1G gives data from observations by Shaper and Wannamethee (1991), who had been examining the relation between physical activity and CHD incidence among 7,630 middle-aged men, randomly chosen from general medical practices in 24 British communities representative of the socioeconomic distribution of men in Great Britain. Using interview techniques, histories of leisure-time physical activities and other life-style habits were obtained. These data were analyzed according to a complex classification scheme of total energy expenditure and its intensity and the men divided into six ordinal groups, where 9% were considered inactive, 31% occasionally active, 23% lightly active, 16% moderately active, 15% moderately vigorous, and 7% vigorous. Follow-up of those 40 to 59 years of age at entry showed CHD risks to be lower with increased physical activity, the rates for moderate or moderately vigorous men being less than half the rates of those for inactive men. Vigorously active individuals experienced higher rates, roughly similar to those for men classified as occasionally or lightly active; however, this finding was based on a small group of men. These results were not adjusted for dietary differences, but total and HDL cholesterol were accounted for, as was cigarette smoking.

This population of British men included 1,916 men with preexisting CHD who were divided into those with and without symptomatic CHD. Men classified as having symptomatic CHD experienced lower rates of CHD recurrence at occasional, light, and moderate levels of energy expenditure but an increased rate at moderately vigorous levels and above. Men with preexisting CHD who entered the study as asymptomatic of CHD experienced a higher rate of CHD recurrence at light and moderate levels than those who were inactive, but those at moderately vigorous and vigorous levels had a lower rate of CHD (not shown). Although based on small numbers, these data suggest that vigorous activities among high-risk men may lead to slightly higher rates of CHD than corresponding rates for less vigorous, regular physical activities.

Overall, the vigorously active men, meaning in large part those who reported sports play at least once weekly, had lower CHD rates than men who played no sports. When sports players were excluded from the analysis (not shown), there remained a significant inverse relation between levels of physical activity (nonvigorous) and CHD incidence, findings contrary to those among British civil servants where a gradient was observed only for vigorous sports (Morris 1990). Again, this difference may have arisen from differences in classification of physical activity, particularly with respect to vigorous exercise.

Other Studies and Comments

Findings to support the concept that physical activity protects against the occurrence of MI and both nonfatal and fatal CHD are corroborated further in recent studies from Finland (Lakka 1994) and Hawaii (Rodriguez 1994).

These data provide good evidence that physical activity does reduce incidence of CHD. The inability to take dietary differences into consideration is a potential limitation of these studies. However, it is unclear whether physically active persons consume healthier diets than those inactive. In a study conducted among men and women in Utah, Slattery et al. (1988b) observed that total caloric consumption, determined using a quantitative food frequency questionnaire, increased with increasing physical activity, although the percentage of total calories consumed as fat, protein, or carbohydrate did not vary across fourths of physical activity. Among Seventh-Day Adventists in California (Lindsted 1991), there was no clear correlation between level of physical activity and a healthy dietary pattern (both self-reported). Several of the studies described previously did adjust for differences in blood lipid profile; however, this might represent "overadjustments," since a favorable change in lipid profile represents one of the proposed mechanisms of benefit for CHD.

A further drawback to these studies is the lack of women included as subjects; the vast majority of studies investigated only men. Findings from Scragg et al. (1987) suggest that observations in women appear to be comparable to men (Table 8.1D). Other studies showing an apparent benefit of physical activity against CHD risk in women include those conducted among Israeli kibbutzim workers in various occupations (Brunner 1974), women insured by the Health Insurance Plan of New York (Shapiro 1965), residents of Framingham, Massachusetts (Kannel 1986), American Cancer Society volunteers (Garfinkel 1988), and women from various regions of Finland (Salonen 1982), and Holland (Magnus 1979).

Physical Fitness: Evidence from Human Studies

While physical activity (a behavior) is a dynamic, ongoing concept, physical fitness (a condition with a heritability of perhaps 10% to 25%) is a static or cross-sectional concept. Yet they are interrelated because fitness establishes limitations for physical activity, and activity modifies fitness from one time to another. A number of studies have revealed important relations of fitness to health. As with physical activity, the evidence for a role of physical fitness in the primary prevention of CHD derives only from observational studies. Findings point in the same direction as the physical activity findings we have just reviewed.

The interrelation between physical activity and fitness was addressed rather effectively in the MRFIT studies (Leon 1987), where baseline physical fitness determined from exercise treadmill tests was compared by thirds of leisure-time physical activity. Both treadmill time and the proportion of subjects achieving a target heart rate were significantly higher with increasing level of leisure-time physical activity, whereas resting and intermediate exercise heart rates were lower. The upper one-third of subjects by physical activity had normal or average estimated mean functional capacity, but the bottom one-third was below average in fitness. Thus the relative risks of CHD in the MRFIT men corresponded to their levels of both physical activity and physical fitness. Findings from recent and representative studies of fitness and CHD or CVD are given in Table 8.2.

Table 8.2. Relative Risks of Coronary Heart Disease (CHD) or Cardiovascular Disease (CVD) by Gradients of Physical Fitness

A. Relative risks of myocardial infarction (MI)[a] among 2,779 Los Angeles public safety officers aged 35–54 years at entry in an 8-year follow-up, 1971–1978, by levels of physical work capacity in high-risk subjects

Age-Matched Men with Selected Characteristic	Work Capacity	No. MI Cases	Relative Risk of MI (95% CI)
Systolic BP above median level	Low	19	5.1 (1.7–21.7)
	High	3	1.0
Serum cholesterol above median level	Low	22	4.4 (1.7–14.9)
	High	4	1.0
Cigarette smoker	Low	22	3.4 (1.4–10.1)
	High	5	1.0
Any two or all three of above	Low	N/A	6.6 (2.3–27.8)
	High	N/A	1.0

B. Rates and relative risks of CHD death[b]* among 2,014 Norwegian industry and government workers aged 40–59 years at entry, in a 7-year follow-up, 1972–1982, by fourths of fitness

Fourths of Fitness	No. CHD Deaths	CHD Death Rate (%)	Relative Risk CHD Death
1 (Low)	29	5.7	1.00
2	12	2.4	0.42
3	11	2.2	0.39
4 (High)	6	1.1	0.19

C. Rates and relative risks of CHD and CVD death[b] among 4,276 Lipid Research Clinics men aged 30–69 years at entry, in an 8.5-year folow-up, 1972–1984, by fourths of fitness

Fourths of Fitness	CHD Death Rate (%)*	CVD Death Rate (%)*	Relative Risk, First Quarter: Fourth Quarter (95% CI) CHD	CVD
1 (Low)	1.69	2.21	6.5 (1.5–28.7)	8.5 (2.0–36.7)
2	0.91	1.56		
3	0.91	1.30		
4 (High)	0.26	0.26		

(continued on following page)

Los Angeles Public Safety Officers

The study by Peters et al. (1983) of physical fitness and risk of MI among 2,779 Los Angeles fire and police personnel touches on a number of relations between fitness and cardiovascular health. Continued employment in these stressful jobs was contingent on maintenance of fitness and avoidance of debilitating disease. Physical fitness testing included spirometry, bicycle ergometry, resting and exercise electrocardiograms, and assessments of flexibility and strength. Below-median physical fitness dou-

Table 8.2. Continued

D. Rates and relative risks of CHD and CVD deaths[b] among 2,431 U.S. railroad workers aged 22–79 years at entry, in a 20-year follow-up, 1957–1977, by treadmill exercise test heart rate

Heart Rate	No. Men	Deaths per 100 Men***		Relative Risk of Death***	
		CHD	CVD	CHD	CVD
128+	526	13.2	18.7	1.00	1.00
116–127	692	11.6	15.7	0.88	0.84
106–115	665	8.7	12.6	0.66	0.67
<106	548	9.1	12.4	0.69	0.66

E. Rates and relative risks of CVD death[b] among 10,244 middle-aged men and 3,120 middle-aged women from the Cooper Clinic in an 8+-year follow-up, by fifths of fitness

Fifths of Fitness	CVD Deaths per 10,000 Man-years	Relative Risk of CVD Death
Men (66 CVD deaths)		
1 (Low)	24.6	1.00
2 to 3	7.8	0.32
4 to 5 (High)	3.1	0.13
Women (7 CVD deaths)		*p* of trend < .05
1 (Low)	7.4	1.00
2 to 3	2.9	0.39
4 to 5 (High)	0.8	0.11
		p of trend > .05

F. Rates and relative risks of CHD death[c] among 4,999 men aged 40–59 years at entry in the Copenhagen Male Study, in a 17-year follow-up, by fifths of fitness and levels of leisure-time physical activity

Fifths of Fitness	High or Medium Physical Activity***			Low Physical Activity**		
	No. Men	CHD Death Rate (%)	Relative Risk CHD Death	No. Men	CHD Death Rate (%)	Relative Risk CHD Death
1 (Low)	732	7.2	1.00	191	10.1	1.00
2	829	5.0	0.69	151	11.7	1.16
3	849	5.8	0.81	143	4.4	0.44
4	877	5.3	0.74	114	10.3	1.02
5 (High)	900	3.7	0.51	77	14.1	1.40

[a]Adjusted for differences in age, and where relevant, cigarette habit, blood pressure, and serum cholesterol.

[b]Adjusted for age differences.

[c]Adjusted for differences in age, cigarette smoking, and social class.

*p of trend <.001.

**p of trend >.05.

***p of trend <.01.

bled the risk of MI during the 8-year follow-up over the risk for men with above-median fitness. Incidence was tripled among 196 men who were unable to complete their exercise tests.

Low physical fitness scores did not predict higher risk of MI unless the men also had above-median levels of systolic blood pressure or serum cholesterol or were smokers (Table 8.2A). Men with low fitness plus two or three of these other adverse characteristics were at 6 or 7 times the risk of experiencing a MI within the next few years of follow-up. Conversely, men with any of those other characteristics were deemed to be protected against MI if they maintained above-average fitness.

Norwegian Industry and Government Workers

Lie and colleagues (1985) studied fitness in relation to incidence of CHD among 2,014 men working in private companies or government agencies in Oslo, Norway, during a 7-year follow-up (Table 8.2B). Subjects in four age groups were categorized into fourths by estimated levels of fitness derived from submaximal ergometer tests rated by cumulative work and body weight, or $km \cdot min^{-1} \cdot kg^{-1}$. Although fitness declined with age, the most fit men in each age group had lower blood pressures, lower heart rates, lower serum lipids, higher maximal heart rates and maximal blood pressures during exercise, and higher spirographic results. Also, they smoked less than did those in lower fitness quartiles. Gradient patterns were generally consistent but not always significant. Interview-assessed physical activity data were considered too fragmentary to establish relations with physical fitness, but leisure-time levels of physical activity and sports play tended to parallel levels of physical fitness by fourths. Although unable to ascertain whether physical fitness modified influences of physical activity on risks of CHD, the investigators concluded that physical fitness as assessed in this study was a very strong inverse predictor of risk of fatal CHD. Because the upper fourth of fitness had a CHD risk as low as that of a comparison group of highly fit expert cross-country skiers (now shown), the possibility of a threshold, or optimum, level of fitness benefit was suggested. Physical activity sufficient to achieve a training effect was advocated for asymptomatic middle-aged men in the belief that it might help maintain a high enough level of fitness to protect against CHD.

Lipid Research Clinics Study

Ekelund et al. (1988) reported an 8.5-year follow-up for CHD and CVD mortality among 4,276 Lipid Research Clinics Study men, aged 30 to 69 at entry, who had undergone treadmill exercise testing and assessment of potential predictors of CHD at baseline. The heart rate at stage 2 of a submaximal exercise test and time-on-treadmill were used as fitness measures. Table 8.2C shows that the cumulative mortality was substantially higher in the fourth of subjects with the lowest level of fitness than in the most fit fourth—6.5 times higher for CHD mortality and 8.5 times higher for all CVD mortality. In multivariate analyses, adjustment for other covariates (cigarette smoking, blood pressure level, and lipoprotein-cholesterol profile) did not change the relative risks meaningfully, indicating that the relations between physical fitness and death from both CHD and CVD were independent of those other variables.

U.S. Railroad Workers

Slattery and Jacobs (1988a) reported a 20-year follow-up for CHD mortality, CVD mortality, and all-cause mortality among 2,431 U.S. railroad workers aged 22 to 79 at entry. They had undergone treadmill fitness tests in 1957–1960 and 1,914 were retested in 1962–1964 (Table 8.2D). Exercise heart rate was the strongest predictor of CVD risk and mortality, but also was most closely related to exercise systolic blood pressure. The investigators decided that the greater CVD risk associated with high exercise heart rate was due largely to the higher blood pressure levels. Like the other recent studies of physical fitness mentioned previously, this one concluded that long-range investigations of the relation between physical activity, physical fitness, and health are needed to determine whether physical activity reduces risks of CHD and premature mortality by enhancing physical fitness, or by some other mechanisms such as metabolic changes.

Cooper Institute for Aerobics Research, Texas

Blair and his colleagues from the Cooper Institute for Aerobics Research in Dallas, Texas, assessed fitness by treadmill performance in 10,244 men and 3,120 women, aged 20–60+. Subjects were followed for an average of 8+ years, totaling 110,482 person-years, for CVD mortality (Blair 1989). During follow-up, 66 such deaths occurred among men, seven in women. CVD mortality rates were lowest (3.1 and 0.8 per 10,000 person-years, respectively, for men and women) among the most fit, and highest (24.6 and 7.4 per 10,000 person-years, respectively, for men and women) among the least fit (Table 8.2E), paralleling closely the results from studies of physical activity levels and mortality. The data in women are based on very small numbers and thus unstable, but appear to reflect findings in men.

Copenhagen Male Study

Hein and his associates in the Copenhagen Male Study (1992) examined the independent and joint effects of leisure-time physical activity and physical fitness on risk of fatal CHD in a 17-year follow-up, 1970–1987. A total of 4,999 men aged 40 to 59 were classified into fifths of fitness measured by maximal bicycle ergometry, and into two levels of leisure-time physical activity: the 15% of men most sedentary and the 85% more active. As seen in Table 8.2F, the CHD death rates for sedentary men were generally higher than for more active men. But death rates were inversely related to fitness fifths only among men who were moderately to highly active. That is, in men with the same level of fitness capacity, only those who were moderately or highly physically active in leisure time had lower CHD mortality experiences, regardless of their fitness level. From these observations it would seem that sedentary living is a more important determinant of cardiovascular health than is cardiopulmonary fitness.

Other Studies and Comments

The findings concerning physical fitness and CHD described here are corroborated by studies in other populations (Gyntelberg 1980; Wilhelmsen 1981; Erikssen 1986;

Sobolski 1987; Sandvik 1993; Lakka 1994). These data suggest that studies of physical fitness should be broadened to whole-body fitness, which involves metabolic and other body systems as well as the cardiovascular system. Many questions about whether and how physical activity influences fitness and health thus might be answered more readily and the mechanisms of each better understood.

As with the studies on physical activity, a potential limitation of the studies on physical fitness is the lack of dietary data, which may confound findings. Further, there are few data on women. Of the studies on physical fitness and risk of CHD or CVD, only Blair et al. (1989) included women as subjects. The number of CVD deaths among women in this study was very small; based on these limited data, findings in women appear to parallel those for men.

Hazards of Exercise

Sudden unexpected cardiac death occasionally occurs during or shortly after an acute bout of exercise, and more commonly than during sedentary periods (Vuori 1978; Thompson 1982). Siscovick and his colleagues (1984) in King County, Washington, compared 133 men without known CHD or other chronic diseases but who suffered primary cardiac arrest, with 133 randomly selected community control subjects as to recent and habitual levels of physical activity. Information provided by wives of decedents and by the controls indicated an increased risk of sudden death during physical activity, with a markedly increased risk among those men who infrequently engaged in moderately vigorous activity in their leisure time. The data indicated a relative risk of 3.6 during activity for men without a habitual pattern of high-intensity activity as compared with men who averaged more than two hours weekly in vigorous activities. More importantly, the rate of sudden cardiac death was considerably lower overall among those men who engaged in more frequent physical activity than the corresponding rate for men less active.

Heavy physical exertion also has been shown capable of precipitating nonfatal MIs, especially in subjects habitually sedentary. Mittelman and his colleagues (1993) interviewed 1,228 MI patients as to the time, kind, and intensity of physical exertion in the 26 hours before onset of MI. The investigators compared the frequencies of exertion at a level of 6 or more metabolic equivalents during each of the 26 hours, at prior times for self-matched MI patients, and at corresponding times for a small sample of population-based control subjects. The overall risk of MI that accompanied heavy exertion in the hour before onset was six times the risk that accompanied heavy exertion at other times, suggesting a triggering effect from exercise. But an inverse graded effect of risk was observed with number of times the men habitually exercised each week, indicating a protective effect of exercise against MI incidence. That is, these data suggest that people who exercise regularly have both a lower overall risk of MI, and a lower risk that any infarction they do sustain would be precipitated by heavy physical exertion.

Similar findings were forthcoming from a study of all MI patients admitted to a large hospital in Berlin and from monitoring the 330,000 residents of Augsburg, Germany, 1989–1991 (Willich 1993). Interviews with 1,194 MI patients and an equal number of control subjects revealed that 7.1% of patients were exerting themselves at a level of 6 or more METs at the onset of infarction, as compared with 3.9% of controls at the corresponding time. Comparison of patients in the hour before infarction with themselves at a prior time showed the same order of relative risk for MI, namely, 2.1. Again, patients who exercised regularly had a significantly lower risk of MI than those who did not, providing further support for the hypothesis of a protective effect from physical activity.

Strength of Evidence of Benefits of Physical Activity and Fitness

All of the above-cited studies are observational in nature, with the established shortcomings generally acknowledged—selection bias, unstudied and unrecognized confounders, small numbers, short periods of follow-up, and other methodological problems in data collection and statistical analysis. It seems unlikely, however, that an analysis of the effect of physical activity or physical fitness on CVD incidence by randomized clinical trials will ever be undertaken. Although this would afford a more rigorous assessment of cause and effect relations, such trials may not be feasible given the ethical issues involved, and the quite intractable problems of high cost and subject noncompliance resulting in risks of misclassification. Given the consistency of these observational data, however, the conclusion that physical activity can reduce risks of CHD seems warranted.

Guidelines for Exercise Prescription

Appendix A contains guidelines for clinicians wishing to prescribe a safe and effective exercise program designed to reduce CHD risk.

When developing an exercise program, the foremost consideration, obviously, is an individual's health status. According to American College of Sports Medicine guidelines (1991), it is unnecessary for asymptomatic, apparently healthy men aged 40 years or younger and women aged 50 years or younger to undergo medical evaluation prior to embarking on a vigorous exercise program. However, such evaluation (medical examination and symptom-limited exercise stress-test) should be performed on higher risk men and women, regardless of age. Higher risk persons are defined as those with two or more of these major coronary risk factors: cigarette smoking, a history of coronary or other atherosclerotic disease in parents or siblings before age 55 years, hypertension, diabetes mellitus, serum cholesterol ≥ 6.20 mmol/l (240 mg/dl). For persons with established cardiac, pulmonary, and metabolic diseases, medical evaluation also should be carried out prior to beginning an exercise program. Medical supervision during the exercise program, if of high intensity, may be necessary for such individuals, and annual exercise testing to monitor patients with coronary artery disease is important (Fletcher 1992).

Ideally, an exercise program is designed to improve health status (including increasing exercise tolerance) and to reduce risk for CHD. However, the biggest challenge may be to ensure that such an exercise program is maintained, and incorporated into a person's lifestyle. To maximize this possibility, the clinician should attempt to identify barriers to exercise—such as previously recommended exercise programs that may have been unenjoyable or unacceptable, time constraints, cultural background, socioeconomic status, etc.—and get the participant to initiate some form of activity that is beneficial to health and, at the same time, acceptable to the participant. In general, *any* physical activity is better than none, and more (to a reasonable limit, which currently is not well defined; see Appendix for details) is better than less. The prior activity status of the participant should be one factor to consider. It is pointless to recommend aerobic exercise at least 3 times a week, for 30 minutes, at 60% to 70% of maximal capacity, to an individual who has been totally sedentary previously; he or she is unlikely to adhere to such a program. A more gradual approach may be more likely to succeed. The participant's goals should also be assessed. For example, someone whose primary goal is to lose weight should be recommended a program that offers aerobic exercise at lower intensity and longer duration (in addition to dietary counseling). However, one who is fit, and whose goal is to develop strength might be recommended a high intensity, short-duration physical training program. Further details are provided in the Appendix. In general, for someone who previously has been sedentary, we recommended starting off prudently and progressing to increasing levels of activity gradually. Persons accustomed to a greater degree of physical activity may start off at a higher level, but progress still should be gradual. Periodic medical evaluation should be made as the health status of an individual changes.

Cost Effectiveness

Of the major personal characteristics that increase CHD risk, physical inactivity is, by far, the most prevalent (Division of Chronic Disease Control and Community Intervention, National Center for Chronic Disease Prevention and Health Promotion 1993; Shephard 1990). Hahn et al. (1990) estimated that of all CHD deaths occurring in 1986, a total of 205,254 were attributable to never or irregularly engaging in physical activity, a number exceeding the 148,879 attributable to cigarette smoking, 171,121 to hypertension, 190,456 to obesity, but fewer than the 253,194 attributed to elevated serum cholesterol. Additionally, the cost to society—including medical services and lost productivity—of physical inactivity was estimated at $5.7 billion, again exceeding the cost of smoking, hypertension, and obesity, but not elevated serum cholesterol. Hatziandreu et al. (1988) performed a cost effectiveness analysis to estimate the economic implications of a physical activity program (specifically, jogging at a level of 2,000 kcal/week) in preventing CHD in two hypothetical cohorts—one inactive, one active—of 1,000 men each, aged 35 years. Over a 30-year period, exercising regularly resulted in 78 fewer CHD deaths and the gain of 1,138 quality-adjusted life-years (QALY). For each QALY gained, the direct cost was $1,395 and the total, $11,313, comparing favorably with other intervention strategies for CHD prevention. The costs factored into these analyses included:

1. Direct cost of exercise: that of equipment for running (clothes, shoes, etc.), and the cost of counseling a patient to exercise during a routine physician visit.
2. Indirect cost of exercise: assumed to be five hours a week of preparation and exercise time. The cost of time was weighted according to the proportion who would enjoy exercise (55%)—assumed without cost, the proportion neutral towards exercise (10%)—$4.50/hour, or half the 1985 hourly wage and the proportion disliking exercise (35%)—$9.00/hour.
3. Direct medial cost of injury sustained during exercise.
4. Indirect cost of injury, or that of time lost.
5. Direct lifetime cost estimates for CHD: including emergency assistance, hospitalization, follow-up care (office visits, tests, medication) and possible coronary angiography and coronary artery bypass grafting.
6. Indirect lifetime cost for CHD, or loss of earnings due to disability and premature death.

In an analysis of the association between physical activity and longevity in men, Paffenbarger et al. (1986a) estimated that for men aged 35 to 70 at study entry, the number of added years of life, truncated at age 80, associated with expending ≥2,000 kcal/week in physical activity, as compared with <500 kcal/week, was more than 2 years. Put in a different way, for these men (again assuming an expenditure of ≥2,000 kcal/week), the estimated hours of life gained per hour of exercise was some 2 to 2½ hours (Paffenbarger 1986b).

Conclusion

The body of epidemiologic data, supported by clinical and laboratory findings, provides strong evidence that the inverse relation between physical activity and risk of CHD represents dominantly a form of "protection" (i.e., a cause of reduced CHD incidence) rather than "selection" (an effect of CHD symptomatology on exercise behavior). The data are clearer for men than women, simply because few studies have been conducted in women. In addition to the relation being plausible biologically, it reflects current understanding of the physiologic and pathologic circumstances concerned. We have come to know that regular rhythmic exercise, especially moderately vigorous endurance activity, leads to improved physiologic fitness, and protects against CHD. The overall strength of evidence supporting a benefit of exercise on CHD may be rated II, and the recommendation that physical activity be included as a preventive measure against CHD may be rated A (US Preventive Services Task Force 1989).

Areas of research where further clarification is needed include the roles that quantity (total amount) of physical activity and intensity of effort may play in prevention of CHD. Findings to date provide no clear picture as to whether both are important, or whether one is more relevant than the other. The interrelationship of physical activity and fitness in preventing CHD also needs elucidation: Is one more important than the other? Finally, all areas of research need to include women; the studies discussed point clearly to the lack of data on women in most studies of physical activity and fitness in relation to CHD risk.

Summary

Quality of available data: A large body of observational data from well-designed prospective cohort studies.

Estimated risk reduction: 35–55% reduction in risk associated with maintenance of an active lifestyle, as compared with a sedentary lifestyle. Data are not available on the role of interventions to increase physical activity in reducing risk of MI.

Comparability of effect in men and women: While fewer data are available on the effects of physical activity or physical fitness on MI risk in women, available evidence suggests benefits comparable with those among men.

Appendix A

Guidelines for Prescribing a Safe and Effective Exercise Program

What kind of exercise, how much, and what intensity is best to reduce the risk of coronary heart disease (CHD)? Answers to these questions may provide the motivation needed to become and remain physically active, especially as one tries to fit exercise into a busy schedule of conflicting commitments. Likewise, knowing at what point further effort becomes fruitless, or even harmful, will help delay discouragement, ''burnout,'' injury, or even worse catastrophes.

Perhaps the failure of Americans to take up and maintain a more active and fit way of life results from the confusing messages they have been receiving over the last two decades, ranging from the ''marathon or else'' to the more recent ''less is more'' and ''fitness without exercise'' recommendations. Now, however, from the epidemiologic evidence available, it seems that expending a total of 1,500 to 2,000 kcal (equivalent to $3^1/_2$ to 6 hours of moderately vigorous, $\geq$4.5 METs, exercise) a week using the long muscles of the legs, arms, and trunk, preferably in sustained, rhythmic fashion will provide most of the protection possible against CHD, both nonfatal and fatal.

Beyond this level of 2,000 kcal, it seems that additional *physical* health benefits come only with increasing effort, and eventually level off at, say, 3,500–4,000 kcal/ week. Yet, while exercising beyond this level may provide few further physical benefits, additional effort may provide significant psychological benefits to some. At every level of energy expenditure up to this 3,500–4,000 kcal benchmark, moderately vigorous exercise ($\geq$4.5 METs) is more protective than activity of less intense effort. Some examples of specific activities and estimates of their MET values are given in the Table, A1. Exercising at 4.5 MET levels and above generally induces a noticeably increased heart rate (60% to 80% of the estimated maximum, or 220 minus age, see below), hard breathing, and at least slight sweating.

These estimates pertain to a 70-kg (155-lb) person of around 72 cm (5 ft 8 in.) in height. A smaller person would require less, a large person more, energy expenditure to achieve these goals.

194

Table A1. Examples of Physical Activities, by Intensities of Effort (MET Scores[a]), as Estimated for Adults

Light <4.5 METS (<5.4 kcal/min)[b]	Moderate 4.5–5.9 METS (5.4-7.0 kcal/min)[b]	Vigorous ≥6.0 METS (>7.0 kcal/min)[b]
Walking <3.5 mph[c]	Brisk walking 3.5–5.0 mph	Fast walking >5.0 mph
Golf in a cart	Golf, pulling or carrying clubs	Stair climbing
Cycling <6 mph	Cycling 6–9 mph	Cycling ≥10 mph
Riding lawnmower	Power lawnmower	Push lawnmower
Snowblower	Shoveling light snow	Shoveling heavy snow
Pruning, weeding	Hoeing	Carrying heavy loads
Coaching	Manual shrub cutting	Jogging or running
Light housekeeping (e.g., dusting, sweeping)	Housework (e.g., floor scrubbing, vacuuming)	Competitive field and court sports
Putting away groceries	Recreational volleyball	Singles tennis
Shuffleboard	Baseball	Rowing machine
Bowling	Canoeing	Fishing in stream
Boating	Badminton, social, singles	Heavy carpentry
Fishing while seated	Housepainting	Fast dancing (folk, square, etc.)
Light home repair	Ballroom dancing	Heavy calisthenics (pushups, situps, pullups)
Self-care	Skiing downhill, light effort	
Games with children	Weight training	
Table tennis	Recreational (leisure) swimming	Aerobic dancing
Trampoline		Splitting wood
Yoga		Lap swimming
Tai chi		Backpacking
		Conditioning exercise
		Judo, karate

Source: Ainsworth (1993), (Passmore (1955).

[a]Ratio of exercise metabolic rate to resting metabolic rate. One MET is defined as the energy expended while sitting quietly, which in the average adult approximates 3.5 ml of oxygen uptake per kilogram of body weight per minute (1.2 kcal/min for 70-kg individual).

[b]For a 70-kg (155-lb) person.

[c]Walking <3.5 mph—casual walking, window shopping, sauntering, strolling, purposeless wandering.

Three Stages to Prevention

Stage One. Not everyone needs a medical evaluation prior to beginning an exercise program, particularly asymptomatic, healthy men aged <40 years and women aged <50 years. But for some men and women over these ages, especially if they have been grossly sedentary or have a serious chronic illness, a medical checkup with EKG monitoring may be advisable before beginning a physical activity or conditioning program (American College of Sports Medicine 1991). The medical examination would preferably include a symptom-limited exercise stress-test either on treadmill or bicycle ergometer. For higher risk men and women, regardless of age, such evaluation also should be carried out. Higher risk persons are defined as those with two or more of these major coronary risk factors: cigarette smoking, a history of coronary or other atherosclerotic disease in parents or siblings before age 55 years, hypertension, diabetes mellitus, serum cholesterol ≥6.20 mmol/l (240 mg/dl). For persons with established cardiac, pulmonary, and metabolic diseases, medical evaluation again should be carried out before beginning an exercise program. Medical supervision during the exercise program, if of high intensity, may be necessary for such individuals, and annual exercise testing to monitor patients with coronary artery disease is important (Fletcher 1992).

At the simplest level, *any* physical activity is better than none, and more is generally better than less. Leisurely walking, gardening, or housework at 1.5 to 4.5 MET level are examples. Progress through this and subsequent stages should be made gradually, with one's comfort level the key to how much and when to increase. It may take several weeks (perhaps 10–20) to reach that level of fitness where health benefits are realized, depending, of course, on one's baseline level.

Stage Two. The U.S. Centers for Disease Control and Prevention and the American College of Sports Medicine (Pate 1995) recently recommended what might be considered a minimal level for health: "Every American adult should accumulate 30 minutes or more of moderate-intensity physical activity on most, preferably all, days of the week." The recommendation suggests that stair-climbing, dancing, intermittent walking, yardwork, and so on might contribute to the total, as might planned exercise or recreational play such as jogging, playing tennis, swimming, and cycling. Regular participation in physical activities that develop and maintain muscular strength and joint flexibility also was recommended (Fletcher 1992). The crux of the plan was to encourage regular, moderate-intensity physical activity, which in fact, might lead to 1,200–1,500 kcal energy expenditure weekly. It is unclear whether the health benefits of, say, three 10-minute bouts of exercise are equivalent to that of one 30-minute workout. Perhaps the recommendation would be improved by calling for 30 minutes each day of uninterrupted physical activity at 4.5 METs or more. However, these recent guidelines were put forth not only to recognize the health benefits of physical activity, but also to recognize that there are significant barriers to participation in physical activity: perhaps one reason so few Americans are physically active may be because previous efforts to promote physical activity have overemphasized the importance of high-intensity exercise.

Stage Three. The recommendation of physical activity that might be considered optimal for health would broaden the minimal level of Stage two and combine it with a regular conditioning or fitness program. A subject should be on his or her feet at least 1 hour of each day moving about. The large muscles, particularly the legs, should be contracting in propelling the body's weight, preferably rhythmically. Moving about in the kitchen or office, climbing stairs, walking to the store or recreationally at noon, looking after children—all such activities count. Again, 30 minutes of this daily hour should be uninterrupted, at an intensity of 4.5 METs or more.

The complementary, conditioning program to achieve optimal health benefits would comprise 30 minutes at least three times a week of moderately vigorous (≥4.5 METs) exercise. Such exercise will increase heart rate to 60–80% of estimated maximum, induce hard breathing (although permit halting conversation), and cause one to break out into a sweat. Unlike moving about, which can be accumulated throughout the day, this more vigorous activity should be sustained for 30 minutes or more. Strengthening exercises to increase muscle power and protect the joints and long bones, together with flexibility or stretching exercises to increase range of motion of joints, should be included. A warm-up period—such as stretching gently or walking slowly for perhaps 5 minutes before increasing the pace to "moderately vigorous" —should precede a workout session. With such a conditioning program, coupled with 7 hours of ambulation, the average-sized person would expend 2,000–3,500 kcal of energy each week and at an intensity protective against CHD.

Pitfalls. In practice, excessive exercise and overtraining infrequently become an issue until one enters into competition, either with one's self or with others. The real issue here is not whether one should exercise or not, but how one should exercise for the greatest benefit with the least risk. It is true that there is some point at which exercise becomes excessive and harmful, but that point is not well-defined. While we can identify with some certainty what is, for all of us, a reasonable level of exercise to protect against CHD, the excessive level depends on one's heritage, prior physical condition, the presence of disease, or even such characteristics as mood, on-the-job or life stress, changes in training routine. Thus, it is up to the individual to exercise prudently, progress slowly, heed the warning signs of impending trouble (for example, chest discomfort, excessive fatigue, undue dyspnea, lightheadedness, or dizziness), and take action—usually to cease exercise and rest. A subject should temporarily stop his program if he develops even a minor illness—the common cold or its equivalent— or if he develops excessive fatigue, insomnia, or persistent muscle soreness. Resumption of activity should begin at a lower level with gradual increase (over a week or two) to the customary level. Perhaps the ideal activity for most older people (aged more than, say, 65 or 70) is moderately brisk walking, say, at about 5 km/h (about 3.5 mph).

Overtraining. The complex of symptoms—some physical, some psychological—that result from overextension of the body's ability to adapt to increases in work load is called "overtraining": the most common cause of injury or discouragement that causes once-active subjects to drop out of an active and fit way of life. Premonitory symptoms of overtraining, indications that one needs rest and time for the body to recover, include mood changes, usually anger or depression; generalized fatigue, a feeling of being "heavy-legged"; lack of interest in training; declining performance; listlessness or languor; anorexia, insomnia, and loss of libido; increased frequency of respiratory illness or worsening allergies; and amenorrhea.

Guidelines. Every safe and effective exercise program carries with it certain cautions:

1. Increase the intensity or amount of exercise no more than 10% per week. Moving from Stage 2 to Stage 3 should occur only after one can walk comfortably for 30 minutes at about 5 km (3.5 miles) per hour.
2. Exercise vigorously (≥ 6.0 METs) for 30 uninterrupted minutes no more than 3 times per week. Risk of injury rises substantially with more frequent heavy workouts. A "hard" day should be followed by an "easy" day.

3. Warm up thoroughly before beginning a workout session. Stretch gently or walk slowly for perhaps 5 minutes before increasing the pace to "moderately vigorous."
4. Cool down slowly, perhaps over 5 minutes, at the end of an exercise program. This helps to protect the heart and the musculoskeletal system from injury.

Both in beginning and maintaining an exercise or conditioning program, the primary elements are to start slowly, exercise prudently, and taper off.

References

Ainsworth BE, Haskell WL, Leon AS, et al. Compendium of physical activities: classification of energy costs of human physical activities. Med Sci Sports Exerc 1993;25:71–80.

American College of Sports Medicine. Guidelines for exercise testing and prescription, 4th ed. Philadelphia: Lea & Febiger, 1991.

Berlin JA, Colditz GA. A meta-analysis of physical activity in the prevention of coronary heart disease. Am J Epidemiol 1990;132:612–28.

Blair SN, Kohl HW III, Paffenbarger RS Jr, et al. Physical fitness and all-cause mortality: a prospective study of healthy men and women. JAMA 1989;262:2395–401.

Blair SN, Kohl HW, Brill PA. Behavioral adaptation to physical activity. In: Bouchard C, Shephard RJ, Stephens T, Sutton JR, McPherson BD, eds. Exercise, fitness, and health: a consensus of current knowledge. Champaign, IL: Human Kinetics Books, 1990: 385–98.

Blomqvist CG, Saltin B. Cardiovascular adaptations to physical training. Annu Rev Physiol 1983;45:169–89.

Brunner D, Manelis G, Modan M, Levin S. Physical activity at work and the incidence of myocardial infarction, angina pectoris and death due to ischemic heart disease: an epidemiologic study in Israeli collective settlements (kibbutzim). J Chron 1974;27: 217–33.

Chapman JM, Goerke LS, Dixon W, et al. The clinical status of a population group in Los Angeles under observation for two to three years. Am J Public Health 1957;47(April suppl):33–42.

Clausen JP. Effect of physical training on cardiovascular adjustments to exercise in man. Physiol Rev 1977;57:779–815.

Curfman GD. The health benefits of exercise: a critical reappraisal. N Engl J Med 1993;328: 574–6.

Donahue RP, Abbott RD, Reed DM, Yano K. Physical activity and coronary heart disease in middle-aged and elderly men: the Honolulu Heart Program. Am J Public Health 1988; 78:683–5.

Division of Chronic Disease Control and Community Intervention, National Center for Chronic Disease Prevention and Health Promotion. Public health focu: physical activity and the prevention of coronary heart disease. MMWR 1993;42:669–72.

Ekelund L-G, Haskell WL, Johnson JL, et al. Physical fitness as a predictor of cardiovascular mortality in asymptomatic North American men: the Lipid Research Clinics Mortality Follow-up Study. N Engl J Med 1988;319:1379–84.

Erikssen J. Physical fitness and coronary heart disease morbidity and mortality: a prospective study of apparently healthy, middle aged men. Acta Med Scand Suppl 1986;711: 189–92.

Ernst E. Fibrinogen, an independent risk factor for cardiovascular disease. Br Med J 1991;303: 597–7.

Fletcher GF, Blair SN, Blumenthal J, et al. Statement on exercise: benefits and recommendations for physical activity programs for all Americans: a statement for health professionals by the Committee on Exercise and Cardiac Rehabilitation of the Council on Clinical Cardiology, American Heart Association. Circulation 1992;86:340–4

Fuster V, Badimon L, Badimon JJ, Chesebro JH. The pathogenesis of coronary artery disease and the acute coronary syndromes. N Engl J Med 1992;326:242–50, 310–18.

Garcia-Palmieri MR, Costa R Jr, Cruz-Vidal M, et al. Increased physical activity: a protective factor against heart attacks in Puerto Rico. Am J Cardiol 1982;50:749–55.

Garfinkel L, Stellman SD. Mortality by relative weight and exercise. Cancer 1988;62: 1844–50.

Gordon DJ, Rifkind BM. High-density lipoprotein: the clinical implications of recent studies. N Engl J Med 1989;321:1311–16.

Gyntelberg F, Lauridsen L, Schubell K. Physical fitness and risk of myocardial infarction in Copenhagen males aged 40–59: a five- and seven-year follow-up study. Scand J Work Environ Health 1980;6:170–8.

Hahn RA, Teutsch SM, Rothenberg RB, Marks JS. Excess deaths from nine chronic disease in the United States 1986. JAMA 1990;264:2654–9.

Hambrecht R, Niebauer J, Marburger C, et al. Various intensities of leisure time physical activity in patients with coronary artery disease: effects on cardiorespiratory fitness and progression of coronary atherosclerotic lesions. J Am Coll Cardiol 1993;22:468–77.

Haskell WL. Exercise-induced changes in plasma lipids and lipoproteins. Prev Med 1984;13: 23–36.

Hatziandreu EL, Koplan JP, Weinstein MC, et al. A cost-effectiveness analysis of exercise as a health promotion activity. Am J Public Health 1988;78:1417–21.

Hein HO, Suadicani P, Gyntelberg F. Physical fitness or physical activity as a predictor of ischaemic heart disease? A 17-year follow-up in the Copenhagen Male Study. J Intern Med 1992;232:471–9.

Kahn HA. The relationship of reported coronary heart disease mortality to physical activity of work. Am J Public Health 1963;53:1058–67.

Kannel WB, Belanger A, D'Agostino R, Israel I. Physical activity and physical demand on the job and risk of cardiovascular disease and death: the Framingham Study. Am Heart J 1986;112:820–5.

Kestin AS, Ellis PA, Barnard MR, et al. Effect of strenuous exercise on platelet activation state and reactivity. Circulation 1993;88:1502–11.

Keys A. Seven countries: a multivariate analysis of death and coronary heart disease. Cambridge, MA: Harvard University Press, 1980.

Kohl HW III, Powell KE, Gordon NF, et al. Physical activity, physical fitness, and sudden cardiac death. Epidemiol Rev 1992;14:37–58.

Kramsch DM, Aspen AJ, Abramowitz BM, et al. Reduction of coronary atherosclerosis by moderate conditioning exercise in monkeys on an atherogenic diet. N Engl J Med 1981; 305:1483–9.

Lakka TA, Venäläinen JM, Rauramaa R, et al. Relation of leisure-time physical activity and cardiorespiratory fitness to the risk of acute myocardial infarction in men. N Engl J Med 1994;330:1549–54.

Lee I-M, Paffenbarger RS Jr, Hsieh C-c. Time trends in physical activity among college alumni, 1962–1988. Am J Epidemiol 1992;135:915–25.

Leon AS, Connett J, Jacobs DR Jr, Rauramaa R. Leisure-time physical activity levels and risk of coronary heart disease and death: the Multiple Risk Factor Intervention Trial. JAMA 1987;258:2388–95.

Lie H, Mundal R, Erikssen J. Coronary risk factors and incidence of coronary death in relation to physical fitness: seven-year follow-up study of middle-aged and elderly men. Euro Heart J 1985;6:147–57.

Lindsted KD, Tonstad S, Kuzma JW. Self-report of physical activity and patterns of mortality in Seventh-Day Adventist men. J Clin Epidemiol 1991;44:355–64.

Magnus K, Matroos A, Strackee J. Walking, cycling, or gardening, with or without seasonal interruption in relation to acute coronary events. Am J Epidemiol 1979;110:724–33.

Menotti A, Puddu V. Ten-year mortality from coronary heart disease among 172,000 men classified by occupational physical activity. Scand J Work Environ Health 1979;5: 100–8.

Mittelman MA, Maclure M, Tofler GH, et al. Triggering of acute myocardial infarction by heavy physical exertion: protection against triggering by regular exertion. N Engl J Med 1993;329:1677–83.

Morris JN, Heady JA, Raffle PAB, et al. Coronary heart disease and physical activity of work. Lancet 1953;2:1053–7, 1111–20.

Morris JN, Chave SPW, Adam C, et al. Vigorous exercise in leisure-time and the incidence of coronary heart disease. Lancet 1973;1:333–9.

Morris JN, Everitt MG, Pollard R, et al. Vigorous exercise in leisure-time: protection against coronary heart disease. Lancet 1980;2:1207–10.

Morris JN, Clayton DG, Everitt MG, et al. Exercise in leisure-time: coronary attack and death rates. B Heart J 1990;63:325–34.

Noakes TD, Higginson L, Opie LH. Physical training increases ventricular fibrillation thresholds of isolated rat hearts during normoxia, hypoxia, and regional ischemia. Circulation 1983; 67:24–30.

Paffenbarger RS Jr, Hale WE. Work activity and coronary heart mortality. N Engl J Med 1975; 292:545–50.

Paffenbarger RS Jr, Wing AL, Hyde RT. Physical activity as an index of heart attack risk in college alumni. Am J Epidemiol 1978;108:161–75.

Paffenbarger RS Jr, Hyde RT, Wing AL, Hsieh C-c. Physical activity, all-cause mortality, and longevity of college alumni. N Engl J Med 1986a;314:605–13.

Paffenbarger RS Jr, Hyde RT, Wing AL, Hsieh C-c. Physical activity and longevity of college alumni. N Engl J Med 1986b;315:399–401.

Paffenbarger RS Jr, Kampert JB, Lee I-M, et al. Changes in physical activity and other lifeway patterns influencing longevity. Med Sci Sports Exerc 1994;26:857–865.

Palatini P. Blood pressure behaviour during physical activity. Sports Med 1988;5:353–74.

Passmore R, Durnin JVGA. Human energy expenditure. Phys Rev 1955;35:801–40.

Pate RR, Pratt M, Blair SN, et al. Physical activity and public health: A recommendation from the Centers for Disease Control and Prevention and the American College of Sports Medicine. JAMA 1995;273:402–7.

Péronnet F, Cléroux J, Perrault H, et al. Plasma norepinephrine response to exercise before and after training in humans. J Appl Physiol 1981;51:812–15.

Peters RK, Cady LD Jr, Bischoff DP, et al. Physical fitness and subsequent myocardial infraction in healthy workers. JAMA 1983;249:3052–6.

Pomrehn PR, Wallace RB, Burmeister LF. Ischemic heart disease mortality in Iowa farmers: the influence of lifestyle. JAMA 1982;248:1073–6.

Powell KE, Thompson PD, Caspersen CJ, Kendrick JS. Physical activity and the incidence of coronary heart disease. Ann Rev Public Health 1987;8:253–87.

Punsar S, Karvonen MJ. Physical activity and coronary heart disease in populations from east and west Finland. Adv Cardiol 1976;18:196–207.

Rauramaa R. Relationship of physical activity, glucose tolerance and weight management. Prev Med 1984;13:37–46.

Richardson PD, Davies MJ, Born GVR. Influence of plaque configuration and stress distribution on fissuring of coronary atherosclerotic plaques. Lancet 1989;2:941–4.

Rodriguez BL, Curb D, Burchfield CM, et al. Physical activity and 23-year incidence of coronary heart disease morbidity and mortality. Among middle-aged men: The Honolulu Heart Program. Circulation 1994;89:2540–4.

Salonen JT, Puska P, Tuomilehto J. Physical activity and risk of myocardial infarction, cerebral stroke and death: a longitudinal study in Eastern Finland. Am J Epidemiol 1982;115: 526–37.

Salonen JT, Slater JS, Tuomilehto J, Rauramaa R. Leisure time and occupational physical activity: risk of death from ischemic heart disease. Am J Epidemiol 1988;127:87–94.

Saltin B. Cardiovascular and pulmonary adaptation to physical activity. In: Bouchard C, Shephard RJ, Stephens T, Sutton JR, McPherson BD, eds. Exercise, fitness, and health: a consensus of current knowledge. Champaign, IL: Human Kinetics Books, 1990:187–203.

Sandvik L, Erikssen J, Thaulow E, et al. Physical fitness as a predictor of mortality among healthy, middle-aged Norwegian men. N Engl J Med 1993;328:533–7.

Scragg R, Stewart A, Jackson R, Beaglehole R. Alcohol and exercise in myocardial infarction and sudden coronary death in men and women. Am J Epidemiol 1987;126:77–85.

Shaper AG, Wannamethee G. Physical activity and ischaemic heart disease in middle-aged British men. Br Heart J 1991;66:384–94.

Shapiro S, Weinblatt E, Frank CW, Sager RV. The HIP study of incidence and prognosis of coronary heart disease: preliminary findings on incidence of myocardial infarction and angina. J Chron Dis 1965;18:527–58.

Shephard RJ. Costs and benefits of an exercising versus a nonexercising society. In: Bouchard C, Shephard RJ, Stephens T, Sutton JR, McPherson BD, eds. Exercise, fitness, and health: a consensus of current knowledge. Champaign, IL: Human Kinetics Books, 1990: 49–60.

Siscovick DS, Weiss NS, Fletcher RH, Lasky T. The incidence of primary cardiac arrest during vigorous exercise. N Engl J Med 1984;311–874–7.

Slattery JL, Jacobs DR. Physical fitness and cardiovascular disease mortality: the U.S. Railroad Study. Am J Epidemiol 1988a;127:571–80.

Slattery ML, Schumacher MC, Smith KR, et al. Physical activity, diet and risk of colon cancer in Utah. Am J Epidemiol 1988b:128:989–99.

Slattery ML, Jacobs DR Jr, Nichaman MZ. Leisure time physical activity and coronary heart disease death: the US Railroad Study. Circulation 1989;79:304–11.

Sobolski J, Kornitzer M, de Backer G, et al. Protection against ischemic heart disease in the Belgian physical fitness study: physical fitness rather than physical activity? Am J Epidemiol 1987;125:601–10.

Stamler J, Lindberg HA, Berkson DM, et al. Prevalence and incidence of coronary heart disease in strata of the labor force of a Chicago industrial corporation. J Chron Dis 1960;11: 405–20.

Taylor HL, Blackburn H, Keys A, et al. Coronary heart disease in seven countries. IV. Five-year follow-up of employees of selected U.S. railroad companies. Circulation 1970; 41(Suppl 1):20–39.

Thompson PD, Funk EJ, Carleton RA, Sturner WQ. Incidence of death during jogging in Rhode Island from 1975 through 1980. JAMA 1982;247:2535–8.

US Preventive Services Task Force. Guide to clinical preventive services: an assessment of the effectiveness of 169 interventions. Report of the US Preventive Services Task Force. Baltimore: Williams & Wilkins, 1989:387–97.

Vuori I, Makarainen M, Jaasheiainer J. Sudden death and physical activity. Cardiology 1978; 83:287–304.

Wilhelmsen L, Bjure J, Ekström-Jodal B, et al. Nine years' follow-up of a maximal exercise test in a random population sample of middle-aged men. Cardiology 1981;68(Suppl 2): 1–8.

Williams RS, Schaible TF, Bishop T, Morey M. Effects of endurance training on cholinergic and adrenergic receptors of the rat heart. J Mol Cell Cardiol 1984;16:395–403.

Willich SN, Lewis M, Löwel H, et al. Physical exertion as a trigger of acute myocardial infarction. N Engl J Med 1993;329:1684–90.

Zukel WJ, Lewis RH, Enterline PE, et al. A short-term community study of the epidemiology of coronary heart disease: a preliminary report on the North Dakota Study. Am J Public Health 1959;49:1630–9.

9

Risk Modification in the Obese Patient

PATRICIA A. DALY, CAREN G. SOLOMON,
AND JOANN E. MANSON

Obesity, defined as a weight 20% or more above desirable levels, afflicts at least 58 million Americans (Kuczmarski 1994) and its prevalence is increasing (Figure 9.1). Women and minorities, including Hispanics, African Americans, American Indians, and Pacific Islanders, are particularly at risk for this condition (Kumanyika 1993). The population risk of coronary heart disease (CHD) mortality attributable to obesity in the United States has been estimated to be 32% (Public Health Focus 1993), and the societal cost of obesity, in terms of medical services and lost productivity, as high as 39.3 billion dollars annually (Colditz 1992). Through its associations with other cardiovascular risk factors, but also independent of these factors, obesity is a major cause of cardiovascular morbidity and mortality.

This chapter first reviews cardiovascular disease risks associated with obesity and weight gain. Insofar as weight reduction appears to be the best means of ameliorating cardiovascular risk in the obese, most of this discussion is devoted to the benefits and risks of available modalities for treating obesity. Management strategies for other cardiovascular risk factors common in the obese, discussed individually in other chapters of this book, are also addressed briefly. Finally, an approach to the initial evaluation and treatment of obesity by the primary care practitioner is presented.

Definitions of Obesity

Several different criteria may be used to classify obesity (Table 9.1). One approach is a comparison with "ideal" body weight (IBW), a standard that is lower than average weight due to the high prevalence of obesity in the U.S. population; body weight 20% or more above IBW is considered obese. Another commonly used measure is body mass index (BMI), also known as Quetelet's index, which corrects weight for height by dividing body weight in kilograms by height in meters squared. While BMI is imperfect as a measure of obesity in that it does not directly reflect adiposity and may be increased in those with higher lean body mass, it allows comparison of the degree

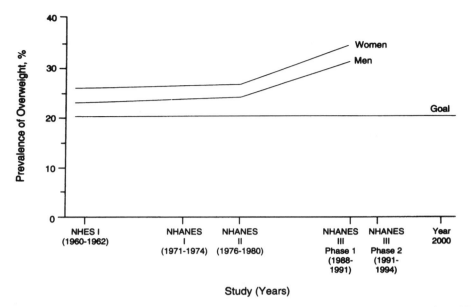

Fig. 9.1. Trends in age-adjusted prevalence of overweight for the US population 20 through 74 years of age, compared with the year 2000 health objective for overweight. NHES indicates National Health Examination Survey; NHANES, National Health and Nutrition Examination Survey. [From Kuczmarski (1990), with permission.]

of obesity of individuals who differ greatly in weight and height, and in most cases is a reasonable surrogate for adiposity. Using this measure, obesity has been defined as a BMI $\geq$ 27.3 kg/m^2 in women and 27.8 kg/m^2 in men (Van Itallie 1985), which corresponds to approximately 20% above ideal body weight according to 1983 Metropolitan Life Insurance Company tables. A BMI $\geq$ 40 kg/m^2, which corresponds to at least 80% above ideal body weight, is considered morbid obesity and is associated with a particularly high risk of obesity-related complications. Table 9.2 shows BMI for a wide range of weights and heights.

While adiposity may be measured more directly, using relatively simple approaches such as skinfold thickness or bioelectric impedance, or more quantitative

Table 9.1. Classification of Obesity

Classification	Relative Weight (% IBW)	BMI (kg/m^2) Men	BMI (kg/m^2) Women
Desirable weight	90–110	20–24	19–23
Overweight	110–120	24–27.8	23–27.3
Obese	120–180	27.8–40	27.3–40
Morbidly obese	≥180	≥40	≥40

Source: Modified from Kanders (1991), with permission.

BMI, body mass index; IBW, ideal body weight. See text for details.

Table 9.2. Body Mass Index (BMI)

BMI (kg/m²)

Height in.	19	20	21	22	23	24	25	26	27.3	27.8	29	30	31	32	33	34	35	36	37	38	39	40
	← Desirable →					← Overweight →		← Obese →													Morbidly Obese →	
											Body Weight, lb											
58	91	95	100	105	110	115	119	124	130	133	138	143	148	153	158	162	167	172	177	181	186	191
59	94	99	104	109	114	119	124	128	135	137	143	148	153	158	163	168	173	178	183	188	193	198
60	97	102	107	112	118	123	128	133	139	142	148	153	158	164	169	174	179	184	189	194	199	204
61	100	106	111	116	121	127	132	137	144	147	153	158	164	169	174	180	185	190	195	201	206	211
62	104	109	115	120	125	131	136	142	149	152	158	164	169	175	180	186	191	196	202	207	213	218
63	107	113	118	124	130	135	141	146	154	157	163	169	175	180	186	192	197	203	208	214	220	225
64	110	116	122	128	134	140	145	151	159	162	169	174	180	186	192	198	203	209	215	221	227	233
65	114	120	126	132	138	144	150	156	164	167	174	180	186	192	198	204	210	216	222	228	234	240
66	117	124	130	136	142	148	155	161	169	172	179	185	192	198	204	210	216	223	229	235	241	247
67	121	127	134	140	147	153	159	166	174	177	185	191	198	204	210	217	223	229	236	242	248	255
68	125	131	138	144	151	158	164	171	179	182	190	197	203	210	217	223	230	236	243	249	256	263
69	128	135	142	149	155	162	169	176	184	188	196	203	209	216	223	230	237	243	250	257	264	270
70	132	139	146	153	160	167	174	181	190	193	202	209	216	223	230	236	243	250	257	264	271	278
71	136	143	150	157	165	172	179	186	195	199	207	215	222	229	236	243	250	258	265	272	279	286
72	140	147	155	162	169	177	184	191	201	205	213	221	228	235	243	250	258	265	272	280	287	294
73	144	151	159	166	174	182	189	197	206	210	219	227	234	242	250	257	265	272	280	287	295	303
74	148	155	163	171	179	187	194	202	212	216	225	233	241	249	256	264	272	280	288	295	303	311
75	152	160	168	176	184	192	200	208	218	222	232	240	248	255	263	271	279	287	295	303	311	319
76	156	164	172	180	189	197	205	213	224	228	238	246	254	262	271	279	287	295	303	312	320	328

Source: Modified from Bray (1988), with permission.

To determine BMI (kg/m²), find the patient's height (in inches) in the lefthand column, move across the row to the patient's weight (in lb). BMI is at the top of the weight column. Cutoff values for "desirable" body weight, overweight, obese, and morbidly obese are shown. Note the slightly different cutoff points for overweight and obese in men vs. women.

approaches such as computed tomography or magnetic resonance imaging, these techniques are costly, not widely used, and not necessary to identify obesity. More recently, increased attention has been given to measures of central fat distribution, particularly the ratio of waist circumference to hip circumference (i.e., waist:hip ratio). A waist: hip ratio greater than 0.95 in men (Bray 1992) and 0.8 in women (Bjorntorp 1987) is consistent with central obesity.

Obesity and Other Cardiovascular Disease Risk Factors

The association between obesity and cardiovascular disease is mediated at least in part by strong links between obesity and several established risk factors for cardiovascular disease, including non-insulin-dependent diabetes mellitus (NIDDM), hypertension, and dyslipidemia. The relative risks of CHD associated with these conditions, as well as that associated with cigarette smoking, is shown in Figure 9.2. These data suggest that the relative risk is highest among individuals with the highest BMI and other concomitant risk factors.

The majority of individuals with NIDDM are obese (Colditz 1990). Prevalence of NIDDM increases directly with BMI; among participants in the National Health and Nutrition Examination Survey, 1976–1980 (NHANES II), NIDDM was almost three

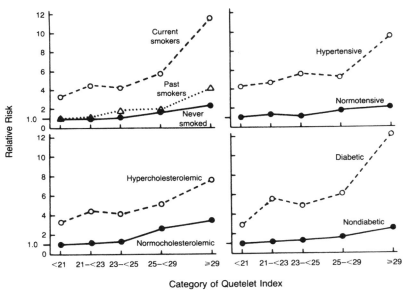

Fig. 9.2. Relative risks of nonfatal myocardial infarction and fatal coronary heart disease (combined) according to category of BMI and the specific coronary risk factors shown (after adjustment for age and smoking status), in women in the Nurses' Health Study. The reference group for each risk factor included women in the leanest BMI category who did not have the specified risk factor. [From Manson (1990), with permission.]

times more common among overweight individuals than among those of normal weight (Van Itallie 1985). Obesity also predicts later risk of NIDDM. Among 115,886 women followed prospectively in the Nurses' Health Study, those who were moderately obese at baseline (BMI 27–28.9 kg/m^2) had ten times the risk of developing diabetes compared with lean women (BMI < 22 kg/m^2), and those with significant obesity (BMI ≥ 35 kg/m^2) more than 60 times the risk (Colditz 1990).

Hypertension is likewise more common in the obese. Obese individuals participating in NHANES had 2.9 times the risk of high blood pressure (>160/95 mmHg) compared with nonobese individuals (Van Itallie 1985). Furthermore, BMI in college-age men has been reported to be a significant predictor of development of hypertension over 32 years of follow-up (Gillum 1982).

In addition, obese individuals commonly have lipid abnormalities which may predispose to cardiovascular disease. Reductions in high density lipoprotein (HDL) (Glueck 1980) and elevations in triglycerides are most common. While low HDL is clearly linked to coronary disease (Gordon 1989), hypertriglyceridemia is controversial as an independent risk factor, but is probably important in combination with obesity and low HDL. Elevations in total cholesterol and low density lipoprotein cholesterol (LDL) have also been reported with overweight by some (Assman 1992), but not all, investigators (Montoye 1966).

Obesity and Coronary Heart Disease

As would be expected based on the observed associations between obesity and several risk factors for cardiovascular disease, risks of CHD morbidity and mortality are significantly increased in obese men and women (see Table 9.3). Compared with lean women (BMI < 21 kg/m^2) participating in the Nurses' Health Study, those with BMI 25–29 kg/m^2 had an age- and smoking-adjusted relative risk for CHD of 1.8; those with BMI ≥ 29 kg/m^2 had a relative risk for CHD of 3.3 (Manson 1990). In this cohort of middle-aged women, risk of CHD was clearly lowest among the leanest women, and 40% of CHD events were attributable to overweight.

The association between relative weight or BMI and CHD mortality has also been demonstrated in several cohorts. An American Cancer Society study of 750,000 men and women revealed a mortality rate from CHD that was 55% greater among those who were 30–40% overweight, and approximately 100% greater among those more than 40% overweight (Lew 1979); similar findings were also reported in an insurance company study involving 4.5 million participants (Build and Blood Pressure Study 1959).

The effect of mild obesity on cardiovascular mortality risk has been more controversial, however. At issue have been studies reporting nadir mortality rates at weights above average (Dyer 1975). These nonlinear associations have been most pronounced for all-cause mortality, but have also been reported in some studies of cardiovascular-specific mortality (Lew 1979). However, the apparent risks associated with leanness in these studies appear to result largely from bias introduced by confounding factors (Manson 1987). For one, failure to control adequately for cigarette smoking, which is associated with both lower BMI and increased mortality, tends to overestimate risks

Table 9.3. Representative Large-Scale Studies of Body Weight and Coronary Heart Disease Morbidity and/or Mortality

Study	Number/ Gender	Age at Entry	Follow-up Period (yr)	Index of Obesity	Association Between Obesity Index and CHD
American Cancer Society (Lew 1975)[a]	336,442 M 419,060 F	30–89	13	Relative weight	M: linear F: J-shaped
Framingham Heart Study (Hubert 1983)	2,252 M 2,818 F	28–62	26	Relative weight	Linear (CHD/CHD mortality in all; MI in F: SD in M)
Nurses' Health Study (Manson 1990)	115,886 F	30–55	8	BMI	Linear
Seventh Day Adventists (Linsted 1991)[a]	8,828 M	52.8 (Mean)	26	BMI	Linear
Harvard Alumni Study (Lee 1993)[a]	19,297 M	46.6 (Mean)	22–26	BMI	Linear
Gothenberg Study of Men Born in 1913 (Ohlson 1985)	792 M	54	13	WHR, BMI, skinfold thickness	Linear for WHR (independent of BMI)
Gothenburg Study of Women (Lapidus 1984)	1,462 F	38–60	12	WHR, BMI, skinfold thickness	Linear for WHR (independent of BMI)
Iowa Women's Health Study (Folsom 1993)[a]	41,837 F	55–69	5	WHR, BMI	Linear for WHR (independent of BMI)

MI, myocardial infarction; SD, sudden death; M, male; F, female; BMI; body mass index; WHR, waist:hip ratio.

[a]Study evaluated CHD mortality only.

of leanness *per se*, and underestimate the true association between weight and mortality. Likewise, failure to recognize preexisting disease, which may underlie weight loss or leanness and also result in mortality, may cause a distortion of the true weight-mortality relationship. Furthermore, inappropriate control for metabolic consequences of obesity, including glucose intolerance, hypertension, and dyslipidemia, may attenuate the association between obesity and cardiovascular mortality.

Of note, when smokers and those who died early in follow-up have been excluded from analyses assessing the association between BMI and subsequent mortality, mortality rates have been lowest among the leanest individuals, and have increased directly with increasing BMI (Lee 1993; Manson 1995). A direct association between BMI and mortality was likewise observed in a study of Seventh Day Adventists, among whom smoking is rare, and leanness is generally a result of lifestyle rather than a consequence of underlying illness. In this population, no increase in mortality was seen even among the very lean (BMI < 20 kg/m^2) (Lindsted 1991).

Moreover, data from Framingham have demonstrated that obesity is a significant independent risk factor for cardiovascular disease, as shown in Figure 9.3. Among 5,209 participants in this study, relative weight on initial examination was a strong predictor of 26-year incidence of CHD, after adjustment for age, cholesterol, blood pressure, smoking, and glucose intolerance (Hubert 1983).

Direct Effects of Obesity on Cardiac Function

Obesity may increase cardiovascular morbidity and mortality in part through direct effects on cardiovascular function. Morbid obesity is associated with volume overload, left ventricular dilatation, and possibly development of eccentric left ventricular hypertrophy, with associated risks of ventricular arrhythmias and sudden death (Messerli 1987). Sleep apnea, which is also associated with obesity, may result in elevated pulmonary pressures with cor pulmonale (Sharp 1980), and may also predispose to hypertension (Hla 1994).

The Role of Insulin Resistance

The effect of obesity on cardiovascular risk may reflect, at least in part, the strong association of obesity with insulin resistance (Peiris 1988). Insulin resistance may

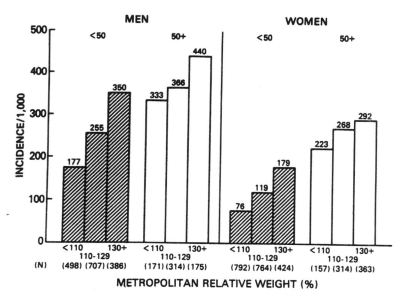

Fig. 9.3. Correlation between the 26-year incidence of cardiovascular disease and relative weight (percentage above ideal weight from the Metropolitan Weight Table) at entry into the Framingham Study. N is the total number of subjects at risk for an event. Incidence rates per 1,000 are shown above each bar. [From Hubert (1983), with permission.]

underlie several obesity-related cardiovascular risk factors, particularly NIDDM (Warram 1990), but also essential hypertension (Ferrannini 1987), and dyslipidemia (Laakso 1990). Of note, insulin resistance or compensatory hyperinsulinemia may promote hypertension by stimulating renal sodium reabsorption (DeFronzo 1975), sympathetic nervous system activity (Rowe 1981), and/or cell membrane cation transport (Doria 1991), and may also result in increased triglyceride production and decreased triglyceride removal (Laakso 1990). Furthermore, insulin resistance may predispose to cardiovascular disease independent of these other risk factors (Laakso 1991), perhaps through augmentation of vascular smooth muscle reactivity, and accelerated atherogenesis (Standley 1993).

The Importance of Fat Distribution

Support for the hypothesis that insulin resistance underlies the adverse effects of obesity derives from data demonstrating that upper body or central obesity, as measured by increased waist:hip ratio, is an even stronger predictor of cardiovascular risk than is body mass index or relative weight (Lapidus 1984). For reasons that are not completely understood, central obesity is closely associated with insulin resistance (Kaplan 1989). Abdominal fat appears to be more lipolytically active than gluteal fat in response to catecholamines and other hormones (Peiris 1986); free fatty acids released from this tissue may contribute to insulin resistance through a direct effect on muscle (Randle 1963), or indirectly by stimulating hepatic glucose production (Reaven 1988) and inhibiting hepatic insulin uptake (Peiris 1986). The relationship between upper body obesity, hyperinsulinemia, and variously metabolic abnormalities is depicted in Figure 9.4. The metabolic profile of individuals with lower body obesity appears to be intermediate between lean and upper body obesity (see Figure 9.5).

Waist:hip ratio correlates directly with blood pressure, with blood glucose levels, glucose-stimulated insulin levels, and triglyceride levels, and inversely with HDL levels (Kalkhoff 1983; Freedman 1990). In prospective studies, a high waist:hip ratio is an independent predictor of NIDDM (Ohlson 1985) and cardiovascular morbidity and mortality (Lapidus 1984; Folsom 1993), even after adjusting for BMI.

Importantly, central adiposity appears to be characteristic of smokers, despite the fact that BMI tends to be lower in smokers than those who have never smoked (Barrett-Connor 1989). Central adiposity has also been reported to increase with age (Shimokata 1989) and to be more common among individuals with histories of "weight cycling" (i.e., repeated loss and regain of weight) (Rodin 1990), although this is controversial (Jeffrey 1992).

The Impact of Early Life Obesity

The adverse effects of obesity on cardiovascular morbidity and mortality become more pronounced with longer duration of follow-up. For example, the association between obesity and myocardial infarction appeared much stronger in later analyses from the Framingham Heart Study than in earlier analyses based on shorter follow-up (Hubert 1983).

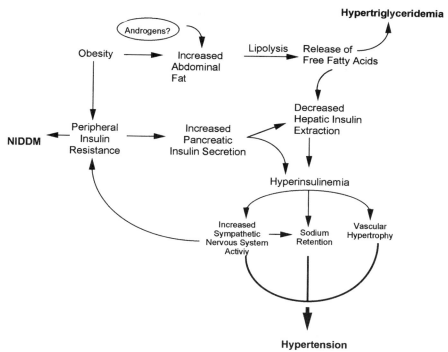

Fig. 9.4. Mechanisms by which upper body obesity, through associated hyperinsulinemia, may promote glucose intolerance, hypertriglyceridemia, and hypertension. [From Kaplan (1989), with permission.]

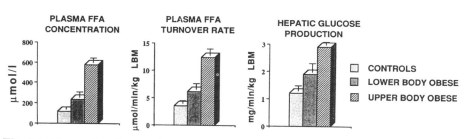

Fig. 9.5. Plasma free fatty acid concentration and turnover, and hepatic glucose production in controls and obese individuals of different body fat distribution patterns. [From Bonadonna (1992), with permission.]

Consistent with a long latency before adverse effects of obesity are obvious, early life obesity has been shown to be a strong predictor of later cardiovascular disease. The Harvard Growth Study, which followed men from adolescent years through middle age, revealed a strong association between baseline obesity and later life all-cause and CHD mortality (Must 1992).

Weight Gain

Weight gain over time also predisposes to other cardiovascular risk factors and to cardiovascular disease, independent of baseline obesity. Among men followed longitudinally in the Framingham Heart Study, each 10% increase in relative weight was associated, on average, with a 6.6 mmHg increase in systolic blood pressure, a 2.5 mg/dl increase in serum glucose, and an 11.3 mg/dl increase in serum cholesterol; rates of CHD increased a corresponding 30–40% (Ashley 1974). Consistent with these observations, weight gain has been reported to be an independent predictor of NIDDM (Colditz 1990) and CHD morbidity and mortality (Manson 1990) among participants in the Nurses' Health Study.

Weight gain is common following smoking cessation, and former smokers are more often obese than current smokers (Comstock 1972; Barrett-Connor 1989). Elevations in lipoprotein lipase have been reported in smokers. This enzyme, which hydrolyzes triglycerides into free fatty acids for uptake into adipocytes, and which appears to play a counterregulatory role to prevent further weight loss in the post-obese, may also contribute to rapid weight gain often seen after smoking is discontinued (Carney 1984).

"Weight Cycling:" an Additional Health Risk in the Obese?

In attempting to become thin, many overweight individuals lose and regain large amounts of weight repeatedly over the years, a process termed "weight cycling." Concerns have been raised about the health risks of this repeated gain and loss, based on epidemiologic, clinical, and animal data, suggesting increased cardiovascular morbidity and mortality in the setting of "weight cycling." Decreases in resting metabolic rate, which makes future weight loss more difficult, increases in the proportion of body fat, particularly abdominal fat (with a corresponding increase in waist-hip ratio), increases in insulin resistance, blood pressure, and lipogenic enzymes have all been suggested (Jeffery 1992; Reed 1993).

Reed and Hill (1993) recently reviewed the animal literature concerning weight cycling, and noted a number of methodologic difficulties. In most studies, longer term metabolic effects of weight change were not distinguished from the acute, transient metabolic effects of weight loss and regain. High-fat diets have generally been employed in studies which have found an excess accumulation of body fat in cycled animals; when animals are cycled using standard diets, no differences in body fat are found between groups. Studies in humans are equally difficult to interpret. Higher body weight, greater body fat content, higher waist:hip ratio, lower resting metabolic rate, and greater difficulty losing weight after regain than initially, have been reported by some investigators (Steen 1988; Blackburn 1989; Rodin 1989) while others have found no such differences (Van Dale 1989; Melby 1990; Wadden 1992a). Until further data are available, concerns about weight cycling should not serve to discourage attempts at weight loss, but rather to increase emphasis on long-term maintenance of weight loss and on prevention of obesity.

Weight Reduction

Rationale for Weight Reduction

Despite the potential risks of weight cycling, it is clear that weight reduction can ameliorate many of the adverse effects of obesity. Significant decreases in serum glucose levels have been reported within days of beginning calorie-reduced diets, and hypoglycemic agents (oral or insulin) can frequently be rapidly decreased or eliminated (Pi-Sunyer 1993). Similarly, weight loss is associated with significant reductions in blood pressure and lipid levels. Decreases in systolic blood pressure of 10–18 mmHg and in diastolic blood pressure of 9–13 mmHg have been reported with weight loss of 8–10 kg (Tuck 1981). Results from a meta-analysis of 70 studies of the effects of weight loss on lipid profile indicate that for every kilogram decrease in body weight, LDL falls by 0.77 mg/dl, and total cholesterol, by 1.93 mg/dl; once weight has stabilized, HDL increases by 0.35 mg/dl per kilogram lost (Dattilo 1992). Consistent with these findings, weight reduction over time among the Framingham population was associated with decreased risks of CHD (Ashley 1974).

Surprisingly, the effect of weight reduction on cardiovascular mortality has not been straightforward. Some studies have reported lower risks of cardiovascular mortality among at least some groups of obese subjects who lost weight as compared with those who remained obese (Hammond 1969; Wannamethee 1990). Others, however, have reported increased cardiovascular mortality with weight loss (Lee 1992; Pamuk 1993). These unexpected observations may be explained, at least in part, by confounding effects of involuntary weight loss due to disease or smoking, or possibly by adverse effects of weight cycling.

Physiology of Weight Reduction

For weight loss to occur, energy expenditure must exceed energy intake. Humans ingest energy as either carbohydrate, protein, fat, or alcohol. Carbohydrate and protein each produce 4 kcal of energy per gram. Fat produces 9 kcal/g and alcohol 7 kcal/g (Shils 1994). Energy expenditure includes the energy required for usual metabolic processes—the resting metabolic rate (RMR)—the energy used to digest and metabolize food—the thermic effect of food—and the energy required for physical activity—the thermic effect of exercise. The RMR accounts for 50–60% of total energy expenditure in sedentary individuals, with the thermic effects of food and exercise each accounting for approximately 20% (Sims 1989; Hill 1993).

In addition to the obligatory expenditure of energy, in each of these "energy compartments," metabolizable energy may also be lost as heat, an adaptive mechanism referred to as facultative thermogenesis (Sims 1989). Facultative thermogenesis, which is driven by sympathetic nervous system activity, and also regulated by insulin and thyroid hormone, allows dissipation of excess calories as heat and thus helps to buffer against weight gain. The capacity for facultative thermogenesis varies significantly between individuals and is thought to account for a greater tendency to develop obesity in some individuals than others (Miller 1967; Ravussin 1988). In situations of markedly decreased caloric intake, a reduction in facultative energy expenditure occurs, preserving energy for other uses. While this response to caloric deprivation has survival advantage in the setting of starvation, it explains in part the diminishing rate of weight loss over time with very low calorie diets, and may play an important role in subsequent regain of lost weight.

Strategies for Weight Reduction

There are a number of available approaches to weight loss, varying from individual efforts to ''cut back'' food consumption to structured commercial programs. At any given time, approximately one-third of American adults are attempting to lose weight (Horm 1993), at a cost of more than $30 billion per year (NIH Technology Assessment Conference 1993). Common techniques are listed in Table 9.4. Each method is described and available information regarding efficacy, advantages, and disadvantages is discussed below.

Changes in Diet Composition

Changing the dietary proportions of nutrients consumed may alter the total caloric intake, or cause significant changes in the amount of energy expended to metabolize food, and thus promote change in body weight. One approach is the fad diet, such as the ''Ice Cream Diet'' or the ''Grapefruit Diet.'' Popular because of simplicity and the promise of rapid weight loss, such diets are nutritionally unbalanced and long-term success rates are low; their use should be discouraged in favor of safer and more effective methods (Atkinson 1993).

Very low-fat diets have gained popularity in recent years, and have several theoretical advantages over simple calorie restriction, including a mild increase in the thermic effect of food and possibly an enhanced sense of satiety in persons ingesting a low fat diets. Epidemiologic data and clinical trials both suggest that higher dietary fat content is associated with higher body weight (Sheppard 1991). Increasing the dietary fiber content has also recently been touted as means of increasing satiety and thus improving adherence to a low-calorie diet (Rigaud 1990). Fiber consists of various indigestible carbohydrates of plant origin, such as cellulose and pectin (Anderson

Table 9.4. Treatment Methods

Decreased Caloric Intake	Increased Caloric Expenditure	Both
Changed diet composition	Exercise	Behavioral Modification
Moderate caloric restriction		Drugs
Severe caloric restriction		
Surgery		

1986). When the fiber content of the diet is increased by substituting grains and vegetables for animal products, the fat content also decreases. It may thus be difficult to assess the independent effects of low fat and high fiber, except when fiber is added to the usual diet as a dietary supplement.

EFFECTIVENESS. Results of clinical trials suggest that even when total calorie intake is unchanged, a decrease in dietary fat content results in weight loss (Kendall 1991; Prewitt 1991; Sheppard 1991), with preferential loss of body fat and possible increase in lean tissue (Prewitt 1991). In studies of obese and normal weight women, when dietary fat was decreased but total caloric intake maintained, weight losses varied from a mean of 2.5 kg in 11 weeks (Kendall 1991) to 3.1 kg in one year (Sheppard 1991). Some weight regain over time is common, with average weight loss after two years of 1.9 kg.

The efficacy of dietary fiber in augmenting weight reduction remains controversial. One placebo-controlled study revealed significantly greater weight loss (5.5 vs 3.0 kg) and decreased hunger after six months when a fiber supplement was added to a hypocaloric diet (Rigaud 1990), but other controlled studies have revealed little or no benefit with fiber supplementation (Atkinson 1989).

ADVANTAGES AND BENEFITS. A diet with decreased fat or increased fiber, without marked caloric restriction, may be easier to tolerate than a reduced calorie diet. Furthermore, decreased fat intake, independent of adiposity, may be associated with decreased risks of breast cancer, colorectal cancer, and heart disease (Liu 1979; Wydner 1986; LaRosa 1990).

In addition to increased satiety, other possible effects of high-fiber diets include decreased blood pressure (Rossner 1988) and improved lipid profile (Sprecher 1993). Also, increased dietary fiber has been associated with decreased risk of colon cancer (Reddy 1980).

DISADVANTAGES AND RISKS. When fiber is provided by increasing fruit, vegetable, and grain consumption, rather than adding a dietary supplement, compliance with the high fiber diet decreases (Atkinson 1989). Increased dietary fiber may cause flatulence, bloating, and abdominal discomfort. Weight losses reported with low-fat or high-fiber diets without caloric restriction are modest and not sufficient to reverse risk factors in individuals with significant obesity.

Moderate Caloric Restriction

Moderate caloric restriction, a mainstay of obesity treatment since the 1950s, is defined as a diet of 800–1,500 kcal/day of conventional foods, usually 1,200 kcal/day for women and 1,500 kcal/day for men (Wadden 1993). The diet may be self-prescribed, prescribed as part of participation in an organized group (Levy 1993), or recommended by a physician or dietitian.

EFFECTIVENESS. As expected, the amount of weight lost varies with the length of time the diet is followed. The usual rate of weight loss is 0.5–1.0% of initial weight per week (Blackburn 1993) for a 10–15% weight loss over 10 to 20 weeks. A recent review reported an average weight loss of 8.5 kg over 20 weeks of moderate caloric restriction (Wadden 1993). Success in the initial weight loss effort, and in weight maintenance, varies with the degree of supervision by the health care provider (Blackburn 1993), concurrent use of behavioral modification techniques, and concurrent participation in an exercise regimen (Wadden 1992c). In the absence of these, one-third of weight is regained in the first year, and most subjects will return to baseline weight within five years (Wadden 1993).

ADVANTAGES AND BENEFITS. Because this diet involves usual foods ingested in smaller portions, it tends to be nutritionally balanced and safe (Wadden 1993). Depending upon the intensity of supervision by the health care provider, it is also a relatively inexpensive method of weight loss. Weight loss in the range usually observed with moderate caloric restriction confers a significant decrease in health risk for overweight individuals (Goldstein 1992).

DISADVANTAGES AND RISKS. The use of the same caloric prescription for all individuals (with a small adjustment based on the patient's sex) leads to markedly different rates of weight loss varying with the patient's size, degree of overweight, and rate of energy expenditure (Wadden 1993). The rate of weight loss may be unacceptably slow for more obese patients, particularly the morbidly obese.

Severe Caloric Restriction

Severe caloric restriction was first prescribed in the 1920s as a safer means of achieving rapid weight loss than total starvation (Wadden 1983). Also referred to as "Very Low Calorie Diets" (VLCDs), these diets provide a maximum of 800 kcal/day. Diets providing approximately 400, 600, and 800 kcal/day result in equivalent amounts of weight loss (Foster 1992). To minimize loss of lean tissue and minimize cardiac complications (as discussed below), such diets should contain sufficient high-quality protein, and adequate vitamins, minerals, and electrolytes. The diet is usually given as a liquid formulation, which completely replaces normal meals for a period of several weeks to months. Food-based diets (lean meat, chicken, or fish) with appropriate supplements are nutritionally equivalent and less expensive than liquid formulations (National Task Force on the Prevention and Treatment of Obesity 1993).

EFFECTIVENESS. When VLCD is prescribed for 12 to 16 weeks, weight losses of 15–25 kg are reported (National Task Force on the Prevention and Treatment of Obesity 1993; Wadden 1983; Wadden 1993). Maintenance of weight loss is less successful, however. While high attrition rates in many studies limit data on long-term follow-up, the majority of patients regain most or all of weight lost within two to five years (Anderson 1991; National Task Force on the Prevention and Treatment of Obesity 1993; Wadden 1993), although the addition of behavior modification and exercise to the diet program appears to reduce the rate of weight regain (Wadden 1989; Phinney 1992).

ADVANTAGES AND BENEFITS. VLCD facilitates reasonably safe, rapid weight loss in motivated, compliant, well-monitored patients with severe obesity (BMI > 30, or 30% or more above ideal body weight). Rapid improvements have been reported in a number of comorbid conditions, including hypertension, hyperlipidemia, diabetes, sleep apnea, right heart failure (Anderson 1991; Wadden 1992b; National Task Force on the Prevention and Treatment of Obesity 1993). VLCD usually leads to a marked decrease in requirements for insulin or oral hypoglycemic therapy in patients with NIDDM, and thus may be a preferred method of weight loss in these patients. Surgical morbidity and mortality, higher in the morbidly obese, is decreased by successful preoperative weight loss with VLCD. The low carbohydrate content of VLCDs leads to the use of fatty acids rather than glucose as the major fuel for metabolic functions, and may lead to preferential mobilization and loss of fat stores rather than lean body tissue (Flatt 1974). In addition, ketone body formation resulting from metabolism of fatty acids may produce anorexia (Felig 1978), and may at least in part underlie the decreases in hunger reported in patients on VLCDs compared to conventional diets (Wadden 1987).

DISADVANTAGES AND RISKS. Adverse effects are common in patients treated with VLCDs for the typically prescribed time periods (12 to 16 weeks) (National Task Force on the Prevention and Treatment of Obesity 1993). Reported side effects include fatigue, weakness, orthostatic dizziness, constipation, diarrhea, nausea, headache, cold intolerance, dry skin, menstrual irregularities, and peripheral neuropathies (Bistrian 1978; Wadden 1983; Anderson 1991). Hyperuricemia may develop, although acute gout is uncommon in patients with no prior history of gout (Atkinson 1989).

While, as noted above, diabetic patients may be particularly responsive to VLCDs, close attention to hypoglycemic therapy is required. Oral hypoglycemic medication should be discontinued at the start of VLCD, and nighttime insulin doses can usually also be discontinued. When fasting glucose values are less than 200 mg/dl, daytime insulin dose can be decreased by 50%. When the total daytime insulin dose is less than 20 units, insulin therapy can be discontinued altogether (Mascioli 1993). Home glucose monitoring is indicated to facilitate insulin adjustment and avoid hypoglycemia.

Gallstones, three times more common in the morbidly obese than in nonobese persons (Anderson 1991), occur with greater frequency in obese individuals undergoing rapid weight loss. Asymptomatic gallstones developed in 11% of patients on VLCDs in one large study (Yang 1992). Symptomatic cholecystitis develops in 2 to 3% of patients during VLCD, and may develop in an equal number of patients during the early refeeding period (Anderson 1991).

Of significant concern with VLCDs is a reported risk of sudden cardiac death, first noted in the 1970s, when numerous cases of fatal arrhythmias occurred in VLCD dieters. Such events have been attributed to poor quality protein, with the resultant cardiac effects of protein-calorie malnutrition, and lack of medical supervision to monitor electrolyte balance (Wadden 1983; National Task Force on the Prevention and Treatment of Obesity 1993). To minimize risk of adverse cardiac events, VLCD should not be prescribed to patients with a history of ventricular arrhythmia, unexplained syncope, prolonged QT interval, unstable angina, or recent myocardial infarction (National Task Force on the Prevention and Treatment of Obesity 1993). Other medical conditions which may contraindicate participation in a VLCD program include systemic infection or other catabolic condition such as active malignancy, recent stroke or transient ischemic attack, decreased renal function, significant hepatic impairment, ongoing lithium or tricyclic antidepressant therapy, active psychosis or substance abuse problems, or a history of bulimia or anorexia (Bistrian 1978; Wadden 1983).

Pregnancy is an absolute contraindication to VLCD, and use of reliable contraceptive method should be ascertained prior to enrolling a woman of childbearing age in a VLCD program (National Task Force on the Prevention and Treatment of Obesity 1993). Data concerning the use of VLCD in the elderly and in children are limited. While VLCD may be appropriate in certain severely obese children and adolescents, concerns about maintaining normal growth and development suggest that extreme care in patient selection and supervision is required (National Task Force on the Prevention and Treatment of Obesity 1993). VLCD may not be appropriate for individuals with milder obesity (BMI < 30 kg/m^2), because greater protein losses during VLCD in these leaner individuals may increase their risk of cardiac events (National Task Force on the Prevention and Treatment of Obesity 1993).

SURGERY. Surgery has been used to treat severe obesity since the early 1950s. Initially, small intestinal bypass procedures were used to induce malabsorption, but such procedures were abandoned in the 1970s because of serious complications (Consensus Development Conference Panel 1991). In the 1980s, intragastric balloons gained popularity, but fell out of use when scientific studies failed to show efficacy (Kral 1988). At present, two surgical procedures, the vertical-banded gastroplasty, and the gastric bypass, are in use in the United States for treatment of morbid obesity, or significant obesity associated with comorbid conditions such as sleep apnea or diabetes mellitus, or in those unresponsive to other methods of weight loss (Kral 1989; Consensus Development Conference Panel 1991). As shown in Figure 9.6 both procedures involve formation of a small (15–30 ml) pouch in the proximal stomach with a restricted outlet. Food passes first into the pouch and then directly into the jejunum after the bypass procedure, or into the distal stomach after the gastroplasty (Gastric operations 1984).

EFFECTIVENESS. Available data indicate that each of these surgical approaches is effective and reasonably safe in an appropriately selected subgroup of obese patients (Consensus Development Conference Panel 1991). Weight loss after surgery averages 55% to 60% of excess weight and occurs primarily within the first six months, with the nadir reached at 12–24 months (Gastric operations 1984; Consensus Development Conference Panel 1991; Lovig 1993). However, an estimated 25–50% of patients regain significant weight between two and five years after surgery (Linner 1982; Lovig 1993). Gastric bypass may result in somewhat greater weight loss than gastroplasty, although the long term complication rate is also higher with this procedure, as discussed below (Linner 1982; Consensus Development Conference Panel 1991).

ADVANTAGES AND BENEFITS. While weight loss may be no greater than that achievable with severe caloric restriction, the rate of weight regain appears to be much lower (Anderson 1984). Long-term improvements in sleep apnea, diabetes mellitus, lipid profile, angina, congestive heart failure, and hypertension have been reported (Kral 1989; Gleysteen 1990; Consensus Development Conference Panel 1991; Pories 1992).

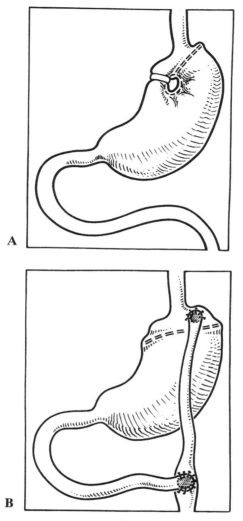

Fig. 9.6. (**A**) Vertical banded gastroplasty. (**B**) Roux-en-Y gastric bypass. [From Consensus Development Conference Panel (1991), with permission.]

DISADVANTAGES AND RISKS. Operative mortality rates range from 0% to 4% and postoperative morbidity may be as high as 14%, with late complications reported in up to 34% (Lovig 1993). Early postoperative complications include wound dehiscence, stomal stenosis, and pneumonia (Consensus Development Conference Panel 1991; Lovig 1993). Later complications include persistent vomiting, ulcers, cholecystitis, electrolyte disturbances, and micronutrient deficiencies, which may occur weeks to months after surgery (Amaral 1984; Benotti 1989; Consensus Development Conference Panel 1991; Lovig 1993). Failure to adhere to the prescribed diet may result in weight regain or obstructive symptoms (Kral 1989). Deficiencies of iron, vitamin B12, and folate are particularly prevalent after the gastric bypass procedure, and may not become apparent until 20 to 60 months postoperatively (Amaral 1984). Other concerns include possible fetal malformations caused by nutritional deficiencies if pregnancy occurs during active weight loss, and reduced absorption of calcium and vitamin D (Amaral 1984; Consensus Development Conference Panel 1991). Careful medical follow-up of these patients must thus continue indefinitely after surgery.

Exercise

Exercise has a number of positive physiologic effects, and is the only nonpharmacologic method of voluntarily increasing energy expenditure. Exercise may suppress the appetite (Segal 1989), and allows preferential loss of fat with preservation of lean tissue. Since resting metabolic rate is proportional to lean body mass, exercise may thus ameliorate the fall in resting metabolic rate which normally occurs with caloric restriction (Pavlou 1989). Exercise as a mitigator of coronary risk is discussed in more detail elsewhere in this text (see Chapter 8).

EFFECTIVENESS. Exercise alone, without concomitant dietary restriction generally does not result in significant weight loss (Dale 1987; Segal 1989) but may expedite the weight loss associated with caloric restriction, or preserve lean body mass with increased loss of fat mass (Pavlou 1989).

ADVANTAGES AND BENEFITS. Even in the absence of weight loss, exercise has been shown to decrease insulin resistance in obese subjects (DeFronzo 1987), which may explain epidemiologic data that risks of diabetes mellitus (Helmrich 1991; Manson 1991), and of coronary disease (Morris 1990) are lower in overweight persons who exercise than in otherwise similar sedentary individuals. A combination of diet and exercise may lead to a greater decrease in WHR than dieting alone (Wood 1991). Participation in an exercise regimen has also been shown to decrease the likelihood of weight regain after a period of caloric restriction (Wadden 1989).

DISADVANTAGES AND RISKS. Vigorous exercise in the absence of prior conditioning has been associated with sudden death (Friedewald 1990). Gradual initiation of an exercise program under medical supervision is thus appropriate in the obese. Osteoarthritis of the knees, more common in the obese (Felson 1988), and general deconditioning may significantly limit participation in an exercise program. With gradual initiation of an appropriate exercise program, such as walking, there are few disadvantages and risks.

Behavioral Modification

Behavioral methods of treating obesity became popular in the early 1970s; since that time more than 100 controlled studies of these methods have been published, and the methods have been incorporated in many popular self-help and commercial diet programs (Brownell 1989). Current programs incorporate one or more of several techniques, with the goal of altering daily habits or behaviors related to eating and exercise. These techniques, reviewed in detail elsewhere (Brownell 1989; Foreyt 1993) are discussed briefly here.

Self-monitoring is a widely used technique in which the patient learns to observe and record his or her own eating behavior, including circumstances related to eating, the amount and types of food consumed, moods, and exercise patterns (Brownell 1989; Foreyt 1993). Increased awareness of behavior is helpful in initiating behavior change and reducing inappropriate eating behavior (Foreyt 1993). *Stimulus control* involves restricting environmental factors associated with inappropriate eating behavior. For example, patients are taught to avoid purchasing or preparing ''problem'' foods, and to avoid eating in association with other activities (such as watching television) which may promote eating excessive amounts or high-calorie foods. *Contingency management or reinforcement* involves rewarding desired eating or exercise patterns. For example, the patient might treat him or herself to a movie, or other non-food-related activity, as a reward for adherence to the exercise program for one week. *Cognitive change* is a method of modifying attitudes and beliefs which may affect treatment success, for example, replacing negative beliefs about the ability to succeed in a weight loss program with a more positive attitude.

EFFECTIVENESS. Behavioral methods are generally used in conjunction with other weight loss methods; the effectiveness of these methods alone is thus difficult to assess (Foreyt 1993). Use of behavioral methods has resulted in weight loss ranging from 3.9 to 10 kg in 8 to 16 weeks (Brownell 1987; Foreyt 1993). The rate of weight regain may be less with behavioral methods than with other techniques; in one study, only one-third of the weight lost was regained after 44 weeks (Brownell 1987).

ADVANTAGES AND BENEFITS. The addition of behavioral techniques to standard weight loss programs appears to increase the amount of weight lost (Wadden 1992c), decrease the rates of attrition and noncompliance (Foreyt 1993), and improve weight maintenance after VLCD or surgery (Brownell 1989; Wadden 1989).

DISADVANTAGES AND RISKS. There are no risks associated with behavioral techniques. In the severely obese, however, these techniques alone are likely to be insufficient to induce significant weight loss (Brownell 1989).

Drug Therapy

Pharmacologic approaches to the treatment of obesity were first reported over 100 years ago. Concerns about the safety of several early approaches (thyroid hormone, dinitrophenol, and later amphetamines) limited the use and acceptance of drug treatment for obesity (Bray 1993). In particular, the abuse potential of amphetamines, appetite suppressants with addictive central nervous system stimulatory effects, led to strict regulation of all antiobesity drugs (Bray 1991). Drug therapy of obesity has been limited even more by common beliefs that obesity is the result of character weakness and self-indulgence, and that antiobesity drugs are only prescribed by ''quacks and charlatans'' (Frank 1993). The concept that pills should ''cure'' rather than control this chronic condition has contributed to regulatory limitations in the availability and duration of treatment with such drugs, and contrasts sharply with the expectations of pharmacologic agents used to treat other chronic conditions such as hypertension, diabetes, gout, and glaucoma (Weintraub 1989; Guy-Grande 1992). While many of the antiobesity agents described below are FDA-approved for treatment of weight loss, regulatory boards within some states limit or forbid prescribing them.

Despite these difficulties, there continues to be considerable interest in drugs that might safely be used in conjunction with other modalities for long-term treatment of obesity. Newer appetite suppressants, thermogenic drugs, hormones such as cholecystokinin, and gastrointestinal enzyme inhibitors such as acarbose, are among the agents studied (Weintraub 1989). The two most widely studied and used classes of antiobesity agents, appetite suppressants and thermogenic drugs, are the focus of the remainder of this section.

APPETITE SUPPRESSANTS. Appetite suppressants appear to work by stimulating CNS noradrenergic pathways or serotonergic pathways. While some noradrenergic agonists, such as amphetamines, have addictive stimulatory effects, those noradrenergic drugs that are currently FDA-approved (e.g., diethylpropion, mazindol, and phentermine, DEA schedule IV drugs) appear to have little abuse potential. Phenylpropanolamine, a common ingredient in over-the-counter cold remedy with little stimulant effect (Greenway 1992), is the only adrenergic appetite suppressant available over the counter.

Serotonergic agonists include fenfluramine, dexfenfluramine (the L-isomer of fenfluramine, active at half the dose), and the antidepressants fluoxetine and sertraline (Bray 1993). Of these, only fenfluramine is FDA-approved for treatment of obesity, and few data are available concerning the efficacy of sertraline for weight loss.

THERMOGENIC DRUGS. Ephedrine, an over-the-counter cold and asthma treatment, is the most widely studied thermogenic drug (Dulloo 1993a). Also a noradrenergic agonist drug with indirect sympathomimetic properties, ephedrine increases sympathetic nervous system activity, driving thermogenesis and modestly increasing energy expenditure. Caffeine, theophylline, and aspirin appear to potentiate these effects *in situ* and *in vivo* (Dulloo 1993b), and ephedrine has been used in varying combinations with these medications. Like other noradrenergic drugs, ephedrine also has some central appetite suppressant effects, but these are probably less important than its thermogenic properties in its long-term effects on body weight.

A promising new class of thermogenic agents has been discovered, which is thought to have a particular affinity to the newly characterized class of β-adrenergic receptors, the β-3 receptor. The β-3 receptor is found in brown adipose tissue, a major site of facultative thermogenesis, and appears to play a crucial role in driving thermogenesis in animal models. By specifically targeting the β-3 adrenoreceptor, it is hoped that these agents will manifest fewer cardiovascular and other side effects related to β-1 and β-2 stimulation (Dulloo 1993a). To date, BRL 26830A is the only β-3 agonist to be used in clinical trials (Connacher 1992).

EFFECTIVENESS. The efficacy of serotonergic appetite suppressants, phenylpropanolamine, and thermogenic drugs in inducing modestly greater weight loss than placebo has been demonstrated in numerous placebo-controlled clinical trials of varying lengths, with and without concomitant caloric restriction (Bray 1993). Table 9.5

Table 9.5. Pharmacotherapy for Obesity: Representative Results of Placebo-Controlled Studies

Drug (Daily dose mg)	Duration (weeks)	Patients (Drug/Placebo)	Mean Weight Loss kg		Dietary Restriction	Reference
			Drug	Placebo		
Fenfluramine (40)	6	44/43	2.4	0.3	None	Dent 1975
Fenfluramine phenteramine (60/15)	28	62/59	9.8	0.7	18–20 kcal/kg IBW	Weintraub 1992
Dexfenfluramine (30)	52	295/268	9.8	7.2	Moderate coloric restriction	Guy-Grande 1989
Phenylpropanolamine (75)	12	53/53	6.1	4.3	16–18 kcal/kg IBW	Weintraub 1986
Ephedrine (150)	8	5/5	2.4	0.6	1000–1400 kcal/d	Pasquali 1987
Ephedrine, caffeine (60/600)	24	24/25	15.9	13.7	1000 kcal/d	Toubro 1993
Ephedrine, caffeine, aspirin (150/150/330)	8	11/13	2.2	0.7	Dietary advice	Krieger 1990
BRL 26830A	18	16/14	15.4	5.4	800 kcal	Connacher 1992

Source: Modified from Bray (1993), with permission.

All studies shown were placebo-controlled trials in which weight loss was statistically significantly greater in drug vs placebo-treated patients.

summarizes several representative studies, all of which have reported a significantly greater weight loss with drug compared to placebo. Recently, a direct comparison between dexfenfluramine (15 mg b.i.d.) and ephedrine/caffeine (20/200 mg t.i.d.) in 100 obese patients, treated with concurrent moderate caloric restriction and exercise for 15 weeks, suggested that the ephedrine caffeine combination may be slightly more effective, particularly in those patients with BMI > 30 kg/m^2 (Breum 1994). As with most methods of weight loss, weight regain is common after cessation of treatment (Douglas 1983). For weight loss to be clinically relevant and sustained, drug treatment must be used as an adjunct, not a substitute for calorie restriction, exercise, and behavioral modification.

ADVANTAGES AND BENEFITS. As discussed above, weight loss appears to be greater when either appetite suppressants or thermogenic agents are added to other weight loss methods. Pharmacotherapy may also play a role in continuing or maintaining weight loss after VLCD (Pasquali 1987a; Finer 1992). Ephedrine and caffeine mixtures may prevent the fall in resting metabolic rate that occurs in response to significant caloric restriction (Pasquali 1987b; Astrup 1991), may prevent the transient decrease in HDL reported with severe caloric restriction (Buemann 1994) and may lead to preferential loss of body fat with preservation of lean tissue (Pasquali 1993; Toubro 1993).

DISADVANTAGES AND RISKS. While little potential for drug addiction exists with fenfluramine and other serotonergic drugs, side effects include fatigue, drowsiness, sedation, diarrhea, nausea, and depression, particularly after acute withdrawal of the drug (Guy-Grande 1992). Some concern persists about addictive potential of noradrenergic appetite suppressants. Increased blood pressure may occur with noradrenergic appetite suppressants (including phenylpropanolamine) and ephedrine; these agents should thus be used cautiously, if at all, in hypertensive individuals. Ephedrine used alone or in combination with caffeine, may have other side effects including tachycardia, tremor, dry mouth, insomnia, and constipation and "withdrawal" symptoms (e.g., fatigue and headache); all of these symptoms are more frequent with high doses of caffeine (600 mg/day) than with ephedrine alone, or ephedrine with aspirin and smaller doses of caffeine (150 mg/day, approximately equivalent to three cups of coffee per day) (Daly 1993; Pasquali 1993; Toubro 1993). β-3 agonists appear to cause few cardiovascular effects, but tremor which persists for the duration of drug treatment occurs in most patients (Connacher 1992). With both the appetite suppressants and the thermogenic agents, side effects generally abate after the first several weeks of treatment (Krieger 1991; Toubro 1993).

Miscellaneous

PSYCHOTHERAPY. Whether the prevalence of psychopathology is greater among the obese than among lean individuals is the subject of some controversy (Rodin 1989; Telch 1994). Obesity may be associated with higher rates of childhood sexual abuse, parental loss or absence, and family alcoholism (Felitti 1991, 1993). The higher prevalence of psychopathology, such as major depression and personality disorder, observed in some studies of obese subjects may be related to the presence or severity of Binge Eating Disorder, and not to obesity *per se* (Yanovski 1993b; Telch 1994). While depression and other psychological distress may not be directly related to the cardiovascular risk imposed by obesity, they are likely to form a barrier to effective treatment of obesity (Felitti 1993). Identifying and treating these conditions may thus play an important role in any successful obesity intervention.

COMMUNITY/WORKPLACE INTERVENTIONS. Because obesity is a widespread problem, a variety of programs targeted at worksites or entire communities have been used, with varying success (Gomel 1993; Jeffery 1993). Such programs aim to screen and educate large populations regarding obesity and other cardiovascular risks. Written materials or group sessions are used to make dietary and exercise recommendations and to instruct individuals in behavioral techniques. Group competitions and positive reinforcement in the form of prizes or small monetary incentives are used to increase participation and compliance. These programs may reach large numbers of overweight individuals, and produce modest weight losses at lower cost than more individualized programs (Geppert 1991). These interventions may be helpful in treating mildly over-weight individuals but are less useful in treatment of severe obesity. They may be best suited for prevention, rather than treatment of obesity (Jeffery 1993).

Cost Effectiveness: Comparison of Weight Reduction Strategies

While several studies have compared the effectiveness of different weight loss strategies, costs have been considered much less commonly. Estimates of "cost per pound" are complicated by variable success in weight reduction and, even more, by high rates of weight regain which are typically ignored in cost estimates. However, a number of authors (Stunkard 1989; Geppert 1991) have emphasized the relative cost savings of group programs administered through the workplace; as compared with clinic or university-based programs (Table 9.6). Because such interventions are less effective in the severely or morbidly obese, more intensive weight-loss strategies, such as VLCD or even surgery, may have economic as well as clinical justification in these and other high risk individuals.

Treatment of Hypertension, Dyslipidemia, and Non-Insulin-Dependent Diabetes Mellitus in the Obese Patient

As previously noted, obesity is associated with abnormalities in blood pressure, lipid profile, and glucose tolerance, all of which improve with weight reduction. While weight loss is a primary approach to all of these disorders in the obese, concomitant pharmacologic treatment of these conditions may be indicated, particularly if weight loss is insufficient. Detailed management strategies for hypertension, hyperlipidemia, and NIDDM are discussed elsewhere in this book. This section notes therapeutic considerations particularly relevant in the obese population.

Table 9.6. Cost Comparison of Various Weight Loss Programs

Program	Cost per 1% Reduction in Percent Overweight
University Clinic	$108.67
Work site program (professional leaders)	$ 33.61
Clinic: VLCD	$ 28.30
Clinic: Behavior therapy	$ 19.62
Work site program (lay leaders)	$ 11.10
Commercial program	$ 7.31
Work site competition	$ 0.92

Hypertension

There is currently no consensus as to which class of antihypertensives is most effective in the setting of obesity. Beta-blockers have been shown to be more effective in controlling hypertension in obese than in lean persons (Schmieder 1983); however, these agents appear to decrease glucose-induced thermogenesis (Acheson 1993), which may hinder weight loss or contribute to weight gain, and may exacerbate abnormalities in lipids (McMahon 1987) and glucose tolerance (Prisant 1992). Because hypertension in the obese is typically a low-renin, volume-overloaded state, diuretics may be more effective, and angiotensin-converting enzyme inhibitors less effective in these individuals. However, thiazides, like beta-blockers, may have adverse effects on lipid profile and glucose tolerance not seen with angiotensin-converting enzyme inhibitors (Pollare 1989). Calcium channel blockers and alpha-blockers, both with few or no adverse metabolic effects, may have some theoretical advantages (Pollare 1988; Weir 1991). In a direct comparison between a calcium channel blocker and a beta-blocker in obesity-related hypertension, however, the former was less effective (Schmieder 1993). The choice of antihypertensive agents in the obese must be individualized, based upon the coexistence of other health risks; in the absence of compelling reasons to choose particular agents, avoiding those agents with adverse metabolic effects is prudent.

Hyperlipidemia

In patients experiencing significant weight loss, as with VLCD, the serum cholesterol decreases significantly in the first four to eight weeks. A transient elevation in total cholesterol, exceeding the patient's baseline value, may be observed several months into VLCD; the serum cholesterol again falls below the baseline value with weight maintenance (Phinney 1991). In individuals with high WHRs, hyperlipidemia may be more responsive to dietary changes (Kanaley 1993). With respect to pharmacotherapy, no information is available to suggest that one class of lipid lowering drug is more effective than another in the obese. Since hypertriglyceridemia and low HDL cholesterol are common in the obese (as discussed above) gemfibrozil, particularly effective at correcting these abnormalities (Manninen 1992), is usually an appropriate agent for treating dyslipidemia in the obese. Niacin is best avoided if diabetes is present, due to the deterioration in glucose tolerance sometimes seen with this agent (Henkin 1991).

NIDDM

As previously noted, obese patients tend to be insulin resistant, and when insulin is required for glucose control, large doses are the norm. In obese NIDDM patients, the method of weight loss may be important for achieving optimal improvement in glucose control. Treatment with VLCD results in a rapid, marked improvement in glucose control (Wadden 1983), significantly greater than that seen with moderate caloric restriction, even when weight loss is comparable (Wing 1994). When VLCD is initiated, oral hypoglycemic agents can immediately be discontinued, and insulin either decreased or stopped altogether in the majority of patients (Anderson 1991).

Obesity Prevention

Given the difficulties of weight loss, high rates of weight regain, and potential dangers of weight cycling, primary prevention of obesity remains the optimal approach to minimizing obesity-related health risks. Many behaviors predisposing to obesity are acquired during childhood and adolescence, and overweight children are at high risk for becoming obese adults (Jackson 1991). Young adults, in turn, are at high risk for significant weight gain. Data from NHANES-I showed that significant weight gain (i.e., ≥ 5 kg/m^2) was most likely to occur in 25- to 34-year-olds, and young women were twice as likely as men to gain (Williamson 1990). Increased parity is also a risk factor for excessive weight gain (Rossner 1992). As noted earlier, several ethnic minority groups, are also at particularly high risk for obesity (Kumanyika 1990). Cultural differences, educational attainment (Kahn 1991), economic factors, and differences in physical activity and in perceptions about health risk may all contribute to risk of weight gain (Wing 1989; Jackson 1991).

Prevention efforts should be targeted particularly at these higher risk groups. Efforts aimed at individuals, families, and communities may be appropriate. Educational programs in the school and workplace may be cost-effective methods of preventing weight gain (Jeffery 1993). The primary health care provider plays an important role, not only in treating obesity and its complications, but also in identifying and educating those at risk.

Cardiovascular Risk Assessment in the Obese Patient

The cardiovascular disease risks associated with obesity and the available modalities for treating obesity have been reviewed above. How can this information be used to greatest effect in the primary care setting? The goal of the medical evaluation is to assess the degree of obesity, to evaluate obesity-related risk factors, and then to begin appropriate therapy.

The initial evaluation should thus include weight history, (prior weight loss attempts and results of those attempts), eating pattern, including binge eating, as well as current dietary intake, current and prior smoking history, and exercise habits. Personal and family history of CHD, hypertension, hyperlipidemia, and diabetes should

Table 9.7. Accurate Measurement of Waist:Hip Ratio

1. **The Waist Measurement**
    - Locate the waist. The waist is defined as the smallest circumference of the torso, and is not necessarily at the umbilicus. In some obese patients, narrowing at the waist may not be present; the waist is then defined as the smallest horizontal circumference between the 12th rib and the iliac crest.
    - Measure the waist. The patient should be standing with abdomen relaxed, arms at sides, feet together, with no clothing at the waist. A flexible, nonstretchable tape measure is placed horizontally at the waist, without compressing the skin.

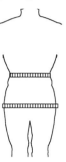

2. **The Hip Measurement**
    - Locate the hip (buttocks). The hip is defined as the circumference at the level of the maximum extension of the buttocks posteriorly, In obese patients, the anterior abdominal wall may sag, and by default, have to be included in the measurement.
    - Measure the hip. The patient should be standing tall but relaxed, with arms at sides, wearing only underwear. The practitioner kneels or squats to be at eye level laterally with the buttocks. A flexible, nonstretchable measuring tape is placed horizontally around the buttocks at the point of maximum circumference without compressing the skin.
3. **The Ratio**
    - Divide the waist circumference by the hip circumference (see Figure 9.7). A WHR of ≤0.95 in men, and ≤0.8 in women is acceptable. Higher ratios indicate increased health risk.

Source: Modified from Yanovski (1993a), with permission.

be ascertained (Yanovski 1993a), as well as any symptoms suggestive of CHD, diabetes or sleep apnea. Current medications, including over-the-counter preparations should be noted. A history of depression, anxiety, bulimia, other psychopathology, past psychiatric medications or treatment, or childhood neglect or abuse may also be relevant.

The physical examination should include weight, height, and measurement of waist and hip circumference, as detailed in Table 9.7. Attention should be given to any signs of end-organ damage from obesity *per se*, or coexisting diabetes or hypertension, for example, the optic fundi, the cardiovascular system, and the peripheral nervous system.

Laboratory evaluation should include fasting glucose, creatinine, lipid profile, and an electrocardiogram (EKG). Liver function testing may also be appropriate depending on the degree of obesity or the presence of symptoms suggesting biliary disease.

Once the overall evaluation is performed, an estimate of the patient's cardiovascular risk can be made. Tables 9.1 and 9.2 may be used to determine BMI and classifying patients accordingly. In all obese patients, particularly those with other asso-

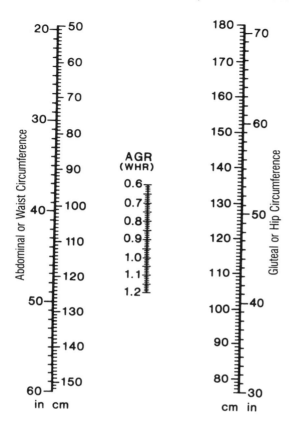

Fig. 9.7. Nomogram for easy determination of WHR. Place a straight edge between the column for waist circumference and the column for hip circumference and read ratio from the point where this straight edge crosses the WHR line. [©Bray (1987), reprinted with permission.]

ciated cardiac risk factors, the importance of moderate exercise and behavioral approaches for successful weight loss and weight maintenance must be emphasized.

Individuals who are overweight and have no other cardiac risk factors are at high risk for additional weight gain, as previously discussed. They should be educated with regard to lifestyle changes, which may lead to moderate weight loss or prevent subsequent weight gain. The patient with an increased waist:hip ratio should be informed of the higher risk of CHD associated with this finding, even in the mildly overweight. Exercise, low fat diet, modest caloric restriction, and participation in community or workplace programs may be useful in these patients.

Individuals who are overweight and have one or more cardiac risk factors should be educated concerning the relationship between weight and the risk factor, and the importance of even modest weight loss in improving these risk factors should be stressed. Institution of a nonstrenuous exercise program (e.g., walking) with appropriate supervision, and referral to a registered dietitian for education and supervision of moderate caloric restriction, with a dietary prescription tailored to each patient's needs, are also indicated in these individuals.

As BMI increases, concurrent cardiac risk factors are more likely to be present. Moderate caloric restriction, exercise, behavioral modification, and pharmacotherapy (where state regulatory boards allow) are all appropriate in the moderately obese. In patients with significant obesity (BMI > 30 kg/m²), VLCD should be considered; in those with morbid obesity (BMI > 40 kg/m²), or significant obesity with concurrent risk factors, particularly with unsuccessful previous weight loss attempts, surgery may be appropriate.

Weight reduction may reduce cardiac risk, and a supervised approach with multidisciplinary involvement of the dietitian, psychologist, physician, nurse, and other primary providers incorporating exercise, behavioral techniques and possibly antiobesity drugs, in addition to appropriate dietary intervention, is required for optimal success. Despite the best efforts of patients and health care providers, maintenance of weight loss is difficult, and weight regain remains relatively common no matter which weight loss approach is used. Continued regular contact with the health care provider and ongoing group support sessions *after* successful weight loss have each been shown to increase the likelihood of maintenance of weight loss (Wadden 1992c).

In addition to the information for patients provided in the Appendix, the American Heart Association (7272 Greenville Ave, Dallas, TX 75231-4596) is a useful resource for low cost pamphlets and patient-oriented educational material concerning diet, weight reduction, exercise, and other risk reduction strategies. Other patient-oriented resources include the books recommended to patients in the appendix, and various lay newsletters, such as the Tufts or Berkeley Nutrition Newsletter.

Conclusions

In this chapter, the direct and indirect associations between obesity and CHD have been detailed, the rationale for weight reduction to ameliorate cardiovascular risk has been outlined, and available approaches to weight reduction have been systematically reviewed, with attention to efficacy, benefits, and risks. The relatively high rates of weight regain with all approaches highlight the difficulties of weight maintenance and emphasizes the importance of primary prevention as the best means of minimizing obesity-related coronary risk.

Summary

Quality of available data: A large body of well-designed observational (prospective cohort) studies.

Estimated risk reduction: 35–55% lower risk associated with maintaining ideal body weight as compared with being 20% or more above desirable weight. Data are not available on the role of sustained weight loss in the prevention of MI.

Comparability of effect in men and women: Effects of obesity on MI risk and the benefits of weight reduction appear comparable in men and women.

Appendix A

Healthy Habits for Lifetime Weight Control

Are you, like many Americans, worried about your weight? While many people worry because of the effects of extra weight on physical appearance, extra pounds are associated with a number of more serious health problems. Diabetes, high blood pressure, high cholesterol, and heart disease are more common in those who are overweight. Fortunately, losing weight can improve all of these problems. The recommendations on this sheet are meant to help overweight individuals lose weight and keep it off, and to prevent the usual weight gain that occurs as normal weight people approach middle age.

How much weight is too much? Obviously, this differs from person to person. The read concern, medically, is too much body fat. A 6-foot, 220-lb athlete may not be overfat even though he is technically overweight. There are several ways of estimating body fat. In the average nonathlete, weight is probably a reasonable reflection of "fatness." Tables of normal weight according to height are available to tell you your "ideal" weight. Using your weight and height, your health care provider may also determine your body mass index, a slightly more accurate measure of overweight and obesity than weight alone. Sophisticated equipment can also be used to determine your body composition—the percentage of fat, muscle, and other lean tissues. While the results of these tests are interesting and may be useful for athletes in training, they are rarely more helpful than weight and height in the average person.

Another important measure of fatness is the distance around your waist (at its narrowest point) divided by the widest distance around your hips. Persons who carry their weight in the "upper body"—abdomen and chest—may not be fatter than those who take their extra weight in the hips, buttocks, and legs, but medical evidence is mounting that upper body obesity is more likely to be associated with high blood pressure, diabetes, high cholesterol, and heart disease.

If you are overweight, there are a number of changes you can make to help lose weight. Before you start, get your doctor or health care provider's "OK." If you take medication for diabetes, high blood pressure, or high cholesterol, these may need to be lowered as weight is lost, so regular checkups are important. In some cases, medication may be discontinued altogether as weight loss occurs.

To lose weight, you must burn off more calories than you eat. There are several ways to do this. Remember, just as weight gain occurs over many months to years, so does weight loss. Weight loss is much more likely to become permanent with small *permanent* changes in your day-to-day lifestyle. Here are some examples:

- Cut down on fat! Did you know that tablespoon for tablespoon, fat has more than twice the calories of sugar? Just by trimming fat from meats, switching from regular to "light" condiments (such as salad dressings), and selecting pretzels instead of chips, you can decrease your total caloric intake without decreasing the overall amount of food you eat.
- Cut down on calories. Have a salad instead of that second helping of lasagna. Snack on carrots and celery or air-popped popcorn rather than cheese and crackers. Calorie content in usually listed on food labels. A registered dietitian can also provide more information and guidelines concerning your caloric needs.
- Increase your activity. A regular exercise program has many benefits besides helping you lose weight. Get your doctor's OK, then start walking! Walking is a great form of exercise, because it requires no special equipment or skills. If the weather is a limiting factor, try walking laps in a nearby mall. Make it a point to increase your activity level throughout the day. Take the stairs rather than the elevator. Park a little further from your destination. As your endurance improves take up other sports, like tennis, bicycling, or cross-country skiing.
- Develop eating awareness. Do you snack in front of TV, or nibble while working in the kitchen? Do you eat when you're nervous, angry, or sad? Many people do. Becoming more aware of these patterns can help change them. Start by keeping a food log, showing where, when, and how much you eat. Measuring portion size may also be helpful. Make a point to limit your eating to designated meal and snack times. Eat only at the table. Eat slowly, savoring the food, and don't read or watch TV while you eat.
- Reward yourself for taking positive steps! Even if your initial goal is to cut out your nightly bag of chips, and walk for 5 minutes three times per week, working toward a reward can help keep you going. The reward can be anything you enjoy—*except* food!
- Learn more about nutrition and exercise. There are many ways to do this. Your health care provider may refer you to a registered dietitian. A number of books, pamphlets, and nutrition newsletters are available, too. Your provider may make specific recommendations. Two helpful books are: *Jane Brody's Nutrition Book* by Jane Brody (W.W. Norton, New York), and *The New American Diet* by Sonja Connor, M.S., R.D., and William Connor, M.D. (Simon & Schuster, New York).

In order to lose weight, and at least as importantly, to maintain weight loss, these new more healthy habits must be incorporated into your daily routine. Developing new habits is a slow and often difficult process. Don't be discouraged if it takes time to see the results of your efforts, and remember that the long-term benefits will make your efforts worthwhile.

References

Acheson K, Jequier E, Wahren J. Influence of beta-adrenergic blockade on glucose-induced thermogenesis in man. J Clin Invest 1983;72:981–6.

Amaral JF, Thompson WR, Caldwell MD, et al. Prospective hematologic evaluation of gastric exclusion surgery for morbid obesity. Ann Surg 1985;201:186–93.

Anderson, JW, Bryant CA. Dietary fiber: diabetes and obesity. Am J Gastroenterol 1986;81: 898–906.

Anderson JW, Hamilton CC, Brinkman-Kaplan V. Benefits and risks of an intensive very-low-calorie diet program for severe obesity. Am J Gastroenterol 1991;87:6–15.

Ashley FW, Kannel WB. Relationship to weight change in atherogenic traits: the Framingham study. J Chron Dis 1974;27:103–14.

Assman G, Schute H. Obesity and hyperlipidemia: results from the Prospective Cardiovascular Munster (PROCAM) Study. In: Bjorntorp P, Brodoff BN, eds. Obesity. New York: JB Lippincott, 1992:502–11.

Astrup A, Toubro S, Cannon S, et al. Thermogenic synergism between ephedrine and caffeine in healthy volunteers: a double-blind, placebo-controlled study. Metabolism 1991;40: 323–9.

Atkinson RL. Low and very low calorie diets. Med Clin North Am 1989;73:203–15.

Barrett-Connor EL. Obesity, atherosclerosis and coronary artery disease. Ann Intern Med 1985; 103:1010–15.

Barrett-Connor E, Khaw K. Cigarette smoking and increased central adiposity. Ann Intern Med 1989;111:783–7.

Benotti PN, Hollingshead J, Mascioli EA, et al. Gastric restrictive operations for morbid obesity. Am J Surg 1989;157:150–5.

Bistrian BR. Clinical use of a protein-sparing modified fast. JAMA 1978;240:2299–302.

Bjorntorp P. Classification of obese patients and complications related to the distribution of surplus fat. Am J Clin Nutr 1987;45:1120–5.

Blackburn GL, Wilson GT, Kanders BS, et al. Weight cycling: the experience of human dieters. Am J Clin Nutr 1989;49:1105–9.

Blackburn GL. Comparison of medically supervised and unsupervised approaches to weight loss and control. Ann Intern Med 1993;119:714–8.

Bonadonna RC, DeFronzo RA. Glucose metabolism in obesity and Type II diabetes. In: Bjorntorp P, Bandoff BN, eds. Philadelphia: JB Lippincott, 1992:492.

Bray GA, Gray DS. Obesity. Part I. Pathogenesis. West J Med 1988;149:429–41.

Bray GA. Barriers to the treatment of obesity. Ann Intern Med 1991;115:152–3.

Bray, GA. An approach to the classification and evaluation of obesity. In: Bjorntorp P, Brodoff BN, eds. Obesity. Philadelphia: JB Lippincott, 1992:294–308.

Bray GA. Use and abuse of appetite-suppressant drugs in the treatment of obesity. Ann Intern Med 1993;119:707–13.

Breum L, Pedersen JK, Ahlstrom F, Frimodt-Moller J. Comparison of an ephedrine/caffeine combination and dexfenfluramine in the treatment of obesity. Int J Obesity 1994;18:99–103.

Brownell KD, Jeffrey RW. Improving long term weight loss: pushing the limits of treatment. Behav Ther 1987;18:353–74.

Brownell KD, Kramer FM. Behavioral management of obesity. Med Clin North Am 1989;73: 185–201.

Buemann B, Marckmann P, Christensen JJ, Astrup A. The effect of ephedrine plus caffeine on plasma lipids and lipoproteins during a 4.1 mJ/day diet. Int J Obesity 1994;18:329–32.

Build and Blood Pressure Study, 1959. Chicago: Society of Actuaries, 1959.

Carney RM, Goldberg AP. Weight gain after cessation of cigarette smoking. A possible role for adipose-tissue lipoprotein lipase. N Engl J Med 1984;310:614–6.

Colditz GA, Willet WC, Stampfer MJ, et al. Weight as a risk factor for clinical diabetes in women. Am J Epidemiol 1990;132:501–13.

Colditz GA. Economic costs of obesity. Am J Clin Nutr 1992;55:503S–7S.

Comstock GW, Stone RW. Change in body weight and subcutaneous fatness related to smoking habits. Arch Environ Health 1972;24:271–6.

Connacher AA, Bennet WM, Jung RT. Clinical studies with the beta-adrenoreceptor agonist BRL 26830A. Am J Clin Nutr 1992;55:258S–61S.

Consensus Development Conference Panel, NIH Conference. Gastrointestinal surgery for severe obesity. Ann Intern Med 1991;115:956–61.

Daly PA, Krieger DR, Dulloo AG, et al. Ephedrine, caffeine, and aspirin: safety and efficacy for treatment of human obesity. Int J Obesity 1993;17(Suppl 1):S73–8.

Dattilo AM, Kris-Etherton M. Effects of weight reduction on blood lipids and lipoproteins: a meta-analysis. Am J Clin Nutr 1992;56:320–8.

DeFronzo RA, Cooke C, Andres R, et al. The effect of insulin on renal handling of sodium, potassium, calcium, and phosphate in man. J Clin Invest 1975;55:845–55.

DeFronzo RA, Sherwin RS, Kraemer R. Effects of physical training on insulin action in obesity. Diabetes 1987;36:1379–85.

Denke MA, Sempos CT, Grundy SM. Excess body weight: an underrecognized contributor to high blood cholesterol levels in white American men. Arch Intern Med 1993;153: 1093–103.

Dent RW, Preston LW. Anorectic effectiveness of various dosages of fenfluramine and placebo: a cooperative study. Curr Ther Res Clin Exp 1975;18:132–43.

Doria A, Fioretto P, Avogaro A, et al. Insulin resistance is associated with high sodium-lithium countertransport in essential hypertension. Am J Physiol 1991;261:E684–91.

Douglas JG, Gough J, Preston PG, et al. Long-term efficacy of fenfluramine in treatment of obesity. Lancet 1983;1:384–6.

Dublin LI. Relationship of obesity to longevity. N Engl J Med 1953;248:971–4.

Dulloo AG. Ephedrine, xanthines and prostaglandin-inhibitors: actions and interactions in the stimulation of thermogenesis. Int J Obesity 1993a;17(Suppl 1):S35–40.

Dulloo AG. Strategies to counteract readjustments toward lower metabolic rates during obesity management. Nutrition 1993b;9:366–72.

Dyer AR, Stamler J, Berkson DM, et al. Relationship of relative weight and body mass index to 14-year mortality in the Chicago Peoples Gas Company Study. J Chron Dis 1975; 28:109–23.

Felig P. Four questions about protein diets. N Engl J Med 1978;298:1025–6.

Felitti VJ. Long-term medical consequences of incest, rape, and molestation. So Med J 1991; 84:328–31.

Felitti VJ. Childhood sexual abuse, depression, and family dysfunction in adult obese patients: a case control study. So Med J 1993;86:732–6.

Felson DT, Anderson JJ, Naimark A, et al. Obesity and knee osteoarthritis. Ann Intern Med 1988;109:8–24.

Ferrannini E, Buzzigoli G, Bonadonna R, et al. Insulin resistance in essential hypertension. N Engl J Med 1987;317:350–7.

Finer N, Finer S, Naoumova R. Drug therapy after very-low-calorie diets. Am J Clin Nutr 1992; 56:195S–8S.

Flatt JP, Blackburn GL. The metabolic fuel regulatory system: implications for protein-sparing therapies during caloric deprivation and disease. Am J Clin Nutr 1974;27:175–87.

Folsom AR, Daye SS, Sellers TA, et al. Body fat distribution and 5-year risk of death in older women. JAMA 1993;269:483–7.

Foreyt JP, Goodrick GK. Evidence for success of behavior modification in weight loss and control. Ann Intern Med 1993;119:698.

Foster GD, Wadden TA, Petersen FJ, et al. A controlled comparison of three very-low-calorie diets: effects on weight, body composition, and symptoms. Am J Clin Nutr 1992;55: 811–7.

Frank A. Futility and avoidance: medical professionals in the treatment of obesity. JAMA 1993; 269:2132–3.

Freedman DS, Jacobsen SJ, Barboriak JJ, et al. Body fat distribution and male/female differences in lipids and lipoproteins. Circulation 1990;81:1498–506.

Friedewald VE, Spence DW. Sudden cardiac death associated with exercise: the risk-benefit issue. Am J Cardiol 1990;66:183–8.

Gastric operations for obesity. Med Let Pharm Ther 1984;26:113–5.

Geppert J, Splett PL. Summary document of nutrition intervention in obesity. J Am Diet Assoc 1991;91:S31–5.

Gillum RF, Taylor HL, Brozek J, et al. Indices of obesity and blood pressure in young men followed 32 years. J Chron Dis 1982;35:211–9.

Gleysteen JJ, Barvoriak JJ, Sasse EA. Sustained coronary-risk-factor reduction after gastric bypass for morbid obesity. Am J Clin Nutr 1990;51:774–8.

Glueck CJ, Taylor HL, Jacobs D, et al. Plasma high-density lipoprotein cholesterol: association with measurement of body mass: the lipid research clinics program prevalence study. Circulation 1980;62:62–9.

Goldstein DJ. Beneficial health effects of modest weight loss. Int J Obesity 1992;16:397–415.

Gomel M, Oldenburg B, Simpson JM, Owen N. Work-site cardiovascular risk reduction: a randomized trial of health risk assessment, education, counseling, and incentives. Am J Public Health 1993;83:1231–8.

Gordon DJ, Probstfield JL, Garrison RJ, et al. High density lipoprotein cholesterol and cardiovascular disease: four prospective studies. Circulation 1989;79:8–15.

Greenway FL. Clinical studies with phenylpropanolamine: a metaanalysis. Am J Clin Nutr 1992;55:203S–5S.

Guy-Grande B, Apfelbaum M, Crepaldi G, et al. International trial of long-term dexfenfluramine in obesity. Lancet 1989;2:1142–5.

Guy-Grande, B. INDEX international dexfenfluramine study: as a model for long-term pharmacotherapy of obesity in the 1990's. Int J Obesity Relat Metab Disord 1992;16:S5–14.

Helmrich SP, Ragland DR, Leung RW, Paffenbarger RS. Physical activity and reduced occurrence of non-insulin-dependent diabetes mellitus. N Engl J Med 1991;325:147–52.

Henkin Y, Oberman A, Hurst DC. Niacin revisited: clinical observations on an important but underutilized drug. Am J Med 1991;91:239–46.

Hill JO, Drougas H, Peters JC. Obesity treatment: can diet composition play a role? Ann Intern Med 1993;119:694–7.

Hla KM, Young TB, Bidwell T, et al. Sleep apnea and hypertension: a population-based study. Ann Intern Med 1994;120:382–8.

Horm J, Anderson K. Who in America is trying to lose weight? Ann Intern Med 1993;119: 672–6.

Hubert HB, Feinleib M, McNamara PM, Castelli, WP. Obesity as an independent risk factor for cardiovascular disease: a 26-year follow-up of participants in the Framingham Heart Study. Circulation 1983;67:968–77.

Jackson YM, Prouix JM, Pelican S. Obesity prevention. Am J Clin Nutr 1991;53:1625S–30S.

Jeffery RW, Wing RR, French SA. Weight cycling and cardiovascular risk factors in obese men and women. Am J Clin Nutr 1992;55:641–4.

Jeffery RW. Minnesota Studies on community-based approaches to weight loss and control. Ann Intern Med 1993;119:719–21.

Kahn HS, Williamson DF, Stevens JA. Race and weight change in US women: the roles of socioeconomic and marital status. Am J Public Health 1991;81:319–23.

Kalkhoff RK, Hartz AH, Rupley D, et al. Relationship of body fat distribution to blood pressure, carbohydrate tolerance, and plasma lipids in healthy obese women. J Lab Clin Med 1983;102:621–7.

Kanaley JA, Andersen-Reid ML, Oenning L, et al. Differential health benefits of weight loss in upper-body and lower-body obese women. Am J Clin Nutr 1993;57:20–6.

Kanders BS, Forse RA, Blackburn GL. Obesity. In: Conn HF, Rakel RE, eds. Conn's current therapy. Philadelphia: WB Saunders, 1991;524–31.

Kaplan NM. The deadly quartet: upper-body obesity, glucose intolerance, hypertriglyceridemia, and hypertension. Arch Intern Med 1989;149:1514–20.

Kendall A, Levitsky DA, Strupp BJ, Lissner L. Weight loss on a low-fat diet: consequences of the control of food intake in humans. Am J Clin Nutr 1991;53:1124–9.

Kissebah AH, Freedman DS, Peiris AN. Health risks of obesity. Med Clin North Am 1989;73: 111–38.

Kral JG. Gastric balloons: a plea for sanity in the midst of balloonacy. Gastroenterology 1988; 95:213–5.

Kral JG. Surgical treatment of obesity. Med Clin North Am 1989;73:51–265.

Krieger DR, Daly PA, Dulloo AG, et al. Ephedrine, caffeine, and aspirin promote weight loss in obese subjects. Trans Assoc Am Phys 1991;103:307–12.

Kuczmarski RJ, Flegal KM, Campbell SM, Johnson CL. Increasing prevalence of overweight US adults: The National Health and Nutrition Examination Surveys, 1960–1991. JAMA 1994;272:205–211.

Kumanyika S. Diet and chronic disease issues for minority populations. J Nutr Educ 1990;22: 89–96.

Kumanyika SK. Special issues regarding obesity in minority populations. Ann Intern Med 1993; 119:650–4.

Laakso M, Sarlund H, Mykkanen L. Insulin resistance is associated with lipid and lipoprotein abnormalities in subjects with varying degrees of glucose tolerance. Arteriosclerosis 1990;10:223–31.

Laakso M, Sarlund H, Salonen R, et al. Asymptomatic atherosclerosis and insulin resistance. Arterioscler Thromb 1991;11:1068–76.

Lapidus L, Bengtsson C, Larsson B, et al. Distribution of adipose tissue and risk of cardiovascular disease and death: a 12-year follow-up of participants in the population study of women in Gothenberg, Sweden. Br Med J 1984;289:1257–61.

LaRosa JC, Hunninghake D, Bush D, et al. The cholesterol facts: a summary of the evidence relating dietary fats, serum cholesterol, and coronary heart disease. Circulation 1990;81: 1721–33.

Lee IM, Paffenbarger RS Jr. Change in body weight and longevity. JAMA 1992;268:2045– 9.

Lee IM, Manson, JE, Hennekens CH, Paffenbarger RS. Body weight and mortality: a 27-year follow-up of middle-aged men. JAMA 1993;270:2823–8.

Levy AS, Heaton AW. Weight control practices of U.S. adults trying to lose weight. Ann Intern Med 1993;119:661–666.

Lew EA, Garfinkel L. Variations in mortality by weight among 750,000 men and women. J Chron Dis 1979;32:563–76.

Lindsted K, Tonstad S, Kuzma JW. Body mass index and patterns of mortality among Seventh-Day Adventist men. Int J Obesity 1990;15:397–406.

Linner JH. Comparative effectiveness of gastric bypass and gastroplasty. Arch Surg 1982;117: 695–700.

Liu K, Stamler J, Moss D, et al. Dietary cholesterol, fat and fibre, and colon-cancer mortality: an analysis of international data. Lancet 1979;2(8146):782–5.

Lovig T, Haffner JFW, Kaaresen R, et al. Gastric banding for morbid obesity: five years of follow-up. Int J Obesity 1993;17:453–7.

MacMahon S, MacDonald G. Treatment of high blood pressure in overweight patients. Nephron 1987;47(Suppl 1):8–12.

Manninen V, Tenkanen L, Koskinen P, et al. Joint effects of serum triglyceride and LDL cholesterol and HDL cholesterol concentrations on coronary heart disease risk in the Helsinki Heart Study: implications for treatment. Circulation 1992;85:37–45.

Manson JE, Stampfer MJ, Hennekens MD, Willett WC. Body weight and longevity: a reassessment. JAMA 1987;257:353–8.

Manson JE, Colditz GA, Stampfer MJ, et al. A prospective study of obesity and risk of coronary heart disease in women. N Engl J Med 1990;322:882–9.

Manson JE, Rimm EB, Stampfer MJ, et al. Physical activity and incidence of non-insulin-dependent-diabetes mellitus in women. Lancet 1991;328:774–8.

Manson JE, Willett WC, Stampfer MJ, et al. Body weight and all-cause mortality among women. N Engl J Med 1995;333:677–85.

Mascioli EA, Bistrian BR. Treatment of obesity. In: Weir GC, and Kahn CR, eds. Joslin's diabetes mellitus, 13th ed. Philadelphia: Lea and Febiger, 1993;363–71.

Melby CL, Schmidt WD, Corrigan D. Resting metabolic rate in weight-cycling collegiate wrestlers compared with physically active, noncycling control subjects. Am J Clin Nutr 1990; 52:409–14.

Messerli FH, Nunez BD, Ventura HO, Synder DW. Overweight and sudden death. Increased ventricular ectopy in cardiopathy of obesity. Arch Intern Med 1987;147:1725–8.

Miller DS, Mumford P, Stock MJ. Gluttony 2. Thermogenesis in overeating man. Am J Clin Nutr 1967;20:1223–9.

Montoye HJ, Epstein FH, Kjelsberg MO. Relationship between serum cholesterol and body fatness: an epidemiologic study. Am J Clin Nutr 1966;18:397–406.

Morris JN, Clayton DG, Everitt MG, et al. Exercise in leisure time: coronary attack and death rates. Br Heart J 1990;63:325–34.

Must A, Jacques PF, Dallal GE, et al. Long-term morbidity and mortality of overweight adolescents: a follow-up of the Harvard Growth Study of 1992 to 1935. N Engl J Med 1992;327:1350–5.

NIH Technology Assessment Conference Panel. Methods of voluntary weight loss and control. Ann Intern Med 1993;199:764–70.

National Task Force on the Prevention and Treatment of Obesity. Very low calorie diets. JAMA 1993;270:967–74.

Ohlson LO, Larsson B, Svardsudd K, et al. The influence of body fat distribution on the incidence of diabetes mellitus: 13.5 years of follow-up of the participants in the study of men born in 1913. Diabetes 1985;34:1055–8.

Pamuk ER, Williamson DF, Serdula MK, et al. Weight loss and subsequent death in a cohort of US adults. Ann Intern Med 1993;119:744–8.

Pasquali R, Cesari MP, Melchionda C, et al. Does ephedrine promote weight loss in low-energy-adapted obese women? Int J Obesity 1987a;11:163–8.

Pasquali R, Cesari MP, Besteghi L, et al. Thermogenic agents in the treatment of obesity: preliminary results. Int J Obes 1987b;11(Suppl 3):23–6.

Pasquali R, Casimirri F. Clinical aspects of ephedrine in the treatment of obesity. Int J Obesity 1993;17(Suppl 1):S65–8.

Pavlou KN, Whatley JE, Jannace PW, et al. Physical activity as a supplement to a weight-loss dietary regimen. Am J Clin Nutr 1989;49:1110–4.

Peiris AN, Mueller RA, Smith GA, et al. Splanchnic insulin metabolism in obesity. J Clin Invest 1986;78:1648–57.

Peiris AN, Struve MF, Mueller RA, et al. Glucose metabolism in obesity: influence of body fat distribution. J Clin Endo Metab 1988;67:760–7.

Phinney SD, Tang AB, Waggoner CR, et al. The transient hypercholesterolemia of major weight loss. Am J Clin Nutr 1991;53:1404–10.

Phinney SD. Exercise during and after very-low calorie dieting. Am J Clin Nutr 1992;56:190S–4S.

Pi-Sunyer FX. Short-term medical benefits and adverse effects of weight loss. Ann Intern Med 1993;119:722–6.

Pollare T, Lithell H, Selinus I, Berne C. Application of prazosin is associated with an increase of insulin sensitivity in obese patients with hypertension. Diabetologia 1988;31:415–20.

Pollare T, Lithell H, Berne C. A comparison of the effects of hydrochlorothiazide and captopril on glucose and lipid metabolism in patients with hypertension. N Engl J Med 1989;321:868–73.

Pories J, MacDonald KG, Morgan EJ, et al. Surgical treatment of obesity and its effect on diabetes: 10-y follow-up. Am J Clin Nutr 1992;55:582S–5S.

Prewitt TE, Schmeisser D, Bowen PE, et al. Changes in body weight, body composition, and energy intake in women fed high- and low-fat diets. Am J Clin Nutr 1991;54:304–10.

Prisant LM, Carr AA. Antihypertensive drug therapy and insulin resistance. Am J Hypertens 1992;5:775–7.

Public health focus: physical activity and the prevention of coronary heart disease. MMWR 1993; 42:669–72.

Ramsay LE. Obesity and hypertension. Nephron 1987;(47 Suppl 1):5–7.

Randle PJ, Hales CN, Garland PB, Newsholme EA. The glucose fatty-acid cycle role in insulin sensitivity and the metabolic disturbances of diabetes mellitus. Lancet 1963;1:787–9.

Ravussin E, Lilloja S, Knowler WC, et al. Reduced rate of energy expenditure as a risk factor for body-weight gain. N Engl J Med 1988;318:467–72.

Reaven GM, Chen YI. Role of abnormal free fatty acid metabolism in the development of non-insulin-dependent diabetes mellitus. Am J Med 1988;85:106–12.

Reddy BS. Dietary fibre and colon cancer: epidemiologic and experimental evidence. Can Med Assoc J 1980;123:850–6.

Reed GW, Hill JO. Weight cycling: a review of the animal literature. Obesity Res 1993;1:392–402.

Rigaud R, Ryttig KR, Angel LA, Apfelbaum M. Overweight treated with energy restriction and a dietary fibre supplement: a 6-month randomized, double-blind, placebo-controlled trial. Int J Obesity 1990;14:763–9.

Rodin J, Schank D, Striegel-Moore R. Psychological features of obesity. Med Clin North Am 1989;73:47–66.

Rodin J, Radke-Sharpe N, Rebuffe-Scrive M, Greenwood MRC. Weight cycling and fat distribution. Int J Obesity 1990;14:303–10.

Rossner S, Anderson RS, Ryttig KR. Effects of a dietary fibre supplement to a weight reduction programme on blood pressure: a randomized, double-blind, placebo-controlled study. Acta Med Scand 1988;223:353–7.

Rossner S. Pregnancy, weight cycling and weight gain in obesity. Int J Obes 1992;16:145–7.

Rowe JW, Young JB, Minaker KL, et al. Effect of insulin and glucose infusions on sympathetic nervous system activity in normal man. Diabetes 1981;30:219–25.

Schmieder RE, Gatzka C, Schachinger H, et al. Obesity as a determinant for response to antihypertensive treatment. Br Med J 1993;307:537–40.

Segal KR, Pi-Sunyer FX. Exercise and obesity. Med Clin North Am 1989; 73:217–36.

Sharp JT, Barrocas M, Chokroverty S. The cardiorespiratory effects of obesity. Clin Chest Med 1980;1:103–18.

Sheppard L, Kristal AR, Kushi LH. Weight loss in women participating in a randomized trial of low-fat diets. Am J Clin Nutr 1991;54:821–8.

Shils ME, Olson JA, Shike M. Modern nutrition, health and disease. Philadelphia: Lea and Febiger, 1994.

Shimokata H, Tobin JD, Muller DC, et al. Studies in the distribution of body fat: I. Effects of age, sex, and obesity. J Gerontol 1989;44:M66–73.

Sims EAH. Storage and expenditure of energy in obesity and their implications for management. Med Clin North Am 1989;73:97–110.

Sprecher DL, Harris BV, Goldberg AC, et al. Efficacy of psyllium in reducing serum cholesterol levels in hypercholesterolemic patients on high- or low-fat diets. Ann Intern Med 1993; 199:545–54.

Standley PR, Bakir MH, Sowers JR. Vascular insulin abnormalities, hypertension, and accelerated atherosclerosis. Am J Kidney Dis 1993;21(Suppl 3):39–46.

Steen SN, Oppliger RA, Brownell KD. Metabolic effects of repeated weight loss and regain in adolescent wrestlers. JAMA 1988;260:47–50.

Stunkard AJ, Cohen RY, Felix MRJ. Weight loss competitions at the worksite: how they work and how well. Prevent Med 1989;18:460–74.

Telch CF, Agras WS. Obesity, binge eating and psychopathology: are they related? Int J Eat Dis 1994;15:53–61.

Toubro S, Astrup AV, Breum L, Quaade F. Safety and efficacy of long-term treatment with ephedrine, caffeine, and an ephedrine/caffeine mixture. Int J Obesity 1993;17(Suppl 1): S69–S72.

Tuck ML, Sowers J, Dornfeld L, et al. The effect of weight reduction on blood pressure, plasma renin activity, and plasma aldosterone levels in obese patients. N Engl J Med 1981;304: 930.

Van Dale DV, Saris WHM, Schoffelen PFM, Ten Hoor F. Does exercise give an additional effect in weight reduction regimens? Int J Obesity 1987;11:367–75.

Van Dale D, Saris WH. Repetitive weight loss and regain: effects on weight reduction, resting metabolic rate, and lipolytic activity before and after exercise and/or diet treatment. Am J Clin Nutr 1989;49:409–16.

Van Itallie T. Health implications of overweight and obesity in the United States. Ann Intern Med 1985;103:983–8.

Wadden TA, Stunkard AJ, Brownell KD. Very low calorie diets: their efficacy, safety, and future. Ann Intern Med 1983;99:675–84.

Wadden TA, Stunkard AJ, Day SC, et al. Less food, less hunger: reports of appetite and symptoms in a controlled study of a protein-sparing modified fast. Int J Obesity 1987;11: 239–49.

Wadden TA, Sternberg, JA, Letizia KA, et al. Treatment of obesity by very low calorie diet, behavioral therapy, and their combination: a five-year perspective. Int J Obesity 1989; 13:39–46.

Wadden TA, Barlett S, Letizia KA, et al. Relationship of dieting history to resting metabolic rate, body composition, eating behavior, and subsequent weight loss. Am J Clin Nutr 1992a;56:203S–8S.

Wadden TA, Foster GD, Letiza KA, Stunkard AJ. A multicenter evaluation of a proprietary weight reduction program for the treatment of marked obesity. Arch Intern Med 1992b; 152:961–6.

Wadden TA, Letizia KA. Predictors of attrition and weight loss in patients treated by moderate and severe caloric restriction. In: Wadden TA, Vanltallie TB, eds. Treatment of the seriously obese patient. New York: Guilford Press. 1992c:398–410.

Wadden TA. Treatment of obesity by moderate and severe caloric restriction: results of clinical research trials. Ann Intern Med 1993;119:688–93.

Wannamethee G, Shaper AG. Weight change in middle-aged British men: implications for health. Eur J Clin Nutr 1990;44:133–42.

Warram JH, Martin BC, Krolewski AS, et al. Slow glucose removal rate and hyperinsulinemia precede the development of type II diabetes in the offspring of diabetic parents. Ann Intern Med 1990;113:909–15.

Weintraub M, Ginsberg G, Stein C, et al. Phenylpropanolamine OROS Acutrim; vs. placebo in combination with caloric restriction and physician-managed behavior modification. Clin Pharmacol Ther 1986;39:501–9.

Weintraub M, Bray GA. Drug treatment of obesity. Med Clin North Am 1989;73:237–49.

Weintraub M. Long-term weight control: the national heart, lung, and blood institute funded multimodal intervention study. Clin Pharmacol Ther 1992;51:581–5.

Weir MR. Impact of age, race, and obesity on hypertensive mechanisms and therapy. Am J Med 1991;90:3S–14S.

Williamson DF, Kahn HS, Remington PL, Anda RF. The 10-year incidence of overweight and major weight gain in US adults. Arch Intern Med 1990;150:665.

Wing RR, Kuller LH, Bundker C, et al. Obesity, obesity-related behaviors, and coronary heart disease risk factors in black and white premenopausal women. Int J Obesity 1989;134: 511–19.

Wing RR, Blair EH, Bononi P, et al. Caloric restriction per se is a significant factor in improvements in glycemic control and insulin sensitivity during weight loss in obese NIDDM patients. Diabetes Care 1994;17:30–36.

Wong FL, Trowbridge FL. Clin Nutr 1984;3:94–9.

Wood PD, Stefanick ML, Williams PT, Haskell WL. The effects on plasma lipoproteins of a prudent weight-reducing diet, with or without exercise in overweight men and women. N Engl J Med 1991;325:461–6.

Wynder EL, Rose DP, Cohen LA. Diet and breast cancer in causation and therapy. Cancer 1986; 58(8 Suppl):1804–13.

Yang H, Petersen GM, Roth MP, et al. Risk factors for gallstone formation during rapid weight loss. Dig Dis Sci 1992;37:912–8.

Yanovski SZ. A practical approach to treatment of the obese patient. Arch Fam Med 1993a;2: 309–16.

Yanovski SZ, Nelson JE, Dubbert BK, Spitzer RL. Association of binge eating disorder and psychiatric comorbidity in obese subjects. Am J Psychol 1993b;150:1472–9.

10

Risk Modification in the Diabetic Patient

JoAnn E. Manson and Angela Spelsberg

Among individuals with insulin-dependent diabetes (IDDM) and non–insulin-dependent diabetes mellitus (NIDDM), atherosclerotic complications, including coronary heart disease (CHD), stroke, and peripheral arterial disease, are major causes of morbidity and mortality (Krolewski 1985). Age-adjusted mortality rates for CHD in population-based studies in the United States are 2–3 times higher among diabetic men and 3 to 7 times higher among diabetic women than among persons without diabetes (Kannel 1979; Heyden 1980; Barrett-Connor 1983; Krolewski 1985; Pan 1986; Manson 1991a). The proportion of CHD attributable to NIDDM among women in the Framingham cohort was 7.7%, as compared with 3.8% among men (Kannel 1985). In the Nurses' Health Study, 13.8% of coronary events in the cohort were attributed to diabetes (Manson 1991a).

Currently, an estimated 16 million persons in the United States have diabetes; the vast majority (more than 90%) are considered to be non–insulin-dependent (Harris 1995). Current combined direct and indirect costs of NIDDM in the United States have been estimated to be at least $40 billion annually (Bransome 1992). In view of the far greater prevalence of NIDDM than IDDM, this chapter only briefly discusses the association of IDDM and CHD, mainly focusing on the complex association of NIDDM and CHD. The impact of currently recognized determinants of CHD, including obesity, dyslipidemia, hypertension, physical inactivity, hyperglycemia, and hyperinsulinemia, are evaluated for the patient with diabetes mellitus. The potential benefits of modifying traditional risk factors for CHD as well as the role of strict glycemic control achieved through diet, oral hypoglycemic agents, and/or insulin are addressed. We also examine the role of aspirin and postmenopausal hormone therapy in the prevention of heart disease among diabetics. Further, the primary prevention of NIDDM through weight loss and physical activity will be addressed. Finally, the cost effectiveness of the different approaches will be examined according to available data.

Mechanisms and Epidemiology of Increased Coronary Heart Disease Risk in Diabetes

Insulin-Dependent Diabetes Mellitus

Traditional cardiovascular risk factors including dyslipidemia, hypertension, and obesity are uncommon in well-controlled IDDM (Ruderman 1984). However, IDDM patients with a strong family history of essential hypertension and diabetes mellitus appear to be at high risk for developing hypertension and renal disease (Viverti 1987); diabetic nephropathy is considered to be the most common cause of hypertension among individuals with IDDM (National High Blood Pressure Education Program Working Group 1994). Data on the natural history of macrovascular complications of IDDM are scant; however, the onset of clinically manifest atherosclerosis occurs at an earlier age in those with IDDM than in the general population and the risk of CHD is markedly elevated after the third decade of life (Krolewski 1987). Table 10.1 summarizes possible atherogenic and hemostatic mechanisms of increased CHD risk in IDDM patients with and without impaired renal function.

In a cohort study of 292 IDDM patients at the Joslin Clinic who were followed for 20–40 years from the onset of IDDM, the cumulative CHD mortality rate by age 55 was 35% in both men and women (Krolewski 1987). This compares to an 8%

Table 10.1. Prevalence of Atherogenic and Potentially Atherogenic Factors in Type I and Type II Diabetes

	Type I		
Factor	Normal Renal Function	Impaired Renal Function	Type II
Hypertension	0	+ + +	+ +
Hypercholesterolemia	0 – +	+ + +	+
Hypertriglyceridemia	0 – +	+ + +	+ + +
Remnant particles	?	+ + +	+ +
Decreased HDL cholesterol	0 – +	+ + +	+ +
Obesity	0	0	+ + +
Hyperinsulinemia	+	+ +	+ +
Immune complexes	+ +	?	0

Alterations in Plasma Lipoproteins in Patients with Types I and II Diabetes

Lipoprotein	Alteration
LDL	Increased plasma level
	Glycosylation
	Modified in arterial wall to enhance uptake by macrophage
	Triglyceride-enriched
HDL	Decreased plasma level
	Glycosylation
	Triglyceride-enriched
VLDL	Increased plasma level
	Impaired degradation leading to remnant accumulation
	Altered composition → endothelial toxicity; increased lipid uptake by macrophages
Chylomicra	Impaired degradation causing remnant accumulation
Remnants	Increased levels in some type II diabetics

Source: Modified from Ruderman and Haudenschild (1984), with permission.

The symbol (+) indicates increased prevalence, with (+++) signifying the greatest increase. A prevalence not different from that of the general population is indicated by 0. Lipid and lipoprotein abnormalities in type I diabetics with normal renal function are usually associated with poor control.

CHD mortality risk in nondiabetic men and 4% in nondiabetic women in the corresponding age groups in the general population as estimated from the Framingham study (Lerner 1986). By age 55, half of the diabetic cohort had already died of CHD or had symptomatic (history of angina or myocardial infarction) or asymptomatic (pathologic Q wave in electrocardiogram or positive stress test) CHD. In the Pittsburgh Insulin-Dependent Diabetes Mellitus Morbidity and Mortality Study, the overall mortality among 25- to 45-year-old IDDM patients was 20 times higher than in the general population (Dorman 1984). In the Danish Steno-Hospital Study, almost 50% of the patients had died after 35 years duration of the disease, irrespective of age at onset. Myocardial infarction (MI) accounted for 25% of all deaths and was the second leading cause of death after renal failure (Deckert 1978). The hypothesis that diabetes promotes existing atherosclerosis rather than initiating atherosclerotic lesions is corroborated by the observation that in countries with low background rates of CHD, the risk of CHD in diabetic patients is also low (West 1983; World Health Organization 1985), and by the finding that risk of atherosclerotic events is not related to age at onset of IDDM (Krolewski 1987).

Non-Insulin-Dependent Diabetes Mellitus

In contrast to IDDM, traditional coronary risk factors as well as clinically manifest cardiovascular disease are present in excess at the time of diagnosis of NIDDM in both men and women (Kannel 1985; Krolewski 1985). Table 10.1 provides an overview of the mechanisms involved in the increased CHD risk in NIDDM patients, including obesity, high blood pressure, decreased high density lipoprotein cholesterol (HDL-C), and high serum triglycerides. In the Framingham Study, the lipid alterations were found to be more pronounced in diabetic women than in diabetic men. After adjusting for age and major cardiovascular risk factors, diabetic men had a 70% increased risk of CHD, and women had a twofold increased relative risk of CHD as compared with nondiabetic individuals of the same gender in the cohort (Kannel 1985). Diabetes appears to be particularly deleterious in women, completely eliminating the usual female advantage with respect to CHD mortality. Sex differences in the relation of diabetes with CHD have been observed in several cohort studies (Kannel 1979; Heyden 1980; Barrett-Connor 1983; Pan 1986; Manson 1991a) with diabetic women having higher relative risks of CHD than diabetic men (Table 10.2).

The increased incidence of MI and vascular mortality among diabetics cannot be fully explained by the presence of traditional coronary risk factors. In recent years, it has become apparent that hemostatic risk factors for acute thrombosis exist (Ridker 1991) and are highly prevalent among diabetics. Diabetes appears to be associated with hyperaggregable platelets (Haluska 1977) as well as impaired fibrinolytic activity (Juhan-Vague 1987; Vague 1989). Further, elevated levels of fibrinogen, which correlate with increasing blood glucose concentrations, may be of particular importance among diabetic women, as suggested by data from the Framingham Study (Kannel 1990). These abnormalities may promote both atherogenesis and thrombosis. Hyperglycemia and glycosylation of tissue proteins may also contribute to atherogenesis and the accelerated CHD risk in diabetes (Ruderman 1984).

Table 10.2. Prospective Population-Based Studies of Coronary Heart Disease Mortality in Predominantly Middle-Aged Diabetic Patients

Study Location	Year	Age	Follow-Up (Years)	Mortality Risk Ratio[a] Males	Mortality Risk Ratio[a] Females
DuPont Company	1970	<20–64[b]	10	2.87[c,d]	
Israel	1977	≥40	5	3.4[c,d]	
Framingham	1979	45–74	20	1.7	3.3[e]
Evans County	1980	≥22	4.5	1.0	2.8[c]
Rancho Bernardo	1983	40–79	7	2.4	3.5[e]
Warsaw	1984	18–68	9.5	1.33	1.65[c]
Tecumseh	1985	40–54	20	7.9	7.7[e]
		55–69		2.6	0.6[e]
		≥70		1.9	5.3[c,e]
Whitehall	1985	40–64	10	2.45[e]	
Chicago	1986	35–64	9	3.8	4.7[e]
Finland	1986	40–69	11	2.0	4.1[c,d]
Nurses' Health Study	1991	30–55	8		3.0[e]

Source: From Barrett-Connor and Orchard (1985); Manson et al. (1991a), with permission; Panzram (1987), with permission.

[a]Rancho Bernardo and Warsaw identified ischemic heart disease; Israel identified myocardial infarction; all others identified coronary heart disease.

[b]Among a total of 370 diabetic patients, only 9 patients were under 40 years old.

[c]Relative risk (observed/expected death proportion, standardized mortality ratio, Cox standardized risk ratio) Evans County and DuPont Company not age-adjusted; all others age-adjusted.

[d]Newly diagnosed diabetic patients.

[e]Multiply adjusted risk, including age and major coronary heart disease risk factors, with interstudy variations in covariates and statistical methods.

Strength of Evidence for Potential Benefit from Glycemic Control

Data concerning the efficacy of strict glycemic control in the prevention of MI among diabetic patients have been sparse. Although favorable effects of strict glycemic control with intensified insulin treatment have been demonstrated for the microvascular complications in IDDM, including retinopathy (Reichard 1993; Diabetes Control and Complications Trial [DCCT] Research Group 1993), nephropathy (Feldt-Rasmussen 1991; KROC Collaborative Study Group 1988; DCCT Research Group 1993) and neuropathy (Service 1985; DCCT Research Group 1993); it remains unclear whether these findings apply to patients with NIDDM or to the natural course of macrovascular complications in either IDDM or NIDDM.

The potential impact of glycemic control on CHD risk was indirectly examined in a recent analysis of the Framingham data where an independent association between chronic hyperglycemia, as assessed by glycosylated hemoglobin (HbA_{1c}) levels, and CHD was found among women. Across increasing quartiles of HbA_{1c}, a significant increase in prevalence of CHD was observed among women aged 66 to 93 years (p_{trend} = .03), but no such association was present among men (Singer 1992). In contrast, blood glucose levels were not associated with CHD risk.

Therapy with exogenous insulin among patients with NIDDM has been shown to induce antiatherogenic changes in serum lipids and lipoproteins by lowering triglyceride levels and increasing adipose tissue lipoprotein lipase (LPL) activity, which leads to redistribution of HDL particles from HDL_3 to HDL_2 (Pfeiffer 1983; Taskinen 1988). In the DCCT, which was conducted among patients with IDDM, intensive insulin therapy reduced the development of hypercholesterolemia (as defined by serum low density lipoprotein cholesterol concentrations >160 mg/dl) by 34% (95% CI: 7% to 54%) (DCCT Research Group 1993). Because of the young age of the participants (age range: 13 to 39 years at baseline), cardiovascular endpoints after 6.5 years of follow-up were rare: 0.5 events per 100 person-years in the intensive treatment group compared with 0.8 events per 100 person-years in the standard treatment group. A 41% reduction in cardiovascular disease (CVD) risk was observed (95% CI, -10% to 68%), which did not attain statistical significance (DCCT Research Group 1993).

The potential adverse effects of intensive insulin therapy regimens, including severe hypoglycemia, peripheral hyperinsulinemia, and weight gain may, however, limit the extent of achievable glycemic control in the elderly NIDDM patient with coexistent CVD; such individuals are more prone to risks of severe hypoglycemia such as fainting, seizures, falls, stroke, silent ischemia, MI, and sudden death (American Diabetes Association 1993b). Furthermore, the long-term effects of peripheral hyperinsulinemia on vascular disease remain unknown. Endogenous hyperinsulinemia, in apparent contrast to exogenous insulin therapy, is associated with adverse CVD risk factor profiles (Reaven 1988; Zavaroni 1989), including dyslipidemia (Tobey 1981; Zavaroni 1985; Castelli 1986; Laakso 1987), hypertension (Modan 1991) and obesity (Lucas 1985), as well as with an increased risk of CHD (Wellborn 1979; Ducimetiere 1980).

The seemingly contradictory effects of exogenous and endogenous hyperinsulinemia on CHD risk factor profiles are perplexing. A possible explanation is that endogenous hyperinsulinemia in NIDDM influences hepatic metabolism, while in IDDM, exogenous insulin therapy induces peripheral hyperinsulinemia (Nikkilä 1981) (Figure 10.1). The peripheral availability of insulin controls lipoprotein lipase activity,

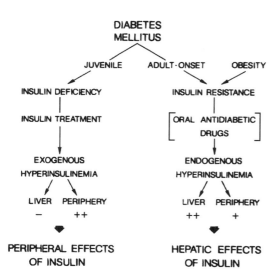

Fig. 10.1. Chart demonstrating the different effects of two types of hyperinsulinemia in diabetes: (1) exogenous hyperinsulinemia produced by administration of insulin in excess of the needs of peripheral tissues (left) and (2) endogenous hyperinsulinemia induced by peripheral insulin resistance (right). [From Nikkilä EA (1981), with permission.]

which increases HDL_2 and total HDL. In insulin-treated IDDM diabetics, a strong positive correlation between postheparin lipoprotein lipase activity and total HDL has been observed (Nikkilä 1978). In insulin-treated NIDDM patients, serum total very low density lipoprotein (VLDL) triglycerides and LDL cholesterol decrease with good glycemic control, and the HDL_2 subfraction increases (Taskinen 1988). At present, there are no prospective or randomized trial data available to assess whether the long-term beneficial effects of insulin therapy on lipoprotein profiles in NIDDM patients may outweigh the potential adverse effects associated with superimposing peripheral hyperinsulinemia on endogenous hyperinsulinemia. It remains to be clarified whether endogenous hyperinsulinemia is a determinant of CHD or is merely a marker of insulin resistance, which may confer increased risk of CHD by still unknown factors.

The only randomized clinical trial of glycemic control and vascular complications in NIDDM was the University Group Diabetes Program (UGDP), which compared oral hypoglycemic agents, standard and variable insulin therapy and placebo (Klimt 1970). This trial revealed an increased risk of cardiovascular death among diabetics treated with oral hypoglycemic agents (tolbutamide and phenformin). The levels of blood glucose achieved in the tolbutamide and standard insulin treatment groups were very similar and lower than in the placebo group; the variable insulin treatment group had the highest proportion of diabetics with good glycemic control (Klimt 1970). Surprisingly, death rates from cardiovascular causes were lowest in the placebo group (3.1%), intermediate in both insulin groups (6.2% and 5.9%), and highest in the oral agent group (12.7%). Although study design, randomization, adherence to treatment, achieved glycemic control, follow-up, and data analytic issues of the trial have been criticized by others (Krall 1985), caution in the use of oral hypoglycemic agents has been recommended as a result of the UGDP (American Diabetes Association 1979; Nathan 1993). With the second generation of oral hypoglycemic agents, including glyburide (glibenclamide), glipizide, and gliclazide, which are safely used worldwide (Krall 1985), and with the recent availability of metformin more potent drugs are available that enhance insulin-mediated glucose metabolism by improving insulin sensitivity and insulin secretion in NIDDM patients (DeFronzo 1983). These medications facilitate the achievement of adequate glucose control (Krall 1985; Nathan 1988) and result in reductions in total cholesterol concentrations (Nathan 1988; Rifkin 1991) and plasma triglycerides (Nathan 1988), as well as elevations in postheparin lipoprotein lipase activity (Pfeiffer 1983).

In summary, strict glycemic control has been proven to prevent or to delay microvascular complications in IDDM, but it remains unclear whether vascular complications in NIDDM are also favorably influenced. Based on available limited evidence, however, it seems likely that glycemic control will benefit both IDDM and NIDDM patients with respect to both microvascular and macrovascular complications.

Intervention Strategies for Maintenance of Strict Glycemic Control

Diet

Normalization or near-normalization of fasting and postprandial glycemia can be achieved with dietary treatment alone and modest to moderate weight loss in most obese NIDDM patients (Henry 1986, 1991; Grundy 1991). In a prospective study of 223 NIDDM patients in Northern Ireland, adequate glycemic control (fasting blood glucose <10 mmol/l) was achieved with dietary therapy alone in 80% of all patients, with favorable alterations of cardiovascular risk factor profiles, including weight and triglyceride levels (Hadden 1986). The prescribed diet contained 42% of calories from carbohydrates, 20% from protein, and 38% from fat, and did not exceed 1,450 kcal (6 MJ). Very low-calorie diets and low-fat/high-carbohydrate diets have been shown to be effective in improving glycemic control via weight loss and favorably modifying blood lipid levels (American Diabetes Association 1989; Henry 1991). Serum triglyceride level reductions of 40 to 60% have been observed with very low calorie diet therapy. However, there seems to be no uniform diet suitable for all NIDDM patients, and dietary failures are common (West 1973; Grundy 1991) (Table 10.3).

Dietary recommendations in NIDDM should take into account whether the patient is obese and loses weight with the weight-reduction diet, and whether β-cell function is severely impaired (Grundy 1991). Determinants of favorable diet response in NIDDM patients include low pretreatment glycemia, less severe β-cell impairment, and body weight <125% of ideal body weight (Henry 1991). Nutritional recommendations of the American Diabetes Association in the past have favored a reduction of daily total fat (<30% of total calories), saturated fat (<10% of total calories) and dietary cholesterol (<300 mg), as well as an increase in fiber and complex carbohydrate intake (American Diabetes Association 1987). Recent data suggest that replace-

Table 10.3. Some Deterrents to Successful Diet Therapy: A Formidable Challenge

1. The diet prescription recommended may lack relevance to patient's preferences and propensities. It may not fit his/her cultural, sociologic, or economic status. The proposed diet may differ from that of the patient's family or friends. The patient may find it difficult to give up calories or specifically proscribed foods (for example, concentrated carbohydrates, alcohol, and animal fat). He/she may not like low-caloric, low-carbohydrate foods in the prescription, such as A and B vegetables. He/she may lack sufficient intelligence, education, incentive, or self-discipline.
2. An insulin-dependent patient may find frequent feedings are not convenient or appealing. He/she may not like to eat the same number of calories every day. He/she may find it difficult to follow the fixed time schedule for meals called for on his/her own prescription, or in any prescription, because of his/her other commitments, or vagaries of preference or appetite. He/she may not like to eat the same ratios and amounts of carbohydrates, proteins, and fats in each meal every day. He/she may not find it convenient to balance periods of unusual exercise with additional carbohydrate in appropriate amounts.
3. The patient and his/her family may misunderstand the general goals and priorities of the diet, or they may not understand either the specific dietary strategies (for example, the principles of the food exchange system) or the specific dietary techniques and alternatives (for example, how much potato is equivalent to one piece of bread).
4. The physician, dietitian, or nurse may have a poor understanding of the principles, strategies, priorities, or methods of diet therapy.
5. The patient education system may be defective because of
   a. limitations of acumen, enthusiasm, and time of health professionals;
   b. limited teaching manpower;
   c. lack of economic incentives for health professionals and institutions to teach patients;
   d. patient education efforts that are seldom sufficiently systematic (for example, responsibilities of physician, dietitian, nurse, and patient may not be clearly and systematically delineated); or
   e. often underestimated general and specific deficiencies in the patient's understanding.

Source: Modified from West (1973), with permission.

ment of carbohydrate with monounsaturated fat may favorably influence glycemic control and blood lipid levels in NIDDM (Garg 1994), but this requires confirmation in future studies. The current nutrition guidelines of the American Diabetes Association emphasize the dependence of dietary therapy on desired glucose, lipid, and weight outcomes in the individual patient (American Diabetes Association 1994a). For individuals with normal lipid levels and reasonable weight, the former recommendations are considered to be appropriate. If weight loss or elevated LDL cholesterol are the primary issues, reduction of dietary fat intake (<30% of calories from total fat, <200 mg/day dietary cholesterol intake, and <7% of total calories from saturated fat) according to the National Cholesterol Education Program Step II guidelines, should be emphasized. If elevated triglycerides and VLDL-cholesterol are the primary problem, weight loss and an increase in physical activity, as well as a modest increase in monounsaturated fat intake (up to 20% of calories from monounsaturated fat, less than 10% from saturated and polyunsaturated fat) and a more moderate intake of carbohydrates may be beneficial (American Diabetes Association 1994b). The goals of medical nutrition therapy in diabetes are provided in the attached appendix.

Oral Hypoglycemic Agents

With the second generation sulfonylureas and with metformin, benefits of oral hypoglycemic therapy include improved insulin sensitivity and insulin secretion (De Fronzo 1983), improved glycemic control, and reductions in hypertriglyceridemia (U.K. Prospective Diabetes Study 1985; Nathan 1988). A randomized clinical trial in NIDDM patients comparing once-per-day NPH insulin and oral hypoglycemic therapy with glyburide revealed a similar degree of glucose control with both, but insulin therapy was associated with higher levels of HDL-C (Nathan 1988). Both glyburide and insulin regimens induced a decrease in serum triglyceride and total cholesterol levels, and caused only minor weight gain, which was not statistically significantly different between the two groups.

The use of a combination of insulin and oral hypoglycemic agents in poorly controlled NIDDM is controversial. In a meta-analysis of 22 clinical trials of combination therapy in NIDDM patients, only slight improvement in glycemic control was achieved in the combination therapy group as well as an increase in peripheral insulin levels (Peters 1991). However, in a recent trial among poorly controlled NIDDM patients receiving oral hypoglycemic agents, the addition of a single dose of NPH insulin in the evening significantly improved glycemic control and dyslipidemia (Yki-Jävinen 1992). Further, combination therapy was not associated with major weight gain as compared with more frequent insulin administration. In patients with secondary failure from sulfonylurea treatment, the addition of insulin and/or biguanides may be effective (Quatrardo 1993). Other drugs such as alpha-glucosidase inhibitors ("starch blockers," i.e., acarbose, which reduces gastrointestinal absorption of carbohydrates), and hydroxychloroquine (a well-known antimalaria agent, which improves glycemic control in some treatment-refractory NIDDM patients) require further study but may offer promising alternatives in the future treatment of therapy-resistant NIDDM by improving glycemic control, insulin sensitivity, and hypertriglyceridemia (Quatraro 1990; Rosak 1990).

Insulin

Strict glycemic control, with improvement of hepatic glucose output and glucose disposal, as well as reductions in serum triglyceride and total cholesterol levels, have been shown to be achievable within one month of intensive conventional split-dose insulin therapy (subcutaneous NPH and regular insulin before breakfast and supper) in the NIDDM patient refractory to dietary and oral hypoglycemic therapy (Henry 1993). However, the large doses of exogenous insulin usually required to overcome insulin resistance may produce significant weight gain and peripheral hyperinsulinemia. Significant weight gain was also observed among IDDM patients assigned to intensive treatment in the DCCT study (DCCT Research Group 1993). The long-term effects of intensive insulin regimens in NIDDM in relation to macrovascular complications are unclear at present (Genuth 1990; Donahue 1992).

For IDDM patients, the DCCT results provide evidence that intensive insulin therapy (average of 6.5 years of follow-up) can prevent long-term microvascular complications. Participants in the intensive treatment group received insulin continuously by subcutaneous insulin infusion or by multiple daily injections to try to achieve chronic normoglycemia (DCCT Research Group 1987). In addition, subjects were encouraged to self-monitor blood glucose at least four times daily and to achieve specified targets (premeal glucose values between 70 and 120 mg/dl [3.9 to 6.7 mmol/l], postmeal levels not exceeding 180 mg/dl [10 mmol/l], and HbA_{1c} levels below 6.05%). Normalization of glucose values, however, was not achieved; the mean glucose values were 40% above these goals. Participants in the intervention group had a two- to threefold increased risk of hypoglycemia as compared with controls (DCCT Research Group 1993). Despite marked reductions in the incidence of microvascular complications (retinopathy, neuropathy, and microalbuminuria) with intensive insulin therapy, it remains to be demonstrated that intensive insulin therapy will also reduce the risk of macrovascular complications in IDDM. For NIDDM, it remains unproven that intensified insulin therapy will be beneficial in the prevention of either microvascular or macrovascular complications.

Modification of Coronary Risk Factors

Dyslipidemia

No randomized clinical trial data are available concerning the potential benefits from modification of traditional coronary risk factors among persons with NIDDM. Two arguments can be made, however, in favor of risk factor prevention or intervention in NIDDM. First, in populations with low background rates of CVD and favorable coronary risk factor profiles, particularly low total and LDL cholesterol levels, morbidity and mortality from CVD are low in both diabetics and nondiabetics (West 1983; World Health Organization Multinational Study of Vascular Disease in Diabetes 1985). Second, no evidence exists that the adverse effects of dyslipidemia, hypertension, obesity, smoking, and physical inactivity in individuals with NIDDM are materially different from the effects in nondiabetics (American Diabetes Association 1989).

Strength of Evidence for Potential Benefit from Control of Dyslipidemia. Evidence from controlled randomized trials demonstrates benefits of reducing total and LDL cholesterol levels in the primary and secondary prevention of MI (see also Chapter 6 on cholesterol lowering). In patients with NIDDM, total and LDL cholesterol levels are not substantially different from those in age- and body weight-matched nondiabetic individuals (American Diabetes Association 1993b). In the U.S. population in 1976 to 1980, the prevalence of high serum cholesterol (≥240 mg/dl or 200–239 mg/dl in the presence of CHD or two or more CHD risk factors) was 70% in individuals with diagnosed diabetes, 77% in undiagnosed diabetics, and 62% among men and 70% among women in the nondiabetic population (Harris 1991). An 8-year follow-up of women in the Nurses' Health Study revealed that diabetics with self-reported high cholesterol levels had nearly double the CHD incidence of diabetics with normal cholesterol levels, triple the CHD incidence of nondiabetic women with high cholesterol, and 12 times the CHD incidence of nondiabetic women with normal cholesterol levels (Manson 1991a). In the Tecumseh Study, hypothetically achievable 8-year reductions in CHD risks of participants with NIDDM were estimated to be 6% in men and 8% in women by reduction of total serum cholesterol as achieved in the Lipid Research Clinics Primary Prevention Trial (Smith 1986). If favorable alterations of other risk factors such as hypertension and cigarette smoking were included in the model, an 18 to 22% reduction in CHD risk after eight years of follow-up was estimated.

The dyslipidemia of NIDDM also includes low HDL-C levels (DeFronzo 1983; Nikkilä 1981; Laakso 1985) and elevated triglyceride levels (DeFronzo 1983; American Diabetes Association 1989). Similarly, small dense particles of LDL cholesterol appear to be elevated and are in part determined by the elevated triglyceride levels (Table 10.1). Body weight, body fat distribution, age, and saturated fat and cholesterol intake appear to be important modifiers of dyslipidemia in both diabetics and nondiabetics. Observational studies in nondiabetic populations have identified low HDL-C levels (≤40 mg/dl) in conjunction with elevated triglyceride levels (≥150 mg/dl) as strong predictors of increased CHD risk (Levy 1988). Although data from diabetic populations have been limited, observational studies have also consistently demonstrated that HDL-C levels and triglyceride levels are independent determinants of CHD risk in NIDDM patients (West 1983; Janka 1985; Pyörälä 1987; Fontbonne 1989). However, in a comparison of CHD risk of diabetic versus nondiabetic women and men, low HDL-C levels and other traditional risk factors could not fully explain the increased CHD risk of individuals with NIDDM (Levy 1988).

Recommendations for individuals at increased CHD risk, including those with diabetes, central obesity, hypertension, peripheral vascular disease, or chronic renal disease, include measurements of lipid subfractions, including LDL-C, HDL-C, and triglyceride levels (NIH Consensus Conference 1993). Nonpharmacological interventions, such as increase of physical activity, cessation of smoking, and dietary changes (Step 1 and Step 2 diet of the National Cholesterol Education Program/American Heart Association) are recommended as initial therapy (NIH Consensus Conference 1993). Although pharmacologic therapy may be indicated to reduce LDL-C levels, the evidence from clinical trials is currently insufficient to establish coronary benefits of modification of triglyceride and/or HDL-C levels by drug therapy (NIH Consensus Conference 1993).

Intervention Strategies for Treatment of Dyslipidemia. Although improved glycemic control favorably influences blood lipid profiles in NIDDM patients, the degree to which dyslipidemia can be normalized by hypoglycemic medication alone remains controversial (Stern 1991). Dietary therapy and exercise should accompany or replace hypoglycemic medication in NIDDM to facilitate weight loss and reduce insulin resistance, a determinant of dyslipidemia (American Diabetes Association 1993b).

Lipid-lowering agents are the next step if lipid abnormalities cannot be controlled by primary measures alone. The choice of the lipid-lowering drug depends on the nature of the blood lipid aberration and on the potential side effects of the drug. In particular, the use of nicotinic acid (niacin) is not recommended in dyslipidemic diabetic patients because of adverse effects on insulin metabolism, including increases in insulin resistance, hyperinsulinemia, and fasting and postprandial hyperglycemia (American Diabetes Association 1993b). Bile acid binding resins carry the risk of severe constipation in older patients or diabetic patients with gastrointestinal autonomic neuropathy. Although they do not interfere with glucose metabolism, they may elevate triglyceride levels. For these reasons, the utility of bile acid binding resins is limited in NIDDM dyslipidemia (American Diabetes Association 1993b). In contrast, 3-hydroxy-3-methylglutaryl coenzyme A (HMG-CoA) reductase inhibitors, which interfere directly with cholesterol biosynthesis, are well tolerated in diabetic patients and are highly effective in the treatment of dyslipidemia (American Diabetes Association 1993b). Reductions in total cholesterol, LDL, and VLDL cholesterol concentrations of 26 to 42% have been documented after 4 weeks of therapy with a reductase inhibitor (lovastatin). In addition, beneficial effects on HDL and triglyceride levels have been documented (Garg 1988).

Because of the lack of clinical trial data in diabetic patients, comparative benefits of specific lipid-lowering therapies in reducing risks of macrovascular complications in NIDDM cannot be directly assessed. However, the evidence from lipid-lowering trials in nondiabetic patients and observational data on the association between blood lipids and CHD risks among NIDDM patients suggest that correction of dyslipidemia is likely to have a favorable effect on the natural history of cardiovascular complications in NIDDM.

Hypertension

Strength of Evidence of Potential Benefit from Control of Hypertension. IDDM, NIDDM, and impaired glucose tolerance are all associated with an increased prevalence of hypertension (Levy 1988). An estimated 3 million Americans have both diabetes and hypertension (American Diabetes Association 1993a). Prevalence of hypertension in the NHANES II data was higher among black diabetics than among whites in each age group below 65 (Harris 1990), and was three times greater among Mexican-Americans than among non-Hispanic whites (Haffner 1989). The overall prevalence of hypertension among diabetics was 63 to 70%; in the general population aged 10 to 74 the prevalence of hypertension was 40%. In the Bedford (Jarrett 1982), Whitehall (Jarrett 1978), Israeli (Hermann 1977), and Framingham (Kannel 1979; Kannel 1985) studies, significantly higher mean systolic and diastolic BP values were observed in diabetic men and women as compared with age-matched nondiabetic subjects. It was estimated that 35 to 75% of diabetic complications can be attributed to hypertension (Bild 1987).

In a recent meta-analysis of 14 randomized clinical trials of antihypertensive drugs in nondiabetic populations (Collins 1990), a 14% overall risk reduction in CHD mortality was achieved with mean reductions of diastolic BP of 5–6 mmHg over five years. Stroke mortality was reduced by 42%. For NIDDM patients, no randomized clinical trial data are available for quantifying the magnitude of CHD risk reductions with hypertension control because most of the trials have excluded participants with diabetes. In the Tecumseh study, the hypothetical lowering of systolic blood pressure among individuals with NIDDM was estimated to translate into an 8% to 10% reduction in CHD risk after 8 years of follow-up; these estimates were based on observed risk reductions in the Hypertension Detection and Follow-Up Program (HDFP) and from estimates from the Framingham Heart Study (Smith 1986). In data from the Nurses' Health Study, diabetic women with hypertension experienced an approximately threefold increase in CHD risk as compared with diabetic women without diagnosed hypertension (Manson 1991a). In light of the substantial benefits of blood pressure lowering in nondiabetics with respect to CHD (see also Chapter 7 on treatment of hypertension), and the high absolute rates of CHD in diabetics with hypertension, the adequate control of blood pressure in the patient with NIDDM is of major importance (American Diabetes Association 1989).

Intervention Strategies for the Treatment of Hypertension. The recently published report on hypertension in diabetes of the National High Blood Pressure Education Program Working Group (1994) recommended lifestyle modifications, including weight management, exercise, control of hyperglycemia, smoking cessation, restriction of dietary saturated fat, salt, and alcohol intake, as the cornerstones of hypertension therapy in individuals with diabetes to achieve a goal BP of < 130/85 mmHg. For pharmacologic treatment, the report has suggested angiotensin converting enzyme (ACE)-inhibitors, calcium channel blockers, or alpha-adrenergic blockers (prazosin), or, alternatively, low-dose thiazide diuretics or β-blockers (Figure 10.2).

These recommendations take into consideration new evidence of benefits of ACE inhibitors, particularly in the patient with diabetic nephropathy, as well as address concerns raised about the potential adverse effects of thiazide diuretics in all diabetic patients, and of cardioselective and nonselective β-blocking agents in insulin-treated diabetics. Potential adverse effects of the latter agents include masking of insulin-induced hypoglycemia, worsening of glucose tolerance, hypokalemia, and dyslipoproteinemia, as well as activation of the renin-angiotensin system in the diabetic patient (Kaplan 1987; Pollare 1989; Davidson 1994). With the availability of new anti-hypertensive drugs including ACE inhibitors, calcium channel blockers, and prazosin,

———→

Fig. 10.2. Suggested approach to hypertension therapy in subjects with diabetes. Treatment goal for people with diabetes is to maintain blod pressure at less than 130/85 mmHg. Diabetic renal disease, autonomic dysfunction, and adverse effects on glucose and lipid metabolism must be considered before the course of therapeutic intervention is chosen. ACE denotes angiotensin converting enzyme. [From National High Blood Pressure Education Program Working Group (1994), with permission.]

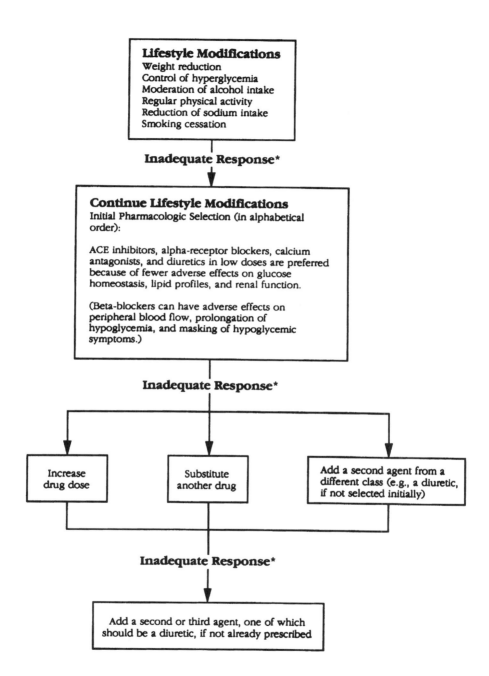

Lifestyle Modifications
Weight reduction
Control of hyperglycemia
Moderation of alcohol intake
Regular physical activity
Reduction of sodium intake
Smoking cessation

Inadequate Response*

Continue Lifestyle Modifications
Initial Pharmacologic Selection (in alphabetical order):

ACE inhibitors, alpha-receptor blockers, calcium antagonists, and diuretics in low doses are preferred because of fewer adverse effects on glucose homeostasis, lipid profiles, and renal function.

(Beta-blockers can have adverse effects on peripheral blood flow, prolongation of hypoglycemia, and masking of hypoglycemic symptoms.)

Inadequate Response*

Increase drug dose

Substitute another drug

Add a second agent from a different class (e.g., a diuretic, if not selected initially)

Inadequate Response*

Add a second or third agent, one of which should be a diuretic, if not already prescribed

*Response means achieved goal blood pressure or considerable progress toward this goal.

these potential side effects can be avoided. ACE inhibitors appear to decrease proteinuria and to preserve glomerular filtration rates in patients with diabetes independent of systemic blood pressure changes (Kasiske 1993). In a recently published randomized, placebo-controlled, clinical trial of an ACE inhibitor (captopril) and the risk of nephropathy among patients with IDDM, a 48% reduction in the risk of doubling of the serum creatinine concentration during a median follow-up of four years was observed with captopril treatment as compared with placebo; the protective effect of captopril was independent of blood pressure changes (Lewis 1993). The use of ACE inhibitors offers a promising approach to hypertension management in the diabetic patient (Pollare 1989). However, no randomized clinical trials among diabetics have been conducted to quantify the reduction in clinical CVD events or the overall benefit: risk ratio of ACE inhibitors or other antihypertensive regimens.

Reduction of Obesity

The importance of obesity in augmenting CHD risk in NIDDM warrants consideration, as obesity is a major determinant of both NIDDM (DeFronzo 1983) and CHD (Hubert 1983; Manson 1990). Obesity is commonly associated with hypertriglyceridemia and decreased levels of HDL-C, and, to a lesser extent, hypercholesterolemia (National Institutes of Health Consensus Development Panel on the Health Implications of Obesity 1985; Wood 1991). Furthermore, obesity, in particular central adiposity, has been linked to glucose intolerance, hyperinsulinemia, and hypertension; insulin resistance has been identified as the mediating factor (Kaplan 1989). Intraabdominal body fat is more metabolically responsive to adrenergic stimulation of lipolysis (Richelsen 1986), and can lead to elevations of free fatty acid concentrations in the portal circulation, insulin resistance, and dyslipidemia.

Weight loss leads to favorable changes in cardiovascular risk factors in nondiabetic individuals, including improvements in glucose tolerance, blood pressure, and lipid abnormalities (Olefsky 1974; Reisin 1978; Tuck 1981; Henry 1986; Kaplan 1989; Henry 1991). Although data are limited concerning the effects of weight loss on cardiovascular risk factor profiles in NIDDM patients, available evidence suggests similar salutary effects (Doar 1975; Hughes 1984; Kaplan 1985; Henry 1986; Amatruda 1988; Wing 1988; Uusitupa 1990) even with moderate weight loss (less than 10% of initial body weight). In a recently published review of 33 weight loss studies among obese subjects with NIDDM, hypertension, or hyperlipidemia, moderate weight loss improved cardiovascular risk factor profiles, including glycemic control in both nondiabetic and diabetic obese individuals (Goldstein 1992). Therefore, aiming for modest or moderate weight loss among both nondiabetic and diabetic patients with obesity seems warranted when larger reductions in body weight are difficult to achieve and/or maintain (Goldstein 1992).

Maintenance of weight reduction is important as weight cycling (phases of weight loss and subsequent weight regain) may increase risk of CHD morbidity and mortality (Lissner 1991). Long-term benefits of weight loss in relation to regional fat distribution and reductions in subsequent cardiovascular and all cause mortality in nondiabetic women and men are still controversial (Technology Assessment Conference Panel 1992). The paucity of data from individuals with sustained weight reduction and the lack of standardization and quality control of the different weight-loss programs limits the assessment of long-term consequences of weight loss. For the obese patient with NIDDM, diet therapy with weight loss likely represents the single most important step towards improved glycemic control (Nuttal 1983; Rifkin 1984). Whether sustained weight reduction will also lead to a reduction in CHD risk remains unclear. The known favorable effects of weight loss on blood lipids, blood pressure, insulin sensitivity, and glycemic control suggest a high probability for this hypothesis. (See Chapter 9 for further discussion of obesity management.)

Cigarette Smoking

Cigarette smoking represents one of the most important risk factors for CHD and other chronic diseases worldwide. In the Nurses' Health Study, cigarette smoking markedly augmented the risk of CHD in both nondiabetic and diabetic women (Manson 1991a). In the Framingham study, cessation of cigarette smoking among diabetics halved the risk of cardiovascular disease as compared with those diabetics who continued smoking, partly due to an accompanying elevation in HDL-C levels (Kannel 1985). The high number of CHD events attributable to smoking among both diabetic and nondiabetic populations supports the conclusion that cessation of cigarette smoking would dramatically reduce CHD morbidity and mortality (American Diabetes Association 1989) (See Chapter 5 for further reference.)

Physical Activity

Strength of Evidence for Potential Benefits from Increase in Physical Activity. Sparse data are available about the actual benefits of physical activity in relation to CHD risk among diabetic individuals. Studies in patients with mild NIDDM have demonstrated a benefit of exercise in increasing insulin sensitivity and glucose tolerance, as well as inducing favorable changes in blood lipids (Ruderman 1979, 1990; Saltin 1979). Exercise as an adjunct to diet regimens produces greater weight loss and higher maintenance rates in obese nondiabetic individuals (Pavlou 1989a) and NIDDM patients (Wing 1988). In combination with weight loss programs, exercise potentially counteracts the decrease in resting energy expenditure observed with dietary treatment, producing greater overall weight reductions and a greater percent fat loss (Kenrick 1974; Donahue 1984; Pavlou 1985; Manson 1992b). Such benefits of exercise have not been consistently reported in all studies, however (Van Dale 1987; Phinney 1988). Methodological differences between the studies, such as the intensity of the applied exercise regimens and differing degrees of control of food intake, may explain the observed inconsistencies (Van Dale 1987). No randomized clinical trials have been conducted to assess the CHD risk reductions in NIDDM patients induced by increased physical activity. Based on the available evidence, however, physical activity may play an important role in the reduction of CHD among diabetic as well as nondiabetic individuals (Schneider 1986) (see also Chapter 8 for further discussion).

Intervention Strategies for Increase in Physical Activity. Exercise is recommended for all patients with NIDDM after a careful exclusion of possible contraindications, including manifest macrovascular and microvascular complications, excessive blood pressure response to exercise, and postorthostatic hypotension (Table 10.4) (Technical Review 1991). In general, rhythmic aerobic exercises (walking, dancing, swimming, jogging), but also resistance exercises (weight lifting), are effective in improving glucose disposal and cardiovascular risk factor profiles (Yki-Järvinen 1983; Goldberg 1989). Depending on the individual's age, condition, and maximum heart rate determined at exercise testing, the optimal range of exercise is considered to be 50% to 70% of VO_{2max} applied for 20 to 45 minutes at least 3 days a week (Table 10.5). Special attention should be given to an adequate warm-up and cool-down phase of 5 to 10 minutes each as well as to appropriate footwear to minimize the risk of musculoskeletal and dermatological injuries. Self-monitoring of blood glucose before, during, and after exercise should be performed if the patient is treated with insulin (Ruderman 1986) or, in some cases, with oral hypoglycemic agents (Kemmer 1987). The value of exercise in the treatment of NIDDM and in the avoidance of its long-term complications remains to be fully assessed. There may be subgroups of diabetic patients who will particularly benefit and others who may experience minimal, if any, benefit. Overall, the benefits of exercise appear to outweigh potential risks for nearly all patients with NIDDM (Technical Review 1991).

Aspirin Treatment

The observed alterations in platelet function and thromboxane release among patients with IDDM and NIDDM implicate a potential role of antiplatelet therapy in diabetes (Early Treatment Diabetic Retinopathy Study [ETDRS] Investigators 1992). So far, only limited randomized clinical trial data are available regarding the reduction of CHD risk in diabetic patients with aspirin treatment. In the ETDRS, a large multicenter study enrolling 3,711 diabetic men and women aged 18 to 70 years, the five-year morbidity and mortality from MI was statistically significantly reduced by 28% in the aspirin group as compared with the placebo group (RR = 0.72; 99% CI: 0.55–.95) (ETDRS Investigators 1992). In secondary prevention, the Antiplatelet Trialists' Collaboration demonstrated a 19% reduction in risk of important vascular events among diabetics in the aspirin treatment group (Antiplatelet Trialists' Collaboration Group 1991). In the Physicians' Health Study, a randomized, double-blind, placebo-controlled trial assessing low-dose aspirin in the primary prevention of cardiovascular disease, diabetic participants assigned to aspirin had a 61% reduction in MI as compared with diabetics in the placebo group (the overall risk reduction with aspirin therapy was 44% for the total study population) (Steering Committee of the Physicians' Health Study Research Group 1989). The effects of aspirin on CHD risk appear not to be substantially different among diabetic and nondiabetic populations. Therefore, aspirin should be considered for the primary and secondary prevention of CHD in IDDM and NIDDM patients, who are at increased risk of developing macrovascular complications (ETDRS Investigators 1992). See Chapter 12 for further discussion of aspirin prophylaxis and therapy.

Estrogen Replacement Therapy

Since estrogen replacement therapy (ERT) is associated with a reduced risk of CHD in most epidemiologic studies (Stampfer 1991a), the use of ERT in postmenopausal

Table 10.4. Potential Beneficial and Adverse Effects of Exercise in Non-Insulin-Dependent Diabetes Mellitus

Potential benefits of exercise
  Increased insulin sensitivity
  Increased glucose tolerance
  Greater weight loss with a given dietary regimen
  Loss of adipose tissue with preservation of lean body mass
  Lowering of blood pressure
  Improved blood lipid profile
Potential adverse effects of exercise
  Cardiovascular
    Cardiac dysfunction and arrhythmias due to ischemic heart disease (often silent)
    Exercise increments in blood pressure during exercise
    Postexercise orthostatic hypotension
  Microvascular
    Retinal hemorrhage
    Increased proteinuria
    Acceleration of microvascular lesions
  Metabolic
    Worsening of hyperglycemia and ketosis
    Hypoglycemia in patients on insulin or sulfonylurea therapy
  Musculoskeletal
    Food ulcers (especially in the presence of neuropathy)
    Orthopedic injury related to neuropathy
    Accelerated degenerative joint disease
    Eye injuries and retinal hemorrhage

Source: Modified from American Diabetes Association (1991), with permission.

Table 10.5. Summary of Exercise Recommendations for Patients with Non-Insulin-Dependent Diabetes Mellitus

Screening	Search for vascular and neurologic complications, including silent ischemic heart disease
	Stress electrocardiogram in patients >35 years old
Exercise program	
Type	Aerobic
Intensity	50–70% of maximum aerobic capacity
Duration	20–60 minutes
Frequency	3–5 times per week
Avoid complications	Warm up and cool down
	Careful selection of exercise type and intensity
	Patient education
	Monitoring of blood glucose by patient and overall program by medical personnel
Compliance	Make exercise enjoyable
	Convenient location
	Positive feedback from involved medical personnel and family

Source: From American Diabetes Association (1991), with permission.

women with NIDDM could be of potential benefit. Estrogen administration in post-menopausal women increases HDL-C concentrations and lowers LDL-C concentrations in postmenopausal women (Stampfer 1991a). (See Chapter 16 for more detailed discussion.) In the Nurses' Health Study, the inverse association between ERT and CHD risk was comparable in nondiabetic and diabetic women, although the latter subgroup was small (Stampfer 1991b). Currently, there are minimal data available regarding the impact of ERT on the risk of CHD among diabetic women. Because of the increased risk of endometrial cancer with unopposed estrogen therapy, the addition of a progestional agent has been recommended; this may be of particular importance for obese women with NIDDM, who are at elevated risk of endometrial cancer (American Diabetes Association 1993b). Less is known, however, about the cardiovascular effects of combined estrogen/progestin therapy than estrogen alone. Due to the high risk of CHD among diabetic women, the epidemiologic evidence that ERT may reduce CHD risk, and the absence of evidence that ERT worsens glucose tolerance or increases risk of NIDDM (Manson 1992a), further research concerning the role of ERT in diabetic women is of great importance.

Primary Prevention of Non-Insulin-Dependent Diabetes Mellitus

Reduction of Obesity

Despite an important role for genetic factors, NIDDM should be considered as a largely preventable disease. Epidemiologic data from Japanese and Chinese migrants support the hypothesis that modern lifestyle factors, including physical activity and diet, exert a powerful impact on the risk of developing NIDDM (Kawate 1979; Dowse 1990). Potentially modifiable determinants of NIDDM that have been identified include body weight, body fat distribution, physical activity, and dietary factors (Manson 1994).

Strength of Evidence for Potential Benefit from Reduction of Obesity. The primary prevention of NIDDM itself may be the most important and promising strategy for reducing diabetes-related vascular disease. Prospective cohort studies have consistently demonstrated that obesity is a strong determinant of NIDDM in both women and men. In the Nurses' Health Study cohort, at least 90% of NIDDM cases among white women were estimated to be attributable to overweight (body mass index > 22 kg/m^2) (Colditz 1990). In this cohort, the risk of NIDDM among women in the highest decile of BMI was more than 60 times higher than among those in the lowest decile. Among a subgroup of women in the Nurses' Health Study with a BMI >27 kg/m^2 at entry, those who lost 5 to 20 kg in the first 4 years of the study had a subsequent 30% reduction in risk of NIDDM compared with women whose weight did not change more than 1 kg during that period (age-adjusted relative risk = 0.7; 95% CI: 0.5–1.1). Although few epidemiologic studies have had the statistical power to assess the influence of weight loss on NIDDM risk, metabolic studies in NIDDM patients have demonstrated beneficial effects of weight loss on glucose tolerance and insulin sensitivity (Doar 1975; Berger 1976; Henry 1988). The totality of available evidence derived from clinical, ecologic, and analytic epidemiologic studies supports an important role of obesity in the genesis of NIDDM. The estimated reduction in the risk of NIDDM associated with maintenance of desirable body weight (BMI ≤ 22.4 kg/m² in women and ≤ 22.7 kg/m² in men), as compared with being obese (≥20% of desirable weight, or BMI ≥ 27.3 kg/m² in women and ≥27.8 kg/m² in men), is estimated to 50% to 75% (Manson 1994).

Intervention Strategies for Reduction of Obesity. The successful long-term treatment of obesity is one of the greatest challenges in medicine and public health. The complex etiology of obesity may partially account for the failures observed for a variety of weight loss regimens (Council on Scientific Affairs 1988). (See Chapter 9 for discussion of weight reduction strategies and their efficacy).

In NIDDM patients, prolonged behavioral treatment emphasizing exercise and low-fat diets has produced weight loss comparable to that in nondiabetic individuals (Wing 1993). In a recent review of eight studies using behavioral treatment alone or in combination with diet and exercise, the achieved reductions in body weight ranged from 2.9 to 16.4 kg (Wing 1993). After one year, maintenance of weight loss was observed primarily among those who used regular exercise regimens and prolonged behavioral treatment. The results were best in studies where behavioral treatment was extended (weekly meetings for at least one year) (Wing 1993). A continuous care approach, including ongoing professional contact, skills training, social support, and exercise, has been proposed to improve long-term maintenance of weight reduction (Perri 1993) (Table 10.6).

The potential effects of obesity reduction through diet and physical activity in the primary prevention of NIDDM have been minimally studied. In a 5-year intervention study among Swedish men aged 47 to 49 at baseline, the investigators compared diet and exercise regimen to no intervention among 41 individuals with newly diagnosed NIDDM and 181 with impaired glucose tolerance (IGT) in the intervention group, and 79 individuals with IGT and 118 normal subjects in the control group, in relation to magnitude of weight loss, cardiovascular risk profiles, and clinical outcome (Eriksson 1991). Body weight was reduced by 2.3% to 3.7% among the intervention group, and the control group experienced an increase in weight of 0.5% to 1.7%. Glucose tolerance was normalized in 54% of newly diagnosed NIDDM cases, and in the IGT group, 76% had normal glucose levels on the oral glucose tolerance test (OGTT) after 5 years of intervention. Only 10.6% of participants with IGT assigned to the intervention group developed NIDDM within 5 years, as compared with 28.6% in the IGT control group (Eriksson 1991). Triglyceride and total cholesterol levels declined in the intervention NIDDM and IGT groups, as well as in the normal control group, while triglyceride levels increased in the IGT control group. These results suggest that sustained modification of lifestyle factors directed at weight loss, including dietary changes and increase in physical activity, are feasible and may help to prevent, or at least postpone, the onset of NIDDM.

Increase in Physical Activity

Strength of Evidence for Potential Benefit from Increase of Physical Activity. An inverse association between physical activity and the risk of NIDDM has been dem-

Table 10.6. Maintenance Strategies for Long-Term
Management of Obesity

Ongoing professional contact
  Purposes
    Continued vigilance regarding key behaviors
    Reinforcement of adherence
    Problem solving of obstacles to maintenance
  Methods
    Personal contacts between patient and professional
    Telephone contacts
    Contact by mail
    Combinations of the above
Skill training
  Purposes
    Identification of high-risk situations
    Training to avoid lapses
    Positive coping with slips and relapse
  Methods
    Review of past patterns of relapse
    Formal training in program solving
    Practice in coping with high-risk situations
    Cognitive restructuring of a lapse
Social support
  Purposes
    Additional guidance
    Emotional support
    Social reinforcement
  Methods
    Couples training
    Buddy systems
    Self-help group
    Telephone networks
Physical activity
  Purposes
    Additional caloric expenditure
    Preservation of lean tissue
    Improved mood and self-concept
  Methods
    Life-style changes
    Aerobic training
    Resistance training
Multicomponent programs
  Purposes
    Effectiveness of multiple methods
    Lack of data for matching strategies to patients
    Interest value of multiple strategies
  Method
    Combinations of strategies listed above

Source: From Perri (1993), with permission.

onstrated in several cross-sectional (King 1984; Taylor 1984; Zimmet 1990; Dowse 1991) and prospective cohort studies (Helmrich 1991; Manson 1991b, 1992b; Burchfiel 1995). The consistently observed reductions in risk of NIDDM among physically active compared with sedentary individuals in these studies suggest that physical inactivity is an important determinant of NIDDM and that regular moderate and/or vigorous exercise may be protective against NIDDM. The estimated reduction in the risk of NIDDM in these studies associated with regular moderate and/or vigorous exercise, as compared with a sedentary lifestyle, is 30 to 50% (Manson 1994).

Based on the data from observational epidemiologic studies, and limited data from clinical trials, there is growing support for the hypothesis that reducing obesity and enhancing physical activity will be beneficial in the prevention of NIDDM, and consequently, in the prevention of CHD. Additional data from prospective studies and randomized clinical trials are needed to quantify the benefits of exercise in the general population and among high-risk groups. Scientific questions of particular interest relate to the intensity, duration, and frequency of physical activity required to reduce the risk of developing NIDDM in both men and women. The efficacy of these exercise regimens among men and women in different age groups and the optimal timing of exercise interventions remain to be determined.

Intervention Strategies for Increasing Physical Activity. The benefits of exercise include an increase in energy expenditure, loss of adipose tissue with preservation of lean body mass, as well as favorable alterations of insulin sensitivity, blood pressure, and lipids (Pavlou 1989b). Weight-bearing exercise, such as walking, jogging, or cross-country skiing, produces an increase in energy expenditure directly related to body weight (Pavlou 1991). The feasibility, safety, and effectiveness of vigorous exercise, however, in severely obese or elderly individuals must be carefully considered (Skarfors 1987; Pavlou 1991). See Chapter 8 for further discussion of risk assessment and strategies for increasing physical activity.

Cost Effectiveness

The impact of diabetes on morbidity and mortality, as well as the economic costs attributable to the disease, are substantial. NIDDM was the seventh leading cause of mortality in the United States in 1986 (National Center for Health Statistics 1986), accounting for 144,000 or 6.8% of all deaths (Huse 1989). Combined direct and indirect costs of NIDDM in the United States have been estimated to be $40 billion annually (Bransome 1992). A recent analysis estimated the total health care costs of diabetes to be as high as $105 billion per year, which is 14.6% of U.S. health care costs in 1992 (Rubin 1994). In the United Kingdom, treatment of diabetes and its complications annually consumes 4% to 5% of total health care expenditure or approximately £1 billion at 1989 prices (Leese 1992).

Cost-effectiveness studies of diabetes management are scant (Persson 1989), including those evaluating new advances in treatment such as insulin pumps, new home glucose-monitoring techniques, and achievement of normalization of chronic gly-

Table 10.7. Elements of Cost-Effectiveness

Costs
  Research
  Screening
  Intervention
  Side effects of intervention
  Treatment of other diseases developing as a result of the increased
    longevity
Cost savings
  Health care for diabetes
  Screening for complications
  Treatment of complications
  Rehabilitation services
  Custodial care
Effectiveness
  Increase in life years
  Improvement in quality of life

Source: From Eastman (1993), with permission.

cemia. Elements of such analyses are given in Table 10.7. A few studies have been conducted on the cost effectiveness of screening procedures and early treatment for microvascular complications in IDDM (Javitt 1991; Siegel 1992). It was estimated that early treatment of microalbuminuria in IDDM patients with ACE inhibitors as compared with usual care would reduce costs by $7,900 to $16,500 per year of life saved (Siegel 1992). Treatment at a later stage, that is, proteinuria, would still improve life expectancy and save health care costs, yet to a lesser extent than early intervention (Siegel 1992). The early detection and treatment of proliferative diabetic retinopathy and clinically significant macular edema were estimated to yield savings of over $167.0 million per year and 79,236 person-years of sight if early intervention could be delivered to all patients with IDDM (Javitt 1991). Similar analyses have not yet been performed for the atherosclerotic complications of NIDDM.

With the results of the DCCT (DCCT Research Group 1993), the clinical effectiveness of tight glycemic control in IDDM has been conclusively demonstrated; however, it remains unclear how cost-effective this approach is when broadly applied. It is also unlikely that every patient with IDDM will have access to a team of endocrinologists, nurses, dietitians, and behavioral specialists who can assist with the development and maintenance of the intensive regimen (DCCT Research Group 1993; Laker 1993). In NIDDM, education programs, as well as diet and exercise regimens, aimed at reduction of obesity have been found to be equally cost effective as compared with other medical interventions (Connor 1984; Kaplan 1988). Screening for and treatment of coexisting coronary risk factors, such as hypertension and dyslipidemia, are clearly indicated and cost effective in the diabetic patient, although formal analyses are lacking. Additional clinical trial data are needed to form the basis of comprehensive and precise cost-effectiveness analyses for interventions in both IDDM and NIDDM.

Summary

Quality of available data: Data are sparse concerning maintenance of normal glycemia and risk of MI among individuals with diabetes.

Estimated risk reduction: The risk reduction associated with maintenance of normal glycemia is unknown. However, available evidence strongly supports modification of traditional CHD risk factors in this extremely high risk group.

Comparability of effect in men and women: Available evidence suggests a stronger influence of diabetes on increased MI risk in women than in men.

Appendix A

Nutrition Therapy for Diabetes Mellitus

Table A1. Goals of Medical Nutrition Therapy

1. Maintenance of as near-normal blood glucose levels as possible by balancing food intake with insulin (either endogenous or exogenous) or oral glucose-lowering medications and activity levels.
2. Achievement of optimal serum lipid levels.
3. Provision of adequate calories for maintaining or achieving reasonable weights for adults, normal growth and development rates in children, increased metabolic needs during pregnancy and lactation, or recovery from catabolic illnesses. Reasonable weight is defined as the weight an individual and health care provider acknowledge as achievable and maintainable, both short- and long-term. This may not be the same as the traditionally defined desirable or ideal body weight.
4. Prevention and treatment of the acute complications of insulin-treated diabetes such as hypoglycemia, short-term illnesses, and exercise-related problems, and of the long-term complications of diabetes such as renal disease, autonomic neuropathy, hypertension, and cardiovascular disease.
5. Improvement of overall health through optimal nutrition. *Dietary Guidelines for Americans*[a] and *The Food Guide Pyramid*[b] illustrate nutritional guidelines and nutrient needs for all healthy Americans, and can be used by people with diabetes and their family members.

Source: From American Diabetes Association (1994b), with permission.

[a]U.S. Department of Agriculture, U.S. Department of Health and Human Services. Nutrition and your health: dietary guidelines for Americans, 3rd ed. Hyattsville, MD: USDA's Human Nutrition Information Service, 1990.

[b]U.S. Department of Agriculture. Hyattsville, MD: The Food Guide Pyramid. USDA's Human Nutrition Information Service, 1992.

Table A2. Historical Perspective of Nutrition Recommendations

Year	Distribution of Calories		
	%Carbohydrate	%Protein	%Fat
Before 1921	Starvation diets		
1921	20	10	70
1950	40	20	40
1971	45	20	35
1986	up to 60	12–20	<30
1994	—[a]	10–20	—[a,b]

Source: Modified from American Diabetes Association (1994), with permission.
[a]Based on nutritional assessment and treatment goals.
[b]Less than 10% of calories from saturated fats.

References

American Diabetes Association. Policy statement: the UGDP controversy. Diabetes Care 1979; 2:1–3.

American Diabetes Association. Recommendations and principles for individuals with diabetes mellitus: 1986. Diabetes Care 1987;10:126–32.

American Diabetes Association. Role of cardiovascular risk factors in prevention and treatment of macrovascular disease in diabetes. Diabetes Care 1989;12:573–9.

American Diabetes Association. Technical review: exercise and NIDDM. Diabetes Care 1991; 14(Suppl):52–6.

American Diabetes Association. Diabetes 1993 vital statistics. Alexandria, VA: American Diabetes Association, 1993a.

American Diabetes Association. Detection and management of lipid disorders in diabetes. Diabetes Care 1993b;16(Suppl 2):106–12.

American Diabetes Association. Technical review: nutrition principles for the management of diabetes and related complications. Diabetes Care 1994a;17:490–518.

American Diabetes Association. Nutrition recommendations and principles for people with diabetes mellitus. Diabetes Care 1994b;17:519–22.

Antiplatelets Trialists' Collaboration Group. Overall effect on major vascular events: subgroup issues and comparison of agents. Diabetes and Heart Disease. Chapt. XVI, 1–41. Read before the 40th Annual Session of the American College of Cardiology; March 6, 1991; Atlanta, Ga.

Armatruda JM, Richeson JF, Welle SL, et al. The safety and efficacy of a controlled low-energy ('very-low-calorie') diet in the treatment of non-insulin-dependent diabetes and obesity. Arch Intern Med 1988;148:873–7.

Barrett-Connor E, Wingard DL. Sex differential in ischemic heart disease mortality in diabetics: a prospective population-based study. Am J Epidemiol 1983;118:489–96.

Barrett-Connor E, Orchard T. In: National Diabetes Group, ed. Diabetes in America. U.S. PHS 85-1468, 16:1–41, Bethesda, MD: National Institutes of Health, 1985.

Berger M, Baumhoff EE, Gries FA. Weight reduction and glucose intolerance in obesity. [In German]. Dtsch Med Wochenschr 1976;101:307–12.

Bild D, Teusch SM. The control of hypertension in persons with diabetes: a public health approach. Public Health Rep 1987;102:522–9.

Bransome ED. Financing the care of diabetes mellitus in the U.S. Diabetes Care 1992;15(Suppl 2):1–5.

Burchfiel CM, Sharp DS, Curb JD, et al. Physical Activity and Incidence of Diabetes: The Honolulu Heart Program. Am J Epidemiol 1995;141:360–8.

Castelli WP, Anderson K. A population risk: prevalence of high cholesterol levels in hypertensive patients in the Framingham Study. Am J Med 1986;30:165–71.

Colditz GA, Wilett WC, Stampfer MJ, et al. Weight as a risk factor for clinical diabetes in women. Am J Epidemiol 1990;132:501–13.

Collins R, Peto R, MacMahon S, et al. Blood pressure, stroke, and coronary heart disease. Part 2, short-term reductions in blood pressure: overview of randomised drug trials in their epidemiologic context. Lancet 1990;335:827–38.

Connor H. Diabetic management and education: costs and benefits. In: Balesi AK, Hide DW, Giles G, eds. Diabetes education. New York: Wiley, 1984.

Consensus Statement. Treatment of hypertension in diabetes. Diabetes Care 1993;16:1394–401.

Council on Scientific Affairs. Council report: treatment of obesity in adults. JAMA 1988;260:2547–51.

Davidson MB. Caveat to recommendations in the consensus statement: treatment of hypertension in diabetes. Diabetes Care 1994;17:345–46.

Deckert T, Poulsen JE, Larsen M. Prognosis of diabetics with diabetes onset before age thirty-one. I. Survival, causes of death, and complications. Diabetologia 1978;14:363–70.

DeFronzo RA, Ferrannini E, Koivisto V. New concepts in the pathogenesis and treatment of noninsulin-dependent diabetes mellitus. Am J Med 1983;74:52–81.

Diabetes Control and Complications Trial (DCCT): Results of feasibility study. Diabetes Care 1987;10:1–19.

The Diabetes Control and Complications Trial Research Group. The effect of intensive treatment of diabetes on the development and progression of long-term complications in insulin-dependent diabetes mellitus. N Engl J Med 1993;329:977–86.

Doar JWH, Wilde CE, Thompson ME, et al. Influence of treatment with diet alone on oral glucose-tolerance test and plasma sugar and insulin levels in patients with maturity-onset diabetes mellitus. Lancet 1975;1:1263–7.

Donahue RP, Lin DH, Kirschenbaum DS, Keesey RE. Metabolic consequences of dieting and exercise in the treatment of obesity. J Consult Clin Psychol 1984;5:827–36.

Donahue RP, Orchard TJ. Diabetes mellitus and macrovascular complications: an epidemiological perspective. Diabetes Care 1992;15:1141–55.

Dorman JS, Laporte RE, Kuller LH, et al. The Pittsburgh Insulin-Dependent Diabetes Mellitus (IDDM) Morbidity and Mortality Study: mortality results. Diabetes 1984/33:271–6.

Dowse GK, Gareeboo H, Zimmet PZ, et al. High prevalence of NIDDM and impaired glucose tolerance in Indian, Creole, and Chinese Mauritians. Diabetes 1990;39:390–6.

Dowse GK, Zimmet PZ, Gareboo H, et al. Abdominal obesity and physical activity as risk factors for NIDDM and impaired glucose tolerance in Indian, Creole, and Chinese Mauritians. Diabetes Care 1991;14:271–82.

Ducimetiere P, Eschwege E, Papoz L, et al. Relationship of plasma insulin levels to the incidence of myocardial infarction and coronary heart disease mortality in a middle-aged population. Diabetologia 1980;19:205–10.

Eastman RC, Silverman R, Harris M, et al. Lessening the Burden of Diabetes. Diabetes Care 1993;16:1095–1102.

EDTRS Investigators. Aspirin effects on mortality and morbidity in patients with diabetes mellitus: early treatment diabetic retinopathy study report 14. JAMA 1992;268:1292–300.

Eriksson KF, Lindgärde F. Prevention of type 2 (non-insulin-dependent) diabetes mellitus by diet and physical exercise. Diabetologia 1991;34:891–8.

Feldt-Rasmussen B, Matthiessen ER, Jensen T, et al. Effect of improved metabolic control on loss of kidney function in type 1 insulin-dependent) diabetic patients: an update of the Steno studies. Diabetologia 1991;34:164–70.

Fontbonne A, Eschwege E, Cambien F, et al. Hypertriglyceridemia as a risk factor of coronary heart disease mortality in subjects with impaired glucose tolerance or diabetes: results from the 11-year follow-up of the Paris Prospective Study. Diabetologia 1989;32:300–4.

Garg A, Grundy SM. Lovastatin for lowering cholesterol levels in non-insulin-dependent diabetes mellitus. N Engl J Med 1988;318:81–6.

Garg A, Bantle JP, Henry RR, et al. Effects of varying carbohydrate content of diet in patients with non-insulin dependent diabetes mellitus. JAMA 1994;271:1421–8.

Genuth S. Insulin use in NIDDM. Diabetes Care 1990;13:1240–64.

Goldberg AP. Aerobic and resistive exercise modify risk factors of coronary heart disease. Med Sci Sports Exercise 1989;21:669–74.

Goldstein DJ. Beneficial effects of modest weight loss. Int J Obesity 1992;16:397–415.

Greenland P, Reicher-Reiss H, Goldbourt U, et al. In-hospital and 1-year mortality in 1,524 women after myocardial infarction: comparison with 4,315 men. Circulation 1991;83:484–91.

Grundy SM. Dietary therapy of diabetes mellitus: is there a single best diet? Diabetes Care 1991;14:796–801.

Hadden DR, Blair ALT, Wilson EA, et al. Natural history of diabetes presenting age 40–69: a prospective study of the influence of intensive dietary therapy. Q J Med 1986;230:579–98.

Haffner SM, Mitchell BD, Pugh JA, et al. Proteinuria in Mexican Americans and non-Hispanic whites with NIDDM. Diabetes Care 1989;12:530–6.

Haluska PV, Luri D, Colwell JA. Increased synthesis of prostaglandin E-like material by platelets from patients with diabetes mellitus. N Engl J Med 1977;297:1306.

Harris MI. Summary In: National Diabetes Data Group, eds. Diabetes in America. National Institutes of Health; NIH publication no. 95-1468. Bethesda, MD; 1995;1–13.

Harris MI. Noninsulin-dependent diabetes mellitus in black and white Americans. Diabetes/Metab Rev 1990;6:71–90.

Harris MI. Hypercholesterolemia in diabetes and glucose intolerance in the U.S. population. Diabetes Care 1991;14:366–74.

Helmrich SP, Ragland DR, Leung RW, Paffenbarger RS. Physical activity and reduced occurrence of non-insulin-dependent diabetes mellitus. N Engl J Med 1991;325:147–52.

Henry RR, Schaeffer L, Olefsky JM. Glycemic effects of intensive caloric restriction and isocaloric refeeding in noninsulin-dependent diabetes mellitus. J Clin Endocrinol Metab 1985;61:917–25.

Henry RR, Wiest-Kent TA, Scheaffer L, et al. Metabolic consequences of very-low-calorie diet in obese non-insulin-dependent diabetic and nondiabetic subjects. Diabetes 1986;35:155–64.

Henry RR, Brechtel G, Griver K. Secretion and hepatic extraction of insulin after weight loss in obese non-insulin-dependent diabetes mellitus. J Clin Endocrinol Metabol 1988;66:979–86.

Henry RR, Gumbiner B. Benefits and limitations of very-low-calorie diet therapy in obese NIDDM. Diabetes Care 1991;14:802–23.

Henry RR, Gumbiner B, Ditzler T, et al. Intensive conventional insulin therapy for type II diabetes. Diabetes Care 1993;16:21–31.

Herman JB, Medalie JH, Goldbourt U. Differences in cardiovascular morbidity and mortality between previously known and newly diagnosed adult diabetics. Diabetologia 1977;13:229–34.

Heyden S, Heiss G, Bartel AG, Hames CG. Sex differences in coronary mortality among diabetics in Evans County, Georgia. J Chron Dis 1980;33:265–73.

Hubert HB, Feinleib M, McNamara PM, et al. Obesity as an independent risk factor for cardiovascular disease: a 26-year follow-up of participants in the Framingham Heart Study. Circulation 1983;249:2199–203.

Hughes TA, Gwynne JT, Switzer BR, et al. Effects of caloric restriction and weight loss on glycemic control, insulin release and resistance, and atherosclerotic risk in obese patients with type II diabetes mellitus. Am J Med 1984;77:7–17.

Huse DM, Oster G, Killen AR, et al. The economic costs of non-insulin-dependent diabetes mellitus. JAMA 1989;262:2708–13.

Janka HU. Five-year incidence of major cardiovascular complications in diabetes mellitus. Horm Metab Res Suppl 1985;15:15–9.

Jarrett RJ, Keen H, McCartney M, et al. Glucose tolerance and blood pressure in two population samples: their relation to diabetes mellitus and hypertension. Int J Epidemiol 1978;63:54–64.

Jarrett RJ, McCartney P, Keen H. The Bedford survey: ten year mortality rates in newly diagnosed diabetics, borderline diabetics and normoglyceamic controls and risk indices for coronary heart disease in borderline diabetics. Diabetologia 1982;22:79–84.

Javitt JC, Aiello LP, Bassi LJ, et al. Detecting and treating retinopathy in patients with type I diabetes mellitus. Ophthalmology 1991;98:1565–74.

Juhan-Vague I, Vague PH, Alessi MC, et al. Relationship between plasma insulin, triglyceride, body mass index, and plasminogen activator inhibitor 1. Diabetes Metab 1987;13:331–6.

Kannel WB, McGee DL. Diabetes and glucose intolerance as risk factors for cardiovascular disease: the Framingham Study. Diabetes Care 1979;2:120–6.

Kannel WB. Lipid, diabetes, and coronary heart disease: insights from the Framingham Study. Am Heart J 1985;110:1100–7.

Kannel WB, D'Agostino RB, Wilson PWF, et al. Diabetes, fibrinogen, and risk of cardiovascular disease: the Framingham experience. Am Heart J 1990;120:672–9.

Kaplan RM, Wilson DK, Hartwell SL, et al. Prospective evaluation of HDL cholesterol after diet and physical conditioning programs for patients with type II diabetes mellitus. Diabetes Care 1985:8:343–8.

Kaplan NM, Rosenstock J, Raskin P. A differing view of treatment of hypertension in patients with diabetics. Arch Intern Med 1987;147:1160–2.

Kaplan RM, Atkins CJ, Wilson DK. The cost-utility of diet and exercise interventions in non-insulin-dependent diabetes mellitus. Health Promotion 1988;2:331–40.

Kaplan NM. The deadly quartet: upper-body obesity, glucose intolerance, hypertriglyceridemia, and hypertension. Arch Intern Med 1989;149:1514–20.

Kasiske BL, Kalil RSN, Ma JZ, et al. Effect of antihypertensive therapy on the kidney in patients with diabetes: a meta regression analysis. Ann Intern Med 1993;118:129–38.

Kawate R, Yamakido M, Nishimoto Y, et al. Diabetes mellitus and its vascular complications in Japanese migrants on the island of Hawaii. Diabetes Care 1979;2:161–70.

Kemmer FW, Tacken M, Berger M. Mechanism of exercise-induced hypoglycemia during sulfonylurea treatment. Diabetes 1987;36:1178–82.

Kenrick M, Ball FM, Canary JJ. Exercise and weight reduction in obesity. Arch Phys Med Rehab 1972;53:232–7.

King H, Zimmet P, Raper LR, Balkau B. Risk factors for diabetes in three pacific populations. Am J Epidemiol 1984;119:396–409.

Klimt CE, Knatterud GL, Meinert CL, Prout TE. The University Group Diabetes Program: a study on the effects of hypoglycemic agents on vascular complications in patients with adult-onset diabetes. Part II. Mortality results. Diabetes 1970;19(Suppl 2):789–830.

Krall P. Oral hypoglycemic agents. In: Marble A, Krall LP, Bradley RF, Christlieb AR, Soeldner JS, eds. Joslin's diabetes mellitus, 12th ed. Philadelphia: Lea & Febiger, 1985:412–52.

The KROC Collaborative Study Group. Diabetic retinopathy after two years of intensified insulin treatment: follow-up of the KROC Collaborative Study. JAMA 1988;260:37–41.

Krolewski AS, Warram JH, Christlieb AR. Onset, course, complications, and prognosis of diabetes mellitus. In: Marble A, Krall LP, Bradley RF, Christlieb AR, Soeldner JS, eds. Joslin's diabetes mellitus. Philadelphia: Lea & Febiger, 1985;251–77.

Krolewski AS, Kosinski EJ, Warram JH, et al. Magnitude and determinants of coronary artery disease in juvenile-onset, insulin-dependent diabetes mellitus. Am J Cardiol 1987;59: 750–5.

Laakso M, Voutilainen E, Sarlund H, et al. Serum lipids and lipoproteins in middle-aged non-insulin-dependent diabetics. Atherosclerosis 1985;56:271–81.

Laakso M, Pyörälä K, Voutilainen E, et al. Plasma insulin levels and serum lipids and lipoproteins in middle-aged non-insulin dependent diabetic and non-diabetic subjects. Am J Epidemiol 1987;123:611–21.

Laker RD. The Diabetes Control and Complications Trial: implications for policy and practice. N Engl J Med 1993;329:1035–6.

Leese B. The costs of diabetes and its complications. Soc Sci Med 1992;35:1303–10.

Lerner DJ, Kannel WB. Patterns of coronary heart disease morbidity and mortality in the sexes: a 26-year follow-up of the Framingham population. Am Heart J 1986;111:383–90.

Levy D, Kannel WB. Cardiovascular risks: new insights from Framingham. Am Heart J 1988; 116:2664–7.

Lewis EJ, Hunsicker LG, Bain RP, Rohde RD for the Collaborative Study Group. The effect of angiotensin-converting-enzyme inhibition on diabetic nephropathy. N Engl J Med 1993;329:1456–62.

Lissner L, Odell PM, D'Agostino RB, et al. Variability of body weight and health outcomes in the Framingham population. N Engl J Med 1991;324:1839–43.

Lucas CP, Estrigarribia JA, Darga LL, Reaven GM. Insulin and blood pressure in obesity. Hypertension 1985;5:702–6.

Manson JE, Colditz GA, Stampfer MJ, et al. A prospective study of obesity and risk of coronary heart disease in women. N Engl J Med 1990;32:882–9.

Manson JE, Colditz GA, Stampfer MJ, et al. A prospective study of maturity-onset diabetes mellitus and coronary heart disease and stroke in women. Arch Intern Med 1991a;151: 1141–7.

Manson JE, Rimm EB, Stampfer MJ, et al. Physical activity and incidence of non-insulin-dependent diabetes mellitus in women. Lancet 1991b;338:774–8.

Manson JE, Rimm EB, Colditz GA, et al. A prospective study of postmenopausal estrogen therapy and subsequent incidence of non-insulin-dependent diabetes mellitus. Ann Epidemiol 1992a;2:665–73.

Manson JE, Nathan DM, Krolewski AS, et al. A prospective study of exercise and incidence of diabetes among U.S. male physicians. JAMA 1992b;268:63–7.

Manson JE, Spelsberg A. The primary prevention of non-insulin-dependent diabetes mellitus. Am J Prev Med 1994;102:172–184.

Modan M, Halkin H. Hyperinsulinemia or increased sympathetic drive as links for obesity and hypertension. Diabetes Care 1991;14:470–87.

Nathan DM, Roussell A, Godine JE. Glyburide or insulin for metabolic control in non-insulin-dependent diabetes mellitus: a randomized, double-blind study. Ann Intern Med 1988; 108:334–40.

Nathan DM. Medical progress: long-term complications of diabetes mellitus. N Engl J Med 1993;328:1676–85.

National Center for Health Statistics. Table B. Advance report of final mortality statistics, 1984. Monthly Vital Statistics Report Vol. 35, No. 6, Supplement 2. U.S. Department of Health and Human Services Publication (PHS) 86-1120. Public Health Service, Hyattsville, Md. September 26, 1986.

National High Blood Pressure Education Program Working Group. National High Blood Pressure Education Program Working Group Report on hypertension in Diabetes. Hypertension 1994;23:145–58.

National Institutes of Health Consensus Development Panel on the Health Implications of Obesity. Health implications of obesity: National Institutes of Health consensus development conference statement. Ann Intern Med 1985;103:1073–7.

National Institutes of Health Consensus Conference. Triglyceride, high-density lipoprotein, and coronary heart disease. JAMA 1993;269:505–10.

Nikkilä EA, Hormila P. Serum lipids and lipoproteins in insulin-treated diabetes: demonstration of increased high-density lipoprotein concentration. Diabetes 1978;27:1087–6.

Nikkilä EA. High density lipoprotein in diabetes. Diabetes 1981;30(Suppl 2):82–7.

Nuttal FQ. Diet and the diabetic patient. Diabetes Care 1983;6:197–207.

Olefsky JM, Reaven GM, Farquhar JW. Effects of weight reduction in obesity: studies of carbohydrate and lipid metabolism. J Clin Invest 1974;41:53:64–76.

Pan WH, Cedres LB, Liu K, et al. Relationship of clinical diabetes to risk of coronary heart disease mortality in men and women. Am J Epidemiol 1986;123:504–16.

Panzram G. Mortality and survival in type 2 (non-insulin-dependent) diabetes mellitus. Diabetologia 1987;30:123–31.

Pavlou KN, Steffee WP, Lerman RH, Burrows BA. Effects of dieting and exercise on lean body mass, oxygen uptake, and strength. Med Sci Sports Exerc 1985;17:466–71.

Pavlou KN, Krey S, Steffee WP. Exercise as an adjunct to weight loss and maintenance in moderately obese subjects. Am J Clin Nutr 1989a;49:1115–23.

Pavlou KN, Whatley JE, Jannace PW, et al. Physical activity as a supplement to weight-loss regimen. Am J Clin Nutr 1989b;49:1110–4.

Perri MG, Sears SF, Clark JE. Strategies for improving maintenance of weight loss: towards a continuous care model of obesity management. Diabetes Care 1993;16:200–9.

Persson U. The economics of diabetes: a review. IHE Working Paper 1989, p 3, Lund, 1989.

Peters AL, Davidson MB. Insulin plus sulfonylurea agent for treating type 2 diabetes. Ann Intern Med 1991;115:45–53.

Pfeiffer MA, Brunzell JD, Best JD, et al. The response of plasma triglyceride, cholesterol, and lipoprotein lipase to treatment in non-insulin-dependent diabetic subjects without familial hypertriglyceridemia. Diabetes 1983;32:525–31.

Phinney SD, LaGrange BM, O'Connell M, Danforth E. Effects of aerobic exercise on energy expenditure and nitrogen balance during very low calorie dieting. Metabolism 1988;37: 758–65.

Pollare T, Lithell H, Selinus I, Berne C. Sensitivity to insulin during treatment with atenolol and metoprolol: a randomised, double blind study of effects on carbohydrate and lipoprotein metabolism in hypertensive patients. Br Med J 1989;298:1152–7.

Pyörälä K, Laakso M, Uusitupa M. Diabetes and atherosclerosis: an epidemiologic view. Diabetes/Metab Rev 1987;3:463–524.

Quatraro A, Consoli G, Magno M, et al. Hydroxychloroquine in decompensated, treatment-refractory non-insulin-dependent diabetes mellitus: a new job for an old drug? Ann Intern Med 1990;112:678–81.

Quatraro A, Giugliano D. The combination of insulin and oral hypoglycemic drugs: a continuous challenge. Diabetes Metab Rev 1993;19:219–24.

Reaven GM. Role of insulin resistance in human disease: Banting lecture 1988. Diabetes 1988: 37:1595–607.

Reichard P, Nilsson BY, Rosenquist U. The effect of long-term intensified insulin treatment of the development of microvascular complications of diabetes mellitus. N Engl J Med 1993;329:304–9.

Reisin E, Abel R, Modan M, et al. Effect of weight loss without salt restriction on the reduction of blood pressure in overweight hypertensive patients. N Engl J Med 1978;298:1–6.

Richelsen B. Increased alpha$_2$: but similar β-adrenergic receptor activities in subcutaneous gluteal adipocytes from females compared with males. Eur J Clin Invest 1986;16:302–9.

Ridker PM, Hennekens CH. Hemostatic risk factors for coronary heart disease. Circulation 1991;83:1098–100.

Rifkin H. The physician's guide to type II diabetes (NIDDM): diagnosis and treatment. New York: Am Diabetes Assoc, 1984.

Rifkin H. Current status of non-insulin-dependent diabetes mellitus (type II): management with gliclazide. Am J Med 1991;90(Suppl 6A):3S–7S.

Rosak C. Glucosidase inhibition and sulphonylurea secondary failure. Diabetes Nutr Metab 1990;3(Suppl 1):59–62.

Rubin RJ, Altmann WM, Mendelson DN. Health care expenditures for people with diabetes mellitus, 1992. J Clin Endocrinol Metab 1994;78:809A–809F.

Ruderman NB, Ganda OP, Johansen K. The effect of physical training on glucose tolerance and plasma lipids in maturity-onset diabetes. Diabetes 1979;28(Suppl):89–94.

Ruderman NB, Haudenschild C. Diabetes as an atherogenic factor. Prog Cardiovasc Dis 1984; 26:373–412.

Ruderman NB, Schneider S. Exercise and the insulin-dependent diabetic. Hosp Pract 1986;21: 41–51.

Ruderman NB, Apelian AZ, Schneider SH. Exercise in therapy and prevention of type II diabetes: implication for blacks. Diabetes Care 1990;13(Suppl):1163–8.

Saltin B, Lindgärde F, Houston M, et al. Physical training and glucose tolerance in middle-aged men with chemical diabetes. Diabetes 1979;28(Suppl):30–7.

Schneider SH, Vitug A, Ruderman NB. Atherosclerosis and physical activity. Diabetes Metab Rev 1986;1:445–81.

Service FJ, Rizza RA, Daube JR, et al. Near normoglycemia improved nerve conduction and vibration sensation in diabetic nephropathy. Diabetologia 1985;28:722–7.

Siegel JE, Krolewski AS, Warram, JH, Weinstein MC. Cost-effectiveness of screening and early treatment of nephropathy in patients with insulin-dependent diabetes mellitus. J Am Soc Nephrol 1992;3(Suppl 4):S111–9.

Singer DE, Nathan DM, Anderson KM, et al. Association of HbA$_{1c}$ with prevalent cardiovascular disease in the original cohort of the Framingham Heart Study. Diabetes 1992;41: 202–8.

Skarfors ET, Wegener TA, Lithell H, Selinus I. Physical training as treatment for type 2 (non-insulin-dependent) diabetes in elderly men: a feasibility study for over 2 years. Diabetologia 1987;30:370–3.

Smith DA. Comparative approaches to risk reduction of coronary heart disease in the Tecumseh non-insulin-dependent diabetic population. Diabetes Care 1986;9:601–8.

Stampfer MJ, Colditz GA. Estrogen replacement therapy and coronary heart disease: a quantitative assessment of the epidemiologic evidence. Prev Med 1991a;20:47–63.

Stampfer MJ, Colditz GA, Willett, WC, et al. Postmenopausal estrogen therapy and cardiovascular disease: ten-year follow-up from the Nurses' Health Study. N Engl J Med 1991b; 325:756–62.

Steering Committee of the Physicians' Health Study Research Group. Final report on the aspirin component of the ongoing physicians' health study. N Engl J Med 1989;321:129–35.

Stern MP, Mitchell BD, Haffner SM, Hazuda H. Does glycemic control type II diabetes suffice to control diabetic dyslipidemia? Diabetes Care 1991;15:638–44.

Taskinen MR, Kuusi T, Helve E, et al. Insulin therapy induces antiatherogenic changes of serum lipoproteins in noninsulin-dependent diabetes. Arteriosclerosis 1988;8:168–77.

Taylor R, Ram P, Zimmet P, et al. Physical activity and prevalence of diabetes in Melanesian and Indian men in Fiji. Diabetologia 1984;27:578–82.

Technology Assessment Conference Panel. Methods for voluntary weight loss and control: Technology Assessment Conference statement. Ann Intern Med 1992;116:942–9.

Tobey TA, Greenfield M, Kraemer F, Reaven GM. Relationship between insulin resistance, insulin secretion, very low density lipoprotein kinetics, and plasma triglyceride levels in normotriglyceride man. Metabolism 1981;31:165–71.

Tuck ML, Sowers J, Dornfield L, et al. The effect of weight reduction on blood pressure, plasma renin activity, and plasma aldosterone levels in obese patients. N Engl J Med 1981;304: 930–3.

U.K. Prospective Diabetes Study. II. Reduction in HbA_{1c} with basal insulin supplement, sulfonylurea, or biguanide therapy in maturity-onset diabetes: a multicenter study. Diabetes 1985;34:793–8.

Uusitupa MJ, Laakso M, Sarlund H, et al. Effects of a very low calorie diet on metabolic control and cardiovascular risk factors in the treatment of obese non-insulin-dependent diabetics. Am J Clin Nutr 1990;51:768–73.

Vague PH, Juhan-Vague I, Chabert V, et al. Fat distribution and plasminogen activator inhibitor activity in non-diabetic obese women. Metabolism 1989;38:913–5.

Van Dale D, Saris WHM, Schoffelen PFM, Ten Hoor F. Does exercise give an additional effect in weight reduction regimens? Int J Obesity 1987;11:367–75.

Viverti GC, Keen H, Wiseman MJ. Raised arterial pressure in parents of proteinuric insulin-dependent diabetics. Br Med J 1987;295:575–77.

Wadden TA, Stunkard AJ, Brownell KD. Very low calorie diets: their efficacy, safety, and future. Ann Intern Med 1983;99:675–84.

Wellborn TA, Wearne K. Coronary heart disease incidence and cardiovascular mortality in Busselton with reference to glucose and insulin concentrations. Diabetes Care 1979;2: 154–160.

West KM. Diet therapy of diabetes: an analysis of failure. Ann Intern Med 1973;79:425–34.

West KM, Ahujy MMS, Bennett PH, et al. The role of circulating glucose and triglyceride concentrations and their interactions with ''other risk factors'' as determinants of arterial disease in nine diabetic population samples from the WHO multinational study. Diabetes Care 1983;6:361–9.

Wing RR, Epstein LH, Paternostro-Bayles M, et al. Exercise in a behavioral weight control programme for obese patients with Type 2 (non-insulin-dependent) diabetes. Diabetologia 1988;31:902–9.

Wing RR. Behavioral treatment of obesity: its application to type II diabetes. Diabetes Care 1993;16:193–99.

Wood PD, Stefanick MI, Williams PT, et al. The effects of plasma lipoproteins of a prudent weight-reducing diet, with or without exercise, in overweight men and women. N Engl J Med 1991;325:461–6.

World Health Organization Multinational Study of Vascular Disease in Diabetes. Prevalence of small vessel and large vessel disease in diabetic patients from centers. Diabetologia 1985;28:615–40.

The Working Group on Hypertension in Diabetes: Statement on hypertension in diabetes. Arch Intern Med 1987;147:830–42.

Yki-Järvinen H, Koivisto VA. Effects of body composition on insulin sensitivity. Diabetes 1983; 32:965–9.

Yki-Järvinen H, Kauppila M, Kujansuu E, et al. Comparison of insulin regimens in patients with non-insulin-dependent diabetes mellitus. N Engl J Med 1992;327:1426–33.

Zavaroni I, Dall'Aglio E, Alpi O, et al. Evidence for an independent relationship between plasma insulin concentration and concentration of high density lipoprotein cholesterol and triglyceride. Atherosclerosis 1985;55:259–66.

Zavaroni I, Bonora E, Pagliara AM. Risk factors for coronary artery disease in healthy people with hyperinsulinemia and normal glucose tolerance. N Engl J Med 1989;320:702–6.

Zimmet P, Dowse G, Finch C, et al. The epidemiology and natural history of NIDDM: Lessons from the South Pacific. Diabetes Metab Rev 1990;6:91–124.

11

Stress, Anger, and Psychosocial Factors for Coronary Heart Disease

ROBERT ALLAN AND STEPHEN SCHEIDT

A relationship between heart and mind has been suspected since the second millenium B.C., the era of Plato and Hippocrates (Plato, 1953, 1871). Early in the twentieth century, Cannon (1932) and Selye (1956) called attention to major physiologic changes brought about by psychological factors. In the past 35 years, a burgeoning body of observational, epidemiologic, and experimental studies has appeared that can be called "cardiac psychology," an evolving pool of knowledge to help foster and support heart-healthy living. Important research findings are now available for a number of psychosocial variables that may well be interdependent "risk factors" for coronary heart disease (CHD), including psychological stress, the Type A behavior pattern (TABP), anger, vital exhaustion, lack of social support, and job strain. Two other psychological variables, cardiac denial and depression, also have relevance for CHD. Each of these is discussed in detail. In addition, apart from age and gender, each of the traditional major risk factors for CHD (currently listed by the American Heart Association as cigarette smoking, hyperlipidemia, hypertension, and sedentary life-style) has a significant behavioral component. This review of the recent literature on stress and other psychosocial risk factors for CHD will summarize the current state of knowledge in the evolving field of cardiac psychology. Much work, however, is needed to clarify the relative importance of each of the psychosocial variables for both primary and secondary prevention of CHD.

Psychological Stress

The word "stress" is an alteration of *distress*, derived from the Old French *estresse*, signifying "oppression."* During the Middle Ages, the term also meant the "pressure

Copyright © 1995 Robert Allan and Stephen Scheidt.
*We are grateful to E. S. C. Weiner, coeditor of the Oxford English Dictionary for assistance with the etymology of the words "stress" and "anger."

exerted on an object" or "the strain of a load." The current Oxford English Dictionary definition of stress is "a condition or adverse circumstance that disturbs, or is likely to disturb, the normal physiologic or psychological functioning of an individual." There has long been a popular belief that stress, physical or psychological, must be deleterious, but this has been difficult to confirm.

The exercise stress test, widely used in clinical cardiology, determines with great precision the effects of physical stress on cardiac function. In contrast, psychological stress is an exceedingly complex phenomenon that has been difficult to define, measure and, hence, study scientifically. In an early attempt to relate psychological stress with cardiac events, the Recent Life Change (RLC) questionnaire, was used to classify the intensity of a variety of frequently occurring life changes. Events such as the death of a spouse, marriage, divorce, and loss of a job are considered highly stressful, while changes in working hours, trouble with in-laws, and vacations are thought to be less stressful. In a 1974 study, the RLC was administered to 279 survivors of myocardial infarction (MI) and spouses of 226 cases of sudden cardiac death in Helsinki, Finland (Rahe 1974). Marked elevations in RLC scores were seen for most cases of either endpoint compared with control subjects during the six months before the event. Data were particularly impressive for sudden cardiac death.

A study in Goteborg, Sweden (Rosengren 1991) followed a group of 6,935 healthy men, aged 47 to 55 at baseline, for a mean of 11.8 years. Subjects rated themselves on a stress scale "conceived on a purely intuitive basis, focusing on various psychological problems such as anxiety, tension and sleeping difficulties." Among the 5,865 men with the lowest four stress ratings, 6% developed a nonfatal MI or died from CHD. Of the 1,070 men with the two highest stress ratings, 10% suffered MI or cardiac death (odds ratio: 1.5; 95% CI: 1.2–1.9). A second, smaller substudy of 1,066 men born in 1933 and living in Goteborg, however, failed to replicate the initial finding using the identical stress scale, but with only 6-year follow-up (ibid).

Currently, there are too few studies of sufficiently large groups to conclude definitively that psychological stress affects cardiac morbidity or mortality. There are, however, a number of studies with convincing evidence that psychological stress has major influences on possible physiologic mechanisms that could link behavioral factors to cardiac event rates (Table 11.1). This section considers available data on the links between psychological stress and serum lipids, experimental coronary atherosclerosis, coronary artery vasomotion, myocardial ischemia, triggers for acute MI, and sudden cardiac death.

Serum Lipids

Cannon's "fight or flight response" (1932), recast in psychological terms by Friedman and Rosenman (1974) as "free-floating hostility" and "time pressure," the major symptoms of the TABP, suggested that chronic overactivation of the sympathetic nervous system with excess secretion of "stress hormones," for example, catecholamines and cortisol, would be atherogenic. A considerable amount of early work examined serum lipids as a mechanism that might link stress and atherosclerosis. Indeed, Friedman and Rosenman (1959) reported seasonal variations in accountants' cholesterol levels that peak with the April 15th tax deadline. In a review (Niaura 1992) of the

Table 11.1. Possible Physiologic Mechanisms Linking Behavioral Factors to Cardiac Dysfunction[a]

1. Increased coronary atherosclerosis via
- increased serum cholesterol due to chronic or subacute stress (Friedman & Rosenman 1959; Niaura et al. 1992)
- decreased serum HDL caused by increased circulating testosterone related to anger
- increased activation of macrophages, increased platelet aggregability, increased release of platelet-derived growth factors, increased thrombosis, all related to increased sympathetic activity, circulating or neural
- increased blood pressure due to acute or chronic stress, including "job strain" (Schnall et al. 1990)
- increased levels of standard atherosclerotic risk factors (including high animal fat diet, more smoking, higher blood pressures) in Type A or hostile individuals
- unknown mechanisms, possibly related to the sympathetic nervous system, in striving individuals in socially unstable situations (Clarkson et al. 1987)

2. Decreased coronary atherosclerosis via
- modification of standard cardiac risk factors and decreased chronic sympathetic activity due to meditation and group support (Ornish et al. 1993)
- decreased chronic sympathetic activity due to reduced Type A behavior (Friedman et al. 1986; Friedman et al. 1987; Burell 1993)
- decreased levels of standard atherosclerotic risk factors *after* CHD diagnosis in Type A individuals who are spontaneously more compulsive about changing lifestyle once diagnosis is made (Ragland & Brand 1988; Barefoot et al. 1989; Ahern et al. 1990)

3. Increased susceptibility to myocardial ischemia via
- increased myocardial oxygen demands from increased heart rate, blood pressure, and myocardial contractility due to increased sympathetic activity with mental stress or anger (Rozanski et al. 1988; Ironson et al. 1992)
- increased myocardial oxygen demands from increased blood pressure, blood volume, and ventricular wall stress due to renin-angiotensin-aldosterone or adrenal cortical system activation related to stress
- increased myocardial oxygen demands from left ventricular hypertrophy related to higher blood pressures in chronic stress or high "job strain" (Schnall et al. 1990)
- increased platelet aggregability and thrombosis due to increased sympathetic activity
- increased or abnormal coronary vasospasm or vasoconstriction, some possibly due to abnormalities in endothelial derived relaxing factor (EDRF), related to increased sympathetic or decreased parasympathetic activity with mental stress (Feigl 1987; Yeung et al. 1991)
- decreased spontaneous fibrinolytic activity

4. Increased susceptibility to cardiac arrhythmia via
- increased sympathetic stimulation (cardiac sympathetic nerves, left stellate ganglion stimulation or circulating catecholamines) from acute or chronic stress causing lower threshold for life-threatening ventricular arrhythmia (Verrier 1987)
- indirect effects of sympathetic stimulation causing beta-1 epinephrine-mediated hypokalemia
- behavioral influences on QT interval
- increased ischemia
- increased free fatty acids from increased catecholamine or cortisol levels
- decreased parasympathetic stimulation
- increased parasympathetic stimulation causing bradyarrhythmias or heart block
- unknown mechanisms wherein chronically depressed individuals may be more prone to acute "triggers" for arrhythmia

5. Increased cardiac death rate via
- slower response to premonitory symptoms of myocardial ischemia or infarction due to denial or depression: increased chance of out-of-hospital sudden cardiac death or larger myocardial infarct due to delay in administering thrombolysis (Fielding, 1991; Sirous, 1992)
- slower response due to lack of social support (no one to consult or help in emergencies) (Ruberman et al. 1984; House et al. 1988; Berkman et al. 1992; Case et al. 1992; Williams et al. 1992; Orth-Gomer et al. 1993)

[a]Some mechanisms have been demonstrated to be operative in cited references.

stress-lipid literature with an emphasis on reseach conducted within the past decade, the authors conclude that

1. The results of 62 recent studies of episodic stressors, such as medical school examinations or military training exercises, show positive, though inconclusive, results.
2. Some studies of personality traits, such as the TABP and hostility, have shown a positive correlation with serum cholesterol levels, although recent studies using the Cook Medley Hostility Scale have not done so.
3. Most studies of chronic occupational stress fail to show a relationship between stress and lipids.
4. Studies of acute laboratory stressors show temporary increases in free fatty acids, although the relationship between such increases and subsequent cholesterol levels is unclear.

Coronary Atherosclerosis and Vasomotion

Ongoing, well-controlled research in primates has provided experimental confirmation for the importance of simulated psychological stress in the development of atherosclerosis (Kaplan 1993). Cynomolgus monkey colonies were subjected to stress by repeatedly reshuffling groups, breaking up a stable social structure of dominant and subordinate individuals (Clarkson 1987). In some experiments high lipid diets were added to promote atherosclerosis; in others the struggle was accentuated by adding a single sexually receptive female to the disorganized group. Dominant monkeys in unstable and stressful groups developed strikingly increased coronary atherosclerosis compared both with subordinates (who presumably did not struggle as hard to achieve dominance) and with dominant monkeys in stable groups. Beta-blockers prevented this tendency to increased atherosclerosis.

Using a similar protocol, Williams and colleagues (1991) studied the effects of chronic social disruption and diet on coronary artery function in cynomolgus monkeys. As expected, quantitative angiography revealed larger plaques in the socially stressed monkeys compared with controls. Socially disrupted monkeys also showed a paradoxical constriction of coronary arteries in response to acetylcholine, normally a vasodilator, compared with socially stable controls. The authors conclude that, in addition to an atherogenic effect, chronic social stress impairs endothelium-dependent vascular responses of coronary arteries in primates.

Coronary artery vasoconstriction has also been demonstrated in humans after psychological stressors, particularly in atherosclerotic coronary artery segments (Feigl 1987) and there has been much interest in the possible role of endothelial-derived relaxing factor (EDRF). Yeung and coworkers (1991) administered a stressful arithmetic task to 30 CHD patients undergoing cardiac catheterization, with a subgroup of patients receiving intracoronary infusion of acetylcholine. As expected, smooth coronary artery segments dilated. In atherosclerotic (stenosed) artery segments, however, there was paradoxical constriction with both mental stress and acetylcholine. These results suggest that abnormal vasomotor response, probably related to endothelial dysfunction, may be an important determinant of emotionally induced ischemia.

Myocardial Ischemia

In general terms, myocardial ischemia occurs whenever myocardial oxygen demand exceeds available supply. A common cause of transient increased myocardial oxygen demands is physical exercise, and many ischemic episodes are classically triggered by exertion. However, psychological stress can also raise myocardial oxygen needs. The three major determinants of such needs—heart rate, blood pressure, and contractility—all increase with stimulation of the sympathetic nervous system, an almost universal response of the body to internal or external stress. What is less certain, but increasingly likely, is that myocardial oxygen supply might also be affected by internal or external stress.

Impressive findings linking emotional stress with ischemia have been reported (Rozanski 1988) among CHD patients and controls subjected to a series of mental and physical tasks: arithmetic, reading, Stroop color word test (in which a subject reads the name of a color from a card of a different color) and "simulated public speaking," a 5-minute talk to two observers in white laboratory coats about one's own "personal faults and undesirable habits." Quite dramatically, the magnitude of ischemic cardiac dysfunction (measured by radionuclide ventriculography) induced by the stressful "simulated public speaking" task was similar to that observed during bicycle exercise. During periods of mental stress, 59% of patients had wall motion abnormalities and 36% had a fall in left ventricular ejection fraction of more than 5%. Psychologically induced ischemia was silent in 83% of patients with wall motion abnormalities and occurred at lower heart rates than exercise-induced ischemia, suggesting that mental stress may cause ischemia by decreasing myocardial oxygen supply, presumably via coronary artery vasoconstriction.

These results suggest a causal association between mental stress and myocardial ischemia, which is often silent, in CHD patients. Rozanski and associates (1988) concluded that, since mental stress occurs more frequently than the stress of exercise in daily life, it may represent an important factor in the precipitation of clinical coronary events.

Acute Psychological "Triggers" for MI

Another area of recent scientific scrutiny raises the hypothesis that acute emotional arousal may serve as a "trigger" for MI. Dobson et al. (1991) reported an unusually high incidence of fatal MI and coronary death (RR = 1.67; 95% CI: 0.72–3.17) in the four-day period following the Newcastle, Australia earthquake, measuring 5.6 on the Richter scale, in 1989. Similarly, Meisel et al. (1991) noted a sharp increase in the incidence of acute MI and sudden coronary death (SCD) during the first week of the Iraqi SCUD missile attacks on Tel Aviv, Israel, compared with five peaceful control periods. Interestingly, coronary event rates returned to normal levels after the first week despite continued attacks, suggesting that cardiac function is remarkably resilient for the vast majority of the population.

Tofler et al. (1990) reported on 849 patients who were asked to identify possible behavioral and psychological "triggers" for their acute MI. Triggers were identified by nearly half the patients, the most common being emotional upset and moderate physical activity. Similarly, Willich and the TRIMM Study Group (1991) reported that 52% of 224 consecutive acute MI patients reported stress or emotional upset prior to hospital admission. In an ongoing study in which 129 controls were matched to MI cases by neighborhood, age, gender, time of day, and day of the week for the case MI (Jacobs 1992), a 9.5 times increased risk of MI was associated with at least one self-rated "extremely meaningful and desirable or undesirable event" (95% CI: 4.1– 22.03; $p = .001$) within the preceding 26 hours.

Sudden Cardiac Death

Through the centuries there has been a fascination with dramatic life events that seem to trigger sudden cardiac death (SCD). In his classic paper, "Voodoo Death," Cannon (1942, 1957) noted that Soares de Souza was, in 1587, the first to report instances of death apparently induced by fright among South American Indians condemned by a "medicine man." Similar observations have been reported by anthropologists in Africa, Australia, Haiti, and the islands of the Pacific.

In the popular mind, sudden death is associated with both intense fear ("scared to death") and anger. One extraordinary example of the latter is the eighteenth century English surgeon John Hunter, who predicted his own apparently anger-induced demise (Home 1794; Adams 1817).

A substantial literature on psychological stress and cardiac arrhythmia ranges from anecdotal cases where stressors as minor as a ringing alarm clock resulted in immediate life-threatening ventricular arrhythmia (Lown 1976) to well-designed studies in dogs where aversive conditioning and/or noxious stimuli decreased the threshold for ventricular fibrillation and had other effects that would likely promote the occurrence of ventricular arrhythmia (Verrier 1987). Although it is presumed that increased sympathetic activity is the physiologic link between stress and ventricular arrhythmia, there are other possibilities, and this subject needs further exploration, given the continuing enormous toll from SCD in Western countries. Furthermore, although serious ventricular arrhythmia is usually considered the *result* of acute myocardial ischemia or infarction, it is possible that in some cases ventricular arrhythmia, with attendant systemic hypotension, decreased coronary perfusion, and major tachycardia increasing myocardial oxygen needs, is actually the *cause* of acute MI.

Although there are several studies that suggest a high incidence of acute or chronic stress before SCD, the results are unconvincing; many such associations may simply be recall bias, where those close to the deceased selectively remember presumably stressful incidents. The alternate point of view, that SCD is a chance event unrelated to psychological stress, has been advanced by Surawicz (1985) and others. SCD is the rare exception even in very stressful conditions, such as soldiers marching into battle and panic situations affecting large groups. Reviewing the data from the Framingham Heart Study, Kannel and Schatzkin (1985) conclude that there are no specific risk factors for SCD independent of those for CHD.

Conclusion

The studies cited above represent a sample of the research on psychological stress and CHD. The "stress" in each of these studies is quite different, including such diverse phenomena as "life changes," scores on an "intuitively created" questionnaire, experimentally manipulated social disruption of monkey colonies, catastrophic events such as an earthquake and war, and a variety of laboratory stressors, including mental arithmetic and simulated public speaking. While each of these variables provides an interesting perspective on some aspect of stress and cardiac function, it is critical to note that the general term "psychological stress" conveys only limited information. The many parameters affected by stress make it difficult to pinpoint pathways that might exert deleterious effects, and it is by no means conclusively proven that psychological stress increases rates of death or other "hard" cardiovascular endpoints in humans.

The Type A Behavior Pattern

In 1897, Sir William Osler was perhaps the first to link a twentieth-century lifestyle with atherosclerosis: ". . . in the worry and strain of modern life, arterial degeneration is not only very common but develops at a relatively early age. For this I believe that the high pressure at which men live and the habit of working the machine to its maximum are responsible. . . ." (Osler 1897). Systematic investigation of the heart and mind connection began in the late 1950s with the pioneering work of Meyer Friedman and Ray Rosenman, two San Francisco cardiologists who originated the concept of the Type A behavior pattern (TABP), now a household term.

The TABP is a complex syndrome. The scientist who is concerned with easily quantifiable, "hard" data is often uncomfortable with this clinically derived diagnosis. Nonetheless, the definition of the TABP is quite specific. As originally formulated by Friedman and Rosenman (1974):

> Type A behavior pattern is an action-emotion complex that can be observed in any person who is aggressively involved in a chronic, incessant struggle to achieve more and more in less and less time, and if required to do so, against the opposing efforts of other things or other persons. It is not psychosis or a complex of worries or fears or phobias or obsessions, but a socially acceptable—indeed often praised—form of conflict. Persons possessing this pattern also are quite prone to exhibit a free-floating but extraordinarily well-rationalized hostility. As might be expected, there are degrees in the intensity of this behavior pattern. . . . For Type A behavior pattern to explode into being, the environmental challenge must always serve as the fuse for this explosion.

Ten years later, Friedman and Ulmer (1984) offered a more psychodynamic formulation of the TABP that is presented in Figure 11.1. A list of the common clinical attributes of the TABP is given in Table 11.2. In the new model, insecurity and inadequate self-esteem form the nucleus of the TABP. The "struggle to achieve more and more in less and less time," from the earlier definition, is thought to be propelled by an unconscious drive for self-esteem. Hence the individual becomes overly identified with personal achievements in a symbolic and unattainable search for self-worth. Typically, the symptoms of time-urgency and free-floating hostility arise out of any perceived interference with self-defining achievements. Positive self-esteem and a

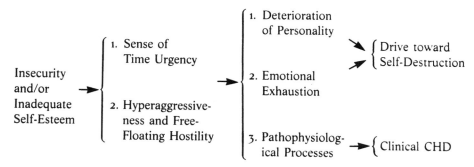

Fig. 11.1. See text.

Table 11.2. Clinical Characteristics of Type A Behavior as Noted on the Videotaped Clinical Examination

Time Pressure Items	Hostility Items
Content	
Spouse says "slow down"	Irritable waiting:
Walks, eats fast, no dawdling	restaurant, traffic, bank
Polyphasic; TV, conversation	
Fetish of being on time	
Difficulty doing nothing	
Substitutes numerals for metaphors	
Behavior, Motor	
Facial tautness expressing tension	Hostile facial set
Tense posture, i.e., clenched fist	Overforceful gestures; fast and jerky
	movements
Motorizations/gestures accompanying responses;	Ticlike drawing back of lips
repetitive hand, arm, leg movements	
Ticlike eyebrow lifting	
Rapid eye blinking	
Expiratory sighing	
Tongue to teeth clicking	
Head nodding	
Behavior, Speech	
Speech hurrying, head nodding when listening	Hostile, jarring laugh
Rapid speech/dysrhythmic, elision of final words	Interrupts interviewer
Sucking in air during speech	loud, explosive, staccato voice
Behavior, Hostile/Competitive Attitudes	
Interviewer challenge: hostile response	Angry generalizations: race, women, doctors
General distrust of others' motives	Competition with children
Exhibits anger at past events	
Physiologic Indicators	
Periorbital pigmentation	
Excessive forehead, upper lip perspiration	

sense of personal security, however, can never be attained solely by accomplishments. Many, in fact, suggest that self-worth is more strongly related to interpersonal connectedness and ''feeling loved'' than with worldly success. Thus, achievement leaves a person unfulfilled when motivated by an unconscious, symbolic quest for self-esteem. For such Type A individuals, frustration often leads to a new round of pursuits that are ''bigger and better.'' Ultimately, time urgency, hyperaggressiveness, and free-floating hostility become pervasive, with a deterioration of personality and physical exhaustion. It is hypothesized that, over the course of several decades, the pathophysiologic processes accompanying the chronic struggle accelerate atherogenesis and lead to premature CHD.

Several questionnaires have been developed for diagnosis of the TABP. The Jenkins Activity Survey (JAS) has been used most extensively, but does not tap into the hostility component. The Framingham Type A scale has been used successfully for the prediction of CHD in the long-running study of the same name (Haynes 1978, 1982) and the Bortner scale has been used often in Europe (Bortner 1989). However, clinical diagnosis of the TABP has been most successful with a videotaped structured interview, now called the videotaped clinical examination (VCE). Detailed instructions for administration and scoring of the VCE were first provided by Friedman and Powell (1984). An updated version that emphasizes the nonverbal, physical signs of the TABP was published by Friedman and Ghandour (1993) and a subscale for insecurity, the presumed nucleus of the TABP, was recently presented by Price et al. (1995). Scores on the VCE are obtained not only from the content responses to a series of questions, but also from the manner in which an individual responds. Motorizations (unconscious movements), facial expressions, and bodily tensions are all scored manifestations. In addition to a global score for the TABP, there are subscales for hostility and time pressure.

The VCE and questionnaires appear to measure different aspects of the TABP. Many of the manifestations of the TABP are beyond the individual's awareness, and thus unlikely to be self-reported.

Evidence Linking the TABP with CHD Risk

A number of studies that have attempted to relate the TABP to CHD are summarized in Table 11.3. The Western Collaborative Group study was the first large-scale prospective investigation (Rosenman 1975), with men classified Type A demonstrating approximately twice the incidence of CHD as those rated Type B (Type B behavior has generally been defined as the absence of the TABP). Similar results were found for both men and women in the Framingham Heart Study in the 1980s (Haynes 1982). The most recent Framingham data, however, report a Type A association only with angina pectoris and not with the harder endpoints of MI or fatal coronary events (Eaker 1989). In one recent study (Williams 1988), the TAB-CHD link was strongest in the youngest (under age 45) of a group of 2,289 patients undergoing coronary arteriography. Several studies, including the Multicenter Post-Infarction Research Program (Case 1985), Aspirin Myocardial Infarction Study (Shekelle 1985a), and the Multiple Risk Factor Intervention Trial (MRFIT) (Shekelle 1985b), all found no relationship between the TABP and CHD in high-risk populations.

Table 11.3. Type A Behavior and Prediction of Coronary Heart Disease: Large-Scale Prospective Clinical Trials

Study	N	Types of Subjects	Follow-up (years)	CHD Incidence Risk Ratio, A:B	Comment
(WCGS, Rosenman et al. 1975)	3,154	Employed California men, aged 35–59	8.5	2.24	
Primary (no prior CHD)					
Framingham (Haynes & Feinleib 1982)	1,330	Subgroup at 8th or 9th biennial exam free of CHD, aged 45–64	10	2.4 men 2.0 women	Angina pectoris only
Framingham (Eaker et al. 1989)	1,289	570 men, 719 women	2	2.2 men 2.6 women	
MRFIT (Shekelle et al. 1985b)	3,110	Subgroup of 12,866 men, age 35–57, in top 10–15% of CHD risk by blood pressure, serum cholesterol	7.1	No relationship between TAB and CHD endpoints using either JAS or SI	
Secondary (in those with diagnosed CHD)					
Multicenter Postinfarct Group (Case et al. 1985)	516	Subgroup of 866 pts within 2 weeks of acute MI	1–3	No difference in mean Type A score of survivors vs deaths	
Aspirin MI Study (Shekelle et al. 1985a)	2,314	Subgroup of 2,698 pts given aspirin for prevention of recurrent CHD 30 days–5 years post-MI	3	No difference in mean Type A score of those with and without coronary events	
WCGS (Ragland & Brand 1988)	231	231 of 257 WCGS subjects who developed angina, silent or symptomatic MI and survived 24 hours	12	Type As had better (RR = 0.58) survival compared with Type Bs	
Duke Univ Med Ctr (Barefoot et al. 1989)	1,478	SI assessment of pts hospitalized for cardiac cath	4–10	Type As with poor left ventricular function had better survival than Type Bs	
CAPS (Ahern et al. 1990)	353	Post-MI pts with arrhythmia assessed with Bortner Type A scale	1	Type As had .70 risk of cardiac death compared to Type Bs for 1 standard deviation in scale score	

CHD, coronary heart disease; MI, myocardial infarction; SI, structured interview; TAB, Type A behavior; JAS, Jenkins Activity Survey; SI, Structured Interview; WCGS, Western Collaborative Group Study; MRFIT, Multiple Risk Factor Intervention Trial; CAPS, Cardiac Arrhythmias Pilot Study.

In a follow-up to the Western Collaborative Group study, Ragland and Brand (1988) showed that individuals diagnosed Type A in 1960, who developed CHD had only 58% of the mortality of those diagnosed Type B over the ensuing 23 years. Rather than a risk factor, Ragland and Brand suggested that the TABP may even be "protective" for subsequent cardiac mortality for those with CHD. Similar results were obtained by Barefoot et al. (1989) in a prospective study of 1,467 symptomatic patients with poor left ventricular function undergoing coronary angiography. Ahern et al. (1990) reported increased cardiac arrest and death among Type Bs, assessed by the Bortner questionnaire, in 353 post-MI patients enrolled in the Cardiac Arrhythmia Pilot Study.

A metanalysis of 83 studies of the TABP and CHD (Booth-Kewley 1987) concluded:

1. The TABP does appear to be a risk factor for CHD, approximately doubling risk.
2. Anger, hostility, and depression also appear to be related to CHD.
3. Structured interviews are more effective for predicting disease endpoints than questionnaires.
4. Cross-sectional studies have been more powerful predictors than prospective studies.
5. The TABP effect has been smaller in studies published more recently than in those done in the early days of the hypothesis.

The inconsistent results of studies attempting to relate the TABP to CHD may be due to a number of factors:

1. Difficulties in diagnostic methodologies: In particular, questionnaires appear less powerful than structured interviews in diagnosing a presumed "virulent core" of the TABP.
2. Diagnostic tools are more effective among general populations than in those at high risk for CHD. Pickering (1985) and Miller et al. (1991) have argued that high-risk populations present an unfavorable environment for discovering a potential relationship between the TABP and CHD for a number of important reasons. First, standard cardiologic risk factors, such as hypertension or serum cholesterol, do not correlate well with angiographic extent of disease in many studies of CHD patients, so that there is no reason to expect the TABP to do so. In addition, groups with CHD may be atypical compared to the general population; current instruments for diagnosis of the TABP are insufficiently sensitive to differentiate among what may be similar personality styles; and beta-blockers, widely used among CHD patients, may blunt the TABP and confound accurate diagnosis.
3. The TABP may have a different effect among those with and without pre-existing CHD (secondary vs primary prevention).
4. Subsets of characteristics of the TABP may not be equally important. As Williams and Barefoot have hypothesized, it may be that hostility is more, and time-pressured behavior less, important as risk factors, and reliance on overall TABP scores may obscure relationships within one subset.

Methodological issues in assessment and treatment of the TABP are complex. Thoresen and Powell (1992) provide the most up-to-date review, with important suggestions for the design of future research and treatment protocols.

Anger

The word "anger" is derived from the Old Norse *angr*, signifying grief, circa 1,000 A.D. The earliest meanings in English were trouble, affliction, vexation, and sorrow. The current Oxford English Dictionary definition, "extreme or passionate displeasure or wrath," was developed in the fourteenth century. Smith (1992) provides a recent and thorough review of the growing literature on anger and disease.

Anger has long been noted as a behavioral precipitant for angina pectoris, and a striking demonstration of the relationship was recently provided by Ironson and co-workers (1992). Subjects were asked to recall an incident that occurred in the past 6 months that still made them "frustrated, angry, irritated or upset." They were also administered a stressful speech task (defending oneself against an accusation of shoplifting), mental arithmetic, and symptom-limited exercise using a bicycle ergometer. Radionuclide ventriculograms showed that, of all conditions, anger recall elicited the greatest impairment (presumably ischemic) in ventricular function, with 7 of 18 CHD patients showing a drop in ejection fraction $\geq 7\%$ (only 4 of the 18 patients had reduction of ejection fraction $\geq 7\%$ during symptom-limited exercise). Most participants felt their reexperienced anger was one-third to one-half as intense as the original experience.

There is a considerable literature on the epidemiology of anger and hostility in the development of CHD. After the initially promising reports of Friedman and Rosenman and others, several studies in the early 1980s failed to demonstrate a relationship between the TABP and CHD. Some investigators searched for a presumed "pathologic core" of the TABP. Williams (1987) coined the term *hostility complex* to describe a coronary-prone behavior pattern thought to be more strongly related to CHD than the global TABP. The hostility complex is marked by a cynical, untrusting, and pessimistic orientation to interpersonal interaction and life in general. The pattern is operationally defined by high scores on the Cook Medley Hostility (Ho) scale of the Minnesota Multiphasic Personality Inventory (MMPI). One should note that the Ho scale was devised to differentiate between school teachers who maintained positive vs negative rapport with students and not to measure hostility, cynicism, or pessimism.

Table 11.4 summarizes the major studies on the relationship between Ho scores and CHD. The results have been inconsistent since the first reported link with degree of atherosclerosis among patients undergoing cardiac catheterization (Williams 1980). Subsequently, the Ho scale predicted CHD- and all-cause mortality in a 25-year study of physicians (Barefoot 1984), although an attempted replication by McCranie and colleagues (1986) failed to support such an association. Among a group of initially healthy Western Electric employees, low Ho scores were associated with the lowest 10-year CHD incidence, and follow-up after 20 years showed Ho scores to be related to subsequent CHD and all-cause mortality (Shekelle 1983). Similar results were found after 28 years of follow-up of a group of law students (Barefoot 1989a). In contrast,

Table 11.4. Relationships between the MMPI Cook-Medley (Ho) Scale and Coronary Heart Disease

Study	N	Description	Results
Williams et al. (1990)	424	CHD patients awaiting cardiac catheterization	Ho score related to degree of atherosclerosis; >70% rate significant CAD with Ho > 10
Barefoot et al. (1984)	255	25-yr follow-up of MDs who completed MMPI in medical school	Ho score predictive of both CHD and all-cause mortality
Shekelle et al. (1983)	1877	Healthy employed men (Western Electric)	Low Ho score (<10) associated with low CHD event rate; highest CHD incidence in middle Ho quintile; Ho score related to 20-year overall mortality
McCranie et al. (1986)	478	MDs who completed MMPI at medical school admission interview	No relation between Ho score and CHD incidence or mortality; may indicate reluctance to admit hostility at time of evaluation for admission
Leon et al. (1988)	280	30-year follow-up of businessmen, mean age 45 at entry	No relation between Ho score and CHD
Hearn et al. (1989)	1399	35-year follow-up of University of Minnesota students who completed MMPI during freshman orientation	No relation between Ho scores and CHD morbidity or mortality
Helmer et al. (1991)	158	CHD patients awaiting cardiac catheterization	No relationship between Ho score and coronary occlusion
Barefoot et al. (1989)	118	Refinement of Cook-Medley Ho scale into 6 subscales; 28-yr follow-up of law students	Total Ho scores associated with mortality; sum 3 subscales (cynicism, hostile affect, aggressive responding) better predicted mortality than full Ho scale
Maruta et al. (1993)	620 (of 1,145) consecutive gen'l med pts		No relationship between Ho score and CHD after controlling for age and gender

MMPI, Minnesota Multiphasic Personality Inventory.

a number of other studies (Leon 1988; Hearn 1989; Helmer 1991; Maruta 1993) all failed to find a link between Ho scores and CHD morbidity or mortality.

It is possible that the inconsistency of these findings may be due to problems such as losses to follow-up or the circumstances under which some questionnaire data were obtained. Barefoot (1992) has identified self-presentation bias as, perhaps, the major limitation of questionnaires attempting to assess hostility. Many individuals are loathe to admit excessive hostility because it is socially undesirable. Another important bias is that questionnaires only access conscious awareness. Many people—perhaps some of the most hostile—are unaware of the extent of their hostility. The environment in which a questionnaire is administered may also have a profound effect (Smith 1993). For example, the medical school applicants in the McCranie study (1986) and job applicants in the Barefoot study (1992) had low Ho scores; in both situations it would seem prudent for subjects to suppress or conceal hostility. In addition, researchers have suggested that a composite hostility score derived from three Cook Medley subscales, "cynicism," "hostile affect," and "aggressive responding," was a better predictor of survival in a group of 118 lawyers than total Ho score (Barefoot 1989a). However, the limitations mentioned previously remained inherent in such an instrument.

Efforts have been made to overcome these limitations by using structured interviews to assess hostility (Table 11.5). Two studies (Dembrowski 1985; MacDougall 1985) scored such interviews using "potential for hostility" (the tendency to become angered during daily activities) and "anger-in" (the inability or unwillingness to express anger) as possible criteria for coronary-prone hostility. Both variables showed predictive ability, suggesting that the amount of hostility in a person's life (e.g., the frequency, intensity, and duration) rather than the extent to which it is expressed, may be most strongly related to CHD.

Two other analyses reexamined structured interview data from large-scale studies of coronary-prone behavior. In MRFIT, 192 subjects showing "potential for hostility" and an "antagonistic interactional style" had 1.5 to 1.7 times the incidence of CHD compared with 384 matched controls (Dembroski 1989). For patients under age 47, interview ratings of hostility more than doubled CHD risk. In a multivariate analysis of 250 CHD cases and 500 matched controls from the Western Collaborative Group Study (Hecker 1988), hostility scored from structured interviews was the single strongest predictor of CHD incidence.

Swan and coworkers (1989) attempted to explain the confusion surrounding the assessment of hostility by comparing scores on the Ho scale with hostility assessed from structured interviews among middle-aged male participants from the National Heart, Lung and Blood Institute Twin Study. Ho ratings differed considerably from those obtained with interviews, demonstrating that hostility assessments derived from interviews and questionnaires share only a limited relationship.

In summary, while some experimental studies reveal dramatic links between anger and short-term effects on cardiac function, epidemiologic studies present a clouded picture, possibly due to the absence of a standardized assessment methodology. Thus, after several decades of intensive investigation, anger or hostility as the presumed "virulent core" of a coronary-prone behavior pattern has not been conclusively validated.

Table 11.5. Structured Interview (SI) Assessment of Hostility and CHD

Study	N	Description	Results
Dembroski et al. (1985)	131	Pts with no or severe CAD at cardiac cath; scoring of SI into speech stylistics, Type A content, hostility, and anger-in	"Potential for hostility" and "anger-in" related to angiographic severity of CAD (see text for definitions)
MacDougall et al. (1985)	125	125 cath pts; retrospective reanalysis of SI tapes from Dimsdale (1979) in which no association had been found between TAB and angiographic	"Potential for hostility" and "anger-in" related to angiographic CAD severity
Dembroski et al. (1989)	192 CHD 384 controls	Reanalysis of interviews from MRFIT, average 7.1-yr follow-up	"Potential for hostility" showed significant relation to CHD; Risk stronger under age 47
Hecker et al. (1988)	250 CHD 500 controls	Reanalysis of SIs from Western Collaborative Group Study, 8.5-yr follow-up	Hostility significantly related to CHD

Vital Exhaustion

Another area of recent interest is the notion of "vital exhaustion" developed in the Netherlands by Appels (1990). According to this hypothesis, a debilitated physical and emotional state may be a precursor of MI. Characteristics that demonstrated a relationship with CHD are described by items of the Maastricht Questionnaire (MQ), developed to assess vital exhaustion. Items on the MQ that were predictive of MI include being tired often, feeling weak, lessened sexual interest, feeling hopeless, and being easily irritated.

Thus far, the vital exhaustion hypothesis has been tested in one prospective study of 3,877 city employees in Rotterdam (Appels 1989). The MQ demonstrated an age-adjusted relative risk of 2.28 for MI over 4.2 years. A subsequent analysis (Appels 1991) revealed that frequently "waking up exhausted" conferred a significant independent additional risk beyond vital exhaustion. Of all the items on the MQ, a positive response to "Do you want to be dead at times?" demonstrated the strongest association with age-adjusted relative risk of MI over four years. Clearly, there is significant overlap between vital exhaustion and chronic psychological stress, the cynicism described by the Ho Scale, and the TABP.

Social Support

Social support, or the degree with which one individual is connected to others, has recently emerged as a risk factor of considerable magnitude, not only for CHD but for morbidity and mortality from all causes. Of all psychosocial factors, social support appears the most consistently positive in the search for a relationship between mind and heart. Early work in the field was focused on higher death rate of widows and widowers compared with the general population (Parkes 1964; Rees 1984). The interested reader is referred to Broadhead et al. (1983) for a review of the early literature. In a recent analysis of five large-scale prospective studies in over 37,000 people on the impact of social relationships and health, House et al. (1988) claim that social support is a variable of major significance, rivaling cigarette smoking in importance as a risk factor for CHD (Figure 11.2).

Studies of social support have relied on questionnaires or brief interviews about the nature and frequency of interpersonal contacts. Efforts are now underway to explore the nature of social support to better understand the underlying mechanisms that may promote health or disease. One study examined the differences between the structure and function of relationships in patients undergoing coronary angiography (Seeman 1987). Structural aspects include the number of relationships and frequency of social contacts while functional aspects refer to the quality of relationships. Results of this study suggest that functional aspects of relationships and feelings of "being loved" appear protective for CHD.

Most recently, for six years, Orth-Gomer et al. (1993) followed 736 men, all 50 years old, all born in Gothenberg, Sweden. Lack of emotional support from very close persons ("attachment") and lack of an extended network of people ("social integra-

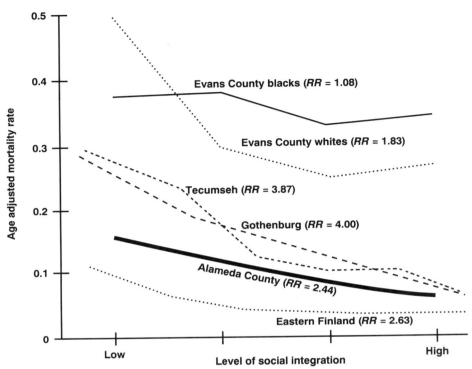

Fig. 11.2. Level of social integration and age-adjusted mortality for males in five prospective studies. RR is the relative risk ratio for mortality at the lowest vs highest level of social integration. Evans County, Georgia; Tecumseh, Michigan; Alameda County, California; Gothenburg, Sweden. [From House et al. (1988), with permission.]

tion'') were significant risk factors in multiple logistic regression analysis as predictors of CHD events (MI or CHD mortality), after controlling for traditional risk factors.

Three large-scale prospective studies have looked at the effects of social isolation on survival after a diagnosis of CHD. Ruberman et al. (1984) were the first to assess social connectedness in a post-MI population. Interviews with 2,315 male survivors in the Beta-Blocker Heart Attack Trial showed that those with both high levels of social isolation and a high degree of life stress had a more than fourfold increased risk of death over the three years following MI. Case et al. (1992) studied living alone and marital disruption in a group of 1,234 patients admitted to coronary care facilities with documented MI. After six months, the recurrent event rate for nonfatal MI or cardiac death was 15.8% for patients living alone vs. 8.8% for those living with a partner. Interestingly, marital disruption (divorce, separation, or widowhood) was not a significant independent risk factor for morbid events. Williams et al. (1992) studied a consecutive sample of 1,368 patients undergoing cardiac catheterization and discovered that unmarried patients without a confidant had a 3.34 increased risk of death within five years compared to patients who were married or had a close friend in whom they confided. A smaller, well-designed study prospectively followed 100 men and 94 women, 65 years of age or older, for six months after hospitalization for acute MI and found lack of emotional support associated with significantly increased mortality (odds ratio: 2.9; 95% CI: 1.2–6.9) (Berkman 1992). These last three studies all examined psychosocial support after controlling for a number of important demographic and physiologic variables, including left ventricular function.

Although the mechanism is poorly understood, social support appears to confer powerful protection against morbid events after a diagnosis of CHD. In an editorial, Ruberman (1992) urges adopting practices that provide social support for isolated cardiac patients, asserting, "for physicians, it is a comforting notion that applying principles to clinical practice that improve the quality of life may yet be shown to extend the length of life as well."

In an attempt to integrate the theory of Type A behavior with social support, Blumenthal et al. (1987) studied the interaction of these two effects on 113 patients undergoing coronary angiography. For Type As, the extent of atherosclerosis was inversely related to perceived social support; that is, Type As with high levels of support had the least atherosclerosis. There was no such relationship for Type Bs. Blumenthal et al. (1987) suggest that results are consistent with the hypothesis that social support moderates the long-term consequences of the TABP. Similarly, Orth-Gomer and Uniden (1990) discovered that lack of social support/social isolation was an independent predictor of mortality over ten years in Type A but not Type B men with CHD.

As with other psychosocial variables, there is an almost total lack of hard data on the mechanism(s) by which social support is linked to decreased cardiac disease. Attractive possibilities include better control of coronary risk factors and/or earlier responses to premonitory symptomatology because of the influences of family or friends. However, the strength of the protective effect, and the often-noted major beneficial influence of social support on noncardiac mortality, suggests that investigations into broader physiologic correlates, possibly autonomic or immunologic, might be fruitful in better understanding this widely acknowledged, apparently protective factor.

Job Strain

Job strain occurs "when individuals have insufficient control over their work situation to be able to satisfactorily deal with the level of demands being placed on them" (Karasek 1988). Job strain is the product of high job demands combined with low decision latitude. For example, firemen, cashiers, and freight handlers have high demands but little variability in decisions and thus, high job strain. Physicians, lawyers, and executives have high demands but also high levels of latitude in decision-making, putatively conferring lower job strain. For assessment, Karasek (1988) has developed both a questionnaire and an "estimation method," which imputes job strain to a number of census-defined occupations. A six-year prospective study of 1,928 Swedish men (Karasek 1981) demonstrated an increased risk of CHD symptoms with a "hectic and psychologically demanding job" and a relative risk of CHD-cardiovascular death of 4. An increased prevalence rate for MI of 2.48 and 3.28, respectively, for two U.S.

populations of 2,409 and 2,424 employed males was found using the imputation method (Karasek 1988). In subsequent research using ambulatory blood pressure monitoring (Schnall 1990), job strain was related to workplace diastolic blood pressure and left ventricular mass. Pieper et al. (1989) published a meta-analysis of five U.S. studies involving 12,555 men, showing that low job decision latitude was related to systolic blood pressure and cigarette smoking, two important risk factors for CHD.

Schnall et al. (1994) provide a recent, thorough review of the job strain literature. According to their findings, 37 studies were published between 1981 and 1993, most of which found a significant correlation between job strain and cardiovascular or all-cause mortality or job strain and risk factors for cardiovascular disease. Thus far, 11 of 13 published studies have found a positive relationship between job strain and cardiovascular disease endpoints. To date, no intervention studies have been attempted.

Cardiac Denial

Denial is a basic psychological defense mechanism that allows people to engage in behavior with little conscious awareness of the consequences. Sometimes, denial is sufficiently powerful to allow negative behavior in spite of some level of awareness, as, for example, in CHD patients who continue to smoke cigarettes. *Cardiac denial* has long been a commonplace expression in clinical cardiology. Because denial of a possible cardiac event may lead to delay in seeking medical care, the implications are profound. With the widespread availability of thrombolysis, the individual who delays seeking treatment risks increased myocardial damage, morbidity, and mortality. The catch phrase ''time is muscle'' captures the essence of this issue. Since approximately 60% of out-of-hospital cardiac deaths occur within two hours of symptoms (Albarran-Sotelo 1988), overcoming the emotional resistance of cardiac denial may lead to reduced morbidity and mortality. In a finding with important clinical implications for secondary prevention, Herlitz et al. (1989) note that, in several studies, previous cardiac history did not result in reduced delay time.

A recent review by Sirous (1992) traced 21 studies on denial in CHD published during the past 25 years and concludes that denial has a long-term negative effect on health outcome. Because of the profound potential benefits of overcoming denial and delay in the era of thrombolytic therapy, this is a subject that deserves the clinician's attention and future research.

Depression

Depression is a frequent precursor of CHD and often accompanies recovery. One meta-analysis (Booth-Kewley 1987) found that depression, more than any other psychological attribute, had the strongest association with CHD. Fielding (1991) provides a recent review of this expanding literature. Writing from a psychiatric perspective, Fernandez (1993) notes that depression is one of the best predictors of recurrent cardiovascular complications as well as poor adherence to lifestyle change after a cardiac event. He suggests that depression is typically underdiagnosed and untreated in the

18% to 44% of cardiac patients whose depression is severe enough to warrant psychiatric intervention.

Most recently, Frasure-Smith et al. (1993) prospectively evaluated the impact of depression on 222 post-MI patients who were discharged from a large university hospital in Montreal, Quebec. Depression was assessed by a modified version of the National Institute of Mental Health Diagnostic Interview Schedule while patients were in the hospital. Major depression was diagnosed in 35 patients (16%). Depression was a significant predictor of mortality, after controlling for previous MI and left ventricular dysfunction (adjusted hazard ratio: 4.29; 95% CI: 3.14–5.44; p = .013), in the first prospective study to demonstrate an association between depression and cardiovascular mortality. In a study at two New York City medical centers, Schleifer et al. (1989) reported that 18% of 283 patients had major and 27% had minor depressive disorder eight to ten days post-MI. At three to four months later, 33% met criteria for major or minor depression. The interested reader is referred to the citations by Fielding and Fernandez for expanded reviews of this literature.

Behavioral Influences on Standard Risk Factors for Coronary Heart Disease

Regardless of one's views on the importance of psychosocial risk factors for CHD, there seems little question that behavioral factors play a major role in the prevalence and severity of the "standard" and well-accepted risk factors in the general population. Figure 11.3 presents our view of the risk factors associated with CHD described with respect to lifestyle. Clearly, cigarette smoking and dietary intake of cholesterol-rich and high saturated fat or high calorie foods are life choices. Hypertension has a lifestyle component for those who are salt-sensitive and/or overweight and inactive. Sedentary lifestyle is also a matter of choice. Thus, each of the "standard" risk factors has a behavioral component. Type A behavior, psychological stress, social support, and weight are also often matters of how we choose to live. Behavior modification, probably responsible for much of the past generation's decline in CHD in this country, still represents a major frontier in preventive cardiology.

Clinical Trials Utilizing Lifestyle Interventions

There have been a number of trials that have attempted to modify CHD with psychological treatment; the total number of subjects has been small, the interventions and outcome measures diverse, and the use of multiple interventions has left us without a clear picture of which factors are most important.

The Lifestyle Intervention Trial (Ornish 1993) has received much recent publicity. In this study, 48 CHD patients were randomized to either a lifestyle intervention program or routine medical care. The program became a major focus in participants' lives: twice-weekly group sessions included exercise, stress management, yoga and meditation, a communal meal, and group therapy. A spouse or significant other was encouraged to attend these 3.5-hour evening meetings. Patients ate a strictly vegetarian diet, much of which was provided by the researchers, with only 6.8% of calories derived from fat. The program required daily meditation for one hour and included visualization exercises of "cleansing" the coronary arteries. Patients underwent coronary arteriograms before entering the program and again after one and four years, with coronary artery lesions analyzed by quantitative angiography. After four years, average stenosis diameter decreased from 43.6% to 39.7% in experimental patients but progressed from 41.6% to 51.4% in the control group. After one year, 82% of experimental subjects showed regression in atherosclerotic lesions, compared to only 42% of controls (Ornish 1990). Patients in the experimental group reported dramatic reductions in frequency, duration, and severity of angina compared to increased symptoms in the control group. Regression of lesions was associated with overall adherence to the program in a dose-response relationship, although none of the individual components demonstrated such a relationship.

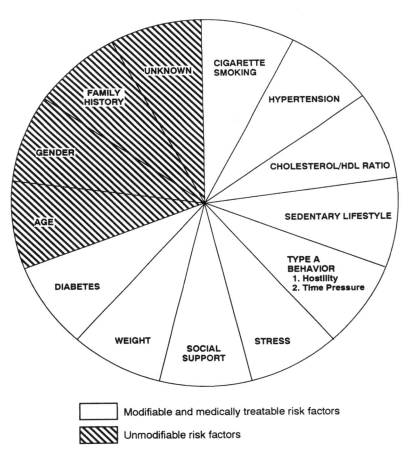

Fig. 11.3. Schematic representation of risk factors for coronary artery disease.

A major criticism of this study is the small number of subjects: 28 patients in the experimental and 20 in the control group. The four-year angiographic results are so far available only in abstract form, and the paper describing the one-year clinical and angiographic findings is quite brief. It is by no means clear that the population at large can be persuaded to adopt a lifestyle so out of keeping with current norms. Nevertheless, Ornish provides a vision of optimal behavior change as one possible direction for the management of CHD.

Schuler et al. (1992) found regression of coronary artery disease with more modest lifestyle change in a group of patients with stable angina pectoris "with no more than average motivation and discipline." A total of 18 patients participated in a treatment program that included a low fat (<20% of calories), low cholesterol (<200 mg/day) diet, and at least three hours of exercise per week. Patients and their spouses participated in four group discussions during the year and opportunities were provided to talk about personal problems after exercise sessions. In this study 18 control subjects received identical instruction about diet and exercise along with the "usual care" of their physicians. At the end of one year, 105 stenoses evaluated by digital angiography revealed significant regression of atherosclerotic lesions in 7 of 18 patients in the treatment group with no change or progression of disease in 11 patients. Regression was detected in only 1 of the 12 patients receiving usual care. Myocardial perfusion during maximal exercise also improved in the treatment group compared with controls and the improvement was independent of regression. The treatment protocol did not require the intense time commitment or much of the psychosocial component provided in Ornish's work, suggesting that regression of coronary lesions may be possible with less radical lifestyle change that should prove more accessible to the general CHD population.

The Recurrent Coronary Prevention Project (RCPP) (Friedman 1986) was the largest behavior modification program for secondary prevention of CHD. This study demonstrated a 44% reduction in recurrent MI for 1,012 patients who received 4.5 years of group counseling for the TABP and cardiac risk factors compared to controls who received counseling about only "standard" risk factors (Figure 11.4). The control group was subsequently offered Type A counseling and showed a similar reduction in MI recurrence rates over an additional year (Friedman 1987). This investigation also determined that Type A counseling was most protective against cardiac death for patients with less severe MI (Powell 1988), suggesting that psychosocial intervention is most effective when individuals are relatively healthy but may provide less benefit when disease is severe and physiologic processes predominate. Finally, there was a significant reduction in sudden, but not nonsudden, cardiac death for Type A individuals (Brackett 1988), providing support for the hypothesis that behavioral factors may be involved in the pathogenesis of lethal arrhythmias.

Burell (1993) randomized 265 nonsmoking post-CABG (coronary artery bypass graft) patients to a group program for modification of the TABP plus cardiac risk factor education vs a usual care control group. During the first year, intervention patients met for 17 three-hour group sessions with five to six "booster sessions" in years 2 and 3. The behavioral treatment was modeled after the RCPP with patients encouraged to reduce anger, impatience, annoyance, and irritation in daily life. At follow-up 4.5 years after surgery, there was a significant difference in total (5 vs 14,

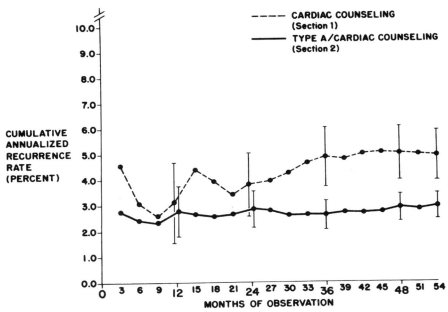

Fig. 11.4. Cumulative annualized recurrence rate of cardiac deaths and nonfatal myocardial infarction in the Recurrent Coronary Prevention Project for participants given Type A and general cardiac risk factor counseling for 4–5 years vs those given general counseling alone. Those given Type A counseling (section 2) have significantly lower recurrence rates at the end of 36 months. [From Friedman et al. (1986), with permission.]

$p = .02$) and cardiovascular (3 vs 9, $p = .05$) deaths between treatment and control patients respectively. There were 8 fatal and nonfatal cardiovascular events in the intervention vs 15 in the control groups ($p = .02$).

A number of other studies have attempted to modify the TABP, many with small numbers of subjects, and some in subjects who did not have CHD. Nunes et al. (1987) provide a meta-analysis of the early work on behavior modification of the TABP.

Hamalainen et al. (1989) studied 275 acute MI patients in Finland, given a comprehensive program that included optimal medical care, physical exercise, smoking cessation, dietary advice, and discussion of psychological problems. The intervention was most intensive during the first three months post-MI, but there was close contact with the treatment team for three years. Controls received care by their own physicians. Patients were followed for ten years, at which time there were 24 sudden cardiac deaths in the intervention group (12.8%) vs 43 (23.0%, $p = .01$) in the control group. The number of nonsudden coronary deaths was similar between groups. Of note, results were significant seven years after all intervention had ceased.

The largest lifestyle modification study was MRFIT (Shekelle 1985a), a primary prevention trial in which 361,662 men were screened to form a cohort of 12,866 high-risk individuals between 35 and 57 years of age without overt CHD who were subsequently assigned at random to either special intervention or usual care. Intervention programs consisted of counseling for cigarette cessation, a stepped-care treatment for hypertension and dietary advice for lowering blood cholesterol levels. In 1982, after an average follow-up of seven years, risk factor levels declined in both groups, but only slightly more for those receiving special intervention. Mortality was 7.1% lower for the intervention group, but this difference was not statistically significant. One explanation offered by the investigators for the disappointing results was the lower than expected mortality of the usual care group. It may be that entry into the study or living in the risk factor-conscious society of that time motivated these men to change health habits, even without special intervention. A high risk subgroup, the 12.5% of participants who had abnormal stress tests at entry, showed more favorable results, with a 57% reduction in CHD mortality ($p = .002$) for intervention versus usual care (Multiple Risk Factor Intervention Trial Research Group 1985). A recent update in 8,012 hypertensive participants after 10.5 years had even more dramatic results, with a reduction of 11% in total and 15% in CHD deaths, and a 36% reduction in total deaths and 50% reduction in CHD deaths for those with diastolic blood pressure $\geq$ 100 mmHg (Multiple Risk Factor Intervention Group 1990) in the intervention group.

The American Heart Association estimates that between 1964 and 1989 mortality from CHD declined over 50%, an improvement thought to result largely from risk factor modification by the general public (American Heart Association 1993). Leaf and Ryan (1991) recently pondered,

> Are we developing ingenious, technologically sophisticated and expensive treatment for established disease and ignoring the fact that the malady is potentially preventable and even reversible? . . . Members of the public will need to accept more responsibility for their own health . . . and be disabused of the fantasy that they can indulge in whatever lifestyle they wish and that medicine will make available a pill or operation to erase the adverse health effects of a lifetime of self-abuse.

Lifestyle change is difficult. Many patients do make substantial changes in health behavior after a diagnosis of CHD, particularly when CHD presents in the dramatic life-threatening setting of acute MI. Sustaining behavioral change, however, is not easy. Many patients revert to former behavior patterns as they feel better and less threatened. The encouraging results of lifestyle change programs indicate that behavioral counseling should be offered to CHD patients far more routinely than current medical practice. We suggest that young, highly stressed Type As with multiple modifiable cardiac risk factors have the most to gain from behavioral intervention—if they can be engaged in treatment. It is here that the physician's influence may be crucial. Many such patients are overly self-reliant and find it difficult to seek help with behavioral issues. The physician's enthusiasm for a risk-reduction program may augment such patients' often marginal motivation. The astute clinician should also be responsive to signs of depression.

Cost of Behavior Modification

Compared with invasive procedures in cardiology, the cost of psychosocial intervention is modest. The cost of the Ornish (1993) program is $4,000 for the first 3 months and $50 per week thereafter, or a total of $5,560 for the first year. In the Recurrent Coronary Prevention Project (Friedman 1986), patients were invited to attend 61 1.5-hour group sessions over 4.5 years, costing $3,050 at $50 per session. The Burrell et al. (1993) study provided 17 three-hour group sessions in the first year and five to six "booster sessions" in years 2 and 3, for an estimated cost of $3,000 per patient for three years. In comparison, at the New York Hospital–Cornell Medical Center in 1992, the average cost was approximately $7,600 for uncomplicated MI (excluding physician fees), $6,800 for cardiac catheterization, $13,000 for PTCA, $43,000 for CABG without cardiac catheterization, and $54,000 for CABG with cardiac catheterization. For secondary prevention, where subjects are known to have CHD and a considerably higher risk than the general population of subsequent death, recurrent CHD event or invasive procedure, it seems reasonable that psychosocial interventions might be cost effective. Cost effectiveness for primary prevention by psychosocial intervention is far more difficult to assess, since many people who will not develop CHD must be treated to reduce morbidity/mortality in a few who are currently hard to identify beforehand.

Conclusion

The association between behavioral, lifestyle, or psychosocial factors and CHD is far from clear, yet there is increasing evidence from many lines of research that there are important links between lifestyle and heart disease. Evidence as diverse as primate studies with social disorganization and prospective follow-up of behavior modification for the TABP in several large clinical trials suggests that particular behavior patterns, perhaps interacting with certain types of external stressors, probably do constitute a substantial risk factor for increased atherosclerosis. Beyond that, however, there may be powerful influences of the mind on short-term or precipitating factors for MI, ventricular arrhythmia or SCD. What remains elusive, though, are the pathophysiologic mechanisms by which psychosocial factors affect cardiac morbidity, the precise psychological patterns or external factors that confer risk or benefit, and thus the best strategies for intervention. The TABP, the first widely known psychosocial risk factor, has been less predictive of CHD in recent research than when first proposed. The search for the "toxic components" of the hostility complex and the TABP is currently muddled by methodological problems in diagnosis. Stress has been considered to have major psychological effects since Hans Selye's "alarm reaction" was formulated more than a half century ago, but the exact definition of stress is still far from clear. Stress may come from outside of the individual, as, for instance, in life changes or job strain or as a response within the individual, as in the hostility complex, the TABP. There are numerous studies that demonstrate an influence of the central nervous system on the propensity for arrhythmia, particularly ventricular tachyarrhythmia. Behavior pattern or stress might increase vulnerabilty to or actually trigger arrhythmia. It seems incontrovertible that mental stress can cause ischemia, and likely that mental stress affects coronary artery tone, at least in persons with coronary atherosclerosis, and the precipitation or exacerbation of myocardial ischemia is another mechanism by which behavioral factors might be associated with clinical manifestations of CHD.

What is evident from recent research is that coronary risk reduction programs that include a psychological component and encourage individualized risk factor modification appear helpful. While efforts continue to refine our understanding of the relationship between behavior and CHD, it is likely that cardiac patients, as well as the general population, will benefit from increased attention to psychosocial factors to help reduce the levels of traditional coronary risk factors and minimize the effects of psychosocial factors on coronary disease by a psychologically prudent lifestyle.

Summary

Quality of available data: Data on the relationship of psychosocial factors with MI are currently insufficient.

Estimated risk reduction: While the role of modification of psychosocial factors on MI risk is unclear, some epidemiologic evidence supports an association between these variables and traditional coronary risk factors, including serum lipids and blood pressure.

Comparability of effect in men and women: Data are insufficient to elucidate gender differences.

Acknowledgment

Supported, in part, by generous grants from The Pinewood Foundation, The Terner Foundation, and The Horace B. Goldsmith Foundation.

Appendix A

Anger Management:
Reducing Unwanted Anger

ROBERT ALLAN

A major theory in behavioral medicine is that excessive anger leads to illness, particularly coronary heart disease (CHD), the United States' leading cause of death and disability. Anger creates stress on the cardiovascular system, increasing demands on the heart. In the late 1950s, two San Francisco cardiologists, Meyer Friedman and Ray Rosenman, described the *Type A behavior pattern* that first connected psychological stress with CHD scientifically [1]. *Free-floating hostility*, the tendency to become easily angered, is one of the major symptoms of Type A behavior. More recently, Dr. Redford Williams, of the Duke University Medical Center, proposed that a "hostility complex," characterized by a hostile, cynical, and untrusting attitude toward people and life in general, is at the core of the heart and mind connection [2]. In addition to free-floating hostility and the hostility complex, unexpressed anger, or *anger-in*, has sometimes been linked to hypertension (high blood pressure) as well as CHD.

Is it better to express or suppress anger? The best answer to this important question is *neither*. It is best not to be angry. Anger triggers the fight or flight response, a natural reaction to danger. During fight or flight, the sympathetic nervous system is activated and "stress hormones" such as adrenalin are secreted, releasing the body's energy reserves. It is thought that chronic, excessive sympathetic nervous system activity contributes to plaque buildup in the coronary arteries. It is also suspected that anger may cause plaques to rupture, leading to myocardial infarction (heart attack) and sudden death. For heart health, it is the *amount* of anger that is of concern—the frequency, intensity, and duration of anger in a person's life. From this point of view, it is best not to be angry. The second best answer to the question of whether or not to express anger is that it is almost always better to *manage* anger, rather than give it free expression. Some people claim that it is "healthy" to express anger, rather than keep it "bottled up." This is untrue, as long as anger is processed and not simply suppressed. Openly expressed anger is often "contagious," leading to arguments and bad feelings.

The Hook

The "hook" is a metaphor to help reduce unwanted anger (Powell 1992, in press). According to the metaphor, we are all like fish, "swimming through the sea of life." Those of us with an overabundance of free-floating hostility are attracted to the 30 or so hassles, or "hooks" that drop before us each day. The "bait" on the hooks is often perceived as *injustice* or *incompetence* and provides a thorough justification for our anger, which most frequently takes the form of blame. For instance, it is very easy to get angry at something or someone who is unfair, immoral, or selfish, three kinds of *injustice*. Similarly, it is easy to become angry at *incompetence*, such as someone who appears unqualified, or even stupid or lazy. Moreover, some people seem to enjoy the "charge" of getting angry along with a feeling of righteous indignation. However, just as a fish who gets "hooked" and pulled out of the water after biting into a tasty-looking bait, we too suffer the negative physiological consequences of getting "hooked" by our own anger. If you recognize a hook for what it is, it is much easier not to bite. If you discover that you have bitten into a hook, let go of your anger as quickly as you can in order to minimize the negative consequences. How many hooks can you avoid today?

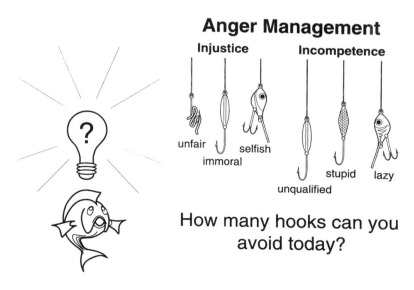

Anger Management

Injustice   Incompetence

unfair   selfish
immoral

stupid   lazy
unqualified

How many hooks can you avoid today?

The "hook" was developed by Dr. Lynda Powell and utilized in the Recurrent Coronary Prevention Project, a study of more than 1,000 post–heart attack patients that reduced *second* heart attack by 44% (Friedman et al. 1986). It was judged by these patients as being the single most important skill they learned during the 4.5-year program.

Appendix References

1. Friedman M, Rosenman RH. Type A behavior and your heart. New York: Knopf, 1974.
2. Williams RB. Refining the Type A hypothesis: emergence of the hostility complex. Am J Cardiol 1987; 60:27J–32J.

References

Adams J. Memoirs of the life and doctrines of John Hunter. London: J. Callow, 1817.

Ahern DK, Gorkin L, Anderson JL, et al. Biobehavioral variables and mortality in the Cardiac Arrhythmia Pilot Study (CAPS). Am J Cardiol 1990;66:59–62.

Albarran-Sotelo R, Flint LS, Kelly KJ. Healthcare provider's manual for basic life support. Dallas, American Heart Association, 1988.

American Heart Association. Dallas: heart and stroke facts statistics, 1993.

Appels A, Mulder P. Fatigue and heart disease: the association between "vital exhaustion" and past, present and future coronary heart disease. J Psychosom Res 1989;33:727–38.

Appels A. Mental precursors of myocardial infarction. Br J Psychiatry 1990;156:465–71.

Appels A, Schouten E. Waking up exhausted as risk indicator of myocardial infarction. Am J Cardiol 1991;68:395–8.

Barefoot JC, Dahlstrom WG, Williams RB. Hostility, CHD incidence, and total mortality: a 25-year follow-up of 255 physicians. Psychosom Med 1984;45:59–63.

Barefoot JC, Dodge KA, Peterson BL, et al. The Cook-Medley Hostility Scale: item content and ability to predict survival. Psychosomatic Med 1989a;51:46–57.

Barefoot JC, Peterson BL, Harrell FE, et al. Type A behavior and survival: a follow-up study of 1467 patients with coronary artery disease. Am J Cardiol 1989b;64:427–32.

Barefoot JC. Developments in the measurement of hostility. In: Friedman HS, ed. Hostility, coping, and health. Washington, DC: American Psychological Association, 1992.

Berkman LF, Leo-Summers L, Horwitz RI. Emotional support and survival after myocardial infarction. Ann Intern Med 1992;117:1003–9.

Blumenthal JA, Burg MM, Barefoot J, et al. Social support, type-A behavior, and coronary artery disease. Psychosom Med 1987;49:331–40.

Booth-Kewley S, Friedman HS. Psychological predictors of heart disease: a quantitative review. Psychol Bull 1987;101:343–62.

Bortner RW. A short rating scale as a potential measure of pattern A behavior. Journal of Chronic Diseases 1969;22:87–91.

Brackett CD, Powell LH. Psychosocial and physiological predictors of sudden cardiac death after healing of acute myocardial infarction. Am J Cardiol 1988;61:979–83.

Broadhead WE, Kaplan BH, James SA, et al. The epidemiologic evidence for a relationship between social support and health. Am J Epidemiol 1983;117:320–5.

Burell G. Behavior modification in secondary prevention of coronary heart disease: a treatment model that can prolong life after myocardial infarction and coronary artery bypass graft surgery. Paper presented at the III Congresso Nazionale, Societa Italiana Di Cardioneu-rologia, Pavia, Italy, September 28, 1993.

Cannon WB. The wisdom of the body. New York: Norton, 1932.

Cannon WB. "Voodoo" death. Am Anthropol 1942:44; reprinted in Psychosom Med 1957;19: 182–90.

Case RB, Heller SS, Case NB, Moss AJ. Type-A behavior and survival after acute myocardial infarction. N Engl J Med 1985;312:737–41.

Case RB, Moss AJ, Case N, et al. Living alone after myocardial infarction: impact on prognosis. JAMA 1992;267:515–19.

Clarkson TB, Kaplan JR, Adams MR, Manuck SB. Psychosocial influences on the pathogenesis of atherosclerosis among nonhuman primates. Circulation 1987;76 (Suppl I):I 29–40.

Cohen S, Tyrell DAJ, Smith, AP. Psychological stress and susceptibility to the common cold. N Engl J Med 1991;325:606–12.

Cottington EM, Matthews KA, Talbott E, Kuller LH. Environmental events preceding sudden death in women. Psychosom Med 1980;42:567–74.

Dembroski TM, MacDougall JM, Williams RB, et al. Components of type A, hostility and anger-in: relationship to angiographic findings. Psychosom Med 1985;47:219–33.

Dembroski TM, MacDougall JM, Costa PT, Grandits GA. Components of hostility as predictors of sudden death and myocardial infarction in the Multiple Risk Factor Intervention Trial. Psychosom Med 1989;51:514–22.

Dimsdale JE, Hackett TP, Hutter AM, et al. Type A behavior and angiographic findings. J Psychosom Res 1979;23:273–6.

Dobson AJ, Alexander HM, Malcolm JA, et al. Heart attacks and the Newcastle earthquake. Med J Aust 1991;155:757–61.

Eaker ED, Abbott RD, Kannell WB. Frequency of uncomplicated angina pectoris in type A compared with type B persons (the Framingham Study). Am J Cardiol 1989;63:1042–5.

Feigl EO. The paradox of adrenergic coronary vasoconstriction. Circulation 1987;76:737–45.

Fernandez F. Depression and its treatment in cardiac patients. Texas Heart Institute Journal. 1993;20:188–197.

Fielding R. Depression and acute myocardial infarction: a review and reinterpretation. Soc Sci Med 1991;32:1017–27.

Frasure-Smith N, Lesperance F, Talajic M. Depression following myocardial infarction. JAMA 1993;270:1819–25.

Friedman M, Ghandour G. Medical diagnosis of type A behavior. Am Heart J 1993;126:607–18.

Friedman M, Rosenman RH. Association of specific overt behavior pattern with blood and cardiovascular findings: blood cholesterol level, blood clotting time, incidence of arcus senilis, and clinical coronary artery disease. JAMA 1959;169:1286–96.

Friedman M, Rosenman RH. Type-A behavior and your heart. New York: Knopf, 1974.

Friedman M, Powell LH. The diagnosis and quantitative assessment of type-A behavior: intro-duction and description of the videotaped structured interview. Integrative Psychiatry 1984;2:123–9.

Friedman M, Ulmer D. Treating type-A behavior and your heart. New York: Knopf, 1984.

Friedman M, Powell LH, Thoresen CE, et al. Effect of discontinuance of type-A behavioral counseling on type-A behavior and cardiac recurrence rate of post myocardial infarction patients. Am Heart J 1987;114:483–90.

Friedman M, Thoresen CE, Gill JJ et al. Alteration of type-A behavior and its effect on cardiac recurrences in post myocardial infarction patients: summary results of the Recurrent Coronary Prevention Project. Am Heart J 1986;112:653–65.

Hamalainen H, Luurila OJ, Kallio V, et al. Long-term reduction in sudden deaths after a multifactorial intervention programme in patients with myocardial infarction: 10-year results of a controlled investigation. Eur Heart J 1989;10:55–62.

Haynes SG, Feinleib M. Type A behavior and the incidence of coronary heart disease in the Framingham Heart Study. Adv Cardiol 1982;29:85–95.

Haynes SG, Feinleib M, Levine S, et al. The relationship of psychosocial factors to coronary heart disease in the Framingham Study. Am J Epidemiology 1978;107:362–83.

Hearn MD, Murray DM, Luepker RV. Hostility, coronary heart disease, and total mortality: a 33-year follow-up study of university students. J Behav Med 1989;12:105–21.

Hecker MH, Chesney MA, Black GW, Farutsch N. Coronary-prone behaviors in the Western Collaborative Group Study. Psychosom Med 1988;50:153–64.

Helmer DC, Ragland DR, Lyme LS. Hostility and coronary artery disease. Am J Epidemiol 1991;133:112–22.

Herlitz J, Blohm M, Hartford M, et al. Delay time in suspected acute myocardial infarction and the importance of its modification. Clin Cardiol 1989;12:370–4.

Home E, in Hunter J. A treatise on the blood and gun shot wounds with a short account of the author's life. London: John Richardson, 1794.

House JS, Landis KR, Umberson D. Social relationships and health. Science 1988;241:540–6.

Ironson G, Taylor CB, Boltwood M, et al. Effects of anger on left ventricular ejection fraction in coronary disease. Am J Cardiol 1992;70:281–5.

Jacobs S, Friedman R, Mittleman M, et al. for the MI Onset Investigators. 9-fold increased risk of myocardial infarction following psychological stress as assessed by a case-control study. Circulation 1992;86 [Suppl I]I:198.

Kannel WB, Schatzkin A. Sudden death: lessons from subsets in population studies. J Am Coll Cardiol 1985;5:141B–149B.

Kaplan JR, Manuck SB, Williams JK, Strawn W. Psychosocial influences on atherosclerosis: evidence for effects and mechanisms in non-human primates. In: Blascovich J, Katkin ES, eds. Cardiovascular reactivity to psychological stress and disease. Washington, DC: American Psychological Association, 1993.

Karasek R, Baker D, Marxer F, et al. Job decision latitude, job demands and cardiovascular disease: a prospective study of Swedish men. Am J Public Health 1981;71:694–705.

Karasek RA, Theorell T, Schwartz JE, et al. Job characteristics in relation to the prevalence of myocardial infarction in the US Health Examination Survey (HES) and the Health and Nutrition Examination Survey (HANES). Am J Public Health 1988;78:910–18.

Leaf A, Ryan TJ. Prevention of coronary heart disease: a medical imperative. N Engl J Med 1991;323:1416–19.

Leon GR, Finn SE, Murray D, Bailey JM. Inability to predict cardiovascular disease from hostility scores or MMPI items related to type A behavior. J Consult Clin Psychol 1988;56:597–600.

Lown B, Temte JV, Reich P, et al. Basis for recurring ventricular fibrillation in the absence of coronary heart disease and its management. N Engl J Med 1976;294:623–9.

MacDougall JM, Dembroski TM, Dimsdale JE, Hackett TP. Components of type A, hostility and anger-in: further relationships to angiographic findings. Health Psychol 1985;4:137–52.

Maruta T, Hamburgen ME, Jennings CA, et al. Keeping hostility in perspective: coronary heart disease and the hostility scale on the Minnesota Multiphasic Personality Inventory. Mayo Clinic Proc 1993;68:109–14.

Matthews KA, Haynes SG. Type-A behavior pattern and coronary disease risk: update and critical evaluation. Am J Epidemiol 1986;123:923–60.

McCranie EW, Watkins LO, Brandsma JM, Sisson BD. Hostility, coronary heart disease (CHD) incidence and total mortality: lack of association in a 25-year follow-up study of 478 physicians. J Behav Med 1986;9:119–25.

McIntosh HD. The stabilizing and unstabilizing influences of neurogenic and vascular activities of the heart as related to sudden cardiac death. J Am Coll Cardiol 1985;5:105B–10B.

Meisel SR, Kutz I, Dayan KI, et al. Effect of Iraqi missile war on incidence of acute myocardial infarction and sudden death in Israeli civilians. Lancet 1991;338:660–1.

Miller TQ, Turner CW, Tindale RS, et al. Reasons for the trend toward null findings in research on type-A behavior. Psychol Bull 1991;110:469–85.

Multiple Risk Factor Intervention Trial Research Group. Exercise electrocardiogram and coronary heart disease mortality in the Multiple Risk Factor Intervention Trial. Am J Cardiol 1985;55:16–24.

Multiple Risk Factor Intervention Group. Mortality after $10^1/_2$ years for hypertensive participants in the Multiple Risk Factor Intervention Trial. Circulation 1990;82:1616–28.

Niaura R, Stoney CM, Herbert N. Lipids in psychological research: the last decade. Biol Psychol 1992;34:1–43.

Nunes EV, Frank KA, Kornfeld DS. Psychologic treatment for the type A behavior pattern and for coronary heart disease: a meta-analysis of the literature. Psychosom Med 1987;48:159–73.

Ornish D, Brown SE, Scherwitz LW, et al. Can lifestyle changes reverse coronary heart disease? Lancet 1990;336:129–33.

Ornish D, Brown SE, Billings JH, et al. Can lifestyle changes reverse coronary atherosclerosis? Four-year results of the Lifestyle Heart Trial. Circulation 1993;88:I-385 [Abstract].

Orth-Gomer K, Uniden AL. Type-A behavior, social support, and coronary risk: interaction and significance for mortality in cardiac patients. Psychosom Med 1990;52:59–72.

Orth-Gomer K, Rosengren A, Wilhelmsen L. Lack of social support and incidence of coronary heart disease in middle-aged Swedish men. Psychosom Med 1993;55:37–43.

Osler W. Lectures on angina pectoris and allied states. New York: Appleton, 1897.

Parkes CM. Effects of bereavement on physical and mental health: a study of the medical records of widows. Br Med J 1964;2:274–9.

Pickering TG. Should studies of patients undergoing coronary angiography be used to evaluate the role of behavioral risk factors for coronary heart disease? J Behav Med 1985;8:203–13.

Pieper C. LaCroix AZ, Karasek RA. The relation of psychosocial dimensions of work with coronary heart disease risk factors: a meta-analysis of five United States data bases. Am J Epidemiol 1989;129:483–94.

Plato. The dialogues of Plato. [Translated by B. Jowett] Oxford: Jowett Copyright Trustees, 1953 (1871).

Powell LH. The cognitive underpinnings of coronary-prone behaviors. Cog Therapy Res 1992;6:123–42.

Powell LH. The hook: a metaphor for gaining control of emotional reactivity. In: Allan R, Scheidt S, eds. Heart and mind: the emergence of cardiac psychology. Washington, DC: American Psychological Association, in press.

Powell LH, Thoresen CE. Effects of type-A behavioral counseling and severity of prior acute myocardial infarction on survival. Am J Cardiol 1988;62:1159–63.

Price VA, Friedman M, Ghandour G. Relation between insecurity and type A behavior. Am Heart J 1995;129:488–91.

Ragland DR, Brand RJ. Type-A behavior and mortality from coronary heart disease. N Engl J Med 1988;318:65–9.

Rahe RH, Romo M, Bennet L, Siltanen P. Recent life changes, myocardial infarction, and abrupt coronary death. Arch Intern Med 1974;133:221−8.

Rees WD, Lutkins SG. Mortality of bereavement. Br Med J 1984;311:552−9.

Rosengren A, Tibblin G, Wilhelmsen L. Self-perceived psychological stress and incidence of coronary artery disease in middle-aged men. Am J Cardiol 1991;68:1171−5.

Rosenman RH, Brand RJ, Jenkins CD, et al. Coronary heart disease in the Western Collaborative Group Study: final follow-up experience of $8^{1}/_{2}$ years. JAMA 1975;233:872−7.

Rozanski A, Bairey CN, Krantz DS, et al. Mental stress and the induction of silent myocardial ischemia in patients with coronary artery disease. N Engl J Med 1988;318:1005−12.

Ruberman W, Weinblatt E, Goldberg J, Chaudhary BS. Psychosocial influences on mortality after myocardial infarction. N Engl J Med 1984;311:552−9.

Ruberman W. Psychosocial influences on mortality of patients with coronary heart disease. JAMA 1992;267:559−60.

Schleifer SJ, Macari-Hinson MM, Coyle DA, et al. The nature and course of depression following myocardial infarction. Arch Intern Med 1989;149:1785−9.

Schleifer SJ, Slater WR, Macari-Hinson MM, et al. Digitalis and B-blocking agents: effects on depression following myocardial infarction. Am Heart J 1991;121:1397−402.

Schnall PL, Pieper C, Schwartz JE, et al. The relationship between ''job strain,'' workplace diastolic blood pressure and left ventricular mass index. JAMA 1990;263:1929−35.

Schnall PL, Landsbergis PA, Baker D. Job strain and cardiovascular disease. Annu Rev Public Health 1994;15:381−411.

Schuler G, Hambrecht R, Schlierf G, et al. Myocardial perfusion and regression of coronary artery disease in patients on a regimen of intensive physical exercise and low fat diet. J Am Coll Cardiol 1992;19:34−42.

Seeman TE, Syme SL. Social networks and coronary artery disease: a comparison of the structure and function of social relations as predictors of disease. Psychosom Med 1987;49: 541−54.

Selye H. The stress of life. New York: McGraw-Hill, 1956.

Shekelle RB, Gale M, Ostfeld AM, Paul O. Hostility, risk of coronary heart disease, and mortality. Psychosom Med 1983;45:109−14.

Shekelle RB, Gale M, Norusis M. Type-A score (Jenkins Activity Survey) and risk of recurrent coronary heart disease in the Aspirin Myocardial Infarction Study. Am J Cardiol 1985a; 56:221−5.

Shekelle RB, Hulley SB, Neaton JD, et al. The MRFIT behavior pattern study II: type-A behavior and incidence of coronary heart disease. Am J Epidemiology 1985b;122:559−70.

Sirous F. Le deni dans la maladie coronarienne. Can Med Assoc J 1992;147:315−21.

Smith TW. Hostility and health: current status of a psychosomatic hypothesis. Health Psychol 1992;11:139−50.

Smith TW, Barefoot JC. The assessment of hostility: implications for research and practice. Paper presented at the annual meeting of the American Psychosomatic Society, Charleston, SC, March 4, 1993.

Surawicz B. Neural control of the heart: summary of discussion. J Am Coll Cardiol 1985;5: 111B−112B.

Swan GE, Carmelli I, Rosenman RH. Psychological correlates of two measures of coronary-prone hostility. Psychosomatics 1989;30:270−8.

Thoresen CE, Powell LH. Type A behavior pattern: new perspectives on theory, assessment and intervention. J Consult Clin Psychol 1992;60;595−604.

Tofler GH, Stone PH, Maclure M, et al. Analysis of possible triggers of acute myocardial infarction (The MILIS Study). Am J Cardiol 1990;66:22−7.

Verrier RL. Mechanisms of behaviorally induced arrhythmias. Circulation (Suppl I) 1987;76: 148–56.

Williams JK, Vita JA, Manuck SB, et al. Psychosocial factors impair vascular responses of coronary arteries. Circulation 1991;84:2146–53.

Williams RB, Haney TL, Lee KL, et al. Type A behavior, hostility and coronary atherosclerosis. Psychosom Med 1980;42:539–49.

Williams RB. Refining the type-A hypothesis: emergence of the hostility complex. Am J Cardiol 1987;60:27J–32J.

Williams RB, Barefoot JC, Haney TL, et al. Type-A behavior and angiographically documented coronary atherosclerosis in a sample of 2,289 patients. Psychosom Med 1988;50:139–52.

Williams RB, Barefoot JC, Califf RM. Prognostic importance of social and economic resources among medically treated patients with angiographically documented coronary artery disease. JAMA 1992;267:520–4.

Willich SN, Lowel H, Lewis M, et al. and the TRIMM Study Group. Association of wake time and the onset of myocardial infarction. Circulation 1991;84[suppl VI];62–7.

Yeung AC, Vekshtein VI, Krantz DS, et al. The effect of atherosclerosis on the vasomotor response of coronary arteries to mental stress. N Engl J Med 1991;325:1551–6.

12

Aspirin

JULIE E. BURING AND CHARLES H. HENNEKENS

In the fifth century B.C., Hippocrates discovered that an extract of willow bark had analgesic properties. The pain-killing effect was the result of salicin, a naturally occurring chemical in willow bark, which is closely related to today's synthetic aspirin, acetylsalicylic acid. It is only quite recently, however—over the past few decades—that attention has focused on the potential role of aspirin in reducing risks of occlusive vascular disease.

Mechanism

The hypothesized mechanism for aspirin's benefit is its ability to decrease platelet aggregation and thereby reduce the risk of thrombotic vascular events. Platelets, platelet products, and thrombosis play key roles in the occurrence of acute occlusive vascular events, such as myocardial infarction (MI) and ischemic stroke. The disruption of platelet- and fibrin-rich atherosclerotic plaque may lead to aggressive platelet deposition and, ultimately, the formation of a thrombus, which can precipitate an acute clinical event. Findings from basic research demonstrate that, in platelets, small amounts of aspirin irreversibly acetylate the active site of cyclooxygenase, which is required for the production of thromboxane A2, a powerful promoter of aggregation (Moncada 1979). This effect is so pronounced that higher doses of aspirin appear to yield no additional benefit. It has, in fact, been hypothesized that far higher doses might even reverse this tendency, due to activation of vessel wall enzymes.

Observational Studies

As regards observational epidemiologic research, several studies, both case-control and prospective cohort, have explored the relationship between aspirin use and primary prevention of cardiovascular disease. The observational evidence in women, among whom there are presently no data from randomized trials, is summarized in Table

12.1. Case-control studies of nonfatal MI have found a protective effect of aspirin use in men and women (Boston Collaborative Drug Surveillance Group 1974) and in men (Jick 1976). In contrast, a case-control study of aspirin use and coronary death in men found no association between aspirin use and fatal coronary disease (Hennekens 1978). Three prospective cohort studies have examined this question. In the Nurses' Health Study, which followed more than 87,000 U.S. women over 6 years, those who reported taking one to six aspirin tablets per week experienced a significant 25% decreased risk of MI compared with women who took no aspirin (Manson 1991). Two other prospective cohort studies, however, found no association between regular aspirin use and risk of MI in men and women (Hammond 1975; Paganini-Hill 1989).

Thus, the observational evidence on this question is not entirely consistent. However, unlike basic research, results of observational epidemiologic investigations are not always precise, since they are based on observations on free-living humans that rarely take place under the tightly controlled conditions possible in the laboratory. For this reason, when a 20% to 30% effect is postulated, as is the case with aspirin and reduction of cardiovascular disease, it is possible that the size of uncontrolled confounding is as large as the hypothesized benefits. Because they are able to control for both known and unknown confounding variables, randomized trials of sufficient sample size are the most reliable study design for detecting such small to moderate effects (Hennekens 1987). Such trials have been carried out testing aspirin in a wide range of patients with and without prior manifestations of cardiovascular disease, and their results provide a firm basis of knowledge concerning the use of aspirin to reduce cardiovascular disease risk.

Randomized Trials

Secondary Prevention Trials

The first randomized trials of aspirin tested its effect among individuals with a prior history of cardiovascular disease. By 1987, 25 trials of antiplatelet therapy in secondary prevention of cardiovascular disease had been conducted among a total of 29,000

Table 12.1. Aspirin in Primary Prevention of CHD in Women

Study	Design	Endpoint	RR[a]
Boston Collaborative Drug Surveillance Program (1974) ($N = 92$)	Case-control	MI	0.74
Nurses' Health Study (1991) ($N = 87,000$)	Prospective cohort	MI	0.75
California Retirement Community Study (1989) ($N = 8,000$)	Prospective cohort	MI	1.06
		IHD	1.70
American Cancer Society Study (1975) ($N = 550,000$)	Prospective cohort	CHD death	1.13

MI, myocardial infarction; IHD, ischemic heart disease; CHD, coronary heart disease.

[a]Relative risk among regular aspirin users compared with nonusers.

patients. Of these 25 trials, 10 were conducted among patients with a prior MI, 13 were among patients with a history of stroke or transient cerebral ischemia, and two were among those with unstable angina pectoris. These trials tested aspirin, dipyridamole, or sulfinpyrazone, either alone or in combination.

While the results of most of the trials suggested a benefit of antiplatelet therapy, they were usually too small in sample size individually to provide reliable results. In such a situation, one means of evaluating the available data on a question is to perform an overview, or meta-analysis. In an overview, the results of several trials are considered in aggregate, with statistical weight given to each trial according to its size. By including larger numbers of subjects, an overview can diminish the play of chance in results and provide a more statistically stable estimate of an effect.

In 1988, with the worldwide collaboration of investigators who had conducted randomized trials of antiplatelet therapy, an overview was published of the 25 completed trials in secondary prevention (Table 12.2) (Antiplatelet Trialists' Collaboration 1988). When all 25 trials were considered, antiplatelet therapy was associated with a 32% reduction in subsequent MI. For nonfatal stroke, there was a 27% decrease in risk, and for total vascular mortality, the reduction was 15%. The overview also considered a combined endpoint termed "important vascular events," which included nonfatal MI, nonfatal stroke, and vascular death. Antiplatelet therapy was associated with a 25% decrease in important vascular events. All these reductions were statistically significant. There was no apparent effect of antiplatelet treatment on nonvascular death, so the significant (p = .0003) benefit observed on total mortality is largely explained by the definite reduction in vascular death.

The trials were also considered separately according to patient entry criteria. In these analyses, the 10 trials of survivors of MI demonstrated statistically significant decreases in risk of 31% for nonfatal reinfarction, 42% for nonfatal stroke, 13% for vascular death, and 22% for important vascular events. The 13 trials of patients with cerebrovascular disease (stroke or transient ischemic attack [TIA]) demonstrated statistically significant reductions of 35% for MI, 22% for subsequent nonfatal stroke,

Table 12.2. Overview of 25 Trials of Antiplatelet Therapy in the Secondary Prevention of Cardiovascular Disease

	Reduction (% ± SD) Among Those Assigned Antiplatelet Therapy			
Endpoint	All (25 trials)	Cerebrovascular[a] (13 trials)	MI[b] (10 trials)	Unstable Angina[c] (2 trials)
Nonfatal MI	32 ± 5	35 ± 12	31 ± 5	35 ± 17
Nonfatal stroke	27 ± 6	22 ± 7	42 ± 11	—[d]
Total vascular mortality	15 ± 4	15 ± 7	13 ± 5	37 ± 19
Important vascular events	25 ± 3	22 ± 5	22 ± 4	36 ± 13

[a]Trials of patients with prior stroke or transient ischemic attacks.

[b]Trials of patients with prior myocardial infarction.

[c]Trials of patients with prior unstable angina.

[d]Too few events reported to permit reliable assessment.

15% for vascular death, and 22% for important vascular events. Finally, for the 2 trials of unstable angina patients, there were statistically significant decreases of 35% in nonfatal MI, 37% in vascular death, and 36% in any vascular event. There were too few strokes in these trials to provide meaningful data.

As regards the different antiplatelet agents tested, there was no clear evidence that aspirin plus dipyridamole was any more effective than aspirin alone, because the indirect comparison between the two risk reductions was not significant, and the overview of the direct comparisons indicated no difference whatsoever. There was also no evidence that daily doses of 900 to 1,500 mg of aspirin were any more effective in reducing vascular events than 300 mg per day, the lowest dose tested.

While this overview provided reliable evidence of the benefit of aspirin therapy in patients with prior MI, stroke, TIA or unstable angina, it did not address directly whether such therapy would benefit other patient populations at increased risk for occlusive vascular disease, such as those with chronic stable angina, peripheral vascular disease, or patients undergoing revascularization procedures. The overview also did not address the question of aspirin's benefit in certain subgroups of high-risk patients, such as women or the elderly, or those with hypertension or diabetes.

To address these questions, the Antiplatelet Trialists' Collaboration has performed an updated overview of the effects of antiplatelet therapy that includes data from trials enrolling a much broader range of high-risk patients (Antiplatelet Trialists' Collaboration 1994). The updated overview utilizes the results of 133 trials of antiplatelet therapy in patients with prior cardiovascular disease. Its results are based on the experience of approximately 53,000 patients, nearly twice the number included in the original overview. The findings among patients with prior MI, stroke, TIA and unstable angina were similar to those of the original 1988 overview.

With respect to new patient populations included in the updated overview, the report includes the experience of approximately 22,000 patients at high-risk for occlusive vascular events due to atrial fibrillation, valve surgery, peripheral vascular disease, chronic stable angina, and coronary revascularization (either coronary artery bypass graft or percutaneous transluminal coronary angioplasty). When analyzed separately according to patient entry criteria, most comparisons of antiplatelet therapy and control failed to achieve statistical significance, due to the small numbers of patients in each patient category. However, when the trials of these various high-risk patients were considered in aggregate, antiplatelet therapy was associated with statistically significant 32% decrease in vascular events.

The updated overview also provides reliable data that antiplatelet treatment in high-risk patients produces vascular event reductions of similar size in various patient subgroups. Specifically, separate data for men and women were available from 29 trials conducted among approximately 40,000 men and 10,000 women. There were comparable benefits on vascular events, with reductions per 1,000 patients treated of 37 events for men (SD 4; $p < .00001$) and 33 events for women (SD 7; $p < .0001$). The data from these 29 trials also demonstrate similar reductions in vascular events for middle-aged as well as older patients, in hypertensives and normotensives, and in diabetics and nondiabetics.

Aspirin was tested in these trials in doses ranging from 75 to 1,500 mg/day. As in the original overview, there was no evidence that higher doses were any more effective in reducing the risk of occlusive vascular events than lower doses. While 300 mg was the lowest daily dose tested in trials in the original overview, the updated analysis includes approximately 5,000 patients randomized in trials testing 75 mg of aspirin per day. When analyzed separately, the trials testing daily doses of 75 mg demonstrated a statistically significant 29% reduction in vascular events associated with aspirin ($p < .0001$).

It has been postulated that doses even lower than 75 mg may confer greater benefit by inhibiting platelet aggregation without blocking the synthesis of prostacyclin, an enzyme with antiplatelet and vasodilative properties. However, even low daily doses appear to depress prostacyclin biosynthesis (Clarke 1991). One strategy that has been proposed to enhance the biochemical selectivity of aspirin for thromboxane A2 while sparing prostacyclin, is the use of a controlled-release aspirin preparation. A small trial comparing a controlled-release 75 mg aspirin preparation with a conventional immediate-release 75 mg preparation has demonstrated the ability of this formulation to inhibit thromboxane A2 production, while decreasing basal prostacyclin biosynthesis only slightly (Clarke 1991). A large-scale trial comparing such a preparation with conventional aspirin will be necessary to determine the clinical value, if any, of preserving prostacyclin during antiplatelet therapy.

In addition to aspirin, dipyridamole, and sulfinpyrazone, which were tested in trials included in the original overview, the updated analysis also includes three trials that tested ticlopidine versus aspirin. As in the original overview, the updated analysis demonstrates no significant differences in effectiveness of the various antiplatelet agents. However, any differences between antiplatelet agents will be much smaller than that between antiplatelet treatment and no antiplatelet treatment, so the results of the overview can not exclude the possibility of a small advantage of one type of agent.

Finally, as regards the optimal duration of treatment in secondary prevention, there is no direct evidence on this question, since no large-scale randomized trials have compared different durations of treatment. For trials of patients with prior MI, stroke, or TIA that provided individual patient data, information is available on events occurring in the first, second, and subsequent years of scheduled treatment. These trials show an apparent trend toward greater effect during the earlier years. However, there are difficulties in interpreting these data, as noncompliance with treatment trends to increase with time (i.e., some in the treatment group will have stopped antiplatelet therapy and others in the control will have initiated such treatment), so an underestimation of the effect of actual treatment will tend to increase over time. In the absence of contrary direct evidence from randomized comparisons of different durations of treatment and contraindications for its use in individual patients, it may be advisable to continue aspirin therapy indefinitely in those patients considered to be at high risk for occlusive vascular events.

Acute Evolving Myocardial Infarction

Because aspirin therapy reduced cardiovascular risks among individuals with a history of MI and those with unstable angina, it was hypothesized that a similar benefit may result if the drug were administered within the first few hours following onset of symptoms of MI. One large-scale placebo-controlled trial has been conducted testing the effects of aspirin during the acute phases of MI. The Second International Study of Infarct Survival (ISIS-2) was a randomized, double-blind, placebo-controlled trial that utilized a 2×2 factorial design in order to assess simultaneously the effects of streptokinase and aspirin in suspected acute MI. ISIS-2 randomized 17,187 patients admitted for suspected evolving MI within 24 hours of symptom onset to either a single intravenous infusion of 1.5 million units of streptokinase over one hour, 162.5 mg aspirin daily for one month, both active treatments, or neither treatment (ISIS-2 Collaborative Group 1988).

Five weeks after randomization, aspirin was associated with 23% reduction in vascular death, a 49% reduction in nonfatal reinfarction, and a 46% reduction in nonfatal stroke (Table 12.3). All of these reductions were statistically significant and provide strong evidence of the benefit of aspirin for the vast majority of patients with suspected evolving MI. There were no significant differences seen between men and women in the effect of aspirin on vascular mortality. There was no increase in hemorrhagic stroke associated with aspirin, and only a slight increase in minor bleeding.

Steptokinase-treated patients experienced a comparable statistically significant 25% reduction in vascular mortality. Streptokinase was associated with a nonsignificant excess of nonfatal reinfarction and had no apparent effect on overall nonfatal stroke, although there was a significant excess of confirmed cerebral hemorrhage. Patients assigned to both aspirin and streptokinase fared best, experiencing a significant 42% decrease in vascular mortality.

About 48 hours are required to achieve maximal inhibition of serum thromboxane B2 with a daily dose of 75 mg of aspirin. For this reason, while doses in this range appear to be as efficacious as higher doses for use in long-term secondary prevention, to achieve a rapid clinical antithrombotic effect in the setting of acute MI requires an initial loading dose of at least 162.5 mg aspirin as in ISIS-2 or 325 mg as in GISSI-2 (Gruppo Italiano per lo Studio della Sopravvivenza Nell Infarto Miocardico).

Despite the clear benefits of aspirin in acute MI, this therapy remains underutilized in this clinical setting. A survey of treatment patterns in the United States before and after publication of the ISIS-2 findings indicates that use of aspirin in acute MI increased substantially, from about 39% of all patients to approximately 72% of those admitted for acute evolving MI (Lamas 1992). While the ISIS-2 results, therefore, appear to have had a marked impact on clinical practice, aspirin could, in fact, be given to nearly all patients with acute MI, as the bleeding risks appear to be minimal and the benefits on fatal and nonfatal vascular events are substantial among this population of high-risk patients. From a public health standpoint, with approximately 1.2

Table 12.3. Results from the Second International Study of Infarct Survival (ISIS-2): Vascular Events in the First 5 Weeks After Suspected Acute MI

Endpoint	Reduction ($\% \pm$ SD) Among Those Assigned Aspirin
Nonfatal reinfarction	49 ± 9
Nonfatal stroke	46 ± 17
Total vascular mortality	23 ± 4

million patients admitted to US hospitals each year with acute MI, increasing the use of aspirin in this setting from 72% of patients to virtually all patients would prevent nearly 8,000 premature deaths each year (Hennekens 1994).

Primary Prevention Trials

The evidence from the secondary prevention trials and ISIS-2 raises, but does not address directly, the possibility that aspirin may also be of a benefit in primary prevention among healthy individuals. Two primary prevention trials of aspirin have been completed, both among male physicians (Table 12.4).

The US Physicians' Health Study utilized a 2 × 2 factorial design to test simultaneously the effects of aspirin in reducing cardiovascular disease and beta-carotene in the prevention of cancer (Hennekens 1983). A total of 22,071 male physicians, aged 40 to 84, were randomized to either 325 mg aspirin on alternate days, 50 mg beta-carotene on alternate days, both agents, or neither.

The aspirin component of the trial was terminated early in 1988, after an average follow-up of 60.2 months, due primarily to the emergence of a statistically extreme benefit on risk of MI. Aspirin was associated with a 44% reduction in risk of a first MI, with significant benefits on fatal and nonfatal events (Steering Committee 1989). As regards stroke, there were insufficient numbers of events upon which to draw firm conclusions. However, the available data did not suggest any reduction in stroke, and there was, in fact, a nonsignificant 19% increase in nonfatal stroke. Because of aspirin's effect on platelet aggregation, a particular concern with its use is a possible increase in hemorrhagic stroke. For this subgroup of strokes in the Physicians' Health Study, although the numbers were small and did not achieve conventional statistical significance, there was the suggestion of a possible increased risk in the aspirin group (23 events vs 12 events, $p = .06$).

The other primary prevention trial was conducted among 5,139 male physicians, aged 50 to 78, in Great Britain. The British trial tested a daily dose of 500 mg aspirin, and the control group was simply asked to avoid aspirin or any aspirin-containing compounds. After six years of treatment and follow-up, there were no significant differences for nonfatal MI, nonfatal stroke, vascular death, or all important vascular events (Peto 1988). It was not possible to distinguish reliably between thrombotic and

Table 12.4. Aspirin in Primary Prevention: U.S. Physicians' Health Study and British Doctors' Trial

| Endpoint | Reduction (% ± SD) Among Those Assigned Aspirin | | |
	U.S. Physicians' Health Study	British Doctors' Trial	Overview
Nonfatal MI	39 ± 9	3 ± 19	32 ± 8
Nonfatal stroke	↑ 19 ± 15	↑ 13 ± 24	↑ 18 ± 13
Total vascular mortality	2 ± 15	7 ± 14	5 ± 10
Important vascular events	18 ± 7	4 ± 12	13 ± 6

↑ = Nonsignificant increased risk of stroke among aspirin-allocated subjects.

hemorrhagic strokes. There was, however, an increase of borderline statistical significance ($p = .05$) in the aspirin group of the subgroup of strokes self-reported as "disabling." It is difficult, however, to know whether this reflects a real increase in such events, which might be more likely to be hemorrhagic in etiology, or is the result of bias in the self-reporting of residual impairment due to the study's open design.

There were several design differences between the two primary prevention trials. While the U.S. trial tested 325 mg on alternate days, the British study used a daily dose of 500 mg. The U.S. trial was double-blind and placebo-controlled, while the British trial was single-blind and had open control. The most striking difference is in sample size, with the U.S. trial more than four times as large.

In order to consider the available primary prevention trial data in aggregate, an overview was performed of the U.S. and British trials (Hennekens 1988). Because the U.S. study was so much larger, the overview demonstrated a highly significant 32% reduction in risk of nonfatal MI. For stroke and vascular death, even when the trials were considered together there were too few endpoints upon which to draw firm conclusions.

Side Effects

Although aspirin's benefits in reducing occlusive vascular events may be approximately equal over the wide dose range tested in trials to date, the principal side effects of the drug appear to be strongly dose-related.

The UK-TIA trial, which tested two daily dosages of aspirin as well as placebo, provides the most informative direct comparison of the side effects of different aspirin dosages (UK-TIA Study Group 1988). This trial, which randomized 2,345 patients with a history of transient ischemic attacks, tested 300 and 1,200 mg/day of aspirin against placebo. For each category of symptom, including indigestion, nausea, or heartburn; constipation; total gastrointestinal bleed; and serious gastrointestinal bleed, the percentage of participants reporting it was lowest in the placebo group, somewhat higher in the group receiving 300 mg/day, and highest among those receiving 1,200 mg daily.

In the ISIS-2 trial of evolving MI, which tested 162.5 mg/day, there were no significant differences between the aspirin and placebo groups for major bleeds, and only a small increase in minor bleeds associated with aspirin. Finally, in primary prevention, in the larger, placebo-controlled U.S. trial, the alternate-day 325-mg aspirin regimen was associated with an excess in ulcer (1.5% vs 1.3%, $p = .08$) and bleeding problems (27.% vs 20.4%, $p < .0001$). Rates of gastrointestinal symptoms other than ulcer were similar (34.8% vs 34.2%). This may have been due partially to the low-dose and alternate-day schedule used in the trial, as well as to a prerandomization run-in period, which eliminated those physicians who reported intolerance to aspirin before they were assigned to study groups.

Strength of the Evidence of Benefits of Aspirin Prophylaxis

In secondary prevention trials there are clear benefits of aspirin for patients with prior cardiovascular disease. The recent update of the overview of antiplatelet trials in secondary prevention indicates that these benefits extend to a much broader range of patients than previously demonstrated, with significant benefits accruing not only to patients with prior MI, stroke, TIA, or unstable angina, but also to patients with peripheral vascular disease, atrial fibrillation, chronic stable angina, valvular disease, and those undergoing revascularization procedures. Among this wide range of patients, aspirin therapy reduces by about 25% the risk of occlusive vascular events, with comparable reductions in men and women. Based on the available data in 1980, the U.S. Food and Drug Administration approved the prescription labeling of aspirin for treatment of men with prior TIAs (FDA Drug Bull 1980), and, in 1985, this was extended to men and women with a prior MI or unstable angina (FDA Drug Bull 1985).

For acute evolving MI, there are clear and conclusive benefits of aspirin on reinfarction, stroke, and vascular death.

In primary prevention, there is a conclusive reduction associated with low-dose aspirin in risk of a first MI in men. However, the evidence concerning stroke and vascular mortality remains inconclusive due to inadequate numbers of endpoints in both primary prevention trials of aspirin as well as in the overview of their findings. With respect to hemorrhagic stroke, the numbers are small but raise the possibility of some excess risk.

The US Preventive Services Task Force (1989) has issued recommendations stating that low-dose aspirin should be considered for men aged 40 and over who are at significantly increased risk of MI and who lack contraindications to the drug.

Because the only randomized trial data in primary prevention are in men, no formal recommendations have been issued on this question for women. The only data available on aspirin use in apparently healthy women derive from observational studies. As summarized above, and as shown in Table 12.1, the findings from these investigations are not entirely consistent, with two studies in women suggesting benefits of aspirin (Boston Collaborative Drug Surveillance Group 1974; Manson 1991) and two reporting no apparent effect (Hammond 1975; Paganini-Hill 1989).

The primary concern in extrapolating findings from trial data in men is that the benefit:risk ratio for prophylactic aspirin use in women may differ, since their risk of MI, the principal outcome that aspirin may prevent, is lower at almost every age, while women and men have roughly comparable rates of stroke, hemorrhagic forms of which aspirin may increase. To evaluate directly the benefits and risks of low-dose aspirin among apparently healthy women, a large-scale randomized trial was begun in 1992. The Women's Health Study will randomize approximately 40,000 U.S. women, aged 45 and older, to alternate-day aspirin (100 mg) or placebo (Buring 1992a,b). The trial will also test the antioxidant vitamins beta-carotene (50 mg on alternate days) and vitamin E (600 IU on alternate days) in the primary prevention of cancer and cardiovascular disease. While awaiting definitive data from this trial, the observational data in women, in conjunction with the definitive randomized trial data in male physicians, suggest that aspirin may be beneficial in primary prevention for those women whose risk of MI is sufficiently high to warrant exposure to any risks of long-term administration of this drug.

It is important to view the potential benefits of aspirin in the context of current knowledge about modification of cardiovascular risk factors. For example, a 10%

decrease in blood cholesterol corresponds to a roughly 20–30% reduction in risks of cardiovascular disease (Peto 1985). For blood pressure, a 5- to 6-mm decrease in diastolic pressure among those with mild-to-moderate hypertension appears to lower risks of coronary heart disease by 14% and stroke by 42% (Collins 1990). Finally, cessation of cigarette smoking results in an approximately 60% decrease in coronary heart disease, perhaps beginning even within a matter of months (Hennekens 1984).

Thus, aspirin should always be viewed as a possible adjunct, not alternative, to control or elimination of other cardiovascular risk factors. Aspirin therapy should be initiated only upon the recommendation of a physician or other primary health care provider. Such a recommendation should be based on an individual clinical judgment that considers the cardiovascular risks of the patient, the adverse effects of the drug, and the documented benefits on various manifestations of cardiovascular disease in different categories of patients (Hennekens 1989).

Clinical Scenarios

While the decision to prescribe aspirin in primary prevention must be based on each individual patient's complete health profile, clinical scenarios may nevertheless provide useful guides as to patients who would appear to be suitable candidates for therapy as well as patients for whom such treatment does not appear warranted or may even be contraindicated.

A 60-year-old woman who is 35 lb over target body weight, has a cholesterol of 260 mg/dl, and has recently been diagnosed with type II diabetes is at elevated risk of MI. A 55-year-old man with a 40 pack-year history of cigarette smoking and cholesterol level of 260 mg/dl is also at substantially increased risk of MI. In the absence of a history of gastrointestinal ulcer or serious bleeding, both patients would be strong candidates for aspirin prophylaxis.

A 42-year-old premenopausal woman whose only cardiovascular risk factor is severe and poorly controlled hypertension (average readings of 160/100 mmHg) is at significantly greater risk of stroke than MI. Because of concern that aspirin may increase the risk of hemorrhagic stroke, aspirin is not indicated, and may be contraindicated, in patients with such as profile. Aspirin may also be contraindicated in a 45-year-old man who has no strong risk factors for cardiovascular disease but suffered a gastrointestinal hemorrhage three years earlier that was severe enough to require blood transfusion.

Cost Effectiveness

Aspirin is a readily available, low-cost drug, whose cost effectiveness in preventing occlusive vascular events compares very favorably with other pharmacologic interventions (Hennekens 1994). This is particularly true in the setting of acute MI, where the risk of fatal and nonfatal vascular events is greatest. Aspirin costs about a penny per standard 325-mg tablet, so the cost of a 30-day course of treatment following acute MI is about 30 cents. In contrast, thrombolytic therapy ranges in cost from about $300 for streptokinase—the lowest priced fibrinolytic agent—to $2,200 for tissue plasminogen activator (tPA). Thus, while aspirin and thrombolytics confer similar mortality reductions of about 25% in acute MI, the cost of aspirin is a tiny fraction of that for thrombolytic drugs, and it has a far greater safety profile than the clot-dissolving drugs. The regular use of aspirin in acute MI would cost just $13 per life saved (Hennekens 1994).

Even in long-term use in secondary prevention, or, where deemed appropriate, in primary prevention, daily aspirin costs less than $5 per year, a remarkably low-cost preventive therapy in this time of increasing concern over the costs of health care. In secondary prevention, among patients with prior MI, stroke, or TIA, aspirin treatment of 1,000 patients for two to three years will prevent about 12 deaths and 32 nonfatal vascular events (Antiplatelet Trialists' Collaboration 1994). At a cost of approximately $10 for two to three years of daily treatment, the costs of secondary prevention with aspirin are roughly $830 per life saved and $310 for each nonfatal vascular event averted. Among patients at somewhat lower, but still substantially elevated risk, such as those with chronic stable angina or peripheral vascular disease, two years of aspirin therapy would be expected to prevent approximately 10 deaths and 20 nonfatal vascular events for every 1,000 patients treated.

In primary prevention, the combined results of the trials in U.S. and British male physicians indicate that five nonfatal MIs will be prevented per 1,000 patients treated over a five-year period (Antiplatelet Trialists' Collaboration 1994). Thus, one nonfatal MI would be prevented per year among 1,000 patients, at a cost of $3,650 per infarct prevented. This is significantly less than the average hospital cost of treating a nonfatal infarction and compares very favorably to the cost effectiveness of other interventions, such as treatment of hypertension. Further, because these figures derive from trials of unusually healthy subjects, who were not selected for study based on predisposing cardiovascular risk factors, the targeted use of aspirin in clinical practice among patients considered at elevated risk would be expected to yield greater absolute reductions in MI and, as a result, have an even more favorable cost-effectiveness profile.

Summary

Quality of available data: Data on primary prevention are derived from two large, well-designed randomized trials.

Estimated risk reduction: Low-dose aspirin is associated with a 30–35% reduction in risk of MI.

Comparability of effect in men and women: Randomized trial data in primary prevention currently include only men; a large, randomized trial of prophylactic aspirin among women is currently ongoing. Benefits of aspirin in secondary prevention appear comparable in men and women.

References

Antiplatelet Trialists' Collaboration. Secondary prevention of vascular disease by prolonged anti-platelet therapy. Br Med J 1988;296:320–32.

Antiplatelet Trialists' Collaboration. Collaborative overview of randomized trials of antiplatelet treatment. Part I: Prevention of vascular death, myocardial infarction and stroke by prolonged antiplatelet therapy in different categories of patients. Br Med J 1994;308: 81–106.

Aspirin for TIA's. FDA Drug Bull 1980;10:2.

Aspirin for heart patients. FDA Drug Bull 1985;15:34–6.

Boston Collaborative Drug Surveillance Group. Regular aspirin intake and acute myocardial infarction. Br Med J 1974;1:440–3.

Buring JE, Hennekens CH, for the Women's Health Study Research Group. The Women's Health Study: summary of the study design. J Myocardial Ischemia 1992;4:27–9.

Buring JE, Hennekens CH, for the Women's Health Study Research Group. Women's Health Study: rationale and background. J Myocardial Ischemia 1992; 4:30–40.

Clarke RJ, Mayo G, Price P, FitzGerald GA. Suppression of thromboxane A2 but not of systemic prostacyclin by controlled-release aspirin. N Engl J Med 1991;325:1137–41.

Collins R, Peto R, MacMahon S, et al. Blood pressure, stroke, and coronary heart disease. Part 2, Short-term reductions in blood pressure: Overview of randomized drug trials in their epidemiological context. Lancet 1990: 335:827–38.

Hammond EC, Garfinkel L. Aspirin and coronary heart disease: findings of a prospective study. Br Med J 1975;2:269–71.

Hennekens CH, Karlson LK, Rosner B. A case-control study of regular aspirin use and coronary deaths. Circulation 1978;58:35–8.

Hennekens CH, Buring JE, Mayrent S. Smoking, aging and coronary heart disease. In: Bosse R, ed. Smoking and Aging, Lexington, MA: DC Heath, 1984.

Hennekens CH, Eberlein K. A randomized trial of aspirin and beta-carotene among U.S. physicians. Prev Med 1985;14:165–8.

Hennekens CH, Buring JE. Epidemiology in medicine. Boston: Little, Brown, 1987.

Hennekens CH, Peto R. Hutchison GB, Doll R. An overview of the British and American aspirin studies. New England Journal of Medicine 1988;318:923–24.

Hennekens CH, Buring JE, Sandercock P, et al. Aspirin and other antiplatelet agents in the secondary and primary prevention of cardiovascular disease. Circulation 1989;80:749–56.

Hennekens CH, Jonas MA, Buring JE. The benefits of aspirin in acute myocardial infarction: still a well-kept secret in the U.S. Arch Int Med 1994;1:37–9.

ISIS-2 (Second International Study of Infarct Survival) Collaborative Group. Randomised trial of intravenous streptokinase, oral aspirin, both, or neither among 17,187 cases of suspected acute myocardial infarction: ISIS-2. Lancet 1988;2:349–60.

Jick H, Miettinen OS. Regular aspirin use and myocardial infarction. Br Med J 1976;1:1057.

Lamas GA, Pfeffer MA, Hamm P, et al. Do the results of randomized clinical trials of cardiovascular drugs influence medical practice? N Engl J Med 1992;327:241–7.

Manson JE, Stampfer MJ, Colditz GA, et al. A prospective study of aspirin use and primary prevention of cardiovascular disease in women. JAMA 1991;266:521–7.

Moncada S, Vanne JR. Arachidonic acid metabolites and the interactions between platelets and blood-vessel walls. N Engl J Med 1979;300:1142–7.

Paganini-Hill A. Chao A, Ross RF, Henderson BE. Aspirin use and chronic diseases: a cohort of the elderly. Br Med J 1989;299;1247–50.

Peto R, Yusuf S, Collins R. Cholesterol-lowering trial results in their epidemiologic context. Circulation 1985;72 (Suppl. III):451.

Peto R, Gray R, Collins R, et al. A randomised trial of the effects of prophylactic daily aspirin among male British doctors. Br Med J 1988;296:313–16.

Steering Committee of the Physicians' Health Study Research Group. Final report on the aspirin component of the ongoing Physicians' Health Study. N Engl J Med 1989;321:129–35.

UK-TIA Study Group. United Kingdom transient ischaemic attack (UK-TIA) aspirin trial interim results. Br Med J 1988;296:316–20.

US Preventive Services Task Force. Aspirin prophylaxis. In: Guide to clinical preventive services: report of the US Preventive Services Task Force. Baltimore, MD: Williams & Wilkins, 1989.

13

Natural Antioxidants

J. Michael Gaziano and Daniel Steinberg

The Role of Oxidation in Atherosclerosis

Current Concepts of Atherogenesis

Natural History of the Atherosclerotic Lesion. Atherosclerosis is an extremely complex, slowly developing chronic disease of the arteries. There is no longer any doubt that hypercholesterolemia is a major causative factor, a conclusion based on a wealth of experimental, clinical epidemiologic, and interventional data (Consensus Conference 1985). Over the past 10 to 15 years there has been a convergence of view with regard to the sequence of events that initiate atherosclerosis and how low density lipoprotein (LDL) plays a role (Ross 1976; Goode 1977; Steinberg 1983; Hansson 1989; Steinberg 1989 Ross 1993) (see Chapter 2.

The first phase of atherogenesis is the development of the fatty streak, which consists of a large number of lipid-loaded cells ("foam cells") lying beneath an intact layer of endothelial cells. Most of the "foam cells" are now known to derive from circulating monocytes that have penetrated between the endothelial cells and taken up residence in the intima. Histochemical studies utilizing monoclonal antibodies specific for monocyte/macrophage protein leave no doubt that most of the foam cells are monocyte-derived, but a few represent smooth muscle cells that have migrated into the intima and taken up lipids. The only other cell type unequivocally identified in atherosclerotic lesions is the T lymphocyte (Hansson 1989).

The second phase of atherogenesis is the conversion of the fatty streak to the fibrous plaque. Experimental and clinical studies, including the recent PDAY Study (Pathological Determinants of Atherosclerosis in Youth Research Group 1993), show that the fatty streak is almost always a necessary precursor of the fibrous plaque. The latter is characterized by the accumulation of connective tissue matrix, the multiplication of smooth muscle cells and the development of a thin layer of connective tissue matrix overlying the lipid-rich core of the lesion.

The third—and most clinically significant—phase of atherosclerosis is the development of the complex lesion. As originally pointed out by Constantinides (1966) and recently extended by the work of Davies and Wolf (1990), the terminal thrombosis

321

generally occurs at the site of a tear in the cap of the lesion, exposing blood to the proatherogenic materials that lie in the lipid core. In the following sections, we will primarily be discussing the role of oxidized LDL (Ox-LDL) in the initiation of atherogenesis (i.e., in the formation of the fatty streak lesion). However, there are a good number of macrophages (and T lymphocytes) in even the most advanced lesions, and the oxidative potential of those macrophages and the proatherogenic effect of oxidized LDL may be relevant to plaque rupture and terminal thrombosis. For example, macrophages are prominent at the shoulders of complex lesions, and we know that these cells can secrete reactive oxygen species and a variety of lytic enzymes. It is easy to see how they could contribute to the thinning of the fibrous cap and to the rupture that sets the stage for a fatal thrombosis. However, hard evidence on this issue is not yet available.

Oxidatively Modified LDL and Foam Cell Formation. The role of LDL as an atherogenic lipoprotein has been well established since the mid-1970s. Brown and Goldstein first identified and described the LDL receptor and demonstrated that more than 70% of the LDL particles leaving the plasma compartment were taken up via that receptor (Brown 1986). However, patients who carry the homozygous form of familial hypercholesteremia and therefore lack LDL receptors, develop atherosclerosis and have lesions that are similar to those in patients with normal LDL receptors. Therefore, the LDL receptor cannot be the sole pathway for the massive accumulation of LDL cholesterol in developing lesions. Goldstein and colleagues (1979) showed that native LDL was not taken up fast enough by macrophages—the major source of foam cells in fatty streak lesions—to become foam cells, because the native LDL receptor downregulates as cholesterol accumulates.

Later studies revealed, however, that LDL could be taken up much more rapidly by macrophages after chemical acetylation. A specific receptor (the acetyl LDL receptor) was identified, and this receptor did not downregulate (Goldstein 1979). Similar chemical modifications could mimic acetylation (Mahley 1979; Fogelman 1980), but there was no evidence that any of these chemical modifications could occur in vivo. Subsequent studies by Henriksen and coworkers (1981) showed that when LDL is incubated with cultured endothelial cells, it is converted to a form that is recognized by the acetyl LDL receptor and that this form of modified LDL could cause cholesterol accumulation in macrophages. The modification of LDL in the presence of cultured endothelial cells, smooth muscle cells or monocyte/macrophages (Henriksen 1981; Cathcart 1985; Parthasarathy 1986; Heinecke 1987) is simply an oxidative process (Morel 1984; Steinbrecher 1984).

Atherogenic Properties of Oxidized LDL. The oxidative modification hypothesis for atherogenesis was originally based on the finding that oxidized LDL enhances foam cell formation. Very quickly, however, a number of additional proatherogenic properties of oxidized LDL were discovered, and the list is now up to more than 15. LDL is cytotoxic to cultured endothelial cells (Henriksen 1979; Jessler 1979) only after oxidative modification (Morel 1984). The cytotoxicity of LDL could provide one of the links between the endothelial injury hypothesis and the oxidative modification hypothesis (Steinberg 1988). An important early step in atherogenesis is the migration of monocytes from the plasma to the subendothelial space, where they will then become resident macrophages and ultimately fat-filled foam cells as they accumulate lipids. The adhesion of circulating monocytes to endothelium, the first step in this process, appears to be aided by the presence of Ox-LDL (Berliner 1990). Following adherence to the endothelium, Ox-LDL enhances migration of monocytes into the subendothelium (Quinn 1985a, 1985b, 1988). Since these discoveries, the many additional atherogenic properties of oxidized LDL have been characterized in detail (Cathcart 1985; Triau 1988; Ardlie 1989; Frostegard 1990; Hamilton 1990; Kugiyama 1990; Simon 1990). Many of these biologic effects are caused by LDL which has undergone only minimal amounts of oxidation (Berliner 1990; Cushing 1990; Rajavashisth 1990; Liao 1991). Which of these atherogenic properties are important in vivo has yet to be determined.

Evidence of Oxidative Modification of LDL In Vivo. Oxidized LDL has been extracted from arterial lesions (both human and rabbit) and characterized (Haberland 1988; Palinski 1989; Rosenfeld 1989; Yla-Herttuala 1989). Autoantibodies that recognize epitopes of oxidized LDL have been demonstrated in the plasma of rabbits and humans (Palinski 1989), implying that either oxidized LDL or something immunochemically closely related to it must be available to act as the antigen in vivo.

The Role of Antioxidants in the Inhibition of Atherosclerosis

Dietary Antioxidants in Humans. Dietary antioxidants represent one of a number of defenses against oxidative damage (Table 13-1). Vitamin C, vitamin E, and beta-carotene are among the most abundant and most widely studied. Vitamin E is a fat-soluble compound composed of the tocopherols and related tocotrienols found in vegetable oils, cereal grains, egg yolk, liver, milk fat, nuts, and green vegetables. Tocopherol, the major component of vitamin E, is the predominant antioxidant in circulating lipoproteins (Esterbauer 1992) and is a strong chain-breaking antioxidant. Carotenoids are found in high concentrations in many fresh fruits and vegetables such as carrots, squash, melons, spinach, and broccoli. Beta-carotene, the most abundant carotenoid, is a vitamin A precursor that can function as a singlet oxygen quencher and a lipid-soluble free radical scavenger (Foote 1970; Burton 1984). Vitamin C (ascorbic acid) is a water-soluble nutrient antioxidant found in many fruits and vegetables. Ascorbic acid is required for a number of biologic processes including collagen metabolism, catechol biosynthesis, and iron absorption. In addition, it can function as

Table 13.1. Natural Defense Mechanisms Against Oxidative Damage

Compartmentalization of oxidative metabolism
Binding of molecular oxygen and reactive species to proteins to prevent random oxidative reactions
Binding of transition metals (iron, copper, etc.) to transport and storage proteins to prevent involvement in free radical reactions
Enzymatic antioxidants (superoxide dismutase, catalase, glutathione peroxidase, etc.)
Nonenzymatic antioxidants (vitaman C, vitamin E, beta-carotene, urate, bilirubin, ubiquinols, etc.)
Mechanisms to repair or dispose of damaged DNA, proteins, lipids, carbohydrates

a water-soluble antioxidant (Frei 1991). Vitamin C has been shown to scavenge peroxyl radicals (Niki 1983; Frei 1991) and superoxide radicals (Som 1983). It represents a water-soluble defense against oxidation of intra- and extracellular biomolecules.

Vitamin E clearly inhibits oxidation of LDL by cells in culture (Steinbrecher 1984); by copper ions when added to isolated LDL (Esterbauer 1992); and by either cultured cells or copper when LDL is purified from plasma of human subjects taking supplemental vitamin E (Esterbauer 1992; Princen 1992; Reaven 1993). Addition of vitamin C to an isolated preparation of LDL in vivo strongly inhibits copper-catalyzed oxidation (Esterbauer 1992; Frei 1993). Vitamin C, being hydrophilic, cannot enter the LDL particle to any extent, but it can act at the surface to regenerate vitamin E that has undergone oxidation (Constantinescu 1993). Thus, maintenance of a high plasma level of vitamin C would be a way to extend the protection afforded by any given level of vitamin E.

The situation with respect to beta-carotene is unclear. Beta-carotene is a good trapping agent for singlet oxygen but has limited potency as a conventional antioxidant. Jialal and colleagues (1991) reported that addition of beta-carotene to LDL in vitro increased its resistance to oxidation. In contrast, a number of investigations (Princen 1992; Reaven 1993; Gaziano 1995a found that LDL from human subjects fed large supplements of beta-carotene (enough to raise plasma levels more than 10-fold) showed no protection against copper-catalyzed or cell-induced oxidation. In view of these findings as well as the protective effect of beta-carotene against coronary heart disease (CHD) observed in some of the studies outlined below, we need to consider that the site of action of beta-carotene may lie elsewhere. Indeed, there is some evidence that carotenoids accumulate in the atherosclerotic lesion (Prince 1988), and that endothelial cells that have taken up beta-carotene are less effective in oxidizing LDL (Navab 1991). Beta-carotene (and vitamin E also) can prevent the endothelial dysfunction that occurs in cholesterol-fed rabbits (Keaney 1993). The normal vasodilatory response in these animals is lost when they are made hypercholesterolemic; there may even be a paradoxical vasoconstriction in response to acetylcholine. This failure to respond to endothelial-derived relaxation factor has been attributed to oxidatively modified LDL (Bossaller 1987), so that the protective effect of beta-carotene or vitamin E may reflect their antioxidant potential in vivo.

Finally, oxidants may act to inhibit platelet aggregation and modulate the synthesis of clotting factors. Vitamin E appears to be a potent inhibitor of platelet aggregation after in vitro and in vivo supplementation (Steiner and Anastasi 1976; Gisinger 1988). Intravenous administration of alpha-tocopherol inhibited coronary thrombosis under experimental conditions in the dog (Oda 1993). Alpha-tocopherol may form a quinone which is a weak competitive inhibitor of vitamin K (Wooley 1945). The clinical implications of these potential effects of antioxidants remains uncertain.

Effectiveness of Antioxidants as Antiatherogenic Agents in Animal Model Studies. If the hypothesis that oxidative modification of LDL plays a significant role in atherogenesis is correct, then use of an antioxidant at the right dose in the right experimental animal could slow the rate of progression of the disease. That indeed appears to be the case. There are now a number of published studies in various animal models, using several different antioxidants, and most have been positive. Table 13.2 sum-

Table 13.2. Effectiveness of Antioxidants in Experimental Atherosclerosis

Animal Model Used	Antioxidant Used	Approximate Percentage Inhibition of Lesion Formation	Reference	Comments
LDL receptor-deficient rabbit	Probucol	50	Carew et al. 1987	Drug started at weaning and continued 7–8 months
		80	Kita et al. 1987	Drug started at 8 weeks and continued for 6 months
LDL receptor-deficient rabbit (regression study)	Probucol	No regression; arrest of progression	Daugherty et al. 1991	Drug started at age 9 months and continued 6 months
Cholesterol-fed rabbit	Probucol	No effect 75	Stein et al. 1989 Daugherty et al. 1989	No clear explanation for different results
	Butylated hydroxytoluene	70	Björkhem et al. 1991	Plasma cholesterol higher in drug-fed group
	N,N'-diphenylphenylenediamine	71	Sparrow et al. 1992	No drop in plasma cholesterol
	Vitamin E	70	Prasad and Kalra 1993	40 mg/kg/d vitamin E; no change in plasma cholesterol
Cholesterol-fed macaques	Vitamin E	35	Verlangieri and Bush 1992	Small numbers of animals
	Probucol	50	Sasahara et al. 1994	Effect only in thoracic-aorta

325

marizes these studies, indicating the animal model, the antioxidant used, and the approximate percentage inhibition of lesion progression obtained.

The first animal studies were carried out using LDL receptor-deficient rabbits as the animal model and treating them with probucol, a cholesterol-lowering agent, as the antioxidant (Carew 1987; Kita 1987). Among animals treated for about 7 months compared with controls given lovastatin (to ensure comparable cholesterol reduction), the extent of atherosclerosis was reduced by 50% in the probucol-treated animals. In a similar study (Kita 1987), the percentage inhibition was even more dramatic (80%), although there was some difference in the cholesterol levels in the two groups. As seen in Table 13.1, several different antioxidant compounds have been used, including probucol, butylated hydroxytoluene, N,N'-diphenylphenylenediamine, and vitamin E. All these compounds have in common their ability to protect LDL against oxidative modification. The possibility that they share, in addition, other properties that make them antiatherogenic seems slim but cannot be completely ruled out. There was only one negative study (Stein 1989), using probucol in cholesterol-fed rabbits. With a very similar protocol, however, Daugherty and colleagues (1989) observed a very significant inhibition of atherogenesis in cholesterol-fed rabbits using probucol. The reason for the different results from these two studies has not been determined.

The overall consistency of these results in LDL receptor-deficient rabbits, in cholesterol-fed rabbits, and in cholesterol-fed monkeys makes a very strong case that oxidative modification of LDL plays a significant role in fatty streak formation. It is noteworthy that in these animal models, plasma cholesterol levels have ranged from 600 to 2,000 mg/dl, constituting a powerful proatherogenic lipoprotein pattern, in view of which the ability of these compounds to inhibit by anywhere from 35% to 80% is impressive. However, several qualifying points need to be kept in mind. First, it is critically important to note that in all of these animal models the lesions studied are almost exclusively at the fatty streak stage; that is, the very earliest stage in atherogenesis. In most of the experiments, the animals have been started on treatment at a very early age and only the very earliest stages in lesion development have been dealt with.

The second point is that the studies in experimental animals have not, for the most part, utilized natural antioxidants, but rather antioxidant drugs, primarily probucol. The one vitamin E trial in monkeys (Verlangieri 1992) involved a very small number of animals, and because of deaths in some of the groups the published data are weak and need to be extended. A few vitamin E trials in rabbits have given conflicting results, in part because vitamin E in some studies lowered cholesterol levels. However, in the recent positive study by Prasad and Kalra (1993) the plasma cholesterol levels were not affected by the vitamin E. Still, we do need additional trials of the natural antioxidants in experimental animals as a guide to what we can hope to accomplish in clinical intervention trials.

Epidemiologic Data on Antioxidants and Risk of Atherosclerosis

Establishing causal relationships in human disease is much more difficult than it is in animal models. A number of researchers, using different methodologies, have provided evidence on the possible role of dietary antioxidants in the prevention of cardiovascular disease (CVD) in humans (Gaziano 1992; 1994a). In the remainder of this chapter, we review the data from descriptive and observational epidemiologic studies as well as randomized trials on the relationship between dietary antioxidants and CVD. We divide this section according to type of methodology (descriptive studies, case-control studies, prospective cohort studies, and randomized trials) and distinguish between studies of dietary intake, on the one hand, and studies of plasma, serum, and tissue levels of antioxidants, on the other.

Descriptive Studies

Population-based descriptive studies deal with characteristics of a population and their relationship to disease rates in that population over time (longitudinal studies) or in comparison with other populations (cross-cultural studies). Several descriptive studies have specifically looked at the role that dietary antioxidants may play in these different disease rates (Table 13.3). Antioxidant exposure has been assessed in terms of estimated intake of foods high in antioxidants for a given population or, alternatively, in terms of the mean plasma or serum level of antioxidant vitamins among randomly selected individuals from a given population. The value of these studies is in the generation of hypotheses that can then be tested with more analytic epidemiologic methodologies such as case-control and prospective cohort studies. The weakness of descriptive studies derives from their inability to control for a large number of potential factors (genetics, other dietary or lifestyle characteristics, availability of health care resources, etc.) that may confound any apparent association.

Dietary Intake Studies. Several descriptive studies have shown an inverse correlation of per capita consumption of fresh fruits and vegetables with population CVD rates. Verlangieri and associates (1985) demonstrated that declining CVD mortality rates in the United States from 1964 to 1978 are inversely correlated with daily per capita fresh fruit and vegetable consumption. Ginter (1979) found a similar inverse relationship of vitamin C supplement intake and U.S. CVD mortality rates. In Israel, as the nation industrialized from 1949 to 1977, CVD mortality rose steadily (Palgy 1981). Specifically, as life expectancy increased from 67.9 years to 73.7 years, there was a rise in ischemic heart and cerebrovascular disease mortality rates, which were highly correlated with increases in fat and meat consumption. Over the same period, an inverse association was found between rates of consumption of vitamin A derived largely from fruit and vegetable sources and changing rates of ischemic heart and cerebrovascular disease mortality rates, after control for other dietary factors. This measure of vitamin A status is also a good marker of carotenoid intake.

Armstrong and associates (1975) reported a strong inverse association of regional consumption of fresh fruits and vegetables with death rates from ischemic heart disease in nine regions in England, Wales, and Scotland (correlation coefficient, $r^2 = -.83$ for men [$p < .05$] and -0.91 for women [$p < .05$]). Finally, the regional consumption of fresh fruits and vegetables was inversely associated with regional cerebrovascular disease mortality rates in a second British study using a similar approach (Acheson and Williams 1983).

Table 13.3 Descriptive Studies of Natural Antioxidants and Population Cardiovascular Disease (CVD) Rates

Reference	Population(s) Studied (Design)	Exposure	Findings
Dietary Intake Studies			
Verlangieri et al. 1985	United States (longitudinal)	Per capita fresh fruits and vegetable consumption	Inverse association with CVD mortality rates
Ginter 1979	United States	Per capita vitamin C production	Inverse association with CVD mortality rates
Plagy 1981	Israel	Per capita vitamin A consumption from fruits and vegetables	Inverse association with CVD mortality rates
Armstrong et al. 1975	9 regions in the United Kingdom	Per capita fruit and vegetable consumption	Inverse association with ischemic heart disease mortality rates
Acheson and Williams 1983	11 regions in the United Kingdom	Per capita fruit and vegetable consumption	Inverse association cerebrovascular disease mortality rates
Blood-Based Studies			
Gey et al. 1987a, 1987b, 1989, 1991	16 European regions	Mean plasma vitamin levels	Inverse association with CVD mortality rates for vitamin E
Riemersma et al. 1990	4 European regions	Mean plasma vitamin levels	Trend toward an inverse association with CVD mortality rates for vitamin E

328

Blood-Based Studies. An alternative to assessing antioxidant status of a population by evaluating fruit and vegetable intake is directly to measure levels of the antioxidants in plasma or serum from a random sample of subjects in a given population. Great care must be taken in handling the samples, since exposure to heat or light or delay in analysis will result in decay of natural antioxidants, particularly vitamin C.

As part of a World Health Organization's MONICA Project, plasma samples were obtained from a random sample of approximately 100 individuals from each of 16 European populations. Gey and associates (1987a, 1987b, 1989, 1991) found that lipid-standardized alpha-tocopherol levels were inversely associated with population ischemic heart disease mortality rates (r^2 = .62; p = .0003), while correlations for vitamin C and carotene were not significant. Using a similar methodology, Riemersma et al. (1990) found an apparent, but nonsignificant, inverse association between vitamin E intake and cardiovascular mortality in four European populations. In this study, cholesterol-adjusted vitamin E levels were lower in the three regions where ischemic heart disease rates were high (southwest Finland, north Karelia, and Scotland) compared with that in Italy, where ischemic heart disease rates are low.

These descriptive studies clearly document interesting trends across populations and within populations over time, particularly with regard to the apparent benefit of fresh fruit and vegetable consumption. However, it is not clear whether the observed trends are due specifically to the intake of dietary antioxidants, as the potential for confounding in these studies is great. It is possible that consumption of fresh fruits and vegetables is protective not because of the antioxidant content of these foods but because of some other substance. Alternatively, the value of consumption of fresh fruits and vegetables may be the result of substitution for and, therefore, reduction in dietary animal fat intake. Finally, fresh fruit and vegetable consumption may merely be a marker for other lifestyle factors which are associated with reduced risk of CVD, such as exercise or decreased rate of smoking.

Case-Control Studies

In contrast to descriptive studies in which only information on a population is collected, in case-control studies, researchers collect information from individuals and therefore attempt to adjust for a wide variety of potential confounders. While there are no case-control studies of dietary intake of antioxidants and CVD, there are several investigations assessing plasma or tissue antioxidant levels (Table 13.4). Two such studies reported significant inverse associations of heart disease with plasma antioxidant level. Riemersma and colleagues (1989, 1991) compared plasma antioxidant levels in patients with angina pectoris with those in healthy controls. Vitamin C, lipid-standardized vitamin E, and beta-carotene levels were significantly lower among cases compared with controls (p = .01, .01, and .001, respectively). The odds ratio for angina between the lowest and highest quintiles of lipid standardized vitamin E level was 2.98 (95% CI: 1.07–6.70) after multivariate adjustment. There were similar trends for vitamin C and beta-carotene; however, adjustment for cigarette smoking significantly attenuated these relationships (odds ratio: 1.63 [0.76–3.49] for vitamin C and 1.41 [0.63–3.13] for beta-carotene). While it is crucial to control for cigarette smoking as an important coronary risk factor, smoking is associated with lower plasma antioxidant

Table 13.4. Case-Control Studies of Natural Antioxidants and Cardiovascular Disease

Reference	Cases and Controls	Exposure	Findings
Riemersma et al. 1989, 1991	110 cases of angina pectoris identified by questionnaire; 394 controls without evidence of angina pectoris	Plasma levels vitamins A, C and E, and β-carotene	Significantly lower vitamin E levels and trends for vitamin C and β-carotene among cases
Ramirez and Flowers. 1980	101 cases of angiographically proven coronary artery disease; 49 controls with normal coronary angiograms	Leukocyte ascorbic acid level	Significantly lower leukocyte ascorbic acid levels in cases
Kardinaal et al. 1993	683 cases of myocardial infarction from 12 European sites; 727 hospital-based controls	Levels of β-carotene and vitamin E in adipose tissue	Significantly lower tissue β-carotene levels in cases and no association for vitamin E

levels. This reduction in antioxidant levels may be at least partially responsible for the coronary risk associated with smoking or smoking may independently increase CVD risk and decrease antioxidant levels. There was no apparent relationship for vitamin A.

Several other case-control studies are worth mentioning. Leukocyte ascorbic acid levels (which may be more stable and more representative of total body ascorbic acid than plasma levels) were significantly lower among those with antiographically documented coronary disease compared with controls ($p < .001$) (Ramirez 1980). In the Scottish Heart Disease study, beta-carotene, vitamin C, and vitamin E intakes were significantly lower among men with previously undiagnosed CHD, while similar though not statistically significant trends were apparent for women (Bolton-Smith 1992). In the Edinburg Artery Study, dietary vitamin E intake was inversely associated with degree of peripheral artery disease independent of smoking effect, while vitamin C was inversely associated among nonsmokers (Donnan 1993).

In a recent case-control study, adipose tissue levels of alpha-tocopherol and beta-carotene were determined in 683 cases of myocardial infarction (MI) and 727 hospital-based controls at 12 sites in Europe and Israel (Kardinaal 1993). Mean adipose levels of beta-carotene were 0.35 μg/g in cases and 0.42 μg/g in controls, while alpha-tocopherol levels were 193 and 192 μg/g for cases and controls, respectively. For beta-carotene the multivariate odds ratio in the lowest quintile of beta-carotene compared with the highest was 1.78 (95% CI = 1.17–2.71) after controlling for a number of potential confounders, with a significant trend across quintiles (p for trend = .001). The associations were strongest among current and ex-smokers. In contrast, there was no apparent increased risk with low alpha-tocopherol levels, with an odds ratio of MI in the lowest compared with the highest category of 0.83 (95% CI: .57 .57–1.21) and no significant trend of alpha-tocopherol tissue levels (p for trend = .27).

In summary, these case-control studies suggest that plasma or tissue antioxidant levels are lower among those with CVD; however, it is difficult to infer causal relationships from these data due to the several inherent weakness of this methodology. Although case-control studies are often efficient and inexpensive (particularly when compared with prospective cohort studies), selection and recall bias as well as change in dietary habits after disease onset may have an impact on risk estimates, since exposure status is ascertained after disease occurrence.

Prospective Cohort Studies

Like case-control studies, prospective cohort studies are less subject to the biases of descriptive studies because exposure data are available for each individual in the study population, thus enabling control for potential confounders. Furthermore, in contrast to case-control studies, in prospective studies the exposure is measured prior to the development of disease, thus minimizing the impact of recall and selection bias, as well as reducing the effects that the disease may have on the exposure, that is, dietary habits or blood antioxidant levels.

Dietary Intake Studies. Several prospective cohort studies have examined the role of dietary intake of antioxidants in relation to subsequent CVD (Table 13.5). The com-

Table 13.5. Prospective Cohort Studies of Intake of Natural Antioxidants and Cardiovascular Disease

References	Study Population	Follow-up Period	Exposure	Endpoint (number)	Findings
Manson et al. 1991, 1992, 1993a, 1993b; Stampfer et al. 1993	89,000 healthy U.S. female nurses	8 years	Vitamins C and E and β-carotene intake from food questionnaire	Coronary heart disease (CHD) (552) ischemic stroke (183)	Inverse association for vitamin E and β-carotene for CHD and stroke; no association for vitamin C.
Rimm et al. 1993	39,000 healthy U.S. male health professionals	4 years	Vitamina C and E and β-carotene intake from food questionnaire	Coronary heart disease (667)	Inverse association for vitamin E and β-carotene; no association for vitamin C.
Enstrom et al. 1992	11,349 U.S. men and women	10 years	Vitamin C intake from food questionnaire	Cardiovascular mortality (929)	Inverse association
Gaziano et al. 1996	1,299 Elderly Massachusetts men and women	5 years	B-carotene score derived from consumption of carotenoid-containing fruits and vegetables	Cardiovascular mortality (151)	Inverse association
Vollset and Bjelke 1983	16,713 Finnish postal workers	11 years	Vitamin C from fruit and vegetable intake	CVD mortality (438)	Inverse association
Lapidus et al. 1986	1,462 Swedish women	12 years	Vitamin C intake from 24-hour diet recall	Myocardial infarction (28) and stroke (13)	No association

monly used methods to assess dietary intake include food diaries or retrospective questionnaires. The food diary involves recording the amount and specific type of everything ingested over several (usually three to seven) days. Questionnaires can be utilized to estimate intake retrospectively. A 24-hour recall questionnaire is used to record dietary intake from the preceding day. This assumes that the subject's recall is accurate and that the preceding 24-hour period is representative of his or her average daily intake. An alternative to the 24-hour recall is a semiquantitative food frequency questionnaire, which inquires about a subject's usual frequency of consuming certain foods on average over the period of several months or a year.

THE NURSES' HEALTH STUDY. The largest prospective dietary intake study to date is the Nurses' Health Study (NHS), examining the relationship of dietary antioxidants with CVD. Researchers with the NHS have followed a cohort of 121,000 U.S. female nurses aged 30–55 at the beginning of this study since 1976 (Manson 1991, 1992a, 1992b, 1993; Stampfer 1993). Biennial questionaires have elicited information about a wide variety of demographic, behavioral, and medical risk factors for CVD. In 1980 and 1984, semiquantitative food frequency questionnaires also asked for data on food intake patterns and supplemental vitamin use. Detailed descriptions of the 61-item 1980 questionnaire and the expanded 116-item 1984 dietary questionnaires, as well as documentation of their reproducibility and validity, have been published (Willett 1985; Salvini 1989). Intake scores were computed by multiplying the frequency of consumption of each unit of food by the nutrient content of the specified portions. Composition values for vitamins were obtained from the U.S. Department of Agriculture and other published sources (Adams 1975; Consumer and Food Economics Institute 1982). Vitamin intake was adjusted for total energy intake (Willett 1986).

The semiquantitative food frequency questionnaire has been extensively validated (Willett 1983; 1985; Stryker 1988; Salvini 1989). Antioxidant micronutrient intakes assessed by food frequency questionnaires correlated well with estimates from food diaries (with r values ranging from .36 to .76) (Willett 1985) and with plasma levels of these nutrients (with r values ranging from .34 to .52) (Willett 1983; Stryker 1988). Correlations substantially less than 1.0 have the impact of attenuating any true relationship that may exist between antioxidant status and CVD. Thus, any estimate of association may underestimate the true relationship.

During 8 years of follow-up in the NHS (671,185 person-years), there were 552 coronary events, including 115 deaths and 437 nonfatal MIs. Women in the highest quintile beta-carotene consumption had a multivariate relative risk (RR) of 0.78 (95% CI: 0.59–1.03; p for trend across quintiles = .02) when compared with women in the lowest quintile after adjustment for age, smoking, and other cardiovascular risk factors. For vitamin E the RR was 0.66 (95% CI: 0.50–0.87) in the highest intake quintile compared with the lowest (p for trend = .001); this association was largely attributed to vitamin E supplementation rather than dietary intake. There was an apparent, though not significant, reduction in risk for the highest intake category of vitamin C (RR = 0.80; 95% CI: 0.58–1.10), and there was no significant trend across quintiles (p for trend = .15) after controlling for vitamin E intake, which was highly correlated with vitamin C consumption. When the intakes of beta-carotene, vitamin E, vitamin C as well as riboflavin were combined into a total antioxidant score by adding the quintile score (1 to 5) for each micronutrient, the RR for coronary disease was 0.54 (95% CI: 0.40–0.73) among those in the highest quintile compared with the lowest (*p* for trend = .001).

In addition to heart disease, the NHS investigated correlations between dietary antioxidants and stroke. During the eight years of follow-up there were 183 ischemic strokes. Among women in the highest quintile of intake (foods plus supplements) compared with those in the lowest, the multivariate RR of ischemic stroke was 0.75 (95% CI: 0.48–1.17) for vitamin C, 0.76 (95% CI: 0.49–1.20) for vitamin E and 0.61 (95% CI: 0.39–0.98) for beta-carotene. For increasing quintiles of a total antioxidant vitamin score, the RRs were 1.0 (referent), 0.93, 0.71, 0.62, 0.46 (*p* for trend = .01) after adjustment for other risk factors.

In the above-mentioned analyses, those with preexisting vascular disease were excluded because the presence of disease may have a significant impact on dietary habits. In a separate analysis of 1,795 subjects with prior CVD, trends similar to those reported above were apparent for subsequent vascular events. Among those in the highest quintile of antioxidant vitamin score, compared with the lowest, the RR was 0.67 (95% CI: 0.36–1.23) for MI and 0.29 (95% CI: 0.09–0.98) for stroke (Manson 1993).

THE HEALTH PROFESSIONALS' FOLLOW-UP STUDY. The Health Professionals' Follow-up Study (HPFS) is a recent prospective cohort study of male dentists, pharmacists, and veterinarians, which has examined dietary antioxidant intake and risk of subsequent CHD during four years of follow-up using methodology identical to that used in the NHS (Rimm 1993). Of approximately 39,000 men who had no history of CVD or other conditions that would have necessitated dietary changes, there were 667 major coronary events (revascularizations, nonfatal MI, and fatal MIs). For beta-carotene, compared with men in the lowest quintile, those in the highest had a RR of 0.75 (95% CI: 0.57–0.99; *p* for trend = .04). Men in the highest quintile of vitamin E consumption had a relative risk of 0.68 (95% CI: 0.51–0.90; *p* for trend = .01) when compared with men in the lowest quintile. Vitamin C intake was not significantly related to risk reduction in this study (*p* for trend = .10).

THE NATIONAL HEALTH AND NUTRITION EXAMINATION SURVEY-I. An observational study of 11,349 U.S. men and women aged 25–74 years, the first National Health and Nutrition Examination Survey (NHANES-I) study, examined vitamin C intake using both food frequency and 24-hour recall questionnaires (Enstrom 1992). Participants were followed for a median period of ten years. Mortality data obtained from death certificates were available for 97% of the men and 94% of the women who died. Cardiovascular rates were 34% lower than expected (RR = 0.66, 95% CI: 0.53–0.82) among participants with the highest vitamin C intake, defined as 50 mg or more from the diet plus regular supplements. One potential limitation of this study was the inability to examine and control for the possible correlation of vitamin C with other vitamin supplementation.

THE MASSACHUSETTS ELDERLY COHORT STUDY. The Massachusetts Elderly Cohort Study also examined dietary information, obtained through in-person interviews (Gaziano 1995b.) The 1,299 participants were followed for an average of 4.75 years through annual mailings, and were interviewed in 1976 and again in 1980. During the follow-up period, 151 died from CVD; 47 of these were from fatal MIs, and the remaining 104 were due to other forms of heart disease, including sudden death and congestive heart failure. The relative risks of cardiovascular death from lowest to highest quartile of beta-carotene intake were 1.00 (referent), 0.75, 0.65, and 0.57, respectively (*p* for trend = .016), after controlling for confounders including age, sex, smoking, alcohol consumption, cholesterol intake, and level of physical functioning. The corresponding relative risks for fatal MI are 1.00 (referent), 0.77, 0.59, 0.32 (*p* for trend = .02). One major problem of this study was the inability to control for several known coronary risk factors such as hypertension and diabetes mellitus. Intake of other antioxidants could not be easily estimated given the brevity of the 41-item questionnaire.

OTHER PROSPECTIVE DIETARY INTAKE STUDIES. Three other dietary studies are worth mentioning. Vollset and Bjelke (1983) reported an inverse association of vitamin C index with cerebrovascular disease mortality rates in a study of 16,713 postal workers who responded to periodic dietary surveys over 11 years of follow-up. Vitamin C index was estimated from fruit and vegetable intake obtained from periodic food questionnaires. In a prospective cohort of 1,462 Swedish women, estimates of vitamin C intake from a 24-hour recall dietary history were not correlated with cardiovascular mortality after 12 years of follow-up after controlling for age (Lapidus 1986). Dietary intake by 24-hour recall may correlate poorly with estimates of average consumption of micronutrients assessed by food diary or food frequency questionnaire. In addition, statistical power to detect small to moderate associations may be lacking because of small sample size. There is no mention of relationship for other antioxidants in these two studies. Finally, in the Caerphilly Prospective Ischemic Heart Disease Study, there was an inverse association of dietary fiber from fruits and vegetables with subsequent ischemic heart disease and a trend for vitamin C (Fehily 1993).

Blood-Based Prospective Studies. There are two main strategies to assess prospectively plasma or serum antioxidant status: nested case-control design and baseline analysis of all samples. In a nested case-control study, blood samples are obtained from a large cohort at the onset of an investigation, and plasma or serum samples are frozen and stored during the follow-up period. At the end of the study or at a point when enough endpoints have accumulated, cases are matched with appropriate controls selected from the remaining disease-free population. Case and control plasma or serum samples are analyzed, and the measured parameters are then compared between cases and controls. The advantage of this strategy is cost-efficiency because only those samples of interest are analyzed. The downside of this strategy is that the particular biochemical parameter of interest may not be stable over time even at subzero temperatures, resulting in levels at the time of measurement that do not accurately reflect baseline values. For example, vitamin C levels are quite unstable and are difficult to measure in stored plasma. An alternative is to measure the biochemical parameter of interest for all subjects at the beginning of the study. While the potential problem of decay can be avoided using this strategy, this costly approach often limits the size of the cohort in question. Results from both types of blood studies are summaried in Table 13.6.

In three nested case-control studies, plasma or serum samples were collected and frozen at baseline. Subjects who later developed CVD were matched with healthy controls, and their baseline blood samples were compared. Street and associates (1991) found a significant inverse association between baseline plasma beta-carotene levels and risk of subsequent MI among 125 incident cases and 125 community- and 125 hospital-based matched controls. Plasma samples in this study had been frozen at $-70°C$ for up to 15 years.

Two other nested case-control studies examined the relationship between serum vitamin A and vitamin E levels and cardiovascular mortality. Kok et al. (1987) compared vitamin A and E levels in sera frozen at $-20°C$ for 6 to 9 years among 84 subjects who died from CVD and 168 age and sex-matched controls. While there was a trend toward increased risk for those with low levels of vitamins A and E, findings were not statistically significant. Specifically, those in the lowest quintile of serum vitamin A had RR = 1.2 (95% CI: 0.6–2.4) compared with those with higher levels and for vitamin E the RR was 1.5 (95% CI: 0.6–3.5). This study lacked statistical power to detect small to moderate effects. Salonen and coworkers (1985) also reported no association between serum vitamin A or E levels and CVD mortality among 92 cases and 92 controls from a cohort of 12,000 men and women. In both these studies serum samples had been stored for over five years at $-20°C$. The early handling of blood samples as well as prolonged storage may have resulted in considerable decay of antioxidants such as vitamin E. Vitamin A is not a powerful antioxidant, and while dietary intake of vitamin A from fruit and vegetable sources is correlated with carotenoid intake, serum vitamin A levels may not accurately reflect an individual's beta-carotene status. For this reason, vitamin A levels in these cohorts may not accurately represent their antioxidant status.

Three studies measured plasma antioxidants levels at baseline for the entire cohort. The Basel Prospective Study measured baseline plasma antioxidants and followed a population of 2,974 middle-aged men (Eichholzer 1992; Gey 1993). An apparent, but not significant, increased risk of death from CHD was observed among those in the lowest quartiles of beta-carotene level (RR = 1.53; 95% CI: 1.07–2.20) and vitamin C level (RR = 1.25; 95% CI: 0.77–2.01) compared with those in the highest quartile. In addition, individuals with low plasma concentrations of both carotene and vitamin C had an elevated risk of ischemic heart disease mortality (RR = 1.96, 95% CI: 1.10–3.50). Results for cerebrovascular death in this study were similar, with substantially increased risks among those with both low beta-carotene and low vitamin C levels (RR = 4.17; 95% CI: 1.68–10.33). There was no apparent relationship of lipid-standardized vitamin E levels with heart disease or stroke death. These results for plasma vitamin E are not consistent with the data from the above-mentioned prospective dietary intake studies (Table 13.5). Gey (1993) suggested that this discrepancy may be due to the relatively high levels of alpha-tocopherol (median = 35 µmol/l) and relatively low variability (first quartile median = 31 µmol/l, last quartile median = 39 µmol/l) in the Basel Study. In contrast, it could be argued that the levels could have been too low to see an effect, since in both the NHS and HPFS, benefit was largely confined to supplement takers, and supplement use was low in the Basel population.

Reference	Study Population	Follow-up	Exposure	Findings
Nested case-control				
Street et al. 1991	125 cases of myocardial infarction and 125 hospital and 125 community-matched controls among a cohort of 26,000 U.S. men and women	14 years	Plasma β-carotene levels in samples levels stored at −70°C	Significant inverse association
Kok et al. 1987	84 cases of cardiovascular disease and 168 matched controls nested in a cohort of 10,000 men and women	6–9 years	Serum levels of vitamin A and E in samples stored at −20°C	No association
Salonen et al. 1984	92 cases of cardiovascular death and 92 matched controls nested in a cohort of 12,000 men and women	5 years	Serum levels of vitamin A and E in samples stored at −20°C	Apparent but nonsignificant increased risk of low vitamin E status
Blood levels analyzed at baseline				
Eicholzer et al. 1992; Grey et al. 1993	Prospective cohort of 2974 middle-aged Swiss men followed for ischemic heart disease (IHD) and stroke	12 years	Plasma vitamins C and E and β-carotene on fresh samples	Significant inverse association for those with both low vitamin C and β-carotene for both IHD and stroke; no association with vitamin E for either IHD or stroke
Morris et al. 1993	Prospective cohort of 1800 subjects enrolled in lipid-lowering trial followed for development of myocardial infarction	14 years	Plasma carotenoid levels	Inverse association
Salonen et al. 1993	Prospective cohort of healthy men followed for the progression of carotid artery wall thickness via serial ultrasound	1 year	Plasma β-carotene and α-tocopherol levels	Inverse association for both α-tocopherol and β-carotene

337

Two additional studies merit mention. After 14 years of follow-up in the Lipid Research Clinic Coronary Primary Prevention Trial, baseline plasma carotenoid levels were inversely correlated with risk of MI after adjustment for age, smoking, HDL, and LDL (Morris 1993). Plasma beta-carotene and vitamin E levels were inversely related to progression of carotid artery wall thickness in the Kupio Ischemic Heart Disease Study (Salonen 1993).

Data from prospective dietary studies suggest a reduction in risk of subsequent cardiovascular events among those who consume higher levels of vitamin E, particularly from supplements, while plasma studies are less convincing concerning the relationship of vitamin E. With regard to beta-carotene, both blood-based and dietary intake studies suggest an inverse relationship, though dietary intake studies are less convincing than those of vitamin E. The apparent relationship of dietary beta-carotene with CVD risk does not include assessment of supplemental beta-carotene, since few subjects were taking beta-carotene supplements at the time these studies were conducted. Results on the association of dietary intake of vitamin C with subsequent CVD are conflicting, and blood-based data are limited because of the difficulty of measuring vitamin C.

Limitations of Observational Epidemiologic Data

While the data from descriptive, case-control and prospective cohort studies are compatible with a possible benefit of antioxidants against CVD, the available observational data are relatively sparse and not uniformly consistent. Additional observational data would certainly make a valuable contribution to the totality of evidence concerning antioxidants and CVD. However, observational investigations in general are limited in their ability to provide reliable data on the most plausible small to moderate benefits of antioxidants. It may be, for example, that greater dietary intake of antioxidants, measured by blood levels or a diet assessment questionnaire, is only a marker for some other dietary practice or even nondietary lifestyle variable that is truly protective. It is, in fact, plausible that intake of antioxidant-rich foods is indeed protective, but the benefit results not from their antioxidant properties, but some other component these foods have in common. In addition, the intakes of individual dietary antioxidants are often highly correlated with each other, making it difficult to determine the specific benefit of any one. For many hypotheses, randomized trials are neither necessary nor desirable; however, when searching for small to moderate effects, the amount of uncontrolled confounding inherent in observational studies may be as large as the likely risk reduction. For this reason data from large-scale randomized trials of adequate dose and duration will be vital in determining the relationship of antioxidant consumption with CVD.

Randomized Trials

Completed Trials. Only limited data from large trials are available on antioxidant use at this time (Table 13.7). Vitamin E has been tested in the treatment of claudication (atherosclerotic disease of the leg arteries) (Livingston 1958; Williams 1971; Haeger

Table 13.7. Completed Randomized, Double-Blind, Placebo-Controlled Trials of Antioxidants in the Treatment or Prevention of Cardiovascular Disease

Reference	Study Population	Treatment	Endpoints	Findings
Anderson et al. 1974	20 patients with angina pectoris	3,200 IU of vitamin E daily for 9 weeks	Angina pain score	Apparent but nonsignificant reduction
Gillilan et al. 1977	52 patients with angina pectoris	1,600 IU of vitamin E daily for 6 months	Exercise tolerance, left ventricular function	No significant improvement
Gaziano et al. 1990	333 male physicians with angina pectoris or bypass surgery	50 mg of synthetic β-carotene on alternate days for 5 years	Major coronary and vascular events	Significant reduction for both endpoints
DeMaio et al. 1992	100 patients following angioplasty	400 IU of vitamin E daily for four months	Restenosis by angiogram or exercise test	Nonsignificant trend toward reduction
Blot et al. 1993	29,000 healthy Chinese men and women at high risk for gastric cancer but at low risk for cardiovascular disease	Cocktail of β-carotene (15 mg), α-tocopherol (30 mg) and selenium (50 μg) daily for 5 years	Gastric cancer and cause specific mortality	Nonsignificant trend toward reduction
The ATBC Cancer Prevention Study Group, 1994	29,000 Finnish male smokers	Factorial design of 20 mg of synthetic β-carotene daily and 50 mg of synthetic α-tocopherol daily for 5 years	Lung cancer and cause specific mortality	No reduction for either antioxidant alone or in combination for CVD mortality

1974). While positive benefits of supplemental vitamin E were observed in each of these studies, cautious interpretation is required due to methodological problems, including small sample size, high dropout rates, and lack of blinding.

In the late 1940s several investigators tested the effects of vitamin E in the treatment of angina pectoris in poorly controlled trials, largely with no effect (Makinson 1948; Donegan 1949; Rinzler 1950). Two more recent trials have evaluated this hypothesis using randomization and double-blinding. There was a nonsignificant trend toward improved angina pain score in a nine-week placebo-controlled trial among stable angina patients consuming 3,200 IU of vitamin E daily compared with placebo (Anderson 1974). Gillilan et al. (1977) tested 1,600 IU of vitamin E daily for six months in a double-blind crossover trial of 52 angina pectoris patients, reporting no apparent benefit of vitamin E treatment as measured by exercise tolerance, symptoms of angina pectoris, or left ventricular function. These studies suggest no apparent benefit of short-term treatment with vitamin E; however, the short duration of treatment and small sample size may have limited the statistical power of these studies to detect small to moderate benefits.

The Physicians' Health Study is a randomized, double-blind, placebo-controlled trial of 22,071 U.S. male physicians aged 40 to 84 testing aspirin in the primary prevention of CVD and beta-carotene in the primary prevention of cancer. A subgroup analysis within the Physicians' Health Study was undertaken among 333 doctors who had a history of chronic stable angina pectoris or who had had a coronary revascularization procedure (defined as coronary bypass surgery or balloon angioplasty) prior to randomization (Gaziano 1990). In this subgroup analysis, two endpoints were defined: major coronary events, including coronary revascularization, fatal coronary disease, and nonfatal MI, and all major vascular events, which included these events as well as nonfatal and fatal stroke. Among subjects who received beta-carotene, there was a 51% reduction (RR = 0.49, 95% CI: 0.29–0.88) in risk of major coronary events, and a 54% reduction (RR = 0.46, 95% CI: 0.24–0.85) in risk of major vascular events. Furthermore, the effect of beta-carotene supplementation was time-dependent, consistent with the hypothesis that antioxidant intake slows the progression of atherosclerosis. Relative risk was analyzed by year of treatment, and there was no effect at the end of the first year, but a risk reduction did appear in the second year and persisted thereafter. However, because these data derive from a subgroup analysis, they cannot be considered a direct test of this hypothesis.

One recent study tested the effect of vitamin E supplementation on subsequent restenosis rates among 100 subjects following percutaneous transluminal coronary angioplasty (DeMaio 1992). For example, the fatty streak lesion develops under an intact endothelium, but angioplasty removes the endothelium completely. Subjects were treated with 400 IU of vitamin E daily following angioplasty. There was an apparent, though not statistically significant, 30% reduction in the risk of restenosis as measured by subsequent catheterization or exercise test. However, restenosis may involve some of the factors contributing to the initiation and progression of atherosclerotic lesion, but it is decidedly not the same process.

A recent large-scale randomized trial of vitamins in the prevention of cancer in Lanxian, China, reported a reduction in overall mortality among those consuming a mixture of beta-carotene (15 mg daily), alpha-tocopherol (30 mg daily), and selenium

(50 μg daily), a result largely due to a reduction in stomach cancer mortality (Blot 1993). Results for cardiovascular mortality were also assessed, although mortality from ischemic heart disease was less than 9% and cerebrovascular mortality 26% of the total. There was an apparent, though nonsignificant, reduction in the risk of cerebrovascular disease mortality (RR = 0.90; 95% CI: 0.76–1.07). It should be noted that in this population the majority of strokes is likely to be hemorrhagic rather than thromboembolic. While the latter type are generally due to atherosclerotic disease, this is not the case for the former. Therefore, the relevance of these findings in terms of atherosclerotic prevention is not clear.

The Alpha-Tocopherol Beta-Carotene Cancer Prevention Trial (ATBC Trial) was the first large-scale randomized trial of antioxidant vitamins in a well-nourished population. This 2 × 2 factorial trial tested the effect of synthetic alpha tocopherol (50 mg daily) and synthetic beta-carotene (20 mg daily) in the prevention of lung cancer among 29,133 Finnish male smokers (ATBC Cancer Prevention Study Group 1994). After adjustment for testing multiple hypotheses, there were no increases or decreases in risk that could not be explained plausibly by chance. Nevertheless, some findings were unexpected. For alpha-tocopherol, there was no clear reduction in risk of ischemic heart disease or ischemic stroke mortality (658 total ischemic deaths among those assigned alpha-tocopherol compared with 704 among those assigned placebo). The apparent benefits among those who took vitamin E in the NHS and the HPFS were largely confined to those who used a dose of 100 IU or more per day, which is higher than the 50 mg used in this trial. There was a possible increase in the risk of hemorrhagic stroke in the alpha-tocopherol treatment group compared with those assigned to placebo (66 vs 44), a finding not compatible with the lower stroke rates among those assigned antioxidant vitamins in the Linxian trial. Hemorrhagic stroke was not a prespecified endpoint, and while this finding is compatible with an antiplatelet effect of vitamin E, it remains plausible that it could be the result of the play of chance. With respect to beta-carotene, there was also no apparent protective effect of supplementation with respect to deaths from ischemic heart disease and stroke; in fact, there were more ischemic deaths in the treated group (721 total ischemic deaths among those assigned beta carotene compared with 641 among those assigned placebo). The ATBC trial results do not disprove the value of antioxidant vitamins, nor do they incriminate them as harmful. They do, however, raise the possibility that some of the previously reported benefits may have been overestimated and that there may be some adverse effects. They also provide support for skepticism and for a moratorium on unsubstantiated health claims.

Ongoing Trials. The available randomized trial data are not yet sufficient to assess fully the risk:benefit ratios for antioxidants. More reliable data from additional large-scale trials should be forthcoming in the near future which will further define the role of antioxidants in the primary and secondary prevention of heart disease. The U.S. National Heart, Lung, and Blood Institute sponsored a conference on ''Antioxidants and the Prevention of Human Atherosclerosis'' (Steinberg 1992). The summary statement supported the need for further large-scale randomized trials examining the role of beta-carotene and vitamins C and E in the primary and secondary prevention of CVD.

Several large-scale randomized trials testing the role of supplemental dietary antioxidants in the prevention of CVD and cancer are currently underway. The Physicians' Health Study is testing synthetic beta-carotene (50 mg on alternate days) in over 22,000 apparently healthy U.S. male physicians with a 12-year period of treatment and follow-up. The Women's Health Study is testing synthetic beta-carotene (50 mg on alternate days) as well as natural vitamin E (600 IU on alternate days) and low-dose aspirin in the primary prevention of CVD and cancer in approximately 40,000 healthy, U.S. female health professionals (Women's Health Study Research Group 1992). A secondary prevention trial of vitamin C (500 mg daily), vitamin E (600 IU on alternate days), and beta-carotene (50 mg on alternate days) in a factorial design is currently underway among 8,000 women excluded from the WHS due to preexisting atherosclerotic disease (Women's Antioxidant CVD Study). The CARET (CARotene plus RETenoic acid) study is testing a combination of beta-carotene (25 mg daily) and retinoic acid (25,000 IU daily) in 18,000 asbestos workers. The Supplementation en Vitamines et Mineraux Antioxidants trial is testing a mixture of lower-dose antioxidant vitamins and minerals (daily doses of 6.0 mg beta-carotene, 15 mg alpha-tocopherol, 120 mg vitamin C, 100 ~g selenium and 20 mg zinc) among 15,000 healthy men and women. Finally, the Heart Protection Study is a 2×2 factorial design trial of Simvastatin, a cholesterol-lowering drug and a cocktail of vitamin E (600 IU), vitamin C (250 mg), and beta-carotene (20 mg).

Cost-Effectiveness

The health benefits of consumption of fresh fruits and vegetables are well documented, and current recommendations of five or more servings per day likely represent a relatively inexpensive means of maintaining good health. Supplemental vitamins represent a multibillion dollar industry. In addition many foods are fortified with vitamins. In the absence of sufficient randomized trial data to quantify adequately the benefits and risks of supplemental dietary antioxidants, estimates on cost effectiveness are premature.

Conclusions

A coherent, plausible hypothesis as to how antioxidants might slow the progression of atherosclerosis has been generated from basic studies in cell biology and subsequent affirmation in animal models of atherosclerosis. However, it is very important to note that all of these studies relate primarily to the very initial stage of atherosclerosis—the generation of the fatty streak lesion. Whether or not antioxidants play any role in the development of the more advanced lesions remains to be tested. Since the fatty streak lesion is the precursor of the more advanced lesions, one might find an effect even if it were limited to the formation of the fatty streak; that is, by reducing the density of fatty streaks, one should ultimately reduce the number of complicated lesions eventually developing. However, that may require either a study of longer duration than is general in intervention studies or the evaluation of earlier lesions than are examined in most clinical trials. The NHLBI workshop (Steinberg 1992) recommended that studies should proceed looking both at coronary events and at effects on lesions. An important study would be one evaluating the development of *new* lesions, for example, by using carotid ultrasound techniques to examine intima/media thickness. A second important point is that there are gaping holes in our understanding of how antioxidants work in vivo. Currently, most investigators measure the extent to which LDL isolated from plasma has been protected against oxidative modification after, for example, feeding a given dose of vitamin E. Yet we know that some of the effects of the antioxidants are exercised within the cells, modifying their capacity to oxidatively modify or to generate lipid peroxides within the cells. In short, we are currently "flying blind" when we design tests of the oxidative modification hypothesis. Nevertheless, as the 1991 Workshop concluded, the hypothesis is sufficiently strong to justify intervention studies, but they should include both long-term trials and those evaluating the generation of early stage lesions. A second rationale for conducting trials testing vitamin antioxidants is the widespread use of these agents. In the United States 64% of U.S. adults report regular multivitamin use and 43% and 34% of adults regularly take vitamins C and E, respectively. Trials of these readily available supplements are necessary to definitively assess potential benefits and risks, since the trend toward increased use seems likely to continue even in the absence of reliable evidence concerning.

Based on the totality of available evidence, antioxidants represent a promising but as yet unproven means to reduce risks of CVD. Nevertheless, many find the prescription of agents to lower risk of CVD more acceptable than eliminating harmful lifestyle practices. It is the avoidance of these harmful lifestyle practices, outlined elsewhere in this text, which will likely provide far greater benefits for which there is already proof beyond a reasonable doubt.

Summary

Quality of available data: Data derive primarily from case-control and cohort epidemiologic studies and a few intervention trials.

Estimated risk reduction: Based on available data, it is not yet possible to determine an estimated risk reduction for antioxidant vitamins.

Comparability of effect in men and women: Data are insufficient to elucidate gender differences.

References

Acheson RM, Williams DRR. Does consumption of fruit and vegetables protect against stroke? Lancet 1993;1:1191–93.

Adams CF. Nutritive values of American foods. Washington, DC: United States Department of Agriculture 1975; (No. 456).

Alpha-Tocopherol, Beta-Carotene Lung Cancer Prevention Study Group. The effect of vitamin E and beta-carotene on the incidence of lung cancer and other cancers in male smokers. N Engl J Med 1994;330:1029–35.

Anderson TW, Reid W. A double-blind trial of vitamin E in the treatment of angina pectoris. Am Heart J 1974;93:444–49.

Ardie NG, Shelley ML, Simons LA. Platelet activation by oxidatively modified low density lipoproteins. Atherosclerosis 1989;76:117–24.

Armstrong BK, Mann JL, Adelstein AM, Eskin F. Commodity consumption and ischemic heart disease mortality, with special reference to dietary practices. J Chronic Dis 1975;36: 673–7.

Berliner JA, Territo MC, Sevanian A. Minimally modified low density lipoprotein stimulates monocyte endothelial interactions. J Clin Invest 1990;85:1260–6.

Bjorkhem I, Henriksson-Freyschuss AH, Breuer O, et al. The antioxidant butylated hydroxytoluene protects against atherosclerosis. Arterioscler Thromb 1991;11:15–22.

Blot WJ, Li J, Taylor PR, et al. Nutritional intervention trials in Linxian, China: supplementation with specific vitamin/mineral combinations, cancer incidence, and disease specific mortality in the general population. J Natl Cancer Inst 1993;85:1483–92.

Bolton-Smith C, Woodward M, Tunstall-Pedoe H. The Scottish heart health study. Dietary intake by food frequency questionnaire and odds ratios for CHD risk. II. The antioxidant vitamins and fiber. Eur J Clin Nutr 1992;46:85–93.

Bossaller C, Habib GB, Yamamoto H, et al. Impaired muscarinic endothelium-dependent relaxation and cyclic guanosine 5'-monophosphate formation in atherosclerotic human coronary artery and rabbit aorta. J Clin Invest 1987;79:170–4.

Brown MS, Goldstein JL. Receptor mediated pathway for cholesterol homeostasis. Science 1986;232:34–47.

Burton GW, Ingold KU. Beta-carotene: an unusual type of lipid antioxidant. Science 1984;224: 569–73.

Carew T, Schwenke D, Steinberg D. Antiatherogenic effect of probucol unrelated to its hypocholesterolemic effect: evidence that antioxidants in vivo can selectively inhibit low density lipoprotein degradation in macrophage-rich fatty streaks and slow the progression of atherosclerosis in the Watanabe heritable hyperlipidemic rabbit. Proc Natl Acad Sci USA 1987;84:7725–9.

Cathcart MK, Morel DW, Chisholm, GM. Monocytes and neutrophils oxidize low density lipoproteins making it cytotoxic. J Leukocyte Biol 1985;38:341–50.

Cathcart MK, Morel DW, Chisolm GM III. Monocytes and neutrophils oxidized low density lipoproteins on formation and inactivation of endothelium-derived relaxing factor. Arterioscler Thromb 1991;11:198–203.

Consensus Conference. Lowering blood cholesterol to prevent heart disease. JAMA 1985;253: 2080–2086.

Constainescu A, Han D, Packer L. Vitamin E recycling in human erythrocyte membranes. J Biol Chem 1993;268:10906–13.

Constantinides P. Plaque fissures in human coronary thrombosis. J Atheroscler Res 1966;6:1.

Consumer and Food Economics Institute. Composition of foods: fruits and fruit juices, raw, processed, prepared. Washington, DC: US Department of Agriculture Handbook 1982; 8–9.

Cushing SD, Berliner JA, Valente AJ. Minimally modified low density lipoprotein induces monocyte chemotactic protein 1 in human endothelial cells and smooth muscle cells. Proc Natl Acad Sci USA 1990;87:5134–8.

Daugherty A, Zweifel BS, Schonfeld G. Probucol attenuates the development of aortic atherosclerosis in cholesterol-fed rabbits. Br J Pharmacol 1989;98:612–18.

Daugherty A, Zweifel BS, Schonfeld G. The effects of probucol on progression of atherosclerosis in mature Watanabe heritable hyperlipidemic rabbits. Br J Pharmacol 1991;103: 1013–18.

Davies MJ. A macro and micro view of coronary vascular insult in ischemic heart disease. Circulation 1990;82(Suppl):I138–46.

DeMaio SJ, King SB III, Lembo NJ, et al. Vitamin E supplementation, plasma lipids and incidence of restenosis after percutaneous transluminal coronary angioplasty (PTCA). J Am Coll Nutr 1992;11:131–8.

Donegan CK, Messer AL, Orgain ES, Ruffin JM. Negative results of tocopherol therapy in cardiovascular disease. Am J Med Sci 1949;217:294–9.

Donnan PT, Thompson M, Fowkes FG, et al. Diet as a risk factor for peripheral arterial disease in the general population: the Edinburg Study. Am J Clin Nutr 1993;57:917–21.

Eichholzer M, Stahelin HB, Gey KF. Inverse correlation between essential antioxidants in plasma and subsequent risk to develop cancer, ischemic heart disease and stroke, respectively: 12-year follow-up of the Prospective Basel Study. In: Emerit I and Chance B, eds. Free radicals and aging. Birkhauser Verlag, Basel, Switzerland 1992;398–410.

Enstrom JE, Kanim LE, Klein MA. Vitamin C intake and mortality among a sample of the United States population. Epidemiology 1992;3:194–202.

Esterbauer H, Gebicki J, Puhl H, Jurgens G. The role of lipid peroxidation and antioxidants in oxidative modification of LDL. Free Radical Biol Med 1992;13:341–90.

Fehily AM, Yarnell JW, Sweetnam PM, Elwood PC. Diet and incident ischaemic heart disease: the Caerphilly Study. Br J Nutr 1993;69:303–14.

Fogelman AM, Schechter JS, Hokom M, et al. Malondialdehyde alteration of low-density lipoprotein leads to cholesterol accumulation in human monocyte-macrophages. Proc Natl Acad Sci USA 1980;77:2214–18.

Foote CS, Denny RW, Weaver L, et al. Quenching of singlet oxygen. Ann NY Acad Sci 1970; 171:139–48.

Frei B. Ascorbic acid protects lipids in human plasma and low-density lipoprotein against oxidative damage. Am J Clin Nutr 1991;54:1113S–18S.

Frostegard J, Nilsson J, Haegerstrand A, et al. Oxidized low density lipoprotein induces differentiation and adhesion of human monocytes and the monocytic cell line U937. Proc Natl Acad Sci USA 1990;87:904–8.

Gaziano JM, Manson JE, Ridker PM, et al. Beta-carotene therapy for chronic stable angina. Circulation 1990;82:Suppl III:III-202.

Gaziano JM, Manson JE, Buring JE, Hennekens CH. Dietary antioxidants in cardiovascular disease. Ann of NY Acad Sci 1992;249–59.

Gaziano JM, Manson JM, Hennekens CH. Dietary antioxidants and cardiovascular disease: Epidemiologic studies and clinical intervention trials. In: Frei B, ed. Natural antioxidants and human disease, Academic Press, 1994.

Gaziano JM, Hatta A, Flynn M, et al. Supplementation with beta-carotene in vivo and in vitro does not inhibit low density lipoprotein (LDL) oxidation. Atherosclerosis 1995a;112: 187–95.

Gaziano JM, Manson JE, Branch LG, et al. Dietary beta-carotene and decreased cardiovascular mortality in an elderly cohort. Annals Epidemiol, 1995b;5:255–60.

Gey KF, Stahelin HB, Puska P, Evans A. Relationship of plasma vitamin C to mortality from ischemic heart disease. Ann NY Acad Sci 1987a;498:110–23.

Gey KF, Brubacher GB, Stahelin HB. Plasma levels of antioxidant vitamins in relation to ischemic heart disease and cancer. Am J Clin Nutr 1987b;45:1368–77.

Gey KF, Puska P. Plasma vitamins E and A inversely correlated to mortality from ischemic heart disease in cross-cultural epidemiology. Ann NY Acad Sci 1989;570:254–82.

Gey KF, Puska P, Jordan P, Moser UK. Inverse correlation between plasma vitamin E and mortality from ischemic heart disease in cross-cultural epidemiology. Am J Clin Nutr 1991;53:326S–34S.

Gey KF, Stahelin HB, Eichholzer M. Poor plasma status of carotene and vitamin C is associated with higher mortality from ischemic heart disease and stroke: prospective Basel study. Clin Invest 1993;71:3–6.

Gillilan RE, Mandel B, Warbasse JR. Quantitative evaluation of Vitamin E in the treatment of angina pectoris. Am Heart J 1977;93:444–9.

Ginter E. Decline of coronary mortality in the United States and vitamin C. Am J Clin Nutr 1979;32:511–21.

Gisinger C, Jeremey J, Speiser P, et al. Effect of vitamin E supplementation on platelet thromboxane A at production in type I diabetic patients. Diabetes 1988;37:1260–4.

Goldstein JL, Ho YK, Basu SK, Brown MS. Binding site on macrophages that mediates uptake and degradation of acetylated low-density lipoprotein, producing massive cholesterol deposition. Proc Natl Acad Sci USA 1979;76:333–7.

Haberland ME, Fong D, Cheng L. Malondialdehyde-altered protein occurs in atheroma of Watanabe heritable hyper-lipidemic rabbits. Science 1988;241:215–18.

Haeger K. Long-time treatment of intermittent claudication with vitamin E. Am J Clin Nutr 1974;27:1179–81.

Hansson GK, Holm J, Jonasson L. Detection of activated T-lymphocytes in the human atherosclerotic plaque. Am J Pathol 1989;135:169–75.

Heinecke JW, Rosen H, Chait A. Iron and copper promote modification of low-density lipoprotein by human arterial smooth muscle cells in culture. J Clin Invest 1987;74:1890–4.

Henriksen T, Evensen SA, Carlander B. Injury to human endothelial cells in culture induced by low-density lipoproteins. Scand J Clin Lab Invest 1979;39:361–8.

Henriksen T, Mahoney EM, Steinberg D. Enhanced macrophage degradation of low-density lipoprotein previously incubated with cultured endothelial cells: Recognition by receptors for acetylated low-density lipoproteins. Proc Natl Acad Sci USA 1981;78:6499–503.

Henriksen T, Mahoney EM, Steinberg D. Enhanced macrophage degradation of biologically modified low density lipoprotein. Arteriosclerosis 1983;3:149–59.

Jessler JR, Robertson AL Jr, Chisholm GM. LDL-induced cytotoxicity and its inhibition by HDL in human vascular smooth muscle and endothelial cells in culture. Arteriosclerosis 1979;32:213–19.

Jialal I, Norkus E, Cristol L, Grundy SM. Beta-carotene inhibits the oxidative modification of low-density lipoprotein. Biochimica et Biophysica Acta 1991;1086:134–8.

Kardinaal AFM, Kok FJ, Ringstad J, et al. Antioxidants in adipose tissue and risk of MI: the EURAMIC study. Lancet 1993;342:1379–84.

Keaney JF Jr, Gaziano JM, Xu A, et al. Dietary antioxidants preserve endothelium-dependent vessel relaxation in rabbits. Proc Natl Acad Sci 1994;90:11,880–11,884.

Kita T, Nagano Y, Yokode M, et al. Probucol prevents the progression of atherosclerosis in Watanabe heritable hyperlipidemic rabbit, an animal model for familial hypercholesterolemia. Proc Natl Acad Sci USA 1987;84:5928–31.

Kok FJ, de Bruijn AM, Vermeeren R, et al. Serum selenium, vitamin antioxidants and cardiovascular mortality: a 9 year follow-up study in the Netherlands. Am J Clin Nutr 1987;45:462–8.

Kugiyama K, Kerns SA, Morrisett JK, et al. Impairment of endothelium-dependent arterial relaxation by lysolecithin in modified low density lipoproteins. Nature 1990;334:160–62.

Lapidus L, Anderson H, Bengtson C, Bosceus I. Dietary habits in relation to incidence of cardiovascular disease and death in women: a 12 year follow-up of participants in the study of women in Gothenberg, Sweden. Am J Clin Nutr 1986;44:444–8.

Lavy A, Amotz AB, Aviram M. Preferential inhibition of LDL oxidation by the all-trans isomer of beta-carotene in comparison with 9-cis beta-carotene. Eur J Clin Chem Clin Biochem 1993;31:83–90.

Liao F, Berliner JA, Mehrabian M. Minimally modified low density lipoprotein is biologically active in vivo in mice. J Clin Invest 1991;87:2253–7.

Livingston PD, Jones C. Treatment of intermittent claudication with vitamin E. Lancet 1958; 2:602–4.

Mahley RW, Innerarity TL, Weisgraber KH, Oh SY. Altered metabolism (in vivo and in vitro) of plasma lipoprotein after selective chemical modification of lysine residues of the apoproteins. J Clin Invest 1979;64:743–50.

Makinson DH, Oleesky S, Stone RV. Vitamin E in angina pectoris. Lancet 1948;1:102.

Malden LT, Ross R, Chait A. Oxidatively modified low density lipoproteins inhibit expression of platelet-derived growth factor by human monocyte-derived macrophages. Immunol 1990;144:2343–50.

Manson JE, Stampfer MJ, Willet WC, et al. A prospective study of antioxidant vitamins and incidence of CHD in women. Circulation 1991;84:Suppl II [Abstract].

Manson JE, Stampfer MJ Willett WC, et al. A prospective study of vitamin C and incidence of CHD in women. Circulation 1992a;85:865.

Manson JE, Stampfer MJ, Willet WC, et al. A prospective study of vitamin C and incidence of CHD in women. Circulation 1992b;85:865 [Abstract].

Manson JE, Stampfer MJ, Willet WC, et al. Antioxidant vitamin score and incidence of CHD in women. Circulation 1992c;84:I-2687 [Abstract].

Manson JE, Stampfer MJ, Willet WC, et al. Antioxidant vitamins and incidence of CHD in women. Circulation 1993;88:I-70 [Abstract].

McCay PB. Vitamin E: Interactions with free radicals and ascorbate. Annu Rev Nutr 1985;5: 323–40.

Morel DW, DiCorleto PE, Chisholm GM. Endothelial and smooth muscle cells alter low density lipoprotein in vitro by free radical oxidation. Arteriosclerosis 1984;4:356–64.

Morris DL, Kritchevsky SB, Davis CE. Serum carotenoids and CHD in the Lipid Research Clinics Coronary Primary Prevention Trial. Circulation 1993;87:2 [Abstract].

Navab M, Imes SS, Hama SY, et al. Monocyte transmigration induced by modification of low density lipoprotein in cocultures of human aortic wall cells is due to induction of mono-cyte chemotactic protein 1 synthesis and is abolished by high density lipoprotein. J Clin Invest 1991;88:2039–46.

Niki E, Saito T, Kamiya Y. The role of vitamin C as an antioxidant. Chem Lett 1983;631–2.

Oda T, Ikeda H, Kuwano K, Nakayama H. Alpha-tocopherol inhibits platelet and neutrophil activation during cyclic flow variations in dogs with coronary stenosis and endothelial injury. Circulation 1993; Abstract 0173, 88(Suppl):1–35.

Packer JE, Slater TF, Wilson RL. Direct observation of a free radical interaction between vi-tamin E and vitamin C. Nature 1979;278:737–8.

Palinski W, Rosenfeld ME, Yla-Herttuala S. Low density lipoprotein undergoes oxidative mod-ification in vivo. Proc Natl Acad Sci USA 1989;86:1372–6.

Parthasarathy S, Printz DJ, Boyd D, et al. Macrophage oxidation of low density lipoprotein generates a modified form recognized by the scavenger receptor. Arteriosclerosis 1986;6:505–10.

Pathobiological Determinants of Atherosclerosis in Youth (PDAY) Research Group. Natural history of aortic and coronary atherosclerotic lesions in youth: findings from the PDAY Study. Atheroscler Thromb 1993;13:1291–8.

Plagy A. Association between dietary changes and mortality rates: Israel 1949–1977: a trend-free regression model. Am J Clin Nutr 1981;34:1569–83.

Prasad K, Kalra J. Oxygen free radicals and hypercholesterolemic atherosclerosis: effect of vitamin E. Am Heart J 1993;125:958–73.

Prince MR, LaMuraglia GM, MacNichol EF. Increased preferential absorption in human atherosclerotic plaque with oral beta carotene: implications for laser endarterectomy. Circulation 1988;78:338–44.

Princen HMG, van Poppel G, Vogelezang C, et al. Supplementation with vitamin E but not beta-carotene in vivo protects low density lipoprotein from lipid peroxidation in vitro: effect of cigarette smoking. Artherioscler Thromb 1992;12:554–62.

Quinn MT, Parthsarathy S, Fong LG, Steinberg D. Oxidatively modified low density lipoproteins: a potential role in recruitment and retention of monocyte/macrophages during atherogenesis. Proc Natl Acad Sci USA 1985a;82:5949–53.

Quinn MT, Parthasarathy S, Steinberg D. Endothelial cell-derived chemotactic activity for mouse peritoneal macrophages and the effects of modified forms of low density lipoprotein. Proc Natl Acad Sci USA 1985b;85:5949–53.

Quinn MT, Parthasarathy S, Steinberg D. Lysophosphatidyl-choline: a new chemotactic factor for human monocytes and its potential role in atherogenesis. Proc Natl Acad Sci USA 1988;85:2805–9.

Rajavashisth TB, Andalibi A, Territo MC. Induction of endothelial cell expression of granulocyte and macrophage colony-stimulating factors by modified low density lipoproteins. Nature 1990;344:254–7.

Ramirez J, Flowers NC. Leukocyte ascorbic acid and its relationship to CHD in man. Am J Clin Nutr 1980;33:2079–87.

Reaven PD, Khouw A, Beltz WF, et al. Effect of dietary antioxidant combinations in humans: protection of LDL by vitamin E but not by beta-carotene. Arterioscler Thromb 1993; 13:590–600.

Riemersma RA, Wood DA, Macintyre CCH, et al. Low plasma vitamin E and C increased risk of angina in Scottish men. Ann NY Acad Sci 1989;570:291–5.

Riemersma RA, Oliver M, Elton MA, et al. Plasma antioxidants and CHD: vitamins C and E and selenium. Eur J Clin Nutr 1990;44:143–50.

Riemersma RA, Wood DA, Macintyre CHH, et al. Risk of angina pectoris and plasma concentrations of vitamins A, C, E, and carotene. Lancet 1991;337:1–5.

Rimm EB, Stampfer MJ, Ascherio A, et al. Dietary intake and risk of CHD among men. N Engl J Med 1993;328:1450–6.

Rinzler SH, Bakst H, Benjamin ZH, et al. Failure of alpha tocopherol to influence chest pain in patients with heart disease. Circulation 1950;1:288–93.

Rosenfeld ME, Palinski W, Yla-Herttuala S, et al. Distribution of oxidation specific lipid-protein adducts and apolipoprotein B in atherosclerotic lesions of varying severity from WHHL rabbits. Arteriosclerosis 1989;10:336–49.

Rosenfeld ME, Yla-Herttuala S, Lipton BA, et al. Macrophage colony-stimulating factor mRNA and protein in atherosclerotic lesions of rabbits and man. Am J Pathol 1992;140:291–300.

Ross R, Glomset J. The pathogenesis of atherosclerosis. N Engl J Med 1976;295:369–77.

Ross R. The pathogenesis of atherosclerosis: A perspective for the 1990's. Nature 1993; 362(6423):801–9.

Salonen JT, Salonen R, Penttila I, et al. Serum fatty acids, apolipoproteins, selenium and vitamin antioxidants and risk of death from coronary artery disease. Am J Cardiol 1985;56:226–31.

Salonen JT, Nyyssonen K, Parviainen MT, et al. Low plasma beta carotene, vitamin E and selenium levels associated with accelerated carotid atherogenesis in hypercholesterolemic eastern Finnish Men. Circulation 1993;87:1.

Salvini S, Hunter DJ, Sampson L. Food-based validation of a dietary questionnaire: the effects of week-to-week variation in food consumption. Int J Epidemiol 1989;18:858–67.

Sasahara M, Raines EW, Carew TE, et al. Inhibition of hypercholesterolemia-induced atherosclerosis in *Macaca nemestrina* by probucol: I. Intimal lesion area correlates inversely with resistance of lipoproteins to oxidation. J Clin Invest 1994; in press.

Sato K, Niki E, Shimasaki H. Free radical-mediated chain oxidation of low density lipoprotein and its synergistic inhibition by vitamin E and vitamin C. Arch Biochem Biophys 1990; 279:402–5.

Simon BC, Cunningham LD, Cohen RA. Oxidized low density lipoproteins cause contraction and inhibit endothelium-dependent relaxation in the pig coronary artery. J Clin Invest 1990;86:75–9.

Smith TL, Kummerow FA. Effect of dietary vitamin E on plasma lipids and atherogenesis in restricted ovulatory chickens. Atherosclerosis 1989;75:105–9.

Som S, Raha C, Chatterje IB. Ascorbic acid: a scavenger of superoxide radical. Acta Amino Enzymol 1983;5:243–50.

Sparrow CP, Doebber TW, Olaszewski J, et al. Low density lipoprotein is protected from oxidation and the progression of atherosclerosis is slowed in cholesterol-fed rabbits by the antioxidant *N,N'*-diphenylphenylene-diamine. J Clinic Invest 1992;86:1885–91.

Stampfer MJ, Hennekens CH, Manson JE, et al. Vitamin E consumption and the risk of coronary disease in women. N Engl J Med 1993;328:1444–9.

Stein Y, Stein O, Delplanque B, et al. Lack of effect of probucol on atheroma formation in cholesterol-fed rabbits kept at comparable plasma cholesterol levels. Arteriosclerosis 1989;75:145–55.

Steinberg D. Lipoproteins and atherosclerosis. Atherosclerosis 1983;3:283–301.

Steinberg D. Metabolism of lipoproteins and their role in the pathogenesis of atherosclerosis. In: Stokes III J, Mancini M, eds. Atheroscler Rev 1988;18:1–23.

Steinberg D, Parthasarathy S, Carew TE, et al. Beyond cholesterol: modifications of low density lipoprotein that increase its atherogenicity. N Engl J Med 1989;320:915–24.

Steinberg D and Workshop Participants. Antioxidants in the prevention of human atherosclerosis: summary proceedings of a National Heart, Lung, and Blood Institute Workshop: September 5–6, 1991. Bethesda MD. Circulation 1992;85:2337–47.

Steinbrecher UP, Parthasarathy S, Leake DS, et al. Modification of low density lipoprotein by endothelial cells involves lipid peroxidation and degradation of low density lipoprotein phosopholipids. Proc Natl Acad Sci USA 1984;81:3883–7.

Steiner M, Anastasi J. Vitamin E an inhibitor of the platelet release reaction. J Clin Invest 1976;57:732–7.

Street DA, Comstock GW, Salkeld RM, et al. A population based case-control study of serum antioxidants and MI. Am J Epidemiol 1991;134:719–20.

Stryker WS, Kaplan L, Stein EA, et al. The relation of diet, cigarette smoking and alcohol consumption to plasma beta-carotene and alpha-tocopherol levels. Am J Epidemiol 1988;127:283–6.

Triau JE, Meydani SN, Schaefer EJ. Oxidized low density lipoprotein stimulates prostacyclin production by adult human vascular endothelial cells. Arteriosclerosis 1988;8:810–18.

Verlangieri AJ, Kapeghian JC, El-Dean S, Bush M. Fruit and vegetable consumption and cardiovascular disease mortality. Med Hypoth 1985;16:7–15.

Verlangieri AJ, Bush M. Effects of *d*-alpha-tocopherol supplementation on experimentally induced primate atherosclerosis. J Am Coll Nutr 1992;11:131–8.

Vollset SE, Bjelke E. Does consumption of fruit and vegetables protect against stroke? Lancet 1983;2:742.

Willett WC, Stampfer MJ, Underwood BA, et al. Validation of a dietary questionnaire with plasma carotenoid and alpha-tocopherol levels. Am J Clin Nutr 1983;38:631–639.

Willett WC, Sampson L, Stampfer MJ, et al. Reproducibility and validity of a semiquantitative food frequency questionnaire. Am J Epidemiol 1985;122:51−65.

Willett WC, Stampfer MJ. Total energy intake: implications for epidemiologic analyses. Am J Epidemiol 1986;124:17−27.

Williams HTG, Fenna D, MacBeth RA. Alpha tocopherol in the treatment of intermittent claudication. Surg Gyn Obstet 1971;132:662−6.

Women's Health Study Research Group. The Women's Health Study: summary of the study design. J Myocardial Ischemia 1992;4:27−9.

Woolley DW. Some biologic effects produced by alpha-tocopherol quinone. J Biol Chem 1945; 275:L430−7.

Yla-Herttuala S, Palinski W, Rosenfeld ME. Evidence for the presence of oxidatively modified low density lipoprotein in atherosclerotic lesions of rabbit and man. J Clin Invest 1989; 84:1086−95.

Yla-Herttuala S, Lipton BA, Rosenfeld ME. Macrophages express monocyte chemotactic protein (MCP-1) in human and rabbit atherosclerotic lesions. Proc Natl Acad Sci USA 1991;88:5252−6.

14

Dietary Factors

WALTER C. WILLETT AND ELIZABETH B. LENART

Until quite recently, the topic of diet and heart disease was almost entirely dominated by discussions of the relationships of saturated and polyunsaturated fat and cholesterol with myocardial infarction (MI). These relationships, which became known as the diet-heart hypothesis, will be considered briefly here as the relevant literature is voluminous and has been discussed in detail elsewhere (Consensus Conference 1985; National Research Council 1989; Willett 1990). Some investigators have long suspected that other aspects of diet may also play an important role in the cause and prevention of coronary heart disease (CHD), in part because these dietary lipids and other established risk factors do not fully explain the international differences in CHD rates or individual differences in risk within populations. Recently, substantial evidence has accumulated, suggesting the importance of several other aspects of diet, some of which are potentially more easily modified than the amounts of dietary fat. These dietary factors are the focus of this chapter. One area of great interest, antioxidant vitamins, is discussed in Chapter 13.

The Classical Diet-Heart Hypothesis

As described by Gordon (1988), early interest in diet and heart disease resulted from the demonstration during the 1930s that dietary cholesterol can cause arterial lesions in animals and that this effect is mediated largely through an elevation in plasma cholesterol (Katz 1953; Anitschkow 1967; Wissler 1975; Grundy 1982). Further development of the diet-heart hypothesis has been influenced heavily by two lines of epidemiologic evidence, the first being ecologic correlations relating diet to rates of heart disease. These data, along with findings from migrant studies and special populations, are discussed under descriptive studies. The other primary line of evidence derives from studies of serum cholesterol. These studies have related dietary factors to serum cholesterol and, in separate investigations, serum cholesterol to the risk of CHD. These are discussed briefly in a separate section as such studies do not directly address the relation of diet to heart disease. The role of serum cholesterol is discussed in detail in Chapter 6.

Descriptive Studies of Diet and Coronary Heart Disease

The most influential descriptive data on diet and CHD was the work of Keys relating the mean intake of dietary factors of 16 defined populations in seven countries to the incidence of heart disease in those same groups (Keys 1980). As shown in Figure 14.1, intake of saturated fat as a percentage of calories was strongly correlated with coronary death rates ($r = .84$). In this instance, the countries with low fat intake and low incidence of CHD were in less economically industrialized populations and are likely to have differed in many ways, particularly in physical activity, obesity, and, at that time, smoking habits. Indeed, the slope of the line relating saturated fat to risk of CHD death is nearly $2^{1}/_{2}$ times greater than would be expected if the effect of saturated fat operated only by raising serum cholesterol. In this same study, the percentage of energy from fat had little relationship with CHD incidence or mortality. Indeed, the countries with the highest fat intake (about 40% of energy) included that with the highest CHD rates (Finland) as well as the area with the lowest rates (Crete). In another type of ecologic study, a strong association ($r = .67$) was observed between the percentage of calories from fat in 12 countries and prevalence of raised atherosclerotic lesions in autopsy cases from the same geographic area (Scrimshaw 1968).

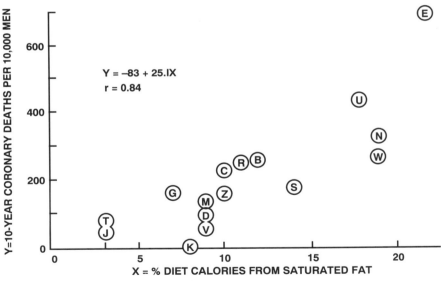

Fig. 14.1. Ten-year coronary death rates of the cohorts plotted against the percentage of dietary calories supplied by saturated fatty acids. *B*, Belgrade; *C*, Crevalcore; *D*, Dalmatia; *E*, east Finland; *G*, Corfu; *J*, Ushibuka; *K*, Crete; *M*, Montegiorgia; *N*, Zutphen; *R*, Rome railroad; *S*, Slavonia; *T*, Tanushimaru; *U*, American railroad; *V*, Velika Krsna; *W*, west Finland; *Z*, Zrenjanin. [From Keys (1980), with permission.]

Little correlation (r = .07), however, was seen with the percentage of total fat from animal fat. As with any correlational study, the possibility of confounding by other risk factors exists. The clearest message from these data and other comparisons (McGill 1968) is that rates of CHD differ dramatically among countries and that the highly developed countries are at highest risk.

Migrant Studies and Secular Trends

CHD incidence rates among three defined Japanese populations living in Japan, Hawaii, and San Francisco have been compared (Kato 1973; Robertson 1977). Saturated fat intake as a percentage of calories in the three populations was found to be 7%, 23%, and 26%, respectively. For these three groups, mean relative weight and serum cholesterol increased in parallel with the saturated fat intake, mean alcohol intake markedly decreased, and dietary cholesterol was similar. Age-adjusted CHD incidence rates were 1.6 per 1,000 person-years in Japan, 3.0 in Hawaii, and 3.7 in San Francisco. These data indicate that the substantial differences in rates of CHD among the three areas cannot be explained by genetic factors and are consistent with the hypothesis that dietary saturated fat may contribute to the difference. However, because other dietary and nondietary factors vary similarly among the groups, such as alcohol intake and obesity, specific casual factors cannot be firmly identified on the basis of this type of data alone.

Data on secular trends in CHD mortality are of interest, but are not consistent with the diet-heart hypothesis. Within North America, CHD mortality rates rose dramatically over the first half of this century (Anderson 1979), although the increase in total and saturated fat consumption was slight. Polyunsaturated fat rose two- to three-fold, largely due to the replacement of animal fats by partially hydrogenated vegetable fat (Friend 1967; Page 1979). Kahn (1970) has estimated that these changes in food consumption would account for only an 8% rise in incidence of CHD.

Since the late 1960s, age-specific mortality rates have decreased steadily (Working Group 1981; Stamler 1985). However, whether CHD *incidence* has also decreased is much less clear, and it is almost certain to have declined to a lesser degree than has mortality. Because of uncertainty about recent time trends in incidence as well as the changes over time in many factors, including smoking habits, exercise, body weights, vitamin supplements, and multiple dietary factors, attribution of secular changes to any particular factor is treacherous. However, the rarity of MI at the turn of this century in the United States and in many parts of the world even today indicates that some combination of diet and lifestyle plays a profoundly important role in the etiology of this disease.

Studies of Diet and Blood Lipids

The clearly established relationship between serum cholesterol and risk of CHD has led to hundreds of controlled metabolic feeding studies to determine the effects of dietary fats on serum cholesterol. Most commonly, such studies have manipulated the proportions in the diet of saturated fat (high in palm oil and most animal fats), polyunsaturated fat (usually as corn oil, but also high in soybean oil and safflower oil), monounsaturated fat (usually as olive oil), and dietary cholesterol. These studies have been summarized as prediction equations by Keys (1984) and Hegsted et al. (1993) (see Table 14.1). These equations indicate that changes in serum cholesterol are directly related to saturated fat intake, to a weaker degree inversely related to polyunsaturated fat intake, and directly related to dietary cholesterol (expressed as the square root of cholesterol in the Keys equation). Monounsaturated fat was not found to influence total cholesterol appreciably relative to carbohydrate intake, and thus was not included in the equations.

A frequent underlying assumption in the use of these equations has been that serum cholesterol represents a surrogate endpoint, and that a dietary factor that changes serum cholesterol will also change risk of CHD in a similar manner. This logic, however, weakened as it became appreciated that total serum cholesterol represents many subcomponents, including the deleterious low density lipoprotein (LDL) fraction as well as the apparently beneficial high density lipoprotein (HDL) component. Thus, the effect of a specific dietary change on total serum cholesterol might increase, decrease, or not influence risk of CHD, depending on which cholesterol components were changed. Thus, more recent metabolic feeding studies have measured a variety of lipid fractions, which have been summarized in new prediction equations by Mensink and Katan (1992) (see Table 14.1). Although the earlier observations by Keys (1984) and Hegsted (1993) for total cholesterol were confirmed, when compared with carbohydrate, saturated fat was shown to raise serum HDL cholesterol almost in proportion to the increase in LDL or total cholesterol. Thus, the ratio of total cholesterol to HDL cholesterol, which appears to summarize reasonably the relation between serum lipids and CHD (Castelli 1983; Stampfer 1991), is little influenced by saturated fat intake. However, when monounsaturated fats are substituted for carbohydrate, HDL increases and LDL changes little. Thus, the lipid pattern on a high monounsaturated fat diet is favorable compared to a diet in which a similar amount of energy is provided by either saturated fat or carbohydrate. Mensink and Katan (1992) also noted that the effect of polyunsaturated fat on serum cholesterol levels appeared to be weak in recent studies; the reason is unclear but could relate to the higher baseline polyunsaturated fat in contemporary diets (about 6% of energy) than in diets conducted in the 1950s when polyunsaturated fat intake was about 3% of energy.

Questions have been raised as to whether the reductions in HDL resulting from a high carbohydrate diet have the same adverse effect as reductions caused by other factors (Brinton 1991). Although this is difficult to address directly, other factors that influence HDL levels, including alcohol, estrogens, obesity, smoking, exercise, and medications, affect CHD risk in the predicted direction (Mannitari 1990; Sacks 1991). The use of the usual cholesterol prediction equations has been further complicated by the recognition that different saturated fats and dairy sources of saturated fat vary in their influence on LDL levels: butter and other dietary fats (high in 14:0, myristic acid) most strongly increase LDL, beef fat (containing palmitic acid, 16:0, and stearic acid, 18:00) raised LDL to a lesser degree, and cocoa butter (containing largely stearic acid) raises LDL only slightly (Denke 1991; Mensink 1992).

The optimal amount of polyunsaturated fat intake in the diet remains uncertain. The earlier metabolic studies predicting total serum cholesterol (Keys 1984; Hegsted

Table 14.1. Equations Predicting Effects of Dietary Fats on Serum Cholesterol

Investigator	Serum Lipid or Lipoprotein Concentration	Predictive Equation
Keys 1984[a]	Total cholesterol	$\Delta SC = 1.3(2\Delta S - \Delta P) + 1.5(\Delta Z)$
Hegsted et al. 1993[b]	Total cholesterol	A. $\Delta SC = 2.10\Delta S - 1.16\Delta P + 0.0670\Delta C$
	LDL cholesterol	B. $\Delta LDL\text{-}C = 1.74\Delta S - 0.766\Delta P + 0.0439\Delta C$
	HDL cholesterol	C. $\Delta HDL\text{-}C = 0.662\Delta S + 0.631\Delta P - 0.0479(S_2P_2 - S_1P_1)$
Mensink & Katan 1992[c]	Total cholesterol	A. $\Delta SC = 1.51(\text{carb}\rightarrow\text{sat}) - 0.12(\text{carb}\rightarrow\text{mono}) - 0.60(\text{carb}\rightarrow\text{poly})$
	LDL cholesterol	B. $\Delta LDL\text{-}C = 1.28(\text{carb}\rightarrow\text{sat}) - 0.24(\text{carb}\rightarrow\text{mono}) - 0.55(\text{carb}\rightarrow\text{poly})$
	HDL cholesterol	C. $\Delta HDL\text{-}C = 0.47(\text{carb}\rightarrow\text{sat}) + 0.34(\text{carb}\rightarrow\text{mono}) + 0.28(\text{carb}\rightarrow\text{poly})$
	Triglyceride	D. $\Delta \text{Triglycerides} = -2.22(\text{carb}\rightarrow\text{sat}) - 1.99(\text{carb}\rightarrow\text{mono}) - 2.47(\text{carb}\rightarrow\text{poly})$

[a] ΔSC is change in serum cholesterol in mg/dl. ΔS is difference between the two diets in % of calories from saturated fat. ΔP is the difference between diets in polyunsaturated fatty acids. ΔZ is the difference between the square roots of the mg of cholesterol/1,000 kcal of diet.

[b] (A) ΔC is change in dietary cholesterol given as mg/1,000 kcal. (B) $\Delta LDL\text{-}C$ is change as mg/dl. (C) $\Delta HDL\text{-}C$ is change in HDL-C in mg/dl. S_iP_i = absolute amounts of saturated and polyunsaturated fatty acids in diets i = 1,2 and R_D^2 = 0.371 and SE_d = 0.100. Authors note that "total equation explains only 40% of variance. The errors in the regression coefficients are large; hence little reliance should be placed on the equation."

[c] All equations predict change expected as a result of 1% daily dietary energy intake as carbohydrate replaced by particular fatty acid. ΔSC, $\Delta LDL\text{-}C$, $\Delta HDL\text{-}C$, Δtriglyceride are mg/dl.

355

1986) suggested that intakes should be maximized, and the American Heart Association recommended intakes of 10% of energy (compared with US averages of about 3% in the 1950s and 6% at present). However, concerns have arisen from animal studies in which omega-6 polyunsaturated fat (typically as corn oil) has promoted tumor growth (Welsch 1992), and the possibility that high intakes of omega-6 relative to omega-3 fatty acids might promote coronary thrombosis (Renaud 1970; Leaf 1988).

The use of cholesterol subfractions instead of simple total cholesterol probably represents an advance in understanding the relations between dietary factors and risk of CHD. However, that these are all surrogate endpoints must be remembered. Dietary fats might influence CHD risk through yet-to-be-defined lipid fractions or by entirely other mechanisms. For example, it had been suggested that dietary fats of all types may increase levels of factor VII, which may be an independent predictor of CHD risk; however, such an effect of dietary fat is not clear (Marckmann 1992). Also, some evidence suggests that higher levels of polyunsaturated fat may reduce the occurrence of sudden death by raising the threshold for ventricular arrhythmias (Hetzel 1989; Charnock 1992). Ideally, these issues are best resolved by observational studies or randomized intervention trials that directly address the relationships between dietary factors and incidence of coronary disease.

Understanding the interrelationships between dietary fats, blood lipids, and CHD risk has been further complicated by the recognition that antioxidants may play a role in preventing atherosclerosis (see Chapter 13). Laboratory evidence suggests that lipid-soluble antioxidants such as vitamin E can block the oxidative modification of LDL, an important step in atherogenesis (Steinberg 1990). Within Europe, countries with higher blood antioxidant levels have lower rates of CHD (Gey 1987), and in two recent prospective studies men and women who consumed the highest amounts of vitamin E (mostly from supplements) had an approximately 40% lower risk of MI compared with those having low vitamin E intakes (Rimm 1993; Stampfer 1993). As liquid vegetable oils, particularly those that are minimally processed, are the primary souce of vitamin E in our diets, reduction of these fats could have adverse effects on CHD risk. Furthermore, LDL particles formed on diets high in monounsaturated fat appear to be relatively resistant to oxidation (Reaven 1993).

Cohort Studies

Despite the long-standing interest in the diet-heart hypothesis, the number of observational studies that have directly addressed associations between dietary fats and risk of CHD is surprisingly small, and these all have major limitations due to their size and/or the methods used to assess dietary intake (Willett 1990). In the prospective studies on this topic, summarized in Table 14.2, the most consistent relationship has been an inverse association between total energy (caloric) intake and risk of CHD. This association is almost certainly due to the protective effect of physical activity, which also increases energy intake. A positive association between saturated fat and CHD risk has been found in only three studies (McGee 1984; Kushi 1985; Goldbourt 1993), and even this may be an artifact because saturated fat was divided by total energy, which will tend to create a positive association simply due to the inverse relationship between energy intake and risk of CHD (Willett 1986). However, existing studies have not been sufficiently large or rigorous to exclude a small association with saturated fat intake. These studies do lend some support to a modest positive association between dietary cholesterol and risk of CHD (Shekelle 1989). However, as the food sources of cholesterol have not been examined in these reports, other components of food high in cholesterol, such as the iron or protein in meat, could contribute to the reported associations with CHD risk. A clear, inverse association between polyunsaturated fat intake and risk of CHD was seen only in the study by Shekelle and colleagues (1981).

Intervention Studies

Ideally, definitive information to confirm or refute dietary hypotheses would be obtained from randomized trials in human populations. Unfortunately, the complexities of conducting primary prevention trials are great due to the problems in maintaining substantial and long-term dietary changes in free-living populations, avoiding similar changes in the control group, and following a sufficiently large study population. Also, in some of the intervention studies, multiple dietary and lifestyle changes were made simultaneously, thus complicating the interpretation of any observed difference in outcome.

Two of the early trials of dietary change were conducted among institutionalized patients (see Table 14.3), one in a Los Angeles Veterans hospital (Dayton 1969) and another in a Finnish mental hospital (Turpeinen 1979), to increase control over the diets. Total fat intake was not reduced in these studies; rather, polyunsaturated fat was greatly increased to about 20% of energy to substitute for saturated fat. In both studies a nonsignificant but suggestive reduction of MI was observed and statistical significance was achieved when less "hard" cardiovascular endpoints were included. In a more recent study of similar design among institutionalized patients, little evidence was seen for a reduction in CHD among the group with modified fat intake (Frantz 1989); however, the duration of follow-up in this study may have been too limited to observe an association.

The diet-heart hypothesis has been evaluated in free-living men as part of two large studies that attempted to reduce several CHD risk factors simultaneously. In the MRFIT study, in which smoking cessation and blood pressure control were also sought, no significant reduction in CHD mortality was seen in the intervention group after 10 years (Multiple Risk Factor Intervention Trial Research Group 1982). Results from the trial conducted among men with very high serum cholesterol (mean: 325 mg/dl) in Oslo, where smoking cessation was also attempted but with little success, were more impressive; after over eight years of follow-up CHD incidence was reduced by about 45% and a significant reduction in total mortality was also found (Hjermann 1986). Even in this study, the interpretation is uncertain as many factors were changed simultaneously. Even apart from some reduction in smoking and some decreases in weight, we cannot be sure whether the benefit was primarily due to an increased intake of polyunsaturated fat or the antioxidants in vegetable oil, or to reductions in saturated fat and cholesterol. Although this may appear to be an arcane distinction, it is relevant

Table 14.2. Prospective Cohort Studies of Dietary Factors in Relation to Risk of Coronary Heart Disease

Study	Population	Dietary Method	CHD Cases	Energy	Sat Fat	Poly	Diet Chol	Lipid[a] Score	Fiber	Fish	Alcohol	Comments
Morris et al. 1977	337 U.K. bank clerks	7-day record, weighted	45	↓	0	—	0	—	↓	—	—	Trend of ↓ risk with high P/S ratio
Shekelle et al. 1981, 1985	1,900 U.S. men	Diet history interview	~200 CHD deaths	—	0	↓	↓	↑	—	↓	—	
Garcia-Palmieri et al. 1980	8,218 Puerto Rican men	24-hour recall	163	↓	0	0	0	—	—	—	↓	Inverse relation with starch intake
Gordon et al. 1981 Dawber et al. 1982	895 Framingham men	24-hour recall	51	↓	0	0	0	—	—	—	↓	No association with egg intake
McGee et al. 1984	7,088 Honolulu men	24-hour recall	309	↓	↑*	0	↑	—	—	—	↓	Dietary fat values were divided by calories
Kromhout et al. 1982, 1984, 1985	857 Zutphen men (Dutch)	Diet history interview	30 CHD deaths	↓	0	0	0	—	↓	↓	0	Inverse relation with fiber not significant when divided by calories
Kushi et al. 1985	1,001 Irish and Boston men	Diet history interview	110 CHD deaths	0	↑*	0	0	↑	↓	—	—	Dietary fat values were divided by calories
Snowdon et al. 1984	25,153 U.S. Seventh Day Adventists	28-item frequency questionnaire	1599	—	—	—	—	—	—	—	—	Positive association with meat intake (RR = 1.5)
Khaw et al. 1987	California men and women	24-hour recall	65 CHD deaths	0	—	—	0	—	↓	—	0	

Reference	Population	Dietary assessment	No. of events							Comments
Burr et al. 1982	10,943 Welsh vegetarians	Short food-frequency questionnaire	585	—	—	—	—	0	—	Vegetarians have lower CHD mortality
Lapidus et al. 1986	1,462 Swedish women	24-hour recall	28 infarctions	↓	—	—	—	—	—	
Norell et al. 1986	10,966 Swedish men and women	?	800 CHD deaths	—	—	—	↓	—	—	
Fraser et al. 1992	31,208 Seventh Day Adventists	65-item food frequency questionnaire	463 incident CHD deaths	—	—	↓	↓	—	—	Those consuming nuts several times per week had significantly lower risk of fatal and nonfatal CHD; inverse relationship for fiber is whole wheat bread vs white bread consumption; attempted to control for food habits associated with increased nut intake
Fehily et al. 1993	2,512 Men from South Wales	50-item food frequency questionnaire	148	↓	0	—	0	—	↓	Total fiber intake lower in those having an incident IHD event, but not independent of total calories
Goldbourt et al. 1993	10,059 Israeli civil service Men	Short dietary questionnaire	1098 CHD deaths	↑*	→	—	—	↓*	—	Independent dietary influence on CHD rates not strong; no difference in CHD for those surviving concentration camps and others from Europe
Dolecek 1992	6,250 Men from usual care group from MRFIT	24 hour dietary recall	175 CHD deaths	↓*	↓*	—	—	↑*	—	Inverse association between polyunsaturated fat intake and CHD marginally significant

Sat, saturated; Poly, polyunsaturated; Chol, cholesterol; IHD, ischemic heart disease; MRFIT, Multiple Risk Factor Intervention Trial.

a Lipid score refers to Keys or Hegsted scores for predicting serum cholesterol.

↓, inverse association; ↑, positive association; 0, no statistically significant association; —, no information.

* Expressed as percent of total calories.

Table 14.3. Dietary Intervention for Prevention of Coronary Heart Disease

Study	Subjects and Duration in Years	N Intervention/ Control	Diets (% Energy)					Outcome MI Events		RR	Comment
			Total Fat	Sat	Poly	Mono	Chol (mg)	Intervention/ Control			
Dayton et al. (1969): high polyunsaturated fat	846 men; up to 8 y	424 422	39 40	— —	20 —	— —	365 653	MI events: 60/78		.77	60 events occurred in intervention and 78 events occurred in control groups. When cerebral and secondary events were included, differences between intervention and control were significant.
Turpeinen et al. (1979): high polyunsaturated fat	676 men; Finnish mental patients; 6-y trials	Approx 250 250	35 34	9 18	13 4	12 11	282 480	CHD mortality: 6/12 Major ECG change or death: 8/26		.49 .33	Intervention crossed over from one hospital to the other after 5 y.
Hjermann et al. (1981): low fat	1,232 men, Oslo 5 y	604 628	28 44	8 18	8 7	— —	289 527	22/39		.56	Intervention included smoking reduction. Marked serum cholesterol and CHD reductions in intervention group. Dietary data from subset of sample.
MRFIT (1982); Cagguila et al. (1981); low fat, cholesterol	12,886 men Minimum of 6 y, up to 10 y	6,248 6,438	35 38	10 14	9 6	— —	250 451	CHD mortality: 115/124		.93	Intervention included blood pressure control and smoking reduction. Intervention and control groups had nearly similar reductions in serum cholesterol levels.
Frantz et al. 1989: high polyunsaturated fat	4393 men, 4664 women; Minnesota; up to 4.5 y	4,541 4,516	38 39	9 18	16 5	14 16	166 446	131/121		1.08	Serum cholesterol levels fell 14.5% in intervention group. No overall differences in CHD events between groups, but short mean duration of follow-up.

Sat, saturated; Poly, polyunsaturated; Mono, monounsaturated; Chol, cholesterol; RR, relative risk.
↓ ↑, Reduced or increased intake-exact amount not given; —, no intake information given.

to some current dietary recommendations to lower all forms of fat, including polyunsaturated fat.

In addition to trials of dietary change among persons without CHD at entry, a number of studies have examined the influence of dietary change among persons with existing CHD (see Table 14.4). Viewed individually, these studies have not provided clear or consistent findings. Law and colleagues (1994) have summarized data from the largest primary and secondary dietary prevention studies by follow-up interval. They estimated that, for a 10% reduction in serum cholesterol (0.6 mmol/l), the risk of nonfatal MI was reduced by 9% in the first two years of follow-up, 14% from year 2 to 5, and by 37% with more than 5 years of follow-up. However, the results for 5 or more years of experience include a total of only 30 events, and are based almost entirely on the Los Angeles Veterans Study, which used a higher fat diet with 20% of energy from polyunsaturated fat.

Several other dietary studies, not reviewed here, have used changes in coronary occlusion assessed by angiography as the endpoint. One such study has been used by Ornish to promote an extremely low fat diet, less than 10% of energy (Ornish 1990). However, the intervention included a complete modification of lifestyle, including exercise, weight and stress reduction, and increased intake of vegetables and fruits; thus attributing any benefit to a single aspect of this package is impossible. Also, the same diet that might be beneficial for patients with coronary artery disease may not necessarily be desirable as a lifelong diet for a population, particularly as high rates of hemorrhagic stroke are seen in populations with diets extremely low in fat and animal protein (Jacobs 1992; Willet 1994).

In a recent randomized trial among patients with unstable angina, a large (70%) reduction was observed among patients assigned to a ''Mediterranean diet'' compared with those receiving an American Heart Association diet (Lorgeril 1994). As the special diet included a high intake of monosaturated fat, high intake of N-3 fatty acids and relatively low intake of N-6 fatty acids, as well as abundant consumption of fruits and vegetables, it is not possible to attribute the findings to a single dietary component. Nevertheless, this study strongly supports further research in alternatives to the American Heart Association recommendations.

Randomized trials that have used drugs rather than diet to modify blood lipids are indirectly important to the diet-heart hypothesis as they have confirmed the importance of both LDL and HDL cholesterol in the etiology of CHD (Mannitari 1990; Law 1994). In the summary by Law and colleagues (1994), reduction of serum cholesterol by 10% by drug treatment reduced CHD events by 21% in years 2 to 5 and by 22% after year 5. Yet, these studies do not directly clarify the effect of saturated fat on CHD risk because of its complicated relationship with blood cholesterol fractions described above.

Other Diet-Heart Hypotheses

In recent years the scope of research on dietary factors that might be related to CHD risk has been expanded greatly. These topics will be described here briefly.

Table 14.4. Dietary Intervention for Secondary Prevention of Coronary Heart Disease

Study	Subjects and Duration in Years	*N* Intervention/Control	Total Fat	Sat	Poly	Mono	Chol (mg)	Intervention/Control	RR	Comment
			Diets (% Energy)					Outcome MI Events		
Morrison 1960 low fat, cholesterol	100 Los Angeles men & women 12 y	50 50	14 80–160	— —	— —	— —	50–70 200–1,800	Total mortality: 31/50	.62	Intervention diet contained 25 g fat. This resulted in low calorie intakes and 15% weight loss by intervention group. Most, not all mortality due to CHD or CVD.
Koranyi (1963) low fat	183 Hungarian men 3 y	45 low fat–no restrictions 45 low fat–no lard or dairy 45 low fat–2/3 animal, 1/3 ed. oil, 45 control	15 19 19 30	— ↓ — —	↑ ↑ ↑ —	— — — —	↓ ↓ ↓ —	Total mortality; (%) 8.7/19.7	.44	Results only from low fat compared to control after 3 years.
Ball et al. (1965) MRC low fat	252 London area men 3 y	123 129	20 43	— —	— —	— —	↓ —	Total mortality: 20/24 New MI or major relapse: 43/44	.83 .98	Overweight were advised to reduce irrespective of group, resulting in 6% and 5% weight loss in intervention and control, respectively.
Rose et al. (1965): corn oil	80 London area men 2 y	26 olive 28 corn 26 control	26 29 33	↓ ↓ —	— ↑ —	↑ — —	↓ ↓ —	CHD mortality: Olive oil, 3; Corn oil, 5; Control, 1 New MI Olive oil, 6; Corn oil, 7; Control, 5	Olive Corn 3.0 5.0 1.2 1.4	Intervention consisted of two groups. One received most fat calories as olive oil and the other as corn oil. Dietary intakes calculated from those still in trial during second year. Both oil groups told to reduce eggs, fatty meats, and other sources of animal fat. Intakes of oil had to be reduced to maintain compliance.

Study	Sample							Outcome	Ratio	Comments
Morris et al. (1968): MRC soya bean oil	393 London area men 5 y (2–6.75)	199 194	46 44	↓ —	↑ —	— —	258 588	CHD mortality 27 25 Major relapse 45 51	1.08 .86	Overweight subjects were put on reducing diets regardless of group (73 Invervention and 90 Control subjects).
Leren (1970): high polyunsaturated fat, low cholesterol	412 Oslo area men 11 y	206 206	39 40	9 —	21 —	10 —	→ —	CHD mortality 79 94 CVD mortality 88 102	.84 .86	About 22% of both groups were already modifying food habits to decrease cholesterol at onset of trial. Intervention diet from subset of 17 in sample. Control diet considered to be average Norwegian intake.
Woodhill et al. (1978); low fat, cholesterol	458 sydney area men 2–7 y	221 237	38 38	10 14	15 9	12 14	248 342	Total mortality 39 28	1.4	63 of 67 deaths were CHD/CVD. Trial became multifactorial. Many in both groups increased physical activity, quit smoking and made dietary changes. Total fat intake was equal in both groups.
Burr et al. (1989): Dart MRC low fat, fish, fiber advice	2,033 men 2 y	Approx 1015 1015	32 35	— —	↑ —	— —	— —	IHD events advice/ nonadvice Fat 132/144 Fish 127/149 Fiber 150/126	.91 .84 1.21	Dietary data given for fat/no-fat advice. 2 × 2 × 2 factorial design with subjects randomized into one of eight categories. Received fat reduction, increased fish consumption, or increased fiber consumption advice, or no advice, or some combination of advice.

Table continues

363

Table 14.4. Continued

Study	Subjects and Duration in Years	N Intervention/Control	Total Fat	Sat	Poly	Mono	Chol (mg)	Outcome MI Events Intervention/Control	RR	Comment
Watts et al. (1992): stars low fat, cholesterol	90 London area men 3 y	26 24	27 —	9 —	8 —	10 —	100/1000kc —	Total cardiac events 3 10	.3	(24 Men consuming intervention diet and taking cholestyramine as well as 16 men not completing trial not included.) Overweight subjects in intervention group were given advice and prescribed a 1,000–1,200 calorie diet. Those in control were told to lose weight but did not get counseling. Marked fall in progression of coronary narrowing in diet group.
Singh et al. (1992): low fat, high fiber, increased antioxidants	505 Indian men and women 1 y	204 (180M) 202 (185M)	24 28	7 11	9 7	8 10	147 287	CHD mortality 20 34 Cardiac events 50 82	.59 .61	Both groups received health advice and diet counseling to replace fats of animal origin or hydrogenated oils with liquid vegetable oil. One group received advice on increasing fruits, vegetables, lentils, nuts, fish.
de Lorgeril et al. (1994): Mediterranean alpha-linolenic acid-rich diet	605 Lyon area men and women 5 y	302 (278M) 303 (271M)	31 33	8 ↑ 12	9 ↑ —	↑ —	217 318	CVD mortality 3 16 New MI 5 17	.24 .27	Experimental groups received counseling and specially formulated margarine (similar in lipid composition to olive oil). Marked decrease in reinfarction and death rate for those on intervention diet.

Total fat, saturated fat, polyunsaturated fat, monounsaturated fat given as percent of energy unless otherwise noted. ↓ or ↑ if decrease or increase was noted. —, if no information was provided.

364

trans-*Fatty Acids*

trans-Fatty acids are produced when lipid vegetable oils, which normally have all double bonds in the *cis* position, are heated in the presence of metal catalysts to form vegetable shortening and margarine. This process was discovered around the turn of the twentieth century, and production increased steadily until about the 1960s as processed vegetable fats displaced animal fats in the U.S. diet, first because of costs and then because of purported health benefits. A similar increase has occurred worldwide; for example, in parts of India, a partially hydrogenated fat containing approximately 60% of fat as *trans* isomers is widely used as a replacement for ghee (Achaya 1987). Per capita consumption of *trans*-fatty acids has decreased slightly in the United States because of the increased use of softer margarine, which typically contains less than the 40% content of these isomers often found in the older stick margarines.

Although concern had existed for some time that *trans*-fatty acids might have adverse effects on CHD risk (Senti 1988), this was greatly heightened by a careful metabolic study conducted by Mensink and Katan (1992). In this study, which used monounsaturated fat as a comparison, a diet with 10% of energy as *trans*-fatty acids raised LDL cholesterol to a similar degree as did saturated fat. However, HDL cholesterol was reduced by *trans* isomers but unaffected by saturated fat. Thus, the increase in the ratio of total cholesterol to HDL cholesterol due to *trans* isomers was about twice that seen with saturated fat. These findings have been reproduced in other metabolic studies (Nestel 1992; Zock 1992; Judd 1994), including adverse effects on blood lipids when *trans*-fatty acids constituted 3% and 6% of energy. See Figure 14.2 for a summary of metabolic studies. Also, *trans*-fatty acids have been found to increase

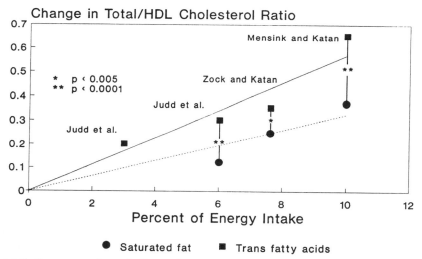

Fig. 14.2. Summary of metabolic studies retaining effect of trans and saturated fatty acids on total/HDL cholesterol ratio.

blood levels of Lp(a), another potential risk factor for CHD, in two metabolic studies (Mensink 1992; Nestel 1992).

Although the uniquely adverse effects of *trans* isomers on blood lipids are alone sufficient to raise serious concern about consumption of these synthetic fats, positive associations between intake of these fats and risk of CHD have also been observed. In the Nurse's Health Study, women with the highest intake of *trans*-fatty acids from processed vegetable fats assessed in 1980 experienced the highest risk of MI during the next eight years (Willett 1993). When those women whose intake of margarine had greatly increased or decreased over the previous 10 years were excluded, the risk was nearly 80% higher for those in the highest 20% of intake compared with those in the lowest 20%. Margarine, cookies, and white bread contributed most to intake and the excess risk of CHD. Similar findings were also seen in a case-control study primarily among men (Ascherio 1994a), and a positive association with the degree of atherosclerosis was also observed in a cross-sectional angiographic study (Siguel 1993). Thus, quite consistent evidence, based on both metabolic and epidemiologic studies, appears to support an adverse effect of partially hydrogenated vegetable fat on CHD risk.

Fish and Omega-3 Fatty Acids

Low rates of CHD in Japan and Greenland have led to speculation that the high consumption of fish in these areas might be protective (Bang 1980; Kagawa 1982). This hypothesis is supported by evidence that long-chain omega-3 fatty acids, which are predominantly provided by cold-water marine fish such as salmon or mackerel, have a variety of presumably favorable physiologic effects. These effects, reviewed by Leaf and Weber (1988), include a potent reduction in very low density lipoprotein cholesterol, inhibition of thromboxane production and increase in prostacyclin synthesis with a resulting reduction in thrombotic tendency, reduction in blood viscosity, increase in fibrinolytic activity, and, perhaps, reduction in blood pressure. However, in a recent meta-analysis (Morris 1993), the effect on blood pressure of even large supplements of omega-3 fatty acids was found to be relatively small. Also, high intake of omega-3 fatty acids appears to increase LDL cholesterol slightly (Kestin 1990).

The hypothesis that intake of fish and omega-3 fatty acids might reduce risk of CHD was supported by the finding that Dutch men consuming more than 30 g of fish per day had only about half the risk of fatal CHD compared with men who consumed none (Kromhout 1985). Lower rates of CHD mortality among men and women who consumed higher amounts of fish were also observed in several prospective studies (Shekelle 1985; Norell 1986; Dolecek 1992), but not in three large studies conducted among Norwegian men (Vollset 1985), Japanese men living in Hawaii (Curb 1985), or U.S. physicians (Morris 1993).

Measurement of long-chain (20- and 22-carbon) omega-3 fatty acids in blood and tissue can provide markers of past fish intake, providing another method to examine the relation between fish intake and risk of CHD. In two small case-control studies, each including fewer than 30 patients with CHD, no significant associations were reported between risk of CHD and long-chain omega-3 fatty acid levels in adipose tissue or platelets (Wood 1984) or in specific serum lipid fractions (Schrade 1961).

Using frozen sera from a prospective study, Miettinen and colleagues (1982) found that phospholipid omega-3 fatty acid levels tended to be lower among the 33 men who subsequently developed MIs than among a series of 64 men who remained free of CHD. The reverse was true, however, for omega-3 fatty acid levels in the triglyceride fraction. Wood and colleagues (1987) measured adipose tissue and platelet fatty acid levels in 80 men with acute MI, 108 men with angina pectoris, and 391 men without CHD. In both adipose and platelets, the long-chain omega-3 fatty acid levels were consistently lower for patients with CHD, and for several comparisons these differences were statistically significant. Whether increased intake of fish or supplements of omega-3 fatty acids reduce the incidence of CHD remains unclear as existing data are incomplete and not consistent.

Fiber

Certain types of fiber in the diet can reduce hyperglycemia (Rivellese 1980; Potter 1981) and may exert a small beneficial effect on blood lipids (Anderson 1984; Behall 1984). Although particularly strong reductions in serum cholesterol have been claimed for oat bran, which is high in soluble fiber, there effects seem to be modest at most, even with extremely high intakes of oat bran (Swain 1990; Jenkins 1993). The relationship between fiber intake and risk of CHD has been reported in four epidemiologic studies and an inverse relationship has been noted in each (Table 14.2). Morris and colleagues (1977) found that men in the highest third of dietary fiber consumption experienced about one-third the risk of CHD during the next 20 years. The protective effect was entirely attributable to fiber from grains; fiber from fruits, vegetables, and other sources was not associated with CHD incidence. Kushi and coworkers (1985), in a follow-up study of Irish siblings, found that those in the highest third of fiber consumption had about only about half the risk of CHD death compared with those in the lowest third. This finding persisted after adjustment for other risk factors, including total serum cholesterol and blood pressure. When adjusted for total energy intake, however, this relationship was no longer statistically significant (Kushi 1987). A similar inverse relationship was seen in the follow-up study of Dutch men conducted by Kromhout and colleagues (1982). Khaw and Barrett-Connor (1987), in a study based on a 12-year follow-up after obtaining a single 24-hour recall, found an inverse relationship between dietary fiber intake and CHD mortality among both men and women.

Although each of these studies of dietary fiber has been quite small, the consistency of the findings is remarkable. Nevertheless, a cautious interpretation of the data would suggest that some aspect of plant products, not necessarily a specific type of fiber, may reduce the risk of CHD. This relationship certainly deserves further examination, with focus on types and sources of fiber as well as a full consideration of other factors in fruits, vegetables, and grains.

The influence of a diet high in fiber on risk of reinfarction was evaluated in a randomized trial among participants who already had experienced a MI (Burr 1989) (see Table 14.4). Despite a substantial increase in dietary fiber, no reduction in risk was seen; if anything, the reinfarction rate was somewhat greater in the high-fiber group.

Folic Acid, Vitamin B_6, and Blood Homocysteine Levels

More than 40 years ago, Rinehart and Greenberg demonstrated that low vitamin B_6 intake produced arterial intimal damage in monkeys (Rinehart 1951). Olszewski (1993), noting the clinical syndrome of homocysteinuria, which is characterized by the homozygous deficiency of cystathionine synthase and fulminant atherosclerosis by age 20, hypothesized that less extreme levels of homocysteinemia might also increase CHD risk. These observations are linked by the roles of vitamin B_6 as a cofactor for cystathionine synthase, the enzyme that metabolizes homocysteine, and of folate and vitamin B_{12}, which are cofactors in another metabolic pathway that converts homocysteine back to methionine. Inadequate levels of any of these vitamins can increase blood homocysteine levels (Figure 14.3). Diet can also influence levels of homocysteine through higher intakes of its precursor, methionine, which is particularly abundant in meat and high-protein dairy products.

A substantial body of evidence supports the role of blood homocysteine level as an independent risk factor of CHD. Positive associations with risk of peripheral and coronary arterial disease have been seen in a number of case-control studies (Kang 1986; Clarke 1991). Also, a positive association was observed between plasma homocysteine level measured in bloods collected at baseline in the Physicians' Health Study and subsequent risk of CHD (Stampfer 1992).

Whether increases in dietary levels of folate and vitamin B_6 will reduce risk of CHD has not been examined directly. However, in the Framingham Heart Study, approximately one-fifth of the population had levels of homocysteine the same as that associated with elevated risk of MI in the Physicians' Health Study (Selhub 1993). Further, these elevated levels were primarily among individuals with lower intakes of vitamin B_6 and folate. At levels of folic acid intake above about 400 µg/day (the 1989 RDA was recently reduced from 400 to 200 µg/day), there appeared to be no further reduction in prevalence of elevated homocysteine levels. Also, supplementation with these water-soluble vitamins can normalize elevated levels, even with amounts similar to those contained in multiple vitamins (Malinow 1990). Thus, assuring adequate intakes of folic acid and vitamin B_6 may be an important means of preventing CHD.

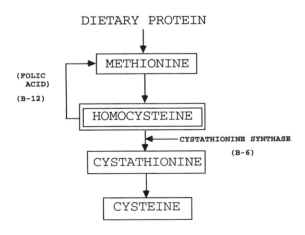

Fig. 14.3. Pathway relating dietary factors to blood homocysteine levels.

Salt

Higher sodium intake, primarily in the form of salt, modestly raises blood pressure, an important determinant of CHD risk, in susceptible individuals. The extensive and somewhat inconsistent literature has recently been reviewed in a series of Law and colleagues (1991). After examining a variety of data sources, these authors conclude that reducing salt (sodium chloride) intake from an average of approximately 8–10 g/day to less than 6g/day will modestly decrease blood pressure. Although the benefit of this reduction would be small for an individual, they estimate that this would reduce the population incidence of CHD by 16% and the incidence of stroke by 22%.

Iron

Iron has been hypothesized to increase risk of CHD, possibly by catalyzing the production of free radicals (Halliwell 1989; Sullivan 1989; McCord 1991). Interest in this relationship was increased by a report from a prospective Finnish study in which serum ferritin levels and iron intake were positively associated with subsequent incidence of CHD (Salonen 1992). A relationship with iron status was not confirmed in a report using serum iron and iron binding capacity in the NHANES follow-up study (Sempos 1994); however, serum iron is not a good indicator of iron stores. In a recent prospective study, nonheme iron, the primary form of this mineral in our diet, was not associated with risk of CHD (Ascherio 1994b). However, intake of heme-iron, primarily from red meat, was related to an increased risk of MI. If tissue iron levels are important with regard to CHD, it is likely that heme iron would play a special role because the absorption of nonheme is greatly downregulated in subjects with adequate iron stores, whereas heme iron is not (Cook 1990).

In contrast, in a recent retrospective autopsy study there was no evidence of increased atherosclerotic disease among those with significant iron-overload (hemochromatosis or multiorgan hemosiderosis) (Miller 1994). In fact, advanced or severe coronary atheroscleroses was present in 12% of iron-overload cases compared with 38% of age-, sex-, and race-matched controls ($p = .01$).

Selenium and Other Minerals

Selenium is an essential trace element and its deficiency has been associated with Keshan disease, a cardiomyopathy described in China. Puska and colleagues (Salonen 1982) reported an association between low selenium levels in prospectively collected blood and subsequent risk of CHD in Finland, a finding that has been confirmed and extended to stroke in a larger study from the same country (Virtamo 1985). In a small study from southern Finland, it was suggested that this inverse association may result from confounding by intake of fish, which, in Finland, is a major source of both long-chain omega-3 fatty acids and selenium (Miettinen 1983). In one U.S. study, an inverse association between blood selenium levels and degree of atherosclerosis has been found among patients undergoing coronary artery angiography (Moore 1984). A case-control study conducted in Holland (Kok 1989) found that higher selenium levels in toenail clippings, which provide an estimate of long-term intake, were associated with a lower risk of CHD. No relationship with serum selenium levels was observed.

Dietary intakes of a number of other minerals, including calcium, magnesium, chromium, copper, and zinc, have been hypothesized to be related to risk of CHD, some through a hypothesized role in the regulation of blood pressure. These relationships, reviewed elsewhere in greater detail (Willett 1990), remain to be clearly established.

Alcohol

Among the various dietary factors that have been examined in epidemiologic studies of CHD, the most consistent association has been an inverse relationship with moderate alcohol intake. This relationship has been reviewed elsewhere (Moore 1986; Stampfer 1988; Ellison 1990; Maclure 1993); reductions in risk at moderate levels of intake have been observed in the vast majority of studies. In general, consumption of one or two drinks of beer, wine, or liquor per day has corresponded to a reduction in risk of approximately 20–40%.

Alcohol increases blood levels of HDL cholesterol, which is likely to be the most important mechanism underlying its protective effect. In two studies in which the HDL levels were statistically controlled in the analysis (Criqui 1987; Gaziano 1993), the suggestion of some inverse relationship with CHD remained, consistent with the possibility that additional causal pathways might be involved. At high alcohol consumption levels, the risk of death attributed to CHD has been found to be similar to or even higher than the risk among nondrinkers (Moore 1986), which may be due to direct myocardial toxicity or the tendency for alcohol to induce arrhythmias, resulting in the assignment of MI as a cause of death. The meta-analysis by Maclure (1993) suggests a persistent effect of lower risks of CHD among heavier drinkers when CHD has been defined clearly as nonfatal MI.

Some have suggested, largely on the basis of the ecologic correlation indicating a low risk in France, that red wine might uniquely or most potently reduce the risk of CHD (Renaud 1992). Also, red wine appeared to reduce the oxidation of LDL cholesterol in a recent metabolic study (Frankel 1993). However, in case-control and cohort studies, in which the influences of confounding factors can be more readily controlled, beer, wine, and distilled beverages have similar inverse associations with risk of CHD (Maclure 1993). Thus alcohol *per se* appears to be the factor primarily responsible for the protective association.

Despite the large body of evidence indicating that moderate alcohol intake is associated with a reduced risk of CHD, some have been reluctant to accept this as a causal relationship (Shaper 1990). One argument has been that nondrinkers include a substantial number of former alcoholics who continue to be at excess risk of CHD, thus creating the perception of elevated risk among this group relative to moderate drinkers. This hypothesis, however, was not supported by the findings of studies that have found a reduction in risk among moderate drinkers relative to lifetime nondrinkers or those who had not been drinking for 10 or more years (Rosenberg 1981; Klatsky 1990; Rimm 1991).

A second argument used against the hypothesis of reduced risk has been that alcohol intake primarily causes an elevation in levels of HDL-3 fraction, although it is HDL-2 rather than HDL-3 that is related to reduced risk of CHD. In general, the use of a hypothetical mechanism as evidence against a large body of empirical data provides a very weak argument. In this instance, the data indicating that alcohol exclusively affects HDL-3 are based on a very small study (Haskell 1984) contradicted by other findings (Camargo 1985; Valimaki 1986). Furthermore, a protective relationship has been observed between HDL-3 and risk of CHD in several studies (Miller 1987; Gaziano 1993).

Overweight

Although a review of the relationship between adiposity and CHD risk is beyond the scope of this chapter and is covered in detail in Chapter 9, this is an important means, by which diet influences risk of this disease. Excessive body fatness, even at average levels for the U.S. population, increases the prevalence of abnormalities in blood lipids, glucose tolerance, and blood pressure (Garrison 1993). Consistent with these metabolic influences, the risk of both CHD incidence (Manson 1987) and mortality (Lew 1979) increases linearly with body weight after adjustment for age, height, and cigarette smoking. Further, persons of average body weight are at increased risk compared to the leanest individuals. Given the high and increasing level of adiposity in our society, its contribution to population rates of CHD is large, and probably more than any single component of the diet. Although energy intake is a critical part of the equation that determines whether an individual loses or gains weight; the importance of regular exercise and the avoidance of extreme inactivity such as television watching is becoming increasingly recognized (Gortmaker 1990).

Overall Strength of the Evidence

As many different hypotheses are encompassed by the relation between diet and CHD, a general statement as to the strength of evidence is not possible. The inverse relationship between alcohol consumption and CHD risk is strongly supported, to a far greater degree than other specific aspects of diet. The implications of this relationship for dietary recommendations are, however, extremely complex because of the adverse effects of alcohol on risks of accidents, numerous cancers, liver disease, and many other conditions, as well as the possibility of addiction. The evidence for an important role of adiposity is also extremely strong and sufficient for taking action on an individual and public health basis.

Available data suggest that the percentage of energy from fat in the diet is not an important determinant of CHD risk, although an effect of extremely low fat intake cannot be excluded. The type of fat in the diet appears more important, even though many details remain unsettled. Randomized intervention studies have done little to resolve these issues as they have either been negative or open to many possible interpretations. Although the evidence is not conclusive, a reduction in fat from land animals, particularly from dairy sources, seems prudent. These fats are not only the major sources of saturated fat in our diets, but also contain few antioxidants or other beneficial micronutrients, thus being a major source of "empty calories." As saturated fat is not an essential nutrient, it is impossible to indicate an optimal level; recommendations have suggested that saturated fat intake should be reduced to 8–10% of energy, but lower intakes will probably reduce CHD risk further. As *trans*-fatty acids from partially hydrogenated fat appear to have uniquely adverse effects on blood lipids, are associated with CHD risk, have other poorly understood effects on critical metabolic pathways, and are not naturally part of the human food supply, prudence would dictate that their intake be eliminated or greatly reduced.

If animal and partially hydrogenated fats are substantially reduced, the practical question is whether their calories should be replaced by carbohydrates or by liquid vegetable oils. The two general directions are characterized by the traditional Asian diet, in which rice or other grains were the primary source of energy, or the Mediterranean diet, in which olive oil was a major energy source. Although the ratio of total cholesterol to HDL cholesterol is clearly better on a diet high in monounsaturated fat, this question remains unresolved, and it may well be that equally health diets can be designed using either strategy. In both regions, CHD has been extremely low and overall life expectancy high, although rates of hemorrhagic stroke have historically been extremely high in Japan and other parts of Asia (Jacobs 1992; Tanaka 1992). Fortunately, an individual does not need to choose one or the other alternative exclusively, thus creating a variety of options for those attempting to improve upon the traditional U.S. diet.

High intake of animal products, particularly eggs and meat, may increase risk of CHD quite apart from the fat content. Cholesterol intake has been associated with risk of CHD in a number of studies, and eggs and meat are the primary sources. Not generally appreciated, the lean component of meat contains the majority of the cholesterol found in this food. Also, meat is a major source of methionine, and high intakes tend to elevate blood homocysteine levels, particularly when diets are suboptimal in folate. Furthermore, red meat is the primary source of dietary heme, which may also increase risk by adding to iron stores that are already replete. None of these mechanisms is proven to be important for CHD risk and further data examining intakes of these foods in relation to CHD risk are needed. However, the overall evidence and prudence suggest that just focusing on low-fat versions of animal products may be inadequate, and that the intakes of eggs and meat should be modest if they are to be consumed at all. A limitation on egg consumption has long been a part of American Heart Association recommendations. However, the current U.S. Dietary Pyramid (U.S. Department of Agriculture 1992), is probably misleading as meat is included in a group with legumes and 2 to 3 servings a day are recommended. Evidence that relatively high levels of fish consumption is beneficial is quite inconsistent at this time, but regular consumption does appear to be at least compatible with excellent health.

An annotated Department of Agriculture dietary pyramid is shown in Figure 14.4, as well as an alternative pyramid based on traditional diets of the Mediterranean that attempts to translate current nutritional knowledge into an attractive eating pattern. Although the healthy features of the Mediterranean diet have been particularly well documented, it is likely that similarly healthy diets can be assembled from other culinary traditions that rely primarily on plant, rather than animal, foods. It should also be noted that these dietary patterns have been suggested for healthy adults in general, and that optimal diets may differ during periods of growth, pregnancy, and lactation.

Evidence regarding the specific roles of folic acid, vitamin B_6, fiber, and dietary antioxidants in the etiology of CHD must be considered inconclusive at present and these are appropriately the topic of much ongoing research. Nevertheless, at the level of food consumption, the collective weight of evidence that generous intakes of fruits and vegetables will reduce risk of CHD is substantial, even if we do not yet fully understand which chemical components are responsible for a beneficial effect. Benefits of high fruit and vegetable intake with respect to incidence of various cancers are also likely and underlie national campaigns to increase intake of these foods.

Whether to take vitamin supplements is a common question of physicians and other individuals. This issue extends beyond the consideration of CHD risk because benefits of folate supplementation in reducing risk of neural tube defects are well established (MRC Vitamin Study Research Group 1991; Werler 1993), and inverse associations with various neoplasms have also been observed (Giovannucci 1993). Also, the recognition that elevated blood homocysteine level is a highly prevalent independent risk factor, as well as evidence that these elevations are frequently related to suboptimal intake of folic acid and vitamin B_6 provides support for the use of vitamin supplements in preventing CHD. Thus, current evidence, although far from complete, suggests that supplements of folate, and possibly other vitamins, at the levels contained in most multivitamin preparations may have substantial benefits for at least an important but unidentified subgroup of the U.S. population. As intakes of folate as well as other micronutrients appear marginal for many Americans (Block 1993), the risks of using multivitamins appear nonexistent, and the cost of supplements is low, the use of a daily or several-times-a-week multiple vitamin appears rational for the majority of Americans given current knowledge. The use of vitamin E and other antioxidant vitamin supplements is discussed in Chapter 13. For other vitamins and minerals there is presently little evidence of benefit of supplements over the RDA levels and, particularly for vitamins A and D, a real risk of harm at high intakes (National Research Council 1989).

Nutrition guidelines for reducing coronary risk are provided in an appendix at the end of this textbook.

Cost Effectiveness

Although the issue has received little formal attention, the cost effectiveness of preventing CHD by dietary means is potentially highly advantageous compared with most medical interventions. A major limitation in undertaking any formal analysis is that many of the benefits are not firmly established or quantified. Nevertheless, most dietary changes that appear likely to reduce risk would be similar or lower in cost than the present American diet. An exception to this may be the desired increase in fruits and vegetables, as these foods are often expensive and, being low in calories, tend to be added to the diet rather than displacing other sources of energy. Thus, this topic deserves further careful examination to identify practices and policies that would fa-

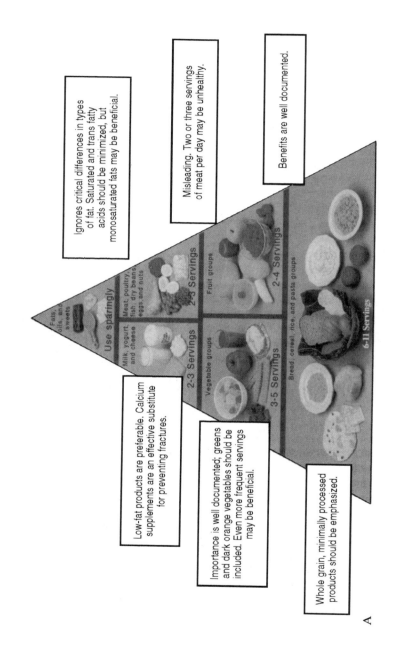

Ignores critical differences in types of fat. Saturated and trans fatty acids should be minimized, but monosaturated fats may be beneficial.

Misleading. Two or three servings of meat per day may be unhealthy.

Benefits are well documented.

Use sparingly

Fats, oils, and sweets

Milk, yogurt, and cheese
2-3 Servings

Meat, poultry, fish, dry beans, eggs, and nuts
2-3 Servings

Fruit groups
2-4 Servings

Vegetable groups
3-5 Servings

Bread, cereal, rice, and pasta groups
6-11 Servings

Low-fat products are preferable. Calcium supplements are an effective substitute for preventing fractures.

Importance is well documented; greens and dark orange vegetables should be included. Even more frequent servings may be beneficial.

Whole grain, minimally processed products should be emphasized.

A

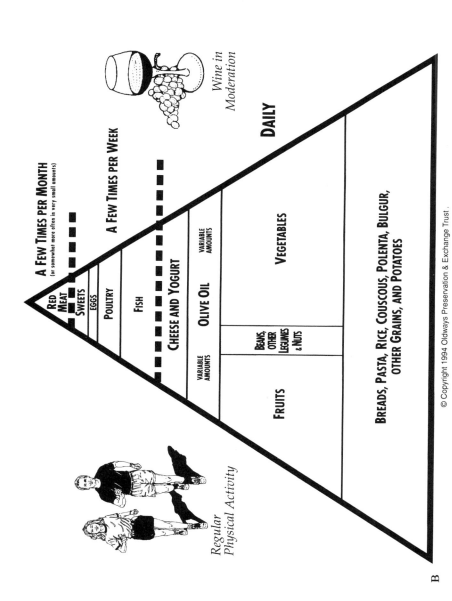

A Few Times Per Month (or somewhat more often in very small amounts)

A Few Times Per Week

DAILY

Red Meat

Sweets

Eggs

Poultry

Fish

Cheese and Yogurt

Olive Oil

Variable Amounts

Vegetables

Fruits

Beans, Other Legumes & Nuts

Breads, Pasta, Rice, Couscous, Polenta, Bulgur, Other Grains, and Potatoes

Wine in Moderation

Regular Physical Activity

B

© Copyright 1994 Oldways Preservation & Exchange Trust.

Fig. 14.4. Annotated United States Department of Agriculture Pyramid (A) and alternative Pyramid (B) based on traditional diets of the Mediterranean. [From Willett, "Diet and Health: what should we eat?" Science (Vol. 264: 532–537), April 22, 1994 © AAAS, reproduced with permission.]

cilitate consumption of these foods, particularly among lower income groups, who typically have the greatest need for improved nutrition.

Summary

Quality of available data: Quality of data varies concerning various dietary factors on risk of MI.

Estimated risk reduction: Available evidence generally supports a reduced risk of MI with increased consumption of fruits and vegetables, fiber, monounsaturated fatty acids, and moderate amounts of alcohol. In contrast, increased dietary intakes of saturated fats and *trans*-fatty acids appear to increase risk of MI.

Comparability of effect in men and women: Data are insufficient to elucidate gender differences in any of these effects.

References

Achaya KT. Fat status of Indians: a review. J. Sci Ind Res 1987;46:112–26.

Anderson JW, Story L, Sieling B, et al. Hypocholesterolemic effects of oat bran or bean intake for hypercholesterolemic men. Am J Clin Nutr 1984;40:1146–55.

Anderson TW. The male epidemic. In: Proceedings of the Conference on the Decline in Coronary Heart Disease Mortality. (R.J. Havlik, M. Feinleib, eds.) U.S. Department of Health, Education, and Welfare, Public Health Service, NIH, Washington, DC (NIH Publ. No. 79-1610, 1979, pp. 42–7.

Anitschkow N. A history of experimentation on arteriosclerosis in animals. In: Blumenthal HT, ed. Cowdry's arteriosclerosis, 2nd ed. New York: Macmillan, 1967:21–44.

Ascherio A, Hennekens CH, Buring JE, et al. *Trans* fatty acids intake and risk of myocardial infarction. Circulation 1994a;89:94–101.

Ascherio A, Rimm EB, Stampfer MJ, et al. Dietary iron intake and risk of coronary disease among men. Circulation 1994b;89:969–74.

Bang HO, Dyerberg J, Sinclair HM. The composition of the Eskimo food in north western Greenland. Am J Clin Nutr 1980;33:2657–61.

Behall KM, Lee KH, Moser PB. Blood lipids and lipoproteins in adult men fed four refined fibers. Am J Clin Nutr 1984;39:209–14.

Block G, Abrams B. Vitamin and mineral status of women of childbearing potential. Ann NY Acad Sci 1993;678:244–54.

Brinton EA, Eisenberg S, Breslow JL. Increased apo A-1 and apo A-11 fractional catabolic rate in patients with low density lipoprotein-cholesterol levels with or without hypertriglyceridemia. J Clin Invest 1991;87:536–44.

Burr ML, Sweetnam PM. Vegetarianism, dietary fiber, and mortality. Am J Clin Nutr 1982;36:873–77.

Burr ML, Fehily AM, Gilbert JF. Effects of changes in fat, fish, fibre intakes on death and myocardial reinfarction: diet and reinfarction trial (DART). Lancet 1989;ii:757–61.

Caggiula AW, Christakis G, Farrand M, et al. The Multiple Risk Factor Intervention Trial (MRFIT). IV. Intervention on blood lipids. Prev Med 1981;10:443–475.

Camargo Jr CA, Williams PT, Vranizan KM, et al. The effect of moderate alcohol intake on serum apolipoproteins A-1 and A-11: a controlled study. JAMA 1985;253:2854–7.

Castelli WP, Abbott RD, McNamara PM. Summary estimation of cholesterol used to predict coronary heart disease. Circulation 1983;67:730–4.

Charnock JS, McLennan PL, Abeywardena MY. Dietary modulation of lipid metabolism and mechanical performance of the heart. Mol Cell Biochem 1992;116:19–25.

Clarke R, Daly L, Robinson D, et al. Hyperhomocysteinemia: an independent risk factor for vascular disease. N Engl J Med 1991;324:1149–5.

Consensus Conference. Lowering blood cholesterol to prevent heart disease. JAMA 1985;253: 2080–6.

Cook JD. Adaptation in iron metabolism. Am J Clin Nutr 1990;51:301–8.

Criqui MH, Cowan LD, Tyroler HA, et al. Lipoproteins as mediators for the effects of alcohol consumption and cigarette smoking on cardiovascular mortality: results from the Lipid Research Clinics Follow-up Study. Am J Epidemiol 1987;126:629–37.

Curb JD, Reed DM. Fish consumption and mortality from coronary heart disease [Letter]. N Engl J Med 1985;313:821.

Dawber TR, Nickerson RJ, Brand FN, Pool J. Eggs, serum cholesterol, and coronary heart disease. Am J Clin Nutr 1982;36:617–25.

Dayton S, Pearce ML, Hashimoto S, et al. A controlled clinical trial of a diet high in unsaturated fat in preventing complications of atherosclerosis. Circulation 1969;40(Suppl II-1).

De Lorgeril M, Renaud S, Mamelle N, et al. Mediterranean alpha-linolenic acid-rich diet in secondary prevention of coronary heart disease. Lancet 1994;343:1454–9.

Denke MA, Grundy SM. Effects of fats high in stearic acid on lipid and lipoprotein concentrations in men. Am J Clin Nutr 1991;54:1036–40.

Dolecek TA. Epidemiologic evidence of relationships between dietary polyunsaturated fatty acids and mortality in the Multiple Risk Factor Intervention Trial. Proc Soc Exp Biol Med 1992;200:177–82.

Ellison RC. Cheers! Epidemiology 1990;1:337–9.

Fehily AM, Yarnell JWG, Sweetnam PM, Elwood PC. Diet and incident ischaemic heart disease: the Caerphilly Study. Br J Nutr 1993;69:303–14.

Frantz ID, Dawson EA, Ashman PL, et al. Test of effect of lipid lowering by diet on cardiovascular risk: the Minnesota coronary survey. Arteriosclerosis 1989;9:129–35.

Fraser GE, Sabaté J, Beeson WL, Strahan TM. A possible protective effect of nut consumption on risk of coronary heart disease: the Adventist Health Study. Arch Intern Med 1992; 152:1416–24.

Friend B. Nutrients in the United States Food Supply: a review of trends, 1909–1913 to 1965. Am J Clin Nutr 1967;20:907–14.

Garcia-Palmieri MR, Sorlie PD, Tillotsen J, et al. Relation of dietary intake to subsequent coronary heart disease incidence: the Puerto Rican Heart Health Program. An J Clin Nutr 1980;33:1818–27.

Garrison RJ, Kannel WB. A new approach for estimating healthy body weights. Int J obesity 1993;17:417–23.

Gaziano JM, Buring JE, Breslow JL, et al. Moderate alcohol intake, increased levels of high-density lipoprotein and its subfractions and decreased risk of myocardial infarction. N Engl J Med 1993;329:1829–34.

Gey KF, Brubacher GB, Stahelin HB. Plasma levels of antioxidant vitamins in relation to ischemic heart disease and cancer. Am J Clin Nutr 1987;45(s):1368–77.

Giovannucci E, Stampfer MJ, Colditz GA, et al. Folate, methionine, and alcohol intake and risk of colorectal adenoma. JNCI 1993;85:875–884.

Goldbourt U, Yaari S, Medalie JH. Factors predictive of long-term coronary heart disease mortality among 10,059 male Israeli civil servants and municipal employees: a 23-year mortality follow-up in the Israeli ischemic heart disease study. Cardiology 1993;82:100–21.

Gordon T, Kagan A, Garcia-Palmieri M, et al. Diet and its relation to coronary heart disease and death in three populations. Circulation 1981;63:500–15.

Gordon T. The diet-heart idea: outline of a history. Am J Epidemiol 1988;127:220–5.

Gortmaker SL, Dietz WH, Cheung LW. Inactivity, diet, and the fattening of America. J Am Diet Assoc 1990;90:1247–52.

Grundy SM, Bilheimer D, Blackburn H, et al. Rationale of the Diet-Heart Statement of the American Heart Association: report of Nutrition Committee. Circulation 1982;65: 839A–54A.

Halliwell B. Current status review: free radicals, reactive oxygen species and human disease: a critical evaluation with special reference to atherosclerosis. Br J Exp Pathol 1989;70: 737–57.

Haskell WL, Camargo Jr C, Williams PT, et al. The effect of cessation and the resumption of moderate alcohol intake on serum high-density-lipoprotein subfractions: a controlled study. N Engl J Med 1984;310:805–10.

Hegsted DM. Serum-cholesterol response to dietary cholesterol: a re-evaluation. Am J Clin Nutr 1986;44:299–305.

Hegsted DM, Ausman LM, Johnson JA, Dallal GE. Dietary fat and serum lipids: an evaluation of the experimental data. Am J Clin Nutr 1993;57:875–83.

Hetzel BS, Charnock JS, Dwyer T, McLennan PL. Fall in coronary heart disease mortality in U.S.A. and Australia due to sudden death: evidence for the role of polyunsaturated fat. J Clin Epidemiol 1989;42:885–93.

Hjermann I, Holme I, Byre KV, Leren P. Effect of diet and smoking intervention on the incidence of coronary heart disease: report from the Oslo Study Group of a randomised trial in healthy men. Lancet 1981;ii:1303–10.

Hjermann I, Holme I, Leren P. Oslo Study Diet and Anti-smoking trial: results after 102 months. Am J Med 1986;80:7–11.

Jacobs D, Blackburn H, Higgins M, et al. Report of the Conference on Low Blood Cholesterol: mortality associations. Circulation 1992;86:1046–60.

Jenkins DJ, Wolever TM, Rao AV. Effect of blood lipids of very high intakes of fiber in diets low in saturated fat and cholesterol. N. Engl J Med 1993;329:21–6.

Judd JT, Clevidence BA, Muesing RA, et al. Dietary *trans* fatty acids: effects on plasma lipids and lipoproteins of healthy men and women. Am J Clin Nutr 1994;59:861–868.

Kagawa Y, Nishizawa M, Suzuki M, et al. Eicosapolyenoic acids of serum lipids of Japanese islanders with low incidence of cardiovascular disease. J. Nutr Sci Vitaminol 1982;28: 441–53.

Kahn HA. Change in serum cholesterol associated with changes in the United States civilian diet 1909–1965. Am J Clin Nutr 1970;23:879–82.

Kang SS, Wong PWK, Cook HY, et al. Protein bound hemocyst(e)ine: a possible risk factor for coronary artery disease. J Clin Invest 1986;77:1482–6.

Kato H, Tillotson J, Nichamen MZ, et al. Epidemiologic studies of coronary heart disease and stroke in Japanese men living in Japan, Hawaii and California: serum lipids and diet. Am J Epidemiol 1973;97:372–85.

Katz LN, Stamler JS. Experimental Atherosclerosis. Springfield, IL: Charles C. Thomas, 1953: 24–32.

Kestin M, Clifton P, Belling GB, Nestel PJ. N-3 fatty acids of marine origin lower systolic blood pressure and triglycerides but raise LDL cholesterol compared with N-3 and N-6 fatty acids from plants. Am J Clin Nutr 1990;51:1028–34.

Keys A. Seven countries: a multivariate analysis of death and coronary heart disease. Cambridge, MA: Harvard University Press, 1980.

Keys A. Serum cholesterol response to dietary cholesterol. Am J Clin Nutr 1984;40:351–9.

Khaw KT, Barrett-Connor E. Dietary fiber and reduce ischemic heart disease mortality rates in men and women: a 12-year prospective study. Am J Epidemiol 1987;126:1093–102.

Klatsky AI, Armstrong MA, Griedman GD. Risk of cardiovascular mortality in alcohol drinkers, ex-drinkers, and nondrinkers. Am J Cardiol 1990;66:1237–42.

Kok FJ, Hofman A, Witteman JC, et al. Decreased selenium levels in acute myocardial infarction. JAMA 1989;261:1161–4.

Korányi A. Prophylaxis and treatment of the coronary syndrome. Ther Hung 1963;12:17–20.

Kromhout D, Bosschieter EB, de Lezenne Coulander C. Dietary fiber and 10-year mortality from coronary heart disease, cancer and all causes: the Zutphen Study. Lancet 1982;ii: 518–21.

Kromhout D, de Lezenne Coulander C. Diet, prevalence and 10-year mortality from coronary heart disease in 871 middle-aged men: the Zutphen Study. Am J Epidemiol 1984:119: 733–41.

Kromhout D, Bosscheiter EB, de Lezenne Coulander C. The inverse relation between fish consumption and 20-year mortality from coronary heart disease. N. Engl J Med 1985; 312:1205–9.

Kushi LH, Lew RA, Stare FJ, et al. Diet and 20-year mortality from coronary heart disease: the Ireland-Boston Diet-Heart Study. N Engl J Med 1985;312:811–18.

Kushi LH. Total energy intake: implication for epidemiologic analyses [Letter]. Am J Epidemiol 1987;126:981–2.

Lapidus L, Anderson H, Bengtsson C, Bosaeus I. Dietary habits in relation to incidence of cardiovascular disease and death in women: a 12-year follow-up of participants in the population study of women in Gothenburg, Sweden. Am J Clin Nutr 1986;44:444–8.

Law MR, Frost CD, Wald NJ. By how much does dietary salt reduction lower blood pressure? Br Med J. 1991;302:811–24.

Law MR, Wald NJ, Thompson SG. By how much and how quickly does reduction in serum cholesterol concentration lower risk of ischaemic heart disease? Br Med J 1994;308: 367–72.

Leaf A, Weber PC. Cardiovascular effects of n-3 fatty acids. N Engl J Med 1988;318:549–57.

Leren P. The Oslo diet-heart study: eleven-year report. Circulation 1970;42:835–942.

Lew EA, Garfinkel L. Variations in mortality by weight among 750,000 men and women. J Chron Dis 1979;32:563–76.

Maclure M. A demonstration of deductive, meta-analysis: ethanol intake and risk of myocardial infarction. Epidemiol Rev 1993;15:328–51.

Malinow MR. Hyperhomocyst(e)inemia: a common and easily reversible risk factor for occlusive atherosclerosis. Circulation 1990;81:2004–6.

Mannitari M, Huttunen JK, Koskinen P, et al. Lipoproteins and coronary heart disease in the Helsinki Heart Study. Eur Heart J 1990;(Suppl H):26–31.

Manson JE, Stampfer MJ, Hennekens CH, Willett WC. Body weight and longevity: a reassessment. JAMA 1987;257:353–8.

Marckmann P, Sandström B, Jespersen J. Effects of total fat content and fatty acid composition in diet on factor VII coagulant activity and blood lipids. Atherosclerosis 1990;80:227–33.

Marckmann P, Sandström B, Jespersen J. Fasting blood coagulation and fibrinolysis of young adults unchanged by reduction in dietary fat content. Arterioscler Thromb 1992;12: 201–5.

McCord JM. Is iron sufficiently a risk factor in ischemic heart disease? Circulation 1991;83: 1112–14.

McGee DL, Reed DM, Yano K, et al. Ten-year incidence of coronary heart disease in the Honolulu Heart Program: relationship to nutrient intake. Am J Epidemiol 1984;119: 667–76.

McGill HC. The geographic pathway of atherosclerosis. Baltimore: Williams & Wilkins, 1968.

Mensink RP, Katan MB. Effect of dietary fatty acids on serum lipids and lipoproteins. Arteriosclerosis and Thrombosis 1992a;12:911−19.

Mensink RP, Zock PL, Katan MB, Hornstra G. Effect of dietary *cis* and *trans* fatty acids on serum lipoprotein [a] levels in humans. J Lipid Res 1992b;33:1493−501.

Miettinen TA, Naukkarinen V, Huttunen JK, et al. Fatty-acid composition of serum lipids predicts myocardial infarction. Br Med J 1982;285:993−6.

Miettinen TA, Alfthan G, Huttunen JK, et al. Serum selenium concentration related to myocardial infarction and fatty acid content of serum lipids. Br Med J 1983;287:517−19.

Miller M, Grover M, Hutchins MD. Hemochromatosis, multiorgan hemosiderosis, and coronary artery disease. JAMA 1994;272:231−3.

Miller NE. Associations of high-density lipoprotein subclasses and apolipoproteins with ischemic heart disease and coronary artherosclerosis. Am Heart J 1987;113:589−97.

Moore JA, Novia R, Wells IC. Selenium concentrations in plasma of patients with arteriographically defined coronary atherosclerosis. Clin Chem 1984;30:1171−3.

Moore RD, Pearson TA. Moderate alcohol consumption and coronary artery disease: a review. Medicine 1986;65:242−67.

Morris JN, Ball KP, Antonis A, et al. Controlled trial of soya-bean oil in myocardial infarction. Lancet 1968;ii:693−700.

Morris JN, Marr JW, Clayton DG. Diet and heart: a postscript. Br Med J 1977;2:1307−14.

Morris MC, Sacks FM, Rosner B. Does fish oil lower blood pressure? A meta-analysis of controlled trials. Circulation 1993;88:523−33.

Morrision LM. Diet in coronary artherosclerosis. JAMA 1960;173:884−8.

MRC. Low-fat diet in myocardial infarction: a controlled trial. Lancet 1965;ii:501−4.

MRC Vitamin Study Research Group. Prevention of neural tube defects: results of the Medical Research Council Vitamin Study. Lancet 1991;338:131−7.

Multiple Risk Factor Intervention Trial Research Group. Multiple Risk Factor Intervention Trial: risk factor changes and mortality results. JAMA 1982;248:1465−77.

National Research Council. Diet and health: implications for reducing chronic disease risk. Washington, DC: National Academy Press, 1989.

Nestel P, Noakes M, Belling B, et al. Plasma lipoprotein and Lp[a] changes with substitution of elaidic acid for oleic acid in the diet. J Lipid Res 1992;33:1029−36.

Norell SE, Ahlbom A, Feychting M, Pedersen NL. Fish consumption and mortality from coronary heart disease. Br Med J 1986;293:426.

Olszewski AJ, McCully KS. Homocysteine metabolism and the oxidative modification of proteins and lipids. Free Radic Biol Med 1993;14:683−93.

Ornish D. Dr. Dean Ornish's program for reversing heart disease. New York: Ballantine, 1990.

Page L, Marston RM. Food consumption pattern: U.S. diet. In: Havlik RJ, Feinleib M, eds. Proceedings of the Conference on the Decline in Coronary Heart Disease Mortality, U.S. Department Health, Education, Welfare, Public Health Service, NIH, Washington, DC (NIH Publ. No. 79-1610), 1979, pp. 236−43.

Potter JG, Coffman KP, Reid RL, et al. Effect of test meals of varying dietary fiber content on plasma insulin and glucose response. Am J Clin Nutr 1981;34:328−34.

Reaven P, Parthasaranthy S, Grasse GJ, Miller E, Steinberg D, Witzum JL. Effects of oleate-rich and linoleate-rich diets on the susceptibility of low density lipoprotein to oxidative modification in mildly hypercholesterolemic subjects. J Clin Invest 1993;91:668−76.

Renaud S, Kuba K, Goulet C, et al. Relationship between fatty-acid composition of platelets and platelet aggregation in rat and man: relation to thrombosis. Cir Res 1970;26:553−64.

Renaud S, de Lorgeril M. Wine, alcohol, platelets, and the French paradox for coronary disease. Lancet 1992;339:1523−6.

Rimm EB, Giovannucci EL, Willett WC, et al. A prospective study of alcohol consumption and the risk of coronary disease in men. Lancet 1991;338:464–8.

Rimm EB, Stampfer MJ, Ascherio A, et al. Vitamin E consumption and the risk of coronary heart disease in men. N Engl J Med 1993;328:1450–6.

Rinehart FJ, Greenberg LD. Pathogenesis of experimental arteriosclerosis in pyridoxine deficiency. Arch Pathol 1951;51:12–18.

Rivellese A, Riccardi G, Giacco A, et al. Effect of dietary fibre on glucose control and serum lipoproteins in diabetic patients. Lancet 1980;ii:447–50.

Robertson TL, Kato H, Rhoads GG, et al. Epidemiologic studies of coronary heart disease and stroke in Japanese men living in Japan, Hawaii and California: incidence of myocardial infarction and death from coronary heart disease. Am J Cardiol 1977;39:239–43.

Rose GA, Thomson WB, Williams RT. Corn oil in treatment of ischaemic heart disease. Br Med J 1965;i:1531–3.

Rosenberg L, Slone D, Shapiro S, et al. Alcoholic beverages and myocardial infarction in your women. Am J Public Health 1981;71:82–5.

Sacks FM, Willett WC. More on chewing the fat—the good fat and the good cholesterol. N Engl J Med 1991;325:1740–42.

Salonen JT, Alfthan G, Huttunen JK, et al. Association between cardiovascular death and myocardial infarction and serum selenium in a matched-pair longitudinal study. Lancet 1982; ii:175–9.

Salonen JT, Nyyssonen K, Korpela H, et al. High stores iron levels are associated with excess risk of myocardial infarction in eastern Finnish men. Circulation 1992;86:803–11.

Schrade W, Biegler R, Boehle E. Fatty-acid distribution in the lipid fractions of healthy persons of different age, patients with atherosclerosis and patients with idiopathic hyperlipidaemia. J Atheroscler Res 1961;1:47–61.

Scrimshaw NS, Guzman MA. Diet and atherosclerosis. Lab Invest 1968;18:623–8.

Selhub J, Jacques PF, Wilson PWF, et al. Vitamin status and intake as primary determinants of homocysteinemia in an elderly population. JAMA 1993;270:2693–8.

Sempos CT, Looker AC, Gillum RF, Makuc DM. Body iron stores and the risk of coronary heart disease. N Engl J Med 1994;330:1119–24.

Senti FR. Health aspects of dietary *trans* fatty acids: August 1985. Federation of American Societies for Experimental Biology (contract No. FDA 223-83-2020). Bethesda, 1988.

Shaper AG. Alcohol and Mortality: a review of prospective studies. Br J Addict 1990;85:837–47.

Shekelle RB, Shyrock AM, Paul O, et al. Diet, serum cholesterol and death from coronary heart disease, the Western Electric Study. N Engl J Med 1981;304:65–70.

Shekelle RB, Missell L, Paul O, Shyrock AM, Stamler J. Fish consumption and mortality from coronary heart disease [Letter]. N Engl J Med 1985;313:820.

Shekelle RB, Stamler J. Dietary cholesterol and ischemic heart disease. Lancet 1989;1:1177–9.

Siguel EN, Lerman RH. *Trans* fatty acid patterns in patients with angiographically documented coronary artery disease. Am J Cardiol 1993;71:916–20.

Singh RB, Rastogi S, Verma R, et al. Randomised controlled trial of cardioprotective diet in patients with recent acute myocardial infarction: results of one year follow-up. Br Med J 1992;304:1015–19.

Snowdon DA, Phillips RL, Fraser GE. Meat consumption and fatal ischemic heart disease. Prev Med 1984;13:490–500.

Stamler J. The marked decline in coronary heart disease mortality rates in the United States, 1968–1981: summary of findings and possible explanations. Cardiology 1985;72:11–12.

Stampfer MJ, Colditz GA, Willett WC, et al. A prospective study of moderate alcohol consumption and the risk of coronary heart disease and stroke in women. N Engl J Med 1988;319:267–73.

Stampfer MJ, Sacks FM, Salvini S, et al. A prospective study of cholesterol, apolipoproteins, and the risk of myocardial infarction. N Engl J Med 1991;325:373–81.

Stampfer MJ, Malinow MR, Willett WC, et al. A prospective study of plasma homocyste(e)ine and risk of myocardial infarction. JAMA 1992;268:877–81.

Stampfer MJ, Hennekens CH, Manson JE, et al. A prospective study of vitamin E consumption and risk of coronary disease in women. N Engl J Med 1993;328:1444–9.

Steinberg D, Witztum JL. Lipoproteins and atherogenesis: current concepts. JAMA 1990;264: 3047–52.

Sullivan JL. The iron paradigm of ischemic heart disease. Am Heart J 1989;117:1177–88.

Swain JF, Rouse IL, Courley CB, Sacks FM. Comparison of the effects of oat bran and low-fiber wheat on serum lipoprotein levels and blood pressure. N Engl J Med 1990;322: 193–5.

Tanaka H, Yamaguchi M, Date C, et al. Nutrition and cardiovascular disease: a brief review of epidemiological studies in Japan. Nutr Health 1992;8:107–23.

Turpeinen O, Karvonen MJ, Pekkarinen M, et al. Dietary prevention of coronary heart disease: the Finnish Mental Hospital Study. Int J Epidemiol 1979;8:99–118.

U.S. Department of Agriculture. The food guide pyramid: home and garden bulletin, No. 252. Washington, DC: GPO, 1992:30 pp.

Valimaki M, Nikkila EA, Taskinen MR, Ylikahri R. Rapid decrease in high density lipoprotein subfractions and postheparin plasma lipase activities after cessation of chronic alcohol intake. Atherosclerosis 1986;59:147–53.

Virtamo J, Valkeila E, Alfthan G, et al. Serum selenium and the risk of coronary heart disease and stroke. Am J Epidemiol 1985;122:276–82.

Vollset SE, Heuch I, Bjelke E. Fish consumption and mortality from coronary heart disease [Letter]. N Engl J Med 1985;313:820–1.

Watts GF, Lewis B, Brunt JNH, et al. Effects of coronary artery disease of lipid-lowering diet, or diet plus cholestyramine, in the St. Thomas' Atherosclerosis Regression Study (STARS). Lancet 1992;339:563–9.

Werler MM, Shapiro S, Mitchell AA. Periconceptional folic acid exposure and risk of occurrent neural tube defects. JAMA 1993;269:1257–61.

Welsch CW. Relationship between dietary fat and experimental mammary tumorigenesis: a review and critique. Cancer Res 1992;52(Suppl 7);2040S–8S.

Willett WC, Stampfer MJ. Total energy intake: implications for epidemiologic analyses. Am J Epidemiol 1986;124:17–27.

Willett WC. Nutritional epidemiology. New York: Oxford University Press, 1990.

Willett WC, Stampfer MJ, Colditz GA, et al. Intake of *trans* fatty acids and risk of coronary heart disease among women. Lancet 1993;341:581–5.

Willett WC. Diet and health: what should we eat? Science 1994;264:532–7.

Wissler RW, Vesselinovitch D. The effects of feeding various dietary fats on the development and regression of hypercholesterolemia and atherosclerosis. Adv Exp Med Biol 1975; 60:65–76.

Wood DA, Butler DS, Riemersma RA, et al. Adipose tissue and platelet fatty acids and coronary heart disease in Scottish men. Lancet 1984;ii:117–21.

Wood DA, Riemersma RA, Butler S, et al. Linoleic and eicosapentaenoic acids in adipose tissue and platelets and risk of coronary heart disease. Lancet 1987;i:117–83.

Woodhill JM, Palmer AJ, Leelarthaepin B, et al. Low fat, low cholesterol diet in secondary prevention of coronary heart disease. Adv Exp Med Biol 1978;109:317–30.

Working Group on Arteriosclerosis of the National Heart, Lung, and Blood Institute. Decline in coronary heart disease mortality, 1963–1978, Vol. 2. Bethesda, MD: National Institutes of Health, 1981:157–258 (DHHS Publication No. (NIH) 82-2035), 1981.

World Health Organization, ''Food and Health Indicators in Europe,'' (Preliminary computer software issued by the WHO Regional Office for Europe, Copenhagen, September 1993).

Zock PL, Katan MB. Hydrogenation alternatives: effects of *trans* fatty acids and stearic acid versus linoleic acid on serum lipids and lipoproteins in humans. J Lipid Res 1992;33: 399–410.

III

PREVENTION OF HEART DISEASE IN WOMEN: SPECIAL ISSUES

15

Gender Differences in Coronary Risk and Risk Factors

NANETTE K. WENGER

Until recently, coronary heart disease (CHD) and its complications were often regarded as a less significant public health problem for women than for men, due to the much lower risk of premature morbidity and mortality from these endpoints among women (Kannel 1987). Specifically, while an equal number of men and women eventually die from CHD, the disease primarily affects middle-aged men and older women. However, in the United States and other industrialized nations, a woman is more likely to die from CHD or a related illness than from any other health problem (Eaker 1993). Not only do women lose their gender protection once they develop overt CHD, but they also suffer more adverse outcomes than their male counterparts; case-fatality rates are higher for women following both myocardial infarction (MI) and myocardial revascularization procedures, with 40% of all coronary events in women being fatal; in addition, 67% of all sudden deaths in women occur in those not known to have CHD (Kannel 1987). Coronary disease is also a leading cause of disability in women (Soldo 1985); 36% of women with CHD aged 55 to 64 years are disabled from their coronary disease, and the percentage increases to 55% at age 75 years and older. The significant decreases in both cardiovascular and CHD mortality rates in such countries during the past several decades have been less pronounced among women than men, as have reductions in the prevalence of coronary risk factors.

In general, risk factors for cardiovascular disease in women are similar to those in men (Bush 1987; Barrett-Connor 1987; Eaker 1987; Higgins 1987; Keil 1987; Stampfer 1987; Wingard 1987), and the correlation of the three major risk factors—cigarette smoking, hypertension, and hypercholesterolemia—with the rates of CHD is comparable for both genders. Additionally, although hypertension and hypercholesterolemia are more prevalent among younger men, there is a male-female crossover effect at older age, most prominent for hypercholesterolemia (Williams 1993) (Figure 15.1). Other risk factors, however, appear to have different effects for women and men, including diabetes, obesity, and body fat distribution, levels of circulating lipoproteins, and gonadal hormone status (Leaf 1990). Most of these modifiable coronary risk factors are also highly prevalent at older ages, with most increasing risk at least through the

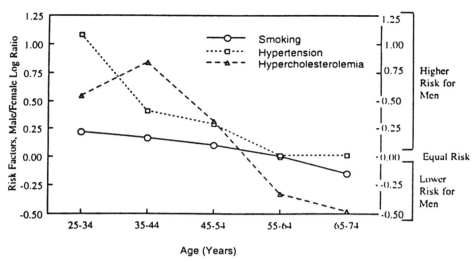

Fig. 15.1. Male/female risk factor prevalence log ratios by age, pooled data from four independent surveys (1979–1986), treatment and control cities combined, Stanford Five-City Project.

eighth decade of life. Although the relative risk of these factors decreases with aging, their absolute risk is increased, owing to the greater prevalence of coronary disease at elderly age. Attenuation of progression, and possibly even regression, of atherosclerosis can occur with coronary risk reduction even at elderly age; thus reduction of coronary risk factors, even in elderly women, offers substantial opportunity to lessen their coronary morbidity and mortality (Kannel 1988).

Nonmodifiable risk factors such as family history should not be overlooked, as women whose mother or siblings had premature coronary disease or stroke were more likely to incur MI than those with a comparable paternal history (Rosenberg 1983). Socioeconomic factors are also important, with cardiovascular mortality in the United States being higher among nonworking women, those with less than a 12th-grade education, those whose family incomes are less than $20,000 annually, unmarried women, and those who live alone (Rogot 1988). Social class–CHD interrelationships are comparable for women in England (Health Update 1993).

Clearly, preventive interventions are warranted to improve the cardiovascular health of women in developed countries. There is also an urgent need for the education of women, particularly those in high-risk socioeconomic groups, regarding their risks of CHD, since unless they are made aware of their vulnerability to CHD, it is unlikely that prevention messages will be appropriately heeded.

Despite the magnitude and serious public health implications of CHD among women, most epidemiologic studies have tended either to exclude women systematically because of their relatively low endpoint rates, or to follow insufficient numbers of women to permit reliable estimates of CHD risk or the efficacy of interventions. Similarly, older age groups, which tend to include a much higher proportion of women, have often been excluded from study because of logistical problems and/or small numbers. It is essential to address these information gaps, as both specific coronary risk factors and the effects of interventions may differ qualitatively and/or quantitatively among women, particularly older women, compared with men.

Cigarette Smoking

Although cigarette smoking was previously far more prevalent among men than among women, rates of smoking cessation have been far greater among men, such that there is currently little gender difference in the prevalence of cigarette smoking in the United States (Fiore 1989). From 1955 to 1990, cigarette smoking by both white and black women in the U.S. decreased by 30% and 36% respectively (National Center for Health Statistics 1991). Nevertheless, almost 23% of women in the United States older than 18 years of age still smoke cigarettes (Heart and Stroke Facts 1993); this represents almost 22 million cigarette-smoking women. Moreover, numbers of cigarettes smoked daily has increased among women, while their age at onset of smoking has decreased. As with men, cigarette smoking predominates among less-educated, lower socioeconomic status women. National cross-sectional data from 1965 to 1990 have identified the greatest increase in the percentage of women who smoked in the age group 65 years or older; this constituted a 45% increase in the adoption of smoking. Women with the greatest reduction in the proportion of smokers were in the age cohort 18 to 44 years. The former figures likely reflect the population of women who began smoking during the 1940s and continued to do so into old age, while the latter likely represent the smaller proportion of younger women who smoked in 1987 compared with 1965 (National Center for Health Statistics 1991).

Smoking cessation is similarly associated with demographic variables, being more likely to occur among Caucasians, married people, and those having a higher socioeconomic status (Coambs 1992). Development of CHD predicted smoking cessation in both genders in the Framingham cohort (Freund 1992). While smoking cessation is most likely to occur in the 65–75 age group, the relative decrease in coronary risk in ex-smokers is comparable above and below 65 years of age.

As regards risk of CHD among smokers, especially among premenopausal women, cigarette smoking imparts a far greater risk of MI than is present in nonsmokers, and the relative excess risk of initial infarction is significantly greater in female than male smokers (Hennekens 1979; Nyboe 1991). Smoking may lower the age at menopause and thereby contribute to the more adverse impact of smoking in women (Hansen 1993). In the Nurses' Health Study (Willett 1987), one of the largest epidemiologic investigations conducted entirely among women, the number of cigarettes smoked daily correlated with the risk of fatal CHD (RR = 5.5 for more than 25 cigarettes daily), nonfatal MI (RR = 5.8), and angina (RR = 2.6). A 2 to 3 times increased risk of fatal CHD and nonfatal MI occurred with smoking 1 to 4 or 5 to 14 cigarettes daily. Women in the Nurses' Health Study who smoked 15 or more cigarettes daily had a 2.6-fold increased risk of incident angina compared with nonsmoking women (Willett 1987). Cigarette smoking imparted the greatest risk to women already at increased risk due to older age, parental history of MI, increased weight, hypertension, hypercholesterolemia, or diabetes, mandating that smoking cessation efforts be particularly targeted at these high-risk subgroups.

A consistent finding across studies is that smoking cessation confers benefit such that former smokers have the same rates of MI and fatal CHD as do women who never smoked; this result suggests that relatively acute mechanisms such as platelet aggregation and clotting factors are implicated in the coronary risk of smoking (Rosenberg 1985; Willett 1987). Smoking cessation has also been documented to improve survival and lessen reinfarction in the presence of established CHD, including following MI (Perkins 1985) and after coronary bypass surgery (Hermanson 1988). This beneficial effect did not diminish with increasing age in patients in the Coronary Artery Surgery Study registry (Hermanson 1988). Thus smoking cessation can importantly lesson coronary morbidity and mortality among women at all ages.

Hypertension

In the United States, hypertension occurs in 50% of white women and 79% of black women over the age of 45 years (National Center for Health Statistics 1991). Among those aged 45–64, prevalence of hypertension is 45%, with the percentage rising to 71% after age 65 (National Center for Health Statistics, National Health Interview Survey, unpublished). After age 65 women of all races have a higher prevalence of hypertension than men. Hypertension is almost as frequent in women across the life span as in men, but cardiovascular complications of hypertension are higher for women than for men (Anastos 1991) (Table 15.1). Despite this widespread prevalence of hypertension, only about 54% of all hypertensive individuals in the United States are aware that they have hypertension, and only about 11% currently receive adequate therapy (1993 Heart and Stroke Facts 1992).

Hypertension, both systolic and diastolic, is the dominant contributor to cardiovascular risk in elderly women. Systolic blood pressure increases disproportionately in women with aging until beyond age 80, in contrast to the systolic blood pressure among men that peaks in middle age and levels off subsequently (Kannel 1988). Isolated systolic hypertension, a finding more prevalent in elderly women than men, results in an excess of heart failure, stroke, angina, and MI. Control of blood pressure by drug treatment, including control of isolated systolic hypertension, has been documented to decrease both stroke and nonfatal and fatal cardiovascular events for both women and men (SHEP 1991); however, the reduction in mortality for men in the European Working Party study was substantially greater than for women (Amery 1985).

Women may respond differently than men to drug therapy, and the best drug regimen for hypertension control in women remains uncertain. Clinical trial data document benefits of drug therapy for black women, but these are not evident for white women, among whom some studies have suggested an adverse effect of therapy (Anastos 1991). Effects of antihypertensive therapy on lipid levels and on sexual dysfunction also have not been assessed among women. In the Hypertension Detection and Follow-up Program trial, 46% of subjects were women and 44% were black. Mortality in the stepped care group decreased with therapy in all men and in black

Table 15.1. Cardiovascular Events according to Hypertensive Status, Gender, and Age (Framingham Data Extrapolated to the White U.S. Population Aged 45 to 74 Years)

	Women, *age*			Men, *age*		
	45–54	55–64	65–74	45–54	55–64	65–74
		$\longleftarrow$		N		$\longrightarrow$
Hypertensive status						
Normal (<140/90)	27,327	63,556	69,720	82,956	143,926	106,533
Hypertensive (>160/95)	98,174	246,930	288,609	227,646	405,021	317,730
Number of events attributable to hypertension ($I_H - I_N$)	70,847	183,374	218,889	144,690	261,095	211,197

Source: From Anastos et al. (1991), with permission.

women but increased in white women; however, the fact that white women had the highest percentage of treatment in the referred care group may account for the difference in outcome in this subgroup analysis (Hypertension Detection and Follow-up Program 1979). In the British Medical Research Council study of Treatment of Mild Hypertension (Medical Research Council 1985), all cause mortality decreased by 15% in treated men but increased by 26% in treated women; 48% of subjects were women and almost all were white. By contrast, the Australian Therapeutic Trial of Mild Hypertension (Report by the Management Committee 1980), in which all subjects were white, showed equal or greater benefit for treated women than treated men; this difference did not reach statistical significance, possibly due to the small number of women in the study.

Cholesterol, Lipoproteins, and Triglycerides

In contrast to the situation at younger ages, high serum cholesterol levels are more prevalent in middle-aged and older women, particularly those who are postmenopausal, than in men (Heart and Stroke Facts 1993) (Figure 15.2). Menopause appears to be associated with potentially adverse lipid and lipoprotein changes that are independent of age and body mass index (Stevenson 1993). From early adolescence through the premenopausal years, women have higher levels of high density lipoprotein (HDL) and lower levels of low density lipoprotein (LDL) cholesterol than men. HDL levels remain unchanged during the menstrual cycle, despite lowering of LDL levels during the luteal phase of the cycle (Kim 1979). Serum total cholesterol levels continue to rise with aging in women, at least to age 70; in the postmenopausal years, although HDL levels remain higher for women than for men, LDL levels rise progressively to exceed those in men (Kannel 1988). However the lack of association between menopause and levels of HDL cholesterol suggests that menopause may not affect coronary risk via HDL cholesterol lowering (Demirovic 1992). The contribution to these gender differences of early death among hyperlipidemic men also requires ascertainment. The total:HDL cholesterol ratio continues to rise in women until at least age 80; in men total and LDL cholesterol levels tend not to rise further beyond age 60 (Kannel 1988). In 1980, data showed that about one-third of all women in the United States had serum cholesterol levels greater than 240 mg/dl, with this percentage rising to more than 50% in women older than 55.

The National Health and Nutrition Examination Survey (NHANES) 1988–1991 data show a continuing substantial decline in cholesterol levels of U.S. adults. Mean total cholesterol level for women aged 20 to 34 was 185 mg/dl, rising to 234 mg/dl at age 65 to 74 (Johnson 1993). Since HDL and LDL levels appear to be better markers for risk among women than is total serum cholesterol, recent national data regarding these subsets are of interest. Mean LDL cholesterol at ages 20 to 34 was 110 mg/dl and 147 mg/dl at ages 65 to 74; comparable HDL levels were 56 mg/dl at both age ranges. Mean triglyceride levels at ages 20 to 34 were 101 mg/dl, rising to 168 at ages 55 to 64 and 155 at ages 65 to 74 (Johnson 1993). Based on a 1988 report, however, only 28% of women in the United States had been told their serum choles-

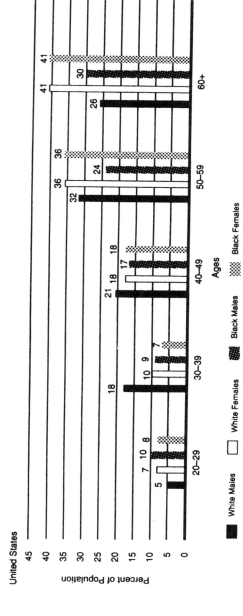

Fig. 15.2. Estimated percentage of adults with serum cholesterol of 240 mg/dl or more, by age, sex and race. [From Centers for Disease Control/National Center for Health Statistics: Unpublished data from Phase I of the National Health and Nutrition Examination Survey III (NHANES III), 1988–91.]

terol level, and only 13.5% of women reported knowing this level (Anda 1990). These data do not differ substantially from those for men.

Elevated serum total cholesterol or LDL levels, as well as decreased HDL levels all impart coronary risk for women; however, the cholesterol-coronary mortality relationship is less prominent among black than white women (Knapp 1992), and the postmenopausal elevation of total cholesterol levels present in white women was not evident among black women (Demirovic 1992). Elevation of triglyceride levels was described to increase risk for women, particularly those older than 50 years, to a greater extent than for men (Castelli 1986). Triglyceride elevation is directly associated with overweight, older age, diabetes melitus, and oral contraceptive use (Castelli 1985). Elevated triglyceride levels and lower levels of high-density lipoprotein cholesterol are described to be more powerful coronary risk factors for women than for men (Castelli 1986; Gordon 1989; LaRosa 1992). It remains uncertain to what extent and by what mechanism elevated triglyceride levels impart risk in women but not in men, but the higher percentage of smaller, more dense LDL fractions, which are more susceptible to oxidation has been implicated; menopause correlated positively with higher levels of LDL cholesterol and decreased LDL particle size, even after adjustment for significant covariates (Campos 1988). However, recent data from the Lipid Research Clinics Follow-up Study (Criqui 1993) show that, although coronary death rates in both genders increased with higher triglyceride levels, after adjustment for covariates, plasma triglyceride levels were not independently associated with coronary mortality. Nor was hypertriglyceridemia found to impart independent risk in the Prospective Cardiovascular Munster (PROCAM) Study cohort in either gender (Assmann 1992). Current recommendations (NIH Consensus 1993) are that HDL and triglyceride levels be measured in those with high total cholesterol levels and in those who have two or more known risk factors for CHD, including age 55 years or older or premature menopause without estrogen replacement therapy (Expert Panel 1993). Patients with diabetes, central obesity, peripheral vascular disease, hypertension, and chronic renal disease (all of which are associated with an increased risk of CHD) are recommended to have triglyceride levels measured. Measurement of HDL and triglyceride levels is recommended for all patients known to have CHD. Nonpharmacologic measures, such as diet, weight loss, smoking cessation, and increased physical activity, are recommended for low HDL or elevated triglyceride levels (NIH Consensus 1993).

In the few primary and secondary prevention clinical trials of cholesterol lowering that included women and where gender comparison was available (Five-year Study 1971; Report by a Research Committee 1971; Miettinen 1972), there was comparable cholesterol-lowering in women and men with clofibrate and with diet, respectively; and comparable gender declines in coronary mortality rates were evident (Rossouw 1990). However, other studies of dietary intervention, both in premenopausal (Mensink 1987; Masarei 1984) and postmenopausal (Barnard 1991) women showed less effect of dietary fat and cholesterol restriction in lowering circulating lipoprotein and triglyceride levels than was evident among men at comparable ages.

Although no primary or secondary prevention trials of cholesterol-lowering with total mortality endpoints have included women, regression of coronary atherosclerosis at coronary arteriography in patients with familial hypercholesterolemia treated with combined drug regimens was comparable in women and men (Kane 1990). In the

Program on the Surgical Control of the Hyperlipidemias, lipid-lowering and coronary arteriography findings of lessened disease progression in women paralleled those of the total study population and of male participants (Buchwald 1992).

Based on data from Framingham and a number of other population studies, increased LDL cholesterol and decreased HDL cholesterol concentrations predict CHD well into the eighth decade (Manolio 1992). Although the attribution of risk is evident, there remains uncertainty as to the role of diet versus drugs in modifying coronary risk, particularly in elderly women, as well as the role of lowering of triglyceride levels in reducing coronary risk (NIH Consensus 1993). Therefore, low-risk primary preventive interventions consisting of diet and lifestyle changes appear appropriate for apparently healthy elderly women. At elderly ages, even these must be individualized, based on general health and functional status, as well as psychosocial and cognitive status, and always with attention to safeguarding overall nutritional intake.

On the other hand, once CHD is documented, more intensive lipid intervention appears reasonable at any age (Expert Panel 1993). Framingham data (Wong 1991) regarding patients recovered from MI identify that the risks of recurrent infarction and coronary and all-cause mortality are increased with elevated cholesterol concentrations. Although the cholesterol-risk association was stronger for men than for women, this association was particularly prominent at elderly ages. However, the role of pharmacotherapy has not been adequately investigated, nor is there evidence as to the best drug regimen; this issue requires evaluation, given the potential greater susceptibility of elderly women to the adverse effects of hypolipidemic agents, such as myopathy and rhabdomyolysis (Goldstein 1990).

Glucose Intolerance and Diabetes Mellitus

Diabetes is a more powerful coronary risk factor for women than for men, negating the protective effect of female gender on CHD risk, even for premenopausal women (Krolewski 1991); diabetic women and diabetic men have comparable rates of coronary disease across the lifespan. Maturity-onset diabetic women in the Nurses' Health Study had a three- to sevenfold increase in cardiovascular events; 14% of coronary events and 15% of cardiovascular deaths were considered a consequence of risk attributable to diabetes (Manson 1991a), and the excess coronary risk due to diabetes was greater in the presence of other coronary risk factors. In addition, more women than men have diabetes mellitus at the time of an initial MI.

The mechanisms by which diabetes imparts excess coronary risk in women remains to be elucidated (Barrett-Connor 1991b) (Figure 15.3), particularly since diabetic women have less unfavorable lipid profiles than do diabetic men (Krolewski 1991). The excess of hypertension in older diabetic women as compared with diabetic men may be a potential contributor to risk (Maggi 1990). Based on Framingham data (Kannel 1990), abnormalities of fibrinogen may adversely influence coronary risk in diabetic women. The contribution of insulin resistance/hyperinsulinemia and its interrelationship with upper-body obesity, hypertension and hypertriglyceridemia to risk suggest that prevention of upper-body obesity warrants attention (Kaplan 1989). These associations in substantial numbers of women with hypertension are likely to influence

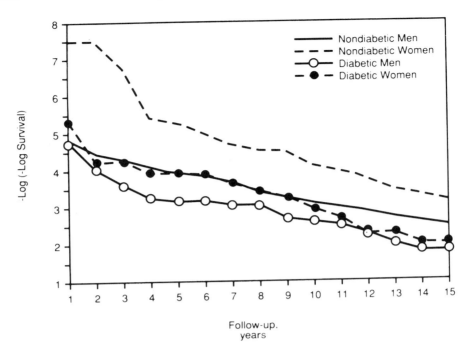

Fig. 15.3. Age-adjusted ischemic heart disease -log (-log survival) by sex and diabetes; Rancho Bernardo, Calif, 1972 through 1988. Curves were estimated by a Cox model blocked on both sex and diabetes status and adjusted for age.

the outcome of pharmacotherapy studies in women in that a variety of antihypertensive agents may alter insulin, glucose, and lipid metabolism. However, other studies describe hyperinsulinemia as a risk factor only for men (Modan 1991). Increased serum uric acid levels are described to correlate better with the presence of CHD in female than in male diabetic patients (Rathmann 1993), independently of hypertension and nephropathy. Although the value of precise blood glucose control in decreasing microvascular complications has been shown for both genders in insulin-dependent diabetes mellitus (American Diabetes Association 1993), this has not been assessed in the more common maturity-onset non-insulin-dependent diabetes. Further, the role of glycemic control in reducing macrovascular complications has been minimally studied in either type of diabetes.

Among the middle-aged women in the Nurses' Health Study, even after adjustment for other risk factors, diabetes exerted an independent effect, with a relative risk of 3.1 (95% CI: 2.3–4.2) for nonfatal MI and for fatal CHD (Manson 1991a). However, this cohort also showed a significant reduction in the incidence of non-insulin-dependent diabetes mellitus among both obese and nonobese women who exercised regularly (Manson 1991b).

Diabetes adversely affects both in-hospital and long-term prognosis for MI, conferring a substantially higher risk of mortality in women than in men (Liao 1993)

(Figure 15.4). In women, as compared with men, diabetes doubled the risk of recurrent infarction; and diabetic women developed cardiac failure four times more often than women without diabetes (Abbott 1988). Diabetes significantly predicted an increased hospital and one-year mortality for women with MI, but not for men (RR = 1.7; 95% CI: 1.10–2.53 vs RR = 0.96; 95% CI: 0.69–1.34) (Greenland 1991). Not only is the female advantage encountered in non-diabetic populations eliminated when diabetes is present (Donahue 1993), but these data and others (Varma 1992) identify diabetic women as a high-risk subset of patients with MI. The higher prevalence of diabetes among women than men who undergo coronary angioplasty and coronary bypass surgery (Eaker 1989) likely contributes to the higher mortality of women who undergo these procedures.

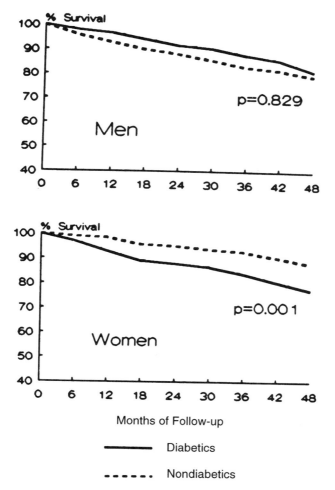

Fig. 15.4. Cumulative survival of patients with angiographically confirmed CHD by sex and diabetic status.

Obesity and Body Fat Distribution

Although obesity has increased in prevalence in the United States for both women and men, the prevalence is greatest among women in general, and among black, Hispanic, and Native American women in particular (Spelsberg 1993). As with cigarette smoking, overweight is inversely related to educational level and family income. Physical inactivity is an important determinant of obesity in women, but obesity may also be a cause of physical inactivity (National Institutes of Health Consensus Development Panel 1985). Based on 1988 data, almost 50% of black women and 30% of white women in the United States were obese (approximately 20% of more above desirable weight) (Barrett-Connor 1985; Manson 1987; National Center for Health Statistics 1991). The average weight gain after age 18 of black women was double that of white women. Based on 26-year follow-up Framingham data, obesity was a significant independent predictor of cardiovascular disease, particularly among women (Hubert 1983). Relative weight in women was positively and independently associated with coronary disease incidence, stroke, congestive failure, and coronary and cardiovascular death. Obesity is associated with triple the risk of CHD as compared with leanness (Manson 1990). Intervention in obesity, in addition to the well-established coronary risk factors, is recommended for the primary prevention of cardiovascular disease. Weight control can substantially improve the cardiovascular risk profile. However, weight loss may prove less effective in lowering LDL and reversing HDL cholesterol levels in women than in men (Brownell 1981).

Although, based on Framingham data, overweight appears to be a more potent risk factor for elderly men than for elderly women, the pattern of body fat distribution may be an important independent risk factor; an increased waist:hip ratio increases risk among both women and men. An increased waist:hip ratio was associated with lower HDL cholesterol and apolipoprotein Al, and higher LDL cholesterol, triglyceride, and apolipoprotein B levels in postmenopausal women. The abdominal fat preponderance in postmenopausal women was thus associated with an atherogenic plasma lipid profile, independent of its association with body mass index (Soler 1988). Upper-body obesity in older women increased the likelihood of angiographically documented coronary disease (Hartz 1990), and has been associated with diabetes, higher triglyceride and insulin levels, as well as increased blood pressure, even in the absence of obesity (Kaplan 1989). In the Goteborg cohort, abdominal body fat distribution or a factor correlated with waist:hip ratio was considered a major explanation for gender difference in the incidence of MI (Larsson 1992).

Despite the uniform agreement as to the need for prevention and reduction of overweight, the optimal approach to weight control has yet to be ascertained (see Chapter 9). Weight loss in women, as well as in men, lowers blood pressure, decreases insulin resistance and glucose intolerance, and improves the lipid profile. Although adipose tissue is a source of estrogen in postmenopausal women (Groden 1973), and the loss of estrogen-producing adipose tissue has been postulated to limit the cholesterol benefits (increased HDL and lowered LDL cholesterol) in postmenopausal women who lose weight as compared with men, the benefits of weight loss in women can be expected to more than offset any benefits of estrogen produced by adipose tissue.

Exercise and Physical Fitness

Although few studies that addressed the relationship between physical activity or physical fitness and CHD report data for women, no evidence was found in either the Framingham (Kannel 1979) or Goteborg (Lapidus 1986) studies that physical activity level was significantly related to coronary death in women. However, potential misclassification of physical activity intensity in women and elderly persons warrants examination (Arroll 1991). Low leisure-time physical activity was related to increased coronary risk in both genders, but was seriously confounded by more frequent smoking in physically inactive persons (Salonen 1988). Nevertheless, other coronary risk factors such as obesity, glucose intolerance, hyperlipidemia, and hypertension are more prevalent in sedentary than in exercising women.

Based on 1988 data, almost 6 of every 10 women in the United States describe a sedentary lifestyle, with the trend toward inactivity increasing (Anda 1990). Physical inactivity is more prominent among less well educated, lower income women. Physical fitness, as measured by maximal treadmill exercise testing, shows a strong, graded, and consistent relationship with lower total mortality rates in both genders (Figure 15.5), a relationship that is not due to confounding by age or other risk factors. The decreased mortality primarily reflected lower rates of cardiovascular disease and of cancer (Blair 1989). It is important to note that the moderate levels of physical fitness described as protective are attainable by most adults. However, a physical fitness in both genders is associated with a more favorable risk profile, with the association more prominent for women than for men (Bovens 1993). Although favorable effects of exercise on circulating levels of lipoproteins have been considered contributory, metanalysis showed that despite lowering of total cholesterol and triglyceride levels, exercise-related lowering of LDL and increase in HDL was not significant for women; losses in body weight with exercise resulted in larger decreases in cholesterol and triglyceride concentrations than did exercise. Women with higher preexercise cholesterol levels responded most favorably to training. All changes were less marked for women than for men (Lokey 1989). In one study of young adults (Donahue 1988), the beneficial effect of physical activity on the lipoprotein profile was evident in men but not in women; sex-hormone-related differences in insulin sensitivity as the mediator of lipoprotein lipid levels were suggested. The favorable effect has been described as greater in postmenopausal than in premenopausal women (Hartung 1984), suggesting that exercise may favorably counteract the adverse effects of menopause and aging on plasma lipids and coronary risk.

Exercise is associated with lower coronary risk even in old age and even after adjustment for other risk factors. Physical activity decreased the cholesterol-related coronary risk in both elderly women and men, as demonstrated in NHANES I. The mechanisms remain unknown, although an increased HDL cholesterol and lower triglyceride levels, as well as lesser body fat, may be operative (Reaven 1990; Paffenbarger 1991). Favorable lipid and lipoprotein levels occurred with moderate exercise intensities attainable by older individuals (Reaven 1990).

The optimal amount of exercise and the preferable exercise modality for women remain undetermined; although both genders have comparable improvements in fitness with exercise training, smaller improvements in total cholesterol/high density lipopro-

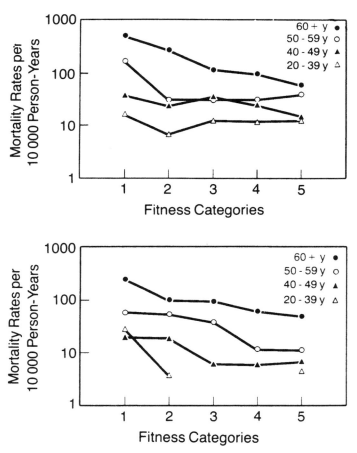

Fig. 15.5. Age-specific, all-cause death rates per 10 000 person-years of follow-up in 10 224 men (top) and 3120 women (bottom) in the Aerobics Center Longitudinal Study, by physical fitness quintiles as determined by maximal treadmill exercise tests.

tein cholesterol occur for women than for men (Lewis 1986). Recent data concerning exercise rehabilitation in elderly patients suggested an excess of injuries in elderly women as compared with men with higher exercise intensity walk-jog activities (Pollock 1991). Reviews and metanalyses of randomized exercise rehabilitation trials after MI showed women to constitute only about 3% of the patients studied, such that gender-specific data cannot be derived (May 1982; O'Connor 1989).

Estrogen Status and Exogenous Gonadal Hormone Therapy

The coronary risk attributes unique to women are menopause, estrogen status, and the gonadal hormones administered for oral contraception and for postmenopausal hormone replacement. An NIH Consensus Conference recommendation (NIH Consensus 1993) is that, although accumulating evidence suggests that the postmenopausal state in women constitutes a risk factor for CHD, recommendations for intervention are deferred until evidence becomes available from prospective trials of estrogen replacement (Martin 1993). However, coronary risk factors increase among women as they become menopausal, independent of age (Stevenson 1993), and insulin is postulated to play a central role (Fontbonne 1991; Razay 1992).

Oral Contraceptives

In the early years of oral contraceptive use, the estrogen-progestin dosage was considerably higher than at present. Women using these oral contraceptives had an increased risk of cardiovascular disease that was accentuated by cigarette smoking (Stadel 1981; Rosenberg 1985; Willett 1987). Current low-dose oral contraceptives impart a lower risk, although most raise LDL and lower HDL cholesterol levels, particularly the cardioprotective HDL_2 fraction (Notelovitz 1989). Adverse effects on glucose tolerance and insulin resistance are similarly less with low-dose formulations. However, oral contraceptives may initiate or intensify hypertension. Despite these changes, there is little evidence that past oral contraceptive use imparts risk, at least for women under age 35 (Stampfer 1988). Some of the newer preparations may even exert a protective effect. A meta-analysis (Stampfer 1990) of both case control and prospective studies found an overall risk of 1.01 for CHD (95% CI: 0.91–1.13) and 1.05 for MI (95% CI: 0.94–1.17) among past oral contraceptive users compared with women who had never used these preparations. Nevertheless, women who smoke cigarettes, particularly those smoking more than 10 cigarettes daily, should probably not use oral contraceptives, although risk has not been demonstrated for newer, lower-dose oral contraceptives. Prostacyclin inhibition and associated increase in platelet-derived thromboxane with resulting increased platelet aggregation are suggested mechanisms (Mileikowsky 1988).

Postmenopausal Hormone Therapy

The higher coronary risk of postmenopausal women (McGee 1973; Matthews 1989; Bush 1990) has been attributed, at least in part, to unfavorable changes in circulating lipoprotein levels, likely mediated by decreased estrogen status, but also influenced by changes in body weight and body fat distribution, among others. Early menopause, regardless of the type of menopause (natural or surgical), increases the risk of infarction, suggesting that increased risk reflects the early cessation of ovulatory function (Palmer 1992). As discussed in detail in chapter 16, most case control and prospective cohort studies show that postmenopausal oral estrogen use is associated with a decreased cardiovascular risk in women, with an approximately 50% reduction in risk of a coronary event (Barrett-Connor 1991a; Stampfer 1991) and a favorable association with cardiovascular and all-cause mortality rates as well (Knopp 1988). These data, despite their consistency, are limited predominantly by the lack of randomized controlled trials; selection bias, particularly related to healthier women being prescribed estrogen by their physicians, may have influenced the results. Self-selection may also play a role in that women who take estrogen, as compared to nonusers, are generally healthier, a leaner, or higher educational level and possibly more compliant with health care and medication use (Manolio 1992).

Other Risk Factors

Having six or more pregnancies was associated in one investigation with a small but consistent increase in coronary and cardiovascular risk; however, the authors emphasize that it is uncertain whether gravity per se reduced lifetime estrogen exposure or whether some unmeasured factor increased risk (Ness 1993), in that most other epidemiologic evidence does not define multiparity as a coronary risk factor. In the Nurses' Health Study, no substantial association was evident between parity and CHD risk.

Epidemiologic studies suggest that alcohol intake reduces the risk of CHD in women (Klatsky 1992), but whether the magnitude of reduction differs between women and men is unknown. The clustering of atherogenic behaviors in both genders associated with coffee consumption, as well as differences in risk factor levels between caffeinated and decaffeinated coffee drinkers, raises questions as to the adverse effect of coffee per se (Puccio 1990).

Based on questionnaire data from female nurses, use of vitamin E supplements by middle-aged women was associated with a reduced coronary risk; the authors emphasize the need for randomized trial data regarding antioxidant vitamin therapy (Stampfer 1993; Steinberg 1993).

Fibrinogen and factor VII levels impart independent coronary risk; based on ARIC data, not only are these levels higher in blacks than in whites and in women than in men, but fibrinogen levels rise with older age, menopause, diabetes, obesity, and smoking; and decrease with physical activity, ethanol intake, and female hormone use (Cook 1990; Folsom 1991; Meilahn 1992). The finding of a lower platelet count in males than in females and in female smokers versus nonsmokers suggests a gender and smoking effect on the hemostatic system that warrants investigation (Green 1992). Antithrombin III levels are lower in premenopausal women than in comparably aged men, but increase following menopause to exceed levels in men of the same age (Meade 1990).

Psychosocial stress among female clerical workers who have blue-collar working husbands, several children, low job mobility, and little control of the work environment is described to increase coronary risk (Haynes 1980). This effect was not found among female executives.

With high stored iron levels, as assessed by a raised serum ferritin concentration, described as a coronary risk factor for Finnish men (Salonen 1992), a question has been raised as to whether menstruation-related iron deficiency decreases tissue oxidation of LDL cholesterol in women.

Preventive Pharmacotherapy

Regular aspirin use may protect against initial MI in women as well as men. In the Nurses' Health Study (Manson 1991c), women taking one to six aspirin weekly had

Table 15.2. Age-Adjusted RR of Nonfatal Myocardial Infarction and Fatal Coronary Heart Disease, According to Aspirin Use, in a Cohort of U.S. Women, 1980 Through 1986[a]

Aspirin per Week No.	Nonfatal Myocardial Infarction			Fatal Coronary Heart Diseases			Nonfatal Infarction and Fatal Coronary Heart Disease		
	Cases	RR	(95% CI)	Cases	RR	(95% CI)	Cases	RR	(95% CI)
0	118	1.00	(Referent)	39	1.00	(Referent)	157	1.00	(Referent)
1–6	59	0.68	(0.49–0.93)	21	0.70	(0.41–1.18)	80	0.68	(0.52–0.89)
1–3	27	0.65	(0.43–0.98)	11	0.81	(0.41–1.57)	38	0.69	(0.48–0.98)
4–6	32	0.71	(0.48–1.05)	10	0.61	(0.31–1.22)	42	0.68	(0.48–0.96)
7–14	30	1.23	(0.82–1.83)	10	1.20	(0.60–2.42)	40	1.22	(0.87–1.73)
≥15	33	0.98	(0.66–1.45)	11	0.83	(0.43–1.61)	44	0.94	(0.67–1.32)

Source: From Manson et al. (1991c), with permission.

[a]Age-adjusted using 5-year age categories. RR indicates relative risk; CI, confidence interval.

Table 15.3. Incidence of CHD, by Age and Sex: 30-Year Follow-up, Framingham Study

	Annual Rate (per 1,000)			
	CHD		MI	
Age (yr)	Men	Women	Men	Women
35–44	5	1	3	—
45–54	11	4	5	1
55–64	19	10	9	3
65–74	23	14	12	6
75–84	30	22	18	8
85+	—	41	—	24
35–64	13	6	6	2
65–94	25	16	13	7

Source: From Kannel and Abbott (1987), with permission.

CHD, coronary heart disease; MI, myocardial infarction.

an age-adjusted relative risk of first MI of 0.68 (95% CI: 0.52–0.89). Risk reduction was most prominent for women who were smokers or had hypercholesterolemia or hypertension. Stroke risk was not altered and risk for cardiovascular death was reduced slightly but not significantly. Although randomized trial data are needed to provide conclusive recommendations, this management should be considered for women whose high risk of MI exceeds that of adverse consequences of long-term aspirin use (Table 15.2).

Summary

CHD is the leading cause of death in American women. Although women develop CHD later in life than do their male counterparts, their outcomes are substantially less favorable both following MI and after myocardial revascularization procedures—coronary bypass surgery and coronary angioplasty (Tables 15.3–15.4; Figure 15.6; Kannel 1987; Heart and Stroke Facts 1993).

Table 15.4. Morbidity After Initial Myocardial Infarction,[a] by Sex: 30-Year Follow-up, Framingham Study

	Rate[b]	
Manifestation	Men	Women
Recurrence of MI	22.0	24.7
Cardiac failure	14.6	16.6
Angina	23.4	16.8
Stroke	7.7	12.7

Source: From Kannel and Abbott (1987), with permission.

[a]Subjects 33 to 87 years of age at first MI.

[b]Age-adjusted 10-year rate per 100 subjects.

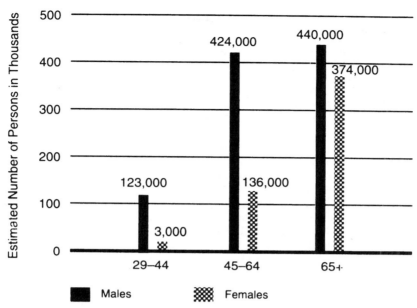

Fig. 15.6. Estimated annual number of Americans, by age and sex, experiencing heart attack. [From Framingham Heart Study, 26-year follow-up.]

Risk factors for CHD are highly prevalent among U.S. women, and risk reduction is important for women of all ages. Because diabetic women have a comparable occurrence of coronary disease to men across the life span, intensive coronary risk reduction is warranted for diabetic women of all ages. Smoking cessation interventions warrant high priority, both for healthy women and for women recovered from MI and after myocardial revascularization. Weight reduction in overweight women is important in that it favorably affects other and potentially more powerful coronary risk attributes—hypertension, glucose intolerance, hyperlipidemia, and the like. Data regarding the coronary benefits of hypertension control are less consistent than those for reduction of stroke risk, for which hypertension control is mandatory. Data on the efficacy of lipid-lowering in decreasing coronary risk are also less powerful, and the independent risk role of hypertriglyceridemia in women remains controversial. Physical fitness, achievable by moderate-intensity leisure exercise, imparts benefit and should be encouraged. Postmenopausal hormone replacement therapy, which addresses a risk attribute unique to women, appears promising, but definitive recommendations must await the results of ongoing clinical trials.

References

Abbott RD, Donahue RP, Kannel WB, Wilson PWF. The impact of diabetes on survival following myocardial infarction in men vs women: the Framingham Study. JAMA 1988; 260:3456–60.

American Diabetes Association. Implications of the diabetes control and complications trial. Clin Diabetes, 1993;July/Aug:91–6.

Amery A, Birkenhager W, Brixko P, et al. Mortality and morbidity results from the European Working Party on High Blood Pressure in the Elderly Trial. Lancet 1985;i:349–54.

Anastos K, Charney P, Charon RA, et al. Hypertension in women: what is really known? The Women's Caucus, Working Group on Women's Health of the Society of General Internal Medicine. Ann Intern Med 1991;115:287–93.

Anda RF, Wallter MN, Wooten KG, Mast EE, Escobedo LG, Sanderson LM. Behavioral risk factor surveillance, 1988. CDC Surveillance Summaries. Morbidity and Mortality Weekly Report. Vol 39, No. SS-2, pp. 1–22, U.S. Department of Health and Human Services, Centers for Disease Control, Atlanta, GA, 1990.

Arroll B, Beaglehole R. Potential misclassification in studies of physical activity. Med Sci Sports Exerc 1991;23:1176–8.

Assmann G, Schulte H. The importance of triglycerides: results from the Prospective Cardiovascular Munster (PROCAM) Study. Eur J Epidemiol 1992;8 (Suppl 1):99–103.

Barnard RJ. Effects of life-style modification on serum lipids. Arch Intern Med 1991;151: 1389–94.

Barrett-Connor EL. Obesity, atherosclerosis and coronary artery disease. Ann Intern Med 1985; 103:1010–19.

Barrett-Connor E, Khaw KT, Wingard DL. A ten-year prospective study of coronary heart disease mortality among Rancho Bernardo women. In: Eaker ED, Packard B, Wenger NK, Clarkson TB, Tyroler HA, eds. Coronary heart disease in women. New York: Haymarket Doyma, 1987:117–21.

Barrett-Connor E, Bush TL. Estrogen and coronary heart disease in women. JAMA 1991a;265: 1861–7.

Barrett-Connor EL, Cohn BA, Wingard DL, Edelstein SL. Why is diabetes mellitus a stronger risk factor for fatal ischemic heart disease in women than in men? JAMA 1991b;265:627–31.

Blair SN, Kohl HW III, Paffenbarger RS Jr, et al. Physical fitness and all-cause mortality: a prospective study of healthy men and women. JAMA 1989;262:2395–401.

Bovens AM, Van Baak MA, Vrencken JG, et al. Physical activity, fitness, and selected risk factors for CHD in active men and women. Med Sci Sports Exerc 1993;25:572–6.

Brownell KD, Stunkard AJ. Differential changes in plasma high-density lipoprotein-cholesterol levels in obese men and women during weight reduction. Arch Intern Med 1981;141: 1142–6.

Buchwald H, Campos CT, Matts JP, Fitch LL, Long JM, Varco RL, the POSCH Group. Women in the POSCH trial: effects of aggressive cholesterol modification in women with coronary heart disease. Ann Surg 1992;216:389–400.

Bush TL, Criqui MH, Cowan LD, et al. Cardiovascular disease mortality in women: Results from the Lipid Research Clinics Follow-up Study. In: Eaker ED, Packard B, Wenger NK, Clarkson TB, Tyroler HA, eds. Coronary heart disease in women, New York: Haymarket Doyma, 1987:106–11.

Bush TL. The epidemiology of cardiovascular disease in postmenopausal women. Ann NY Acad Sci 1990;592:263–71.

Campos H, McNamara JR, Wilson PWF, Ordovas JM, Schaefer EJ. Differences in low density lipoprotein subfractions and apolipoproteins in premenopausal and postmenopausal women. J Clin Endocrinol Metab 1988;67:30–5.

Castelli WP. The triglyceride issue: a view from Framingham. Am Heart J 1986;112:432–7.

Coambs RB, Li S, Kozlowski LT. Age Interacts with heaviness of smoking in predicting success in cessation of smoking. Am J Epidemiol 1992;135:240–6.

Cook NS, Ubben D. Fibrinogen as a major risk factor in cardiovascular disease. TIPS Reviews 1990; 11:444–51.

Criqui MH, Heiss G, Cohn R, et al. Plasma triglyceride level and mortality from coronary heart disease. N Engl J Med 1993;328:1220–5.

Demirovic J. Sprafka JM, Folsom AR, Laitinen D, Blackburn H. Menopause and serum cholesterol: differences between blacks and whites: the Minnesota Heart Survey. Am J Epidemiol 1992;136:155–64.

Donahue RP, Orchard TJ, Becker DJ, Kuller LH, Drash AL. Physical activity, insulin sensitivity, and the lipoprotein profile in young adults: the Beaver County study. Am J Epidemiol 1988;127:95–103.

Donahue RP, Goldberg RJ, Chen Z, Gore JM, Alpert JS. The influence of sex and diabetes mellitus on survival following acute myocardial infarction: a community-wide perspective. J Clin Epidemiol 1993;46:245–52.

Eaker ED, Castelli WP. Coronary heart disease and its risk factors among women in the Framingham Study. In: Eaker ED, Packard B, Wenger NK, Clarkson TB, Tyroler HA, eds. Coronary heart disease in women. New York: Haymarket Doyma, 1987;122–30.

Eaker ED, Kronmal R, Kennedy JW, Davis K. Comparison of the long-term, postsurgical survival of women and men in the Coronary Artery Surgery Study (CASS). Am Heart J 1989;117:71–81.

Eaker ED, Chesebro JH, Sacks FM, Wenger NK, Whisnant JP, Winston M. Cardiovascular disease in women. Circulation 1993;88:1999–2009.

Expert Panel on Detection, Evaluation, and Treatment of High Blood Cholesterol in Adults. Summary of the second report of the National Cholesterol Education Program (NCEP) Expert Panel on Detection, Evaluation, and Treatment of High Blood Cholesterol in Adults (Adult Treatment Panel II). JAMA 1993;269:3015–23.

Fiore MC, Novotny TE, Pierce JP, Hatziandreu EJ, Patel KM, Davis RM. Trends in cigarette smoking in the United States: the changing influence of gender and race. JAMA 1989; 261:49–55.

Five-year Study by a Group of Physicians of the Newcastle upon Tyne Region. Trial of clofibrate in the treatment of ischaemic heart disease. Br Med J 1971;4:767–5.

Folsom AR, Wu KK, Davis CE, Conlan MG, Sorlie PD, Szklo M. Population correlates of plasma fibrinogen and factor VII, putative cardiovascular risk factors. Atherosclerosis 1991;91:191–205.

Fontbonne A. Insulin. A sex hormone for cardiovascular risk? Circulation 1991;84:1442–4.

Freund KM, D'Agostino RB, Belanger AJ, Kannel WB, Stokes J III. Predictors of smoking cessation: the Framingham Study. Am J Epidemiol 1992;135:957–64.

Goldstein MR. Myopathy and rhabdomyolysis with lovastatin taken with gemfibrozil. JAMA 1990;264:2991.

Gordon DJ, Probstfield JL, Garrison RJ, et al. High-density lipoprotein cholesterol and cardiovascular disease: four prospective American studies. Circulation 1989;79:8–15.

Green MS, Peled I, Najenson T. Gender differences in platelet count and its association with cigarette smoking in a large cohort in Israel. J Clin Epidemiol 1992;45:77–84.

Greenland P, Reicher-Reiss H, Goldbourt U, Behar S, and the Israeli SPRINT Investigators. In-hospital and 1-year mortality in 1,524 women after myocardial infarction: comparison with 4,315 men. Circulation 1991;83:484–91.

Grodin JM, Siteri PK, MacDonald PC. Source of estrogen production in postmenopausal women. J Clin Endocrinol Metab 1973;36:207–14.

Gurwitz JH, Col NF, Avorn J. The exclusion of elderly and women from clinical trials in acute myocardial infarction. JAMA 1992;268:1417–22.

Hansen EF, Andersen LT, Von Eyben FE, Cigarette smoking and age at first acute myocardial infarction, and influence of gender and extent of smoking. Am J Cardiol 1993;71: 1439–42.

Hartung GH, Moore CE, Mitchell R, Kappus CM. Relationship of menopausal status and exercise level to HDL cholesterol in women. Exp Aging Res 1984;10:13–18.

Hartz A, Grubb B, Wild R, et al. The association of waist hip ratio and angiographically determined coronary artery disease. Int J Obesity 1990;14:657–65.

Haynes SG, Feinleib M, Kannel WB. The relationship of psychosocial factors to coronary heart disease in the Framingham Study. III. Eight-year incidence of coronary heart disease. Am J Epidemiol 1980;111:37–58.

Health Update. Coronary Heart Disease. Health Education Authority, London, 1993.

Heart and stroke facts: 1994 statistical supplement. American Heart Association, Dallas, TX, 1993.

Hennekens CH, Evans D, Peto R. Oral contraceptive use, cigarette smoking and myocardial infarction. Br J. Fam Plan 1979;5:66–7.

Hermanson B, Omenn GS, Kronmal RA, Gersh BJ, and Participants in the Coronary Artery Surgery Study. Beneficial six-year outcome of smoking cessation in older men and women with coronary artery disease: results from the CASS Registry. N Engl J Med 1988;319:1365–9.

Higgins M. Keller JB, Ostrander LD. Risk factors for coronary heart disease in women: Tecumseh Community Health Study, 1959 to 1980. In: Eaker ED, Packard B. Wenger NK, Clarkson TB, Tyroler HA, eds. Coronary heart disease in women. New York: Haymarket Doyma, 1987:83–9.

Hubert HB, Feinleib M, McNamara PM, Castelli WP. Obesity as an independent risk factor for cardiovascular disease: a 26-year follow-up of participants in the Framingham Heart Study. Circulation 1983;67:968–77.

Hypertension Detection and Follow-up Program Cooperative Group. Five-year findings of the Hypertension Detection and Follow-up Program. II. Mortality by race-sex and age. JAMA 1979;242:2572–7.

Johnson CL, Rifkind BM, Sempos CT, et al. Declining serum total cholesterol levels among US adults: the National Health and Nutrition Examination Surveys. JAMA 1993;269: 3002–8.

Kane JP, Malloy MJ, Ports TA, Phillips NR, Diehl JC, Havel RJ. Regression of coronary atherosclerosis during treatment of familial hypercholesterolemia with combined drug regimens. JAMA 1990;264:3007–12.

Kannel WB, Sorlie P. Some health benefits of physical activity: the Framingham Study. Arch Intern Med 1979;139:857–61.

Kannel WB, Garrison RJ, Wilson PWF. Obesity and nutrition in elderly diabetic patients. Am J Med 1986;80 (Suppl 5A):22–30.

Kannel WB, Abbott RD. Incidence and prognosis of myocardial infarction in women: the Framingham Study. In: Eaker ED, Packard B, Wenger NK, Clarkson TB, Tyroler HA, eds. Coronary heart disease in women. New York:; Haymarket Doyma, 1987:208–14.

Kannel WB. Nutrition and the occurrence and prevention of cardiovascular disease in the elderly. Nutr Rev 1988;46:68–78.

Kannel WB, D'Agostino RB, Wilson PWF, Belanger AJ, Gagnon DR. Diabetes, fibrinogen, and risk of cardiovascular disease: the Framingham experience. Am Heart J. 1990;120: 672–6.

Kaplan NM. The deadly quartet: upper-body obesity, glucose intolerance, hypertriglyceridemia, and hypertension. Arch Intern Med 1989;149:1514–20.

Keil JE, Gazes PC, Loadholt CB, et al. Coronary heart disease mortality and its predictors among women in Charleston, South Carolina. In: Eaker ED, Packard B, Wenger NK, Clarkson TB, Tyroler HA, eds. Coronary heart disease in women, New York: Haymarket Doyma, 1987:90–8.

Kim H-J, Kalkhoff RK. Changes in lipoprotein composition during the menstrual cycle. Metabolism 1979;28:663–8.

Klatsky AL, Armstrong MA, Friedman GD. Alcohol and mortality. Ann Intern Med 1992;117: 646–54.

Knapp RG, Sutherland SE, Keil JE, Rust PF, Lackland DT. A comparison of the effects of cholesterol on CHD mortality in black and white women: twenty-eight years of follow-up in the Charleston Heart Study. J Clin Epidemiol 1992;45:1119–29.

Knopp RH. The effects of postmenopausal estrogen therapy on the incidence of arteriosclerotic vascular disease. Obstet Gynecol 1988;72 (Suppl 5):23S–30S.

Krolewski AS, Warram JH, Valsania P, Martin BC, Laffel LMB, Christlieb R. Evolving natural history of coronary artery disease in diabetes mellitus. Am J Med 1991;90 (Suppl 2A): 56S–61S.

Lapidus L, Bengtsson C. Socioeconomic factors and physical activity in relation to cardiovascular disease and death: a 12-year follow-up of participants in a population study of women in Gothenberg, Sweden. Br Heart J 1986;55:295–301.

LaRosa JC. Lipids and cardiovascular disease: do the findings and therapy apply equally to men and women? Women's Health Issues 1992;2:102–13.

Larsson B, Bengtsson C, Bjorntorp P, et al. Is abdominal body fat distribution a major explanation for the sex difference in the incidence of myocardial infarction? The study of men born in 1913 and the study of women, Goteborg, Sweden. Am J Epidemiol 1992;135:266–73.

Leaf DA. Women and coronary artery disease: gender confers no immunity. Postgrad Med 1990;87:55–60.

Lewis DA, Kamon E, Hodgson JL. Physiological differences between genders. Implications for sports conditioning. Sports Med 1986;3:357–69.

Liao Y, Cooper RS, Ghali JK, Lansky D, Cao G, Lee J. Sex differences in the impact of coexistent diabetes on survival in patients with coronary heart disease. Diabetes Care 1993;16:708–13.

Lokey EA, Tran ZV. Effects of exercise training on serum lipid and lipoprotein concentrations in women: a meta-analysis. Int J Sports Med 1989;10:424–9.

Maggi S, Bush TL, Hale WE. Diebetes and other cardiovascular risk factors in an elderly population. Age Ageing 1990;19:173–8.

Manolio TA, Pearson TA, Wenger NK, Barrett-Connor E, Payne GH, Harlan WR. Cholesterol and heart disease in older persons and women: review of an NHLBI workshop. Am J Epidemiol 1992;2:161–76.

Manson JE, Stampfer MJ, Hennekens CH, Willett WC. Body weight and longevity: a reassessment. JAMA 1987;257:353–8.

Manson JE, Colditz GA, Stampfer MJ, et al. A prospective study of obesity and risk of coronary heart disease in women. N. Engl J Med 1990;322:882–9.

Manson JE, Colditz GA, Stampfer MJ, et al. A prospective study of maturity-onset diabetes mellitus and risk of coronary heart disease and stroke in women. Arch Intern Med 1991a; 151:114–7.

Manson JE, Rimm EB, Stampfer MJ, et al. Physical activity and incidence of non-insulin dependent diabetes mellitus in women. Lancet 1991b;338:774–8.

Manson JE, Stampfer MJ, Colditz GA, et al. A prospective study of aspirin use and primary prevention of cardiovascular disease in women. JAMA 1991c;266:521–7.

Martin KA, Freeman MW. Postmenopausal hormone-replacement therapy. N Engl J Med 1993; 328:1115−17.

Masarei JRL, Rouse IL, Lynch WJ, Robertson K, Vandongen R, Beilin LJ. Effects of a lacto-ovo vegetarian diet on serum concentrations of cholesterol, triglyceride, HDL-C, HDL₂-C, HDL₃-C, apoprotein-B, and Lp(a). Am J Clin Nutr 1984;40:468−79.

Matthews KA, Meilahn E, Kuller LH, Kelsey SF, Caggiula AW, Wing RR. Menopause and risk factors for coronary heart disease. N. Engl J Med 1989;321:641−6.

May GS, Eberlein KA, Furberg CD, Passamani ER, DeMets DL. Secondary prevention after myocardial infarction: a review of long-term trials. Prog Cardiovasc Dis 1982;24:331−52.

McGee D. Probability of Developing Certain Cardiovascular Diseases in Eight Years at Specified Values of Characteristics. Washington, DC, 1973. U.S. Department of Health, Education, and Welfare Publication NIH 74-618.

Meade TW, Dyer S, Howarth DJ, Imeson JD, Stirling Y. Antithrombin III and procoagulant activity: sex differences and effects of the menopause. Br J Haematol 1990;74:77−81.

Medical Research Council Working Party. MRC trial of treatment of mild hypertension: principal results. Br Med J 1985;291:97−105.

Meilahn EN. Hemostatic factors and risk of cardiovascular disease in women: an overview. Arch Pathol Lab Med 1992;116:1313−17.

Mensink RP, Katan MB. Effect of monounsaturated fatty acids versus complex carbohydrates on high-density lipoproteins in healthy men and women. Lancet 1987;i:22−5.

Miettinen M, Turpeinen O, Karvonen MJ, Elosuo R, Paavilainen E. Effect of cholesterol-lowering diet on mortality from coronary heart-disease and other causes. Lancet 1972;2:835−838.

Mileikowsky GN, Nadler JL, Huey F, Francis R, Roy S. Evidence that smoking alters prostacyclin formation and platelet aggregation in women who use oral contraceptives. Am J Obstet Gynecol 1988;159:1547−1552.

Modan M, Or J, Karasik A, et al. Hyperinsulinemia, sex, and risk of atherosclerotic cardiovascular disease. Circulation 1991;84:1165−1175.

National Center for Health Statistics. National Health Interview Survey, 1986−88, 1988−90. Unpublished data.

National Center for Health Statistics. Health: United States, 1990, U.S. Public Health Service, Centers for Disease Control, Hyattsville, MD, 1991.

National Institutes of Health Consensus Development Panel on the Health Implications of Obesity. Health implications of obesity. National Institutes of Health Consensus Development Conference Statement. Ann Intern Med 1985;103:147−51.

Ness RB, Harris T, Cobb J, et al. Number of pregnancies and the subsequent risk of cardiovascular disease. N Engl J Med 1993;328:1528−33.

NIH Consensus Development Panel on Triglyceride, High-Density Lipoprotein, and Coronary Heart Disease. Triglyceride, high-density lipoprotein, and coronary heart disease. JAMA 1993;269:505−10.

Notelovitz M. Feldman EB, Gillespy M, Gudat J. Lipid and lipoprotein changes in women taking low-dose, triphasic oral contraceptives: a controlled, comparative, 12-month clinical trial. Am J Obstet Gynecol 1989;160:1269−80.

Nyboe J, Jensen G, Appleyard M, Schnohr P. Smoking and the risk of first acute myocardial infarction. Am Heart J 1991;122:438−47.

O'Connor GT, Buring JE, Yusuf S, et al. An overview of randomized trials of rehabilitation with exercise after myocardial infarction. Circulation 1989;80:234−44.

Paffenbarger RS Jr, Hyde RT, Hsieh C-C, Wing AL. Physical activity, other life-style patterns, cardiovascular disease and longevity. Acta Med Scand 1991;711(Suppl):85−91.

Palmer JR, Rosenberg L. Shapiro S. Reproductive factors and risk of myocardial infarction. Am J. Epidemiol 1992;136:408–16.

Perkins J, Dick TBS. Smoking and myocardial infarction: secondary prevention. Postgrad Med J 1985;61:295–300.

Pollock ML, Carroll JF, Graves JE, et al. Injuries and adherence to walk/jog and resistance training programs in the elderly. Med Sci Sports Exerc 1991;23:1194–200.

Puccio EM, McPhillips JB, Barrett-Connor E, Ganiats TG. Clustering of atherogenic behaviors in coffee drinkers. Am J Public Health 1990;80:1310–13.

Rathmann W, Hauner H, Dannehl K, Gries FA. Association of elevated serum uric acid with coronary heart disease in diabetes mellitus. Diabetes Metab 1993;19 (1 Pt 2):159–66.

Razay G, Heaton KW, Bolton CH. Coronary heart disease risk factors in relation to the menopause. Q J Med 1992;85:889–96.

Reaven PD, McPhillips JB, Barrett-Connor EL, Criqui MH. Leisure time exercise and lipid and lipoprotein levels in an older population. J Am Geriatr Soc 1990;38:847–54.

Report by the Management Committee. The Australian Therapeutic Trial in Mild Hypertension. Lancet 1980;1:1261–7.

Report by a Research Committee of the Scottish Society of Physicians. Ischaemic heart disease: a secondary prevention trial using clofibrate. Br Med J 1971;4:775–84.

Rogot E, Sorlie PD, Johnson NJ, Glover CS, Treasure DW. A mortality study of one million persons by demographic, social, and economic factors: 1979–1971 follow-up. U.S. Longitudinal Mortality Study. U.S. Department of Health and Human Services, Public Health Service, NIH Publication No. 88–2896, March, 1988.

Rosenberg L, Miller DR, Kaufman DW, et al. Myocardial infarction in women under 50 years of age. JAMA 1983;250:2801–6.

Rosenberg L, Kaufman DW, Helmrich SP, Miller DR, Stolley PD, Shapiro S. Myocardial infarction and cigarette smoking in women younger than 50 years of age. JAMA 1985; 253:2965–9.

Rossouw JF. International trials (abstract). Presented at Cholesterol and Heart Disease in Older Persons and in Women, June 18–19, 1990, National Heart, Lung, and Blood Institute, National Institutes of Health, Bethesda, MD, Program and Abstracts Book, p. 22.

Salonen JT, Slater JS, Tuomilehto J, Rauramaa R. Leisure time and occupational physical activity: risk of death from ischemic heart disease. Am J. Epidemiol 1988;127:87–94.

Salonen JT, Nyyssonen K, Korpela H, Tuomilehto J, Seppanen R, Salonen R. High stored iron levels are associated with excess risk of myocardial infarction in Eastern Finnish men. Circulation 1992;86:803–11.

SHEP Cooperative Research Group. Prevention of stroke by antihypertensive drug treatment in older persons with isolated systolic hypertension: final results of the Systolic Hypertension in the Elderly Program (SHEP). JAMA 1991;265:3255–64.

Soldo BJ, Manton KG. Health status and service needs of the oldest old: current patterns and future trends. Milbank Memorial Fund Q Health Soc 1985;63:286–319.

Soler JT, Folsom AR, Kushi LH, Prineas RJ, Seal US. Association of body fat distribution with plasma lipids, lipoproteins, apolipoproteins Al and B in postmenopausal women. J Clin Epidemiol 1988;41:1075–81.

Spelsberg A, Ridker PM, Manson JE. Carbohydrate metabolism, obesity, and diabetes. In: Douglas P, ed. Cardiovascular health and disease in women. Philadelphia: WB Saunders, 1993.

Stadel BV. Oral contraceptives and cardiovascular disease. N Engl J Med 1981;305:612–18.

Stampfer MJ, Willett WC, Colditz GA, Speizer FE, Hennekens CH. A prospective study of past use of oral contraceptive agents and risk of cardiovascular diseases. N Engl J Med 1988;319:1313–17.

Stampfer MJ, Willett WC, Colditz GA, Speizer FE, Hennekens CH. Past use of oral contraceptives and cardiovascular disease: a meta-analysis in the context of the Nurses' Health Study. Am J Obstet Gynecol 1990;163 (Pt 2):285–91.

Stampfer MJ, Colditz GA, Willett WC, et al. Postmenopausal estrogen therapy and cardiovascular disease. Ten-year follow-up from the Nurses' Health Study. N Engl J Med 1991; 325:756–2.

Stampfer MJ, Hennekens CH, Manson JE, Colditz GA, Rosner B, Willett WC. Vitamin E consumption and the risk of coronary disease in women. N Engl J Med 1993;328: 1444–9.

Steinberg D. Antioxidant vitamins and coronary heart disease. N Engl J Med 1993;328:1487–9.

Stevenson JC, Crook D, Godsland IF. Influence of age and menopause on serum lipids and lipoproteins in healthy women. Atherosclerosis 1993;98:83–90.

Varma VK, Murphy PL, Hood WP Jr, et al. Are women with acute myocardial infarction managed differently from men? J Am Coll Cardiol 1992;19:20A [Abstract].

Wenger NK. Exclusion of the elderly and women from coronary trials: is their quality of care compromised? JAMA 1992;268:1460–1.

Willett WC, Green A, Stampfer MJ, et al. Relative and absolute excess risks of coronary heart disease among women who smoke cigarettes. N. Engl J Med 1987;317:1303–9.

Williams EL, Winkleby MA, Fortmann SP. Changes in coronary heart disease risk factors in the 1980s: evidence of a male-female crossover effect with age. Am J Epidemiol 1993; 137:1056–67.

Wingard DL, Cohn BA. Coronary heart disease mortality among women in Alameda County, 1965 to 1973. In: Eaker ED, Packard B, Wenger NK, Clarkson TB, Tyroler HA, eds. Coronary heart disease in women. New York: Haymarket Doyma, 1987:99–105.

Wong ND, Wilson PWF, Kannel WB. Serum cholesterol as a prognostic factor after myocardial infarction: the Framingham Study. Ann Intern Med 1991;115:687–93.

16

Postmenopausal Hormone Therapy

FRANCINE GRODSTEIN, JOANN E. MANSON, AND MEIR J. STAMPFER

Cardiovascular diseases remain the leading cause of death in American women. Several lines of evidence suggest that estrogen is an important mediator of women's risk of heart disease. Rates of coronary heart disease (CHD) are relatively low among premenopausal women, but rise sharply with age. Furthermore, the ratio of rates between men and women grows narrower with increasing age (Figure 16.1). In addition, there is evidence of an increased risk of CHD among young women with bilateral oophorectomy (Stampfer 1990), unless they are treated with estrogen. Finally, accumulating data demonstrate that women who use estrogen replacement therapy (ERT) after menopause have lower rates of heart disease. In this chapter we review these data, including possible biologic mechanisms, and comment on the risk and benefit calculations which take into account all of the potential advantages and disadvantages of hormone use.

Possible Mechanisms of Action

Lipids

There are substantial biologic data supporting a role for estrogen in preventing CHD. The best established mechanism is estrogen's impact on the lipid profile. In experimental studies among postmenopausal women, estrogen reduced low density lipoprotein (LDL) and raised high density lipoprotein (HDL) levels (Bush 1986; Miller 1991). In summarizing estrogen's influence on lipids, Bush and Miller reviewed a substantial body of experimental work and found that, on average, 0.625 mg/day of conjugated estrogens led to a 10% increase in HDL and a 4% decrease in LDL (Bush 1986). Walsh et al. (1991) found that this regimen increased HDL an average of 16% and reduced LDL an average of 15% and that other forms of oral estrogen had generally similar effects. A 1 mg/dl increase in HDL is associated with approximately 3% decrease in risk of coronary disease, and 1 mg/dl decrease in LDL is associated with about 2% decline in risk; hence the changes induced by estrogen could lead to a relatively large decrease in risk (Gordon 1989).

413

DEATH RATE (per 100,000)

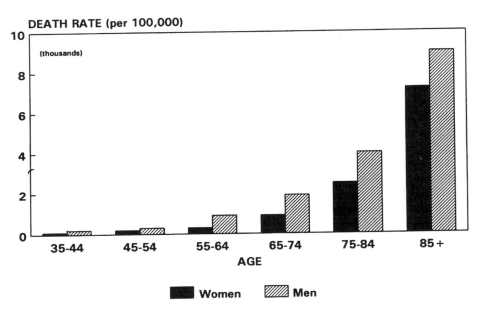

Fig. 16.1. Mortality from CHD in United States white men and women.

In a study of estrogen use among women presenting for angiography, women with no stenosis were more often estrogen users than those with evidence of greater than 70% occlusion (Gruchow 1988); the investigators attempted to examine possible mechanisms by controlling for total cholesterol, triglyceride levels, and HDL-cholesterol in a regression model. Usually, it is inappropriate to adjust for these variables, since they are in the causal pathway. When such variables are included in the model, it is equivalent to asking what the residual effect of estrogen use is on coronary risk above and beyond its effect on lipid levels. In the Gruchow study, adjusting for total cholesterol and triglyceride level had little influence on the results, but after adding HDL levels to the regression model, the observed association between estrogen and stenosis was substantially reduced. This suggests that an elevation in HDL is a probable mechanism of action for a large part of the apparent benefit of estrogen. The data from this study represent concurrent assessment of estrogen use and HDL levels.

Bush and others (1987) have conducted an analysis similar to Gruchow's using longitudinal data from the Lipid Research Clinic follow-up study. In an early examination, much of the apparent benefit of estrogen was attributable to HDL. In later analyses with further follow-up, however, adjustment for HDL had only a modest impact on the association between estrogen and CHD; estrogen use remained a strong, statistically significant predictor of reduced risk even after adjustment for baseline HDL levels. This observation implies that only a small part of the estrogen effect in this cohort, perhaps 25%, could be attributed to changes in HDL. However, there is substantial measurement error when using a single, baseline HDL value to represent HDL status over a period as long as 15 years, and such an interpretation ignores the effects of this error. Hence this analysis probably markedly underestimates the proportion of estrogen's benefits attributable to changes in the lipid profile.

Experimental studies provide substantial evidence that estrogen can protect against heart disease, and suggest additional mechanisms by which this may occur. In several randomized trials in monkeys, estrogen's influence on HDL and LDL levels appeared to be a small or negligible part of its benefits. Adams et al. (1990b) conducted a randomized trial of ovariectomized monkeys fed a moderately atherogenic diet, and reported that the extent of coronary atherosclerosis in monkeys given estrogens was only half as great as in those given placebo, yet there were only modest changes in lipid levels. Similarly, ovariectomized monkeys fed an atherogenic diet and randomized to estrogen supplements had a 70% reduction in LDL uptake and products of LDL degradation in the coronary arteries, despite no significant difference in plasma lipids compared with monkeys given placebo (Wagner 1991). This important finding suggests that estrogen may reduce atherosclerosis by preventing modification of LDL and thereby decreasing the avidity of its uptake in the vessel wall to form atherosclerotic lesions. In addition, cholesterol-fed female rabbits treated with hormones had one-third the aortic accumulation of cholesterol of untreated rabbits, which could only partly be explained by differences in cholesterol levels (Haarbo 1991).

Blood Flow and Vascular Tone

Estrogen receptors are present in the muscularis of arteries (McGill 1989), and increasing evidence, from both animal and human studies, demonstrates that estrogen improves blood flow. Williams et al. (1990) infused the coronary arteries of ovariectomized monkeys with acetylcholine. This caused arterial constriction in the monkeys with no estrogen supplementation, but no constriction and actually minimal dilation of the arteries was observed in those given estrogen. Similarly, decreased systemic vascular resistance was found when estrogen was administered to ewes (Magness 1989), and estrogen led to a hyperpolarization of the coronary vascular smooth muscle membrane in dogs (Harder 1979).

Furthermore, in postmenopausal women observed before and after transdermal estradiol, reduced arterial impedance and decreased vascular tone was reported in uterine arteries after 6 weeks of treatment (Bourne 1990). Increased hyperemic response and a correlated, expanded vasodilator reserve were also found in an observational study of women taking and not taking estrogen (Sarrel 1992). Pines and colleagues (1991) performed Doppler echocardiography on the aorta of postmenopausal women and found that central and peripheral hemodynamic parameters, including peak flow velocity, mean acceleration and ejection time, improved significantly in women after 2.5 months of estrogen use, compared with controls who were not taking estrogen over the same time period. When Doppler ultrasound was used to measure the pulsatility index, or impedance to blood flow, in the internal carotid artery of women before and after treatment with transdermal estradiol, a significant reduction in impedance was observed after 9 weeks of estrogen treatment (Gangar 1991). The beneficial effects on blood flow and vasodilation may explain the recent findings from a placebo-controlled trial that acute administration of estrogen can prolong the treadmill time and decrease symptoms in women with coronary artery disease (Rosano

1993). In addition, Collins et al. (1993) have recently suggested that estrogen may have calcium antagonist effects and act as a calcium-channel blocker.

Other Mechanisms

Estrogen may also reduce CHD by affecting other aspects of the vasculature. Steinleitner et al. (1989) compared prostacyclin levels in the uterine arteries of postmenopausal and premenopausal women, with the hypothesis that estrogen influences production of vasodilators. These investigators observed markedly lower levels of prostacyclin among the postmenopausal women, although the addition of estrogen did not change prostacyclin production.

Estrogen may influence carbohydrate metabolism, although this issue is still controversial. Oral contraceptives have been associated with impaired glucose tolerance, but studies of noncontraceptive estrogen have been inconsistent. In some, increased blood glucose has been observed, but in most studies no significant change has been found in carbohydrate tolerance (Barrett-Connor 1990). A recent observational study, and one of the few which controlled for confounding factors such as age and obesity, found lower levels of insulin and no evidence of impaired glucose tolerance among 194 estrogen-treated women compared with 275 women not using estrogen (Barrett-Connor 1990). Similarly, after adjusting for diabetes risk factors including obesity in a prospective study of 21,028 postmenopausal women, no increase was observed in the incidence of non-insulin-dependent diabetes among estrogen users (RR = 0.80, 95% CI: 0.67–0.96 for current users, and RR = 1.07, 95% CI: 0.93–1.23 for past users) (Manson 1992). A recent clinical trial of 875 women randomized to placebo, estrogen alone, or estrogen with progestin found no significant difference between the groups' levels of postchallenge insulin (PEPI 1995).

In a recent report (Sack 1994), ERT significantly reduced susceptibility of LDL to oxidation. Women given estrogen for 3 weeks had a 16% prolongation of the lag time of LDL oxidation ($p < .01$ compared with pretreatment); after cessation of therapy, the lag time returned to baseline levels.

In addition, in clinical trials, estrogen has been asssociated with reduced blood pressure among postmenopausal women (Coronary Drug Project Research Group 1980), although a recent trial found no change in blood pressure after three years for women on placebo compared to those on estrogen or estrogen with progestin (PEPI 1995).

Evidence For and Against Benefit

Observational Data in Humans

Several epidemiologic approaches have been used to study the association between estrogen and the risk of CHD. Case-control studies compare estrogen use in women with CHD and those without CHD; cross-sectional studies of women undergoing angiography compare the extent of coronary disease in estrogen users and nonusers; and cohort studies compare rates of CHD among women taking estrogen with those not taking estrogen.

The hospital-based case-control studies have provided the least convincing evidence of a protection against heart disease in estrogen users. The relative risk estimates from these studies range from 4.2 to 0.5, with most showing no association (Rosenberg 1976; Jick 1978a, 1978b; Rosenberg 1980; Szklo 1984; LaVecchia 1987). A meta-analysis summarizing these studies yielded a pooled relative risk of 1.33 (95% CI: 0.93–1.91) (Figure 16.2) (Grodstein 1995). Of all the study designs, however, the hospital-based case-control studies carry the greatest likelihood of bias, primarily because of problems in the selection of controls. Women with diseases related to estrogen use must be eliminated from the control group, and this can be difficult. For example, in some hospital-based studies, many of the controls were patients admitted for fracture, a condition which can be prevented by ERT. Such controls would therefore be less likely to have taken estrogen than comparably aged women in the general population. Even in other hospitalized patients, physicians may be reluctant to prescribe estrogens to avoid the possibility of interactions with other medications or simply to reduce the patient's burden of medications. Thus, use of hospital controls tends to obscure the full protective effect of estrogens on CHD.

In contrast, population- or community-based case-control studies do not have this problem in the control selection process, and as expected, they show consistent, protective associations between estrogen and CHD, with relative risks from 0.3 to 0.9 (Talbott 1977; Pfeffer 1978; Adam 1981; Bain 1981; Ross 1981; Beard 1989; Thompson 1989; Rosenberg 1993). The summary relative risk, pooling all the population and community-based case-control studies, is 0.80 (95% CI: 0.68–0.97) (Figure 16.2).

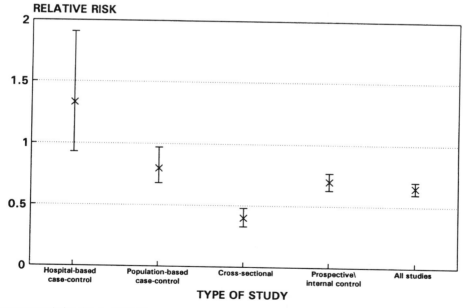

x = summary relative risk, I = 95% CI

Fig. 16.2. Summary of studies of coronary heart disease and estrogen, ever use.

In the cross-sectional studies (Gruchow 1988; Sullivan 1988; McFarland 1989; Hong 1992), the risk estimates for the effect of estrogen on heart disease are among the lowest reported. The summary relative risk from the angiographic studies, comparing women with occlusion and those without, was 0.40 (95% CI: 0.33–0.48). However, estrogen users tend to have greater contact with the health care system and may be more likely to have angiography than nonusers with the same equivocal symptoms. Thus, there may be a higher probability, *a priori*, of finding no evidence of stenosis among the estrogen users in these investigations, perhaps leading to an exaggeration of the benefit of estrogen use on the risk of CHD. In one study (Gruchow 1988), however, no difference was observed in the distribution of symptoms among users and nonusers, suggesting the absence of such a bias. Furthermore, if this bias existed, its magnitude could explain only a small fraction of the apparent benefit of estrogen use.

All of the prospective studies (Potocki 1971; Burch 1974; McMahon 1978; Hammond 1979; Nachtigall 1979; Bush 1983; Lafferty 1985; Stampfer 1985b 1991b; Wilson 1985; Bush 1987; Eaker 1987; Hunt 1987; Petitti 1987; Criqui 1988; Henderson 1988; Croft 1989; Avila 1990; Hunt 1990; Sullivan 1990; Henderson 1991; Wolf 1991; Falkeborn 1992), have observed a protective effect of estrogens on CHD and mortality, although the results from the Framingham Study (Wilson 1985; Eaker 1987) are equivocal (Stampfer 1991a). Furthermore, in several studies (Burch 1974; McMahon 1978; Hunt 1987; Hunt 1990), all participants were estrogen users, and their mortality experience was compared with national mortality statistics. The relative risks in those studies range from approximately 0.3 to 0.4, and the summary relative risk is 0.34 (95% CI: 0.26–0.45). However, patients given estrogen generally are healthier than the general population since they are in contact with the health care system and tend to have a higher socioeconomic status. Thus, such comparisons will overestimate the benefit of ERT. When the results of these studies were excluded from the prospective data, the meta-analysis for the cohort studies using internal controls, comparing ever versus never users, yielded a pooled relative risk of 0.70 (95% CI: 0.63–0.77) (Figure 16.2).

The Nurses' Health Study is the largest prospective study, with 48,470 postmenopausal women free of cardiovascular disease at baseline, among whom 293 nonfatal myocardial infarctions and 112 confirmed coronary deaths were identified after 10 years of follow-up (Stampfer 1991b). Current estrogen users had about half the risk of heart disease, compared to nonusers (age-adjusted RR = 0.51; 95% CI: 0.37–0.70), while among past users, the relative risk was 0.91 (95% CI: 0.73–1.14). Further adjustment for a wide array of cardiovascular risk factors had little effect on these estimates, reflecting the very modest differences in the risk profile of estrogen users and nonusers in this cohort (for current use, multivariate RR = 0.56; 95% CI: 0.40–0.80, and for past use RR = 0.83; 95% CI: 0.65–1.05). There was no marked effect of either duration of use or dosage, although some increase in risk was observed among women using more than 1.25 mg daily (RR = 2.8; 95% CI: 0.9–8.2). However, relatively few women reported using estrogens at this high dose.

Overall Strength of Epidemiologic Evidence Supporting Benefit

Overall, we would assign a grade of B+ to the evidence supporting a protective effect of estrogen on heart disease, with consideration of the following issues. Our meta-analysis of all of the epidemiologic studies assessing ever versus never use, with relative risks ranging from 0.17 to 4.2, resulted in a summary relative risk of 0.65 (95% CI: 0.60–0.70) (Figure 16.2). However, evidence from many of these studies indicates that current estrogen users enjoy greater protection against heart disease than past users. Thus, combining investigations of current, past, and ever use in a summary estimate such as this may be misleading because the results will be directly affected by the proportion of each in the studies included. In general, the summary estimates tend to obscure the stronger protective effect among current users of hormones. We recalculated summary estimates based on analyses of current use, where such data were provided, and as expected, these estimates were lower than those provided by combining studies of any estrogen use (Figure 16.3). For the population-based case-control studies (Talbott 1977; Pfeffer 1978; Adam 1981; Bain 1981; Thompson 1989; Rosenberg 1993), the pooled relative risk for current estrogen use was 0.69 (95% CI: 0.50–0.95); for the cross-sectional studies) Gruchow 1988; Sullivan 1988; Hong 1992), it was 0.39 (95% CI: 0.31–0.48), and for the internally controlled prospective studies (Nachtigall 1979; Lafferty 1985; Criqui 1988; Avila 1990; Henderson 1991; Stampfer 1991b), the summary estimate was 0.55 (95% CI: 0.44–0.70). The pooled relative risk for current estrogen use, combining all three types of studies was 0.49 (95% CI; 0.43–0.56).

Nonetheless, virtually all of the evidence accumulated to date is from observational studies. No large clinical trials of estrogen use and CHD have been conducted, but several have recently been initiated and those data will be forthcoming: the Women's

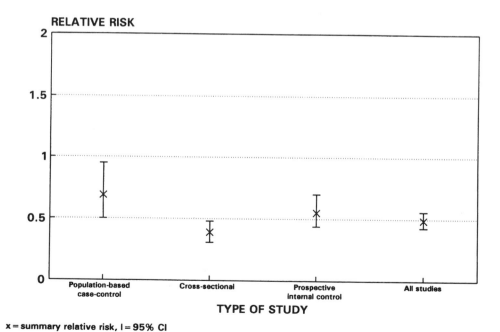

x = summary relative risk, I = 95% CI

Fig. 16.3. Summary of studies of coronary heart disease and estrogen, current use.

Health Initiative, a large trial of estrogen use and estrogen with progestin will be examining the effect of hormone replacement therapy on several disease outcomes, and the Heart and Estrogen-Progestin Replacement Study is investigating secondary prevention of heart disease. In the observational studies, it is the participants and their physicians who decide whether to use estrogen therapy. Often the health status of the patient has an important influence on this decision and on the results of studies that include these patients. Women who use estrogen see a physician more regularly than those who do not, and this increased medical care may decrease their risk of CHD. Furthermore, women who choose to use estrogen may also choose to lead generally healthier lifestyles than those who do not take such medication. Compliance with estrogen therapy (as among current users) might further identify an otherwise lower risk group of women.

Thus, some have argued that estrogen use is merely a marker, rather than a cause, of good health. Most of the studies reviewed here have provided some information bearing on this critical point. One approach is to examine results of studies in which all the women were initially judged eligible by their physicians to receive estrogens. In two such studies of CHD (Nachtigall 1979; Lafferty 1985), the summary relative risk was 0.22 (95% CI: 0.06–0.88), although both investigations were somewhat small.

In the Nurses' Health Study (Stampfer 1991b), the investigators tried to evaluate whether increased medical care among estrogen users could be responsible for the benefit observed. Only women who reported a physician visit in 1978 (65% of the cohort) were included in the analysis, and the results were similar to those found in all subjects: the age-adjusted relative risk for major coronary heart disease was 0.45 (95% CI: 0.31–0.66) for current use. Morever, another subanalysis in that cohort limited to women free from major CHD risk factors (cigarette smoking, hypertension, diabetes, high serum cholesterol, obesity) showed a relative risk for current use of 0.5 (95% CI: 0.3–0.9).

Several studies have compared the CHD risk factor profile of estrogen users and nonusers (Table 16.1). In general population studies, estrogen users appear to have a more favorable cardiac risk profile than nonusers, even apart from hormone use. Barrett-Connor (1991) observed that, in a cohort of upper-middle-class postmenopausal women, those taking estrogens reported better health-care behavior, including more screening tests such as blood cholesterol measurement and mammograms. Similarly, among 9,704 women in a study of osteoporotic fractures (Cauley 1990), users tended to be better educated and less obese, and drank alcohol and participated in sports more often than nonusers. However, these differences were small and can explain only a small portion of the large reduction in risk among estrogen users. Furthermore, in many of the large studies, the subjects tend to be quite homogeneous, chosen because of their common profession or community. In the Nurses' Health Study, the distribution of coronary risk factors was similar among current and never users of estrogens (Stampfer 1991b), although the users tended to be somewhat leaner and more physically active. The same findings were observed in the Lipid Research Clinics Follow-up Study (Bush 1987) and the Leisure World Study (Henderson 1991). In these investigations, multivariate control for numerous risk factors had little impact on the relative risk estimates for estrogen and heart disease, implying an equivalent risk status

Table 16.1. Risk Factor Profiles of Estrogen Users and Nonusers

Study of Osteoporotic Fractures (Cauley, 1990)				Nurses' Health Study (Stampfer, 1991b)				Lipid Research Clinics Program (Bush, 1987)		
	Percent				Percent				Percent	
Profile	Current	Past	Never	Profile	Current	Past	Never	Profile	Current/Past	Never
High school education	15.8	18.2	27.0	Current smoker	11.2	14.7	14.5	< High school education	16	25
Ever smoker	43.2	43.5	37.0	Hypertension	23.2	25.0	21.8	Smoker	33	31
Physical activity in past week	75.5	73.5	63.0	Diabetes	2.7	3.8	3.5	Regular exercise	12	10
Drink alcohol	76.1	74.8	66.4	High serum cholesterol	9.9	11.2	7.6	Alcohol	82	79
BMI ≥27.3 (kg/m²)	28.6	36.2	41.1	Parental MI before age 60	10.6	10.0	9.3	BMI (kg/m²) (mean)	24.7	25.7
Waist:hip ratio >0.84	28.1	29.8	33.5	Vigorous physical activity ≥ once per week	48.2	43.1	42.4	Age	53.8	52.6
				BMI ≥29 (kg/m²)	9.8	13.3	15.0	Systolic blood pressure	129.0	127.7
								Diastolic blood pressure	79.9	79.5
								Cholesterol	234.8	235.2

BMI, body mass index.

for users and nonusers. In the Nurses' Health Study, adjustments for age, cigarette smoking, hypertension, high serum cholesterol level, parental MI before age 60, body mass index, and past use of oral contraceptives yielded a relative risk of 0.56, compared with 0.51 adjusted for age alone. In the Leisure World Study (Henderson 1991), the age-adjusted relative risk of all-cause mortality was 0.80 (95% CI: 0.70–0.87) for estrogen users compared to nonusers; after further adjustment for high blood pressure, history of angina, MI, or stroke, alcohol use, smoking, Quetelet's index, and age at menopause, the relative risk was virtually the same (RR = 0.79, 95% CI: 0.71–0.88). In summary, to explain the benefit as a result of confounding, one would have to presume unknown risk factors, which are extremely strong predictors of CHD and very closely associated with estrogen use.

Both Barrett-Connor (1991) and Horwitz et al. (1993) have pointed out that estrogen users are compliant users of medication and that this characteristic may itself be a marker for low risk. In two clinical trials of drug therapy for secondary prevention of myocardial infarction (MI) in men, trial subjects who were compliant placebo takers had a better outcome than noncompliant placebo subjects (Coronary Drug Project Research Group 1980; Horwitz 1990): however, it is unclear to what extent these findings from drug therapy trials can be extended to observational studies of primary prevention in women, particularly studies in relatively homogeneous populations. It is possible, for example, that clinical trial participants with symptoms of preclinical disease may selectively stop taking their randomly assigned regimen.

Intervention Strategies

Several aspects of estrogen use and characteristics of users may be considered when prescribing estrogen. Data on the effects of dosage are sparse, but the available evidence does not seem to support a substantial change in CHD risk by estrogen dose within the range commonly prescribed (Ross 1981; Henderson 1991; Stampfer 1991b). However, doses above 1.25 mg of conjugated estrogen may have an adverse effect (Stampfer 1991b); such high doses were common in the Framingham population (Wilson 1985) and may explain why this was the only prospective study to report an increased risk of heart disease in estrogen users. Although age has been suggested as a possibly important modifier of the impact of ERT, this is not supported by most studies. The Framingham study observed a nonsignificant protective effect in younger women, and a nonsignificant adverse effect in those over age 60. However, in the Leisure World Study (Henderson 1988; Henderson 1990), where the median age was 73, there was a substantial decrease in coronary and all-cause mortality among estrogen users. Stampfer et al. (1991b) reported a decreased risk of CHD with estrogen use among younger postmenopausal women (with a small, nonsignificant increase in the oldest age group, 60–64 years), and Bush et al. (1987) found a benefit at all ages. In addition, the benefits of estrogen have been observed regardless of the type of menopause in most studies, although some found a stronger effect among women with a surgical menopause (Bush 1983; Szklo 1984; Stampfer 1985; McFarland 1989). Smoking may alter the effect of estrogen therapy, but conflicting results have been reported (Wilson 1985; Criqui 1988).

A recently identified, controversial issue regarding the most effective intervention strategy for estrogen is the use of combination estrogen and progestin therapy. Progestins are often prescribed along with estrogens in women with a uterus, to reduce or eliminate the excess risk of endometrial cancer due to unopposed estrogen; both cyclic (10-mg or 5-mg doses of medroxyprogesterone acetate [MPA]) and continuous (2.5-mg doses of MPA) regimens provide this benefit (Grady 1992). However, progestins tend to raise LDL and lower HDL (Bush 1986), and may thus detract from the beneficial effect of estrogens on the lipid profile. Moreover, progestins also tend to oppose the effect of estrogen on arterial dilation and blood flow (Sarrel 1994). Progestin use was quite uncommon during the period that most of the epidemiologic studies were conducted, and data on its effect on CHD risk are relatively sparse; similarly, current knowledge of the effect of dose of progestin and the specific regimen used (i.e., cyclic vs continuous) is limited. Overall, estrogen-progestin therapy was beneficial in the uncontrolled cohort study of Hunt (1990), but null findings were observed in the population-based case-control study of Thompson (1989). In these British studies, compounds other than conjugated estrogen were used by a substantial number of the women studied. The best-controlled, prospective epidemiologic data with direct information is the recent cohort study in Uppsala, Sweden (Falkeborn 1992), in which women taking an estradiol-levonorgestrel combination of hormone replacement therapy had a 50% decrease in their risk of MI (RR = 0.50; 95% CI: 0.28–0.80) compared with the general population of Uppsala. In women using estrogen alone, this risk was 0.74 (95% CI: 0.61–0.88).

More data are available from experimental studies. In one trial (Miller 1991), cyclical progestin added to estrogen supplementation attenuated the estrogen-induced increase in HDL from 14%–17% but had little effect on the reduction of LDL. In another trial (Sherwin 1989), HDL and the ratio of HDL to LDL increased in the group given estrogen with a placebo and the group given estrogen plus 5 mg cyclic MPA after one year of treatment. However, the group given progestin experienced smaller increases in both parameters; HDL rose 13.7% in the women taking 0.625 mg estrogen alone but only 4.3% in the added progestin group, and the ratio of HDL to LDL in women taking 0.625 mg estrogen alone rose 13.6%, while in the estrogen/progestin group it rose 7.3%. Soma et al. (1993) found that women given conjugated estrogen with 10 mg of medroxyprogesterone cyclically had a 50% reduction in mean plasma levels of lipoprotein(a) compared to controls, in addition to a decrease in total cholesterol and LDL and an increase in HDL. Women given ethinyl estradiol with a nonandrogenic progestin had increased prostacyclin (and HDL), while those taking a more androgenic progestin experienced a decrease in prostacyclin (Ylikorkala 1987). The Postmenopausal Estrogen/ Progestin Interventions Trial (PEPI) provides the most extensive information on added progestin and cholesterol levels (PEPI 1995). Five groups of 175 women each were randomized for three years to placebo, oral estrogen alone, oral estrogen plus cyclic MPA, oral estrogen plus consecutive MPA, or oral estrogen with cyclic micronized progesterone (MP). Significant increases in HDL and decreases in LDL were found for all treatment groups compared to placebo; for LDL similar decreases were observed for all hormone regimens (by 0.37 to 0.46 mmol/L), although for HDL, the elevation among users of MPA (by 0.03 to 0.04 mmol/L) was not as great as for users of estrogen alone (increase of 0.14 mmol/l) or estrogen with MP (0.11 mmol/l).

In animal studies, monkeys given either estrogen alone or estrogen and cyclic progestin had a very similar reduction (by about half) in the extent of coronary atherosclerosis after 30 months, as compared with those given placebo (Adams 1990a). In addition, comparable decreases in aortic accumulation of cholesterol were found in cholesterol-fed female rabbits given estrogen alone and those given estrogen with continuous progestin relative to rabbits given placebo (Haarbo 1991). Taken together, the sparse data available at present suggest that added progestin, either cyclical or continuous, will not eliminate the benefits of estrogen on cardiovascular disease, but it may possibly attenuate the benefit.

However, other effects of the added progestin should also be considered, including the continuation of regular menstrual bleeding when taken cyclically, unpredictable bleeding for most women at the start of a continuous estrogen/progestin regimen, and side effects such as breast tenderness and bloating. Furthermore, the likelihood of patients following specific regimens is an important component.

Risks, Benefits, and Cost

The decision to use estrogen is perhaps the most complex medical decision that any normal healthy menopausal woman typically faces. Because estrogen is relatively inexpensive (one year therapy with 0.625 mg of Premarin costs approximately $140), the issue is complicated more by the potential risks and benefits than by the cost of using estrogen. The benefits of reducing menopausal symptoms and decreasing bone loss are well-established (Grady 1992), and the evidence that estrogen protects against heart disease is quite strong. However, estrogen increases the risk of endometrial cancer (unless progestin is added) and gallstones, and may increase the risk of breast cancer. Grady and colleagues (1992) conducted a metanalysis of studies of heart disease, hip fractures, breast cancer, and endometrial cancer; they found a summary relative risk of 0.65 for CHD (similar to the results of our metanalysis), 0.75 for osteoporosis, 1.25 for breast cancer, and 8.22 for endometrial cancer (Table 16.2).

Table 16.2. Relative Risk of Selected Conditions for a 50-Year-Old White Woman Treated with Long-Term Hormone Replacement

Condition	Relative Risk[a]	
	Estrogen Therapy	Estrogen plus Progestin
Coronary heart disease	0.65	0.65–0.80
Stroke	0.96	0.96
Hip fracture	0.75	0.75
Breast cancer	1.25	1.25–2.00
Endometrial cancer	8.22	1.00

Source: From Grady et al. (1992) with permission.

[a] "Best" estimates of the relative risk for developing each condition in long-term hormone users compared with nonusers. These estimates were used in the model of the risks and benefits of hormone therapy. The same relative-risk estimate was used for dying of each condition in long-term users compared with nonusers except for endometrial cancer, where a relative risk of 3.0 was used.

Based on these risks, they estimated that the use of estrogen could add from 0.7 to 2.1 years to the life expectancy of a 50-year old white woman, while the use of estrogen with progestin could either add from 0.8 to 2.2 years or detract 0.5 years from the life expectancy, depending on her baseline risk of endometrial cancer, heart disease, breast cancer, and osteoporosis and the estimated magnitude of the adverse impact of added progestin on the cardiovascular benefits (Table 16.3). The largest benefits of both estrogen and estrogen with progestin are for women with the greatest risk of heart disease. In particular, women with clinical evidence of existing cardiovascular disease (and at high risk for recurrence) would be most likely to benefit. Also, because of its effects on lipids, estrogen may be especially useful for women with high LDL or low HDL. The least benefit is projected for those at higher risk for breast cancer, particularly if they are at low risk for CHD by virtue of their risk factor profile. However, these projections tend to underestimate the probable net benefit of ERT because they are based on a pooled relative risk of CHD for ever use, rather than the more pronounced benefit observed for current use. Also, although the fear of an increased risk of breast cancer is mostly for long duration of use, the excess risk in these projections is applied when use begins. Nonetheless, although cardiovascular disease accounts for approximately 10 times as many deaths as breast cancer, the fear of breast cancer should also be considered, together with the knowledge that many interventions are available to reduce the risk of cardiovascular disease.

In a similar analysis, Henderson et al. (1986) estimated a 41% decrease in mortality among women aged 50 to 75 if moderate-dose estrogen therapy (without progestin) were used. As expected, the substantial decrease among estrogen users in their risk of CHD, the leading cause of mortality among women, provides the driving force behind these calculations. Finally, however, each individual woman differs in her

Table 16.3. Net Change in Life Expectancy for a 50-Year-Old White Woman Treated with Long-Term Hormone Replacement

Variable	Life Expectancy (years)	Net Change in Life Expectancy (years)		
		Estrogen	E + P[a]	E + P[b]
No risk factors	82.8	+0.9	+1.0	+0.1
With hysterectomy	82.8	+1.1		
With history of coronary heart disease	76.0	+2.1	+2.2	+0.9
At risk for coronary heart disease	79.6	+1.5	+1.6	+0.6
At risk for breast cancer	82.3	+0.7	+0.8	−0.5
At risk for hip fracture	82.4	+1.0	+1.1	+0.2

Source: from Grady et al. (1992), with permission.

[a]Assuming that the addition of a progestin to the estrogen regimen does not alter any of the relative risks for disease seen with estrogen therapy, except to prevent the increased risk due to endometrial cancer (relative risk for endometrial cancer estimated to be 1.0). E + P, estrogen plus progestin.

[b]Assuming that the addition of a progestin to the estrogen regimen provides only two-thirds of the coronary heart disease risk reduction afforded by estrogen therapy (relative risk for coronary heart disease), and that the relative risk for breast cancer in treated women is 2.0.

particular risks and benefits and careful consideration of each woman's unique situation is required.

Patient counselling materials concerning the benefits and risks of hormone replacement therapy are provided in an appendix at the end of this textbook.

Summary

Quality of available data: A large number of well-designed observational (case-control and prospective cohort) studies of ERT.

Estimated risk reduction: Approximately 40–50% reduction of MI risk among current vs never users of ERT. Randomized trials of hormone replacement therapy are currently ongoing.

Comparability of effect in men and women: Not applicable.

References

Adam S. Williams V, Vessey MP. Cardiovascular disease and hormone replacement treatment; a pilot case-control study. Br Med J 1981;282;1277–8.

Adams MR, Kaplan JR, Manuck SB, et al. Inhibition of coronary artery atherosclerosis by 17-beta estradiol in ovariectomized monkeys: lack of an effect of added progesterone. Arteriosclerosis 1990a;10:1051–7.

Adams MR, Clarkson TB, Shively CA, et al. Oral contraceptives, lipoproteins, and atherosclerosis. Am J Obstet Gynecol 1990b;163;1388–93.

Avila MH, Walker AM, Jick H. Use of replacement estrogens and the risk of myocardial infarction. Epidemiology 1990;1:128–33.

Bain C. Willett WC, Hennekens CH, et al. Use of postmenopausal hormones and risk of myocardial infarction. Circulation 1981;64:42–6.

Barrett-Connor E. Putative complications of estrogen replacement therapy: hypertension, diabetes, thrombophlebitis, and gallstones. In: Korenman SG, ed. The menopause. Norwell, MA: Serono Synposia, 1990:199–209.

Barrett-Connor E, Laakso M. Ischemic heart disease risk in postmenopausal women: effects of estrogen use on glucose and insulin levels. Arteriosclerosis 1990;10:531–4.

Barrett-Connor E. Postmenopausal estrogen and prevention bias. Ann Int Med 1991;115:455–6.

Beard CM, Kottke TE, Annegers JF, Ballard DJ. The Rochester Coronary Heart Disease Project: effect of cigarette smoking, hypertension, diabetes, and steroidal estrogen use on coronary heart disease among 40–59 year old women, 1960–82. Mayo Clinic Proc 1989; 64:1471–80.

Bourne T. Hillard TC, Whitehead MI, et al. Oestrogens, arterial status, and postmenopausal women. Lancet 1990;335:1470–1.

Burch JC, Byrd BF, Vaughn WK. The effects of long-term estrogen on hysterectomized women. Am J Obstet Gynecol 1974;188:778–2.

Bush TL, Cowan LD, Barrett-Connor E, et al. Estrogen use and all-cause mortality: preliminary results from the Lipid Research Clinics Program Follow-up Study. JAMA 1983;249: 903–6.

Bush TL, Miller VT. Effects of pharmacologic agents used during menopause. Impact on lipids and lipoproteins. In Mishell D, ed. menopause: physiology and pharmacology. Chicago: Year Book Medical Publishers, 1986:187–208.

Bush TL, Barrett-Connor E, Cowan LD, et al. Cardiovascular mortality and noncontraceptive use of estrogen in women: results from the Lipid Research Clinics Program Follow-up Study. Circulation 1987;75:1102–9.

Cauley JA, Cummings SR, Black DM, et al. Prevalence and determinants of estrogen replacement therapy in elderly women. Am J Obstet Gynecol 1990;163:1438–44.

Collins P, Rosano GM, Jiang C. et al. Cardiovascular protection by estrogen—a calcium antagonist effect? Lancet 1993;341:1264–5.

Coronary Drug Project Research Group. Influence of adherence to treatment and response of cholesterol on mortality in the coronary drug project. N Engl J Med 1980;303:1038–41.

Criqui MH, Suarez L, Barrett-Connor E, et al. Postmenopausal estrogen use and mortality. Am J Epidemiol 1988;128:606–14.

Croft P, Hannaford PC. Risk factors for acute myocardial infarction in women: evidence from the Royal College of General Practitioners' oral contraceptive study. Br Med J 1989; 298:165–9.

Eaker ED, Castelli WP. Coronary heart disease and its risk factors among women in the Framingham Study. In: Eaker E, Packard B, Wenger NK, Clarkson TB, Tyroler HA, eds. Coronary heart disease in women. New York: Haymarket Doyma, 1987:122–32.

Falkeborn M, Persson I. Adami HO, et al. The risk of acute myocardial infarction after oestrogen and oestrogen-progestogen replacement. Br J Obstet Gynecol 1992;99:821–8.

Gangar KF, Vyas S. Whitehead M, et al. Pulsatility index in internal carotid artery in relation to transdermal oestradiol and time since menopause. Lancet 1991;338:839–842.

Gordon DJ, Probstfield JL, Garrison RJ, et al. High-density lipoprotein cholesterol and cardiovascular disease: four prospective American studies. Circulation 1989;79:8–15.

Grady D. Rubin SM, Petitti DB, et al. Hormone therapy to prevent disease and prolong life in postmenopausal women. Ann Intern Med 1992;117:1016–37.

Grodstein F. Stampfer MJ. Menopause and coronary heart disease: what is the role of estrogen replacement therapy. Am J Med 1995; in press.

Gruchow HW, Anderson AJ, Barboriak JJ, Sobocinski KA, Postmenopausal use 101of estrogen and occlusion of coronary arteries. Am Heart J 1988;115:954–63.

Haarbo J, Leth-Espensen P, Stender S, Christiansen C. Estrogen monotherapy and combined estrogen-progestogen replacement therapy attenuate aortic accumulation of cholesterol in ovariectomized cholesterol-fed rabbits. J Clin Invest 1991;87:1274–9.

Hammond CB, Jelovsek FR, Lee LK, et al. Effects of long-term estrogen replacement therapy. I. Metabolic effects. Am J Obstet Gynecol 1979;133:525–36.

Harder DR, Coulson PB. Estrogen receptors and effects of estrogen on membrane electrical properties of coronary vascular smooth muscle. J Cell Physiol 1979;100:375–82.

Henderson BE, Ross RK, Paganini-Hill A, Mack TM. Estrogen use and cardiovascular disease. Am J Obstet Gynecol 1986;154:1181–6.

Henderson BE, Paganini-Hill A, Ross RK. Estrogen replacement therapy and protection from acute myocardial infarction. Am J Obstet Gynecol 1988;159:312–17.

Henderson BE, Paganini-Hill A. Ross RK. Decreased mortality in users of estrogen replacement therapy. Arch Int Med 1991;151:75–8.

Hong MK, Romm PA, Reagan K, et al. Effects of estrogen replacement therapy on serum lipid values and angiographically defined coronary artery disease in postmenopausal women. Am J Cardiol 1992;69:176–78.

Horwitz RI, Viscoli CM, Berkman L, et al. Treatment adherence and risk of death after a myocardial infarction. Lancet 1990;336:542–5.

Horwitz RI, Horwitz SM. Adherence to treatment and health outcomes. Arch Intern Med 1993; 153:1863–8.

Hunt K, Vessey M, McPherson K, Coleman M. Long-term surveillance of mortality and cancer incidence in women receiving hormone replacement therapy. Br J Obstet Gynecol 1987; 94:620–35.

Hunt K, Vessey M, McPherson K. Mortality in a cohort of long-term users of hormone replacement therapy: an updated analysis. Br J Obstet Gynecol 1990;97:1080–86.

Jick H, Dinan B, Rothman KJ. Noncontraceptive estrogens and nonfatal myocardial infarction. JAMA 1978a;239:1407–8.

Jick H, Dinan B, Herman R, Rothman KJ. Myocardial infarction and other vascular diseases in young women: role of estrogens and other factors. JAMA 1978b;240:2548–452.

Lafferty FW, Helmuth DO. Postmenopausal estrogen replacement: the prevention of osteoporosis and systemic effects. Maturitas 1985;7:147–59.

La Vecchia C, Franceschi S, Decarli A, et al. Risk factors for myocardial infarction in young women. Am J Epidemiol 1987;125:832–43.

Magness RR, Rosenfeld CR. Local and systemic estradiol-17 beta: effects on uterine and systemic vasodilation. Am J Physiol 1989;256:536–42.

Manson JE, Rimm EB, Colditz GA, et al. A prospective study of postmenopausal estrogen therapy and subsequent incidence of non-insulin-dependent diabetes mellitus. Ann Epidemiol 1992;2:665–73.

McFarland KF, Boniface ME, Hornung CA, et al. Risk factors and noncontraceptive estrogen use in women with and without coronary disease. Am Heart J 1989;117:1209–14.

McGill HC. Sex steroid hormone receptors in the cardiovascular system. Postgrad Med 1989: 64–8.

McMahon B. Cardiovascular disease and noncontraceptive oestrogen therapy. In: Oliver MF, ed., Coronary heart disease in young women. New York: Churchill Livingstone, 1978: 197–207.

Miller VT, Muesing RA, LaRosa JC, et al. Effects of conjugated equine estrogen with and without three different progestogens on lipoproteins, high-density lipoprotein subfractions, and apolipoprotein A-1. Obstet Gynecol 1991;77:235.

Nachtigall LE, Nachtigall RH, Nachtigall RD, Beckman EM. Estrogen replacement therapy II: a prospective study in the relationship to carcinoma and cardiovascular and metabolic problems. Obstet Gynecol 1979;54:74–9.

Petitti DB, Perlman JA, Sidney S. Noncontraceptive estrogens and mortality: long-term follow-up of women in the Walnut Creek Study. Obstet Gynecol 1987;70:289–93.

Pfeffer RI, Whipple GH, Kurosaki TT, Chapman JM. Coronary risk and estrogen use in postmenopausal women. Am J Epidemiol 1978;107:479–87.

Pines A. Fisman EZ, Levo Y, et al. The effects of hormone replacement therapy in normal postmenopausal women: measurements of Doppler-derived parameters of aortic flow. Am J Obstet Gynecol 1991;164:806–812.

Potocki J. Wplyw leczenia estrogenami na niewydolnose wiencowa u kobiet po menopauzie. Pol Tyg Lek 1971;117:1209–14.

Postmenopausal Estrogen/Progestin Interventions (PEPI) Trial Writing Group. Effects of estrogen/progestin regimens on heart disease risk factors in postmenopausal women. JAMA 1995;273:199–203.

Rosano GMC, Sarrel PM, Poole-Wilson PA, Collins P. Beneficial effect of oestrogen on exercise-induced myocardial ischaemia in women with coronary artery disease. Lancet 1993; 342:133–6.

Rosenberg L, Armstrong B, Jick H. Myocardial infarction and estrogen therapy in postmenopausal women. N Engl J Med 1976;294:1256–9.

Rosenberg L, Stone D, Shapiro S, et al. Noncontraceptive estrogens and myocardial infarction in young women. JAMA 1980;244:339–42.

Rosenberg L, Palmer JR, Shapiro S. A case-control study of myocardial infarction in relation to use of estrogen supplements. Am J Epidemiol 1993;137:54–63.

Ross RK, Paganini-Hill A, Mack TM, et al. Menopausal oestrogen therapy and protection from death from ischaemic heart disease. Lancet 1981;1:858–60.

Sack MN, Rader DJ, Cannon RO. Estrogen and inhibition of oxidation of low- density lipoproteins in postmenopausal women. Lancet 1994;343:269–70.

Sarrel PM, Lindsay D, Rosano GMC, Poole-Wilson PA. Angina and normal coronary arteries in women: gynecologic findings. Am J Obstet Gynecol 1992;167:467–72.

Sarrel PM. Blood flow. In: Lobo R, ed. Treatment of the postmenopausal women. New York: Raven Press, 1994:251–62.

Sherwin BB, Gelfand MM. A prospective one-year study of estrogen and progestin in postmenopausal women: effects on clinical symptoms and lipoprotein lipids. Obstet Gynecol 1989;73:759–66.

Soma MR, Osnago-Gadda I, Paoletti R, et al. The lowering of lipoprotein(a) induced by estrogen plus progesterone replacement therapy in postmenopausal women. Arch Intern Med 1993;153:1462–8.

Stampfer MJ, Willett WC, Colditz GA, et al. A prospective study of postmenopausal estrogen therapy and coronary heart disease. N. Engl J Med 1985;313:1044–9.

Stampfer MJ, Colditz GA, Willett WC. Menopause and heart disease: a review. Ann NY Acad Sci 1990;592:193–203.

Stampfer MJ, Colditz GA. Estrogen replacement therapy and coronary heart disease: a quantitative assessment of the epidemiologic evidence. Prev Med 1991a;20:47–63.

Stampfer MJ, Colditz GA, Willett WC, et al. Postmenopausal estrogen therapy and cardiovascular disease: ten-year follow-up from the Nurses' Health Study. N Engl J Med 1991b; 325:756–62.

Steinleitner A, Stanczyk FZ, Levin JH, et al. Decreased in vitro production of 6-keto-prostaglandin F_1 by uterine arteries from postmenopausal women. Am J Obstet Gynecol 1989; 161:1677–81.

Sullivan JM, Zwagg RV, Lemp GF, et al. Postmenopausal estrogen use and coronary atherosclerosis. Ann Intern Med 1988;108:358–63.

Sullivan JM, Zwaag VR, Hughes J, et al. Effect of estrogen replacement and coronary artery disease on survival in postmenopausal women. Arch Int Med 1990;150:2557–62.

Szklo M, Tonascia J, Gordis L, Bloom I. Estrogen use and myocardial infarction risk: a case-control study. Prev Med 1984;13:510–16.

Talbott E, Kuller LH, Detre K, Perper J. Biologic and Psychosocial risk factors of sudden death from coronary disease in white women. Am J Cardiol 1977;39:858–64.

Thompson SG, Meade TW, Greenberg G. The use of hormonal replacement therapy and the risk of stroke and myocardial infarction in women. J Epidemiol Comm Health 1989;43:173–8.

Wagner JD, Clarkson TB, St Clair RW, et al. Estrogen and progesterone replacement therapy reduces low density lipoprotein accumulation in the coronary arteries of surgically postmenopausal cynomolgus monkeys. J Clin Invest 1991;88:1995–2002.

Walsh BW, Schiff I, Rosner B, et al. Effects of postmenopausal estrogen replacement on the concentration and metabolism of plasma lipoproteins. N Engl J Med 1991;325:1196–204.

Williams JK, Adams MR, Klopfenstein HS. Estrogen modulates responses of atherosclerotic coronary arteries. Circulation 1990;81:1680–7.

Wilson PW, Garrison RJ, Castelli WP. Postmenopausal estrogen use, cigarette smoking, and cardiovascular morbidity in women over 50: the Framingham Study. N Engl J Med 1985;313:1038–43.

Wolf PH, Madans JH, Finucane FF, et al. Reduction of cardiovascular disease-related mortality among postmenopausal women who use hormones: evidence from a national cohort. Am J. Obstet Gynecol 1991;164:489–94.

Ylikorkala O, Kuusi T, Tikkanen MJ, Viinikka L. Desogestrel- and levonorgestrel-containing oral contraceptives have different effects on urinary excretion of prostacyclin metabolites and serum high density lipoproteins. J Clin Eendocrinol Metab 1987;65:1238–42.

IV

INTERVENTIONS IN CHILDHOOD AND ADOLESCENCE

17

Pediatric Preventive Cardiology

WILLIAM B. STRONG AND STEVEN H. KELDER

The idea that atherosclerosis begins in childhood first arose from the observation of atherosclerotic lesions in young autopsied patients in 1915 (Saltykow 1915). More than 40 years later Holman (1961) reported similar observations and suggested a nutritional origin for atherosclerosis. His colleagues began to accumulate autopsy data that formed the basis for a natural history model of atherosclerosis (Figure 17.1) and provided the stimulus for the international research efforts of the next four decades (Strong 1962).

Reismann (1965) was one of the first clinicians to recognize atherosclerosis as a pediatric problem. Two major longitudinal, epidemiologic studies in the United States have confirmed that origins of atherosclerosis in the young and identified the precursor risk factors for coronary artery disease (CAD) in children (Berenson 1981; 1991; Lauer 1975, 1982, 1988, 1989). Hyperlipidemia in the young has also been explored (Glueck 1974; Kwiterovich 1989). Although there had been controversy as to the earliest lesions of atherosclerosis in the coronary arteries, doubt no longer exists. The Pathobiological Determinants of Atherosclerosis in Youth (PDAY) research group (PDAY 1990) has amply confirmed the earlier studies of Korean (Enos 1955) and Vietnam (McNamara 1971) battle casualties, which demonstrated significant coronary atherosclerosis in young soldiers. In addition, the prospective studies of Newman and colleagues (1986) have shown the relationship of risk factors in young men with coronary lesions observed at the autopsies of these youths, who generally had traumatic deaths. The extent of the surface covered by atherosclerosis correlated with serum lipoprotein cholesterol concentrations, cigarette smoking habit, and blood pressure level.

Background and Rationale for Intervening in the Young

The authors of preceding chapters have cited the risk factors that are associated with clinically manifest CAD in adulthood. They have also demonstrated that many of these factors are related to lifestyle behaviors, and as such, should potentially be

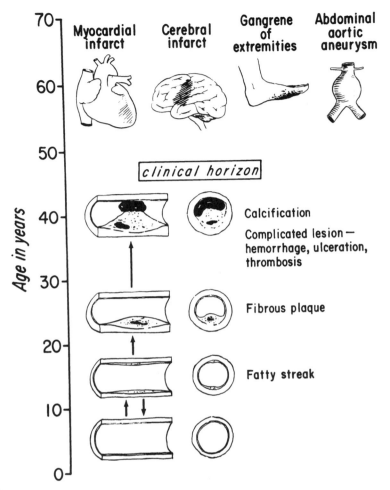

Fig. 17.1. Diagrammatic concept of the natural history of atherosclerosis. [With permission of Academic Press, reprinted with slight modification from H. C. McGill, Jr., et al. Natural history of human atherosclerotic lesions. In: M. Sandler and G. H. Bourne, eds. *Atherosclerosis and its origin*. New York: Academic Press, 1963.]

modifiable. Figure 17.2 illustrates the commonly acknowledged risk factors for adult CAD. On the right side are the interventions, and the risk factors they affect are listed on the left.

The major premises of pediatric preventive cardiology are that these lifestyle behaviors are initiated in childhood and that altering childhood behaviors will have an impact on adult behaviors. These beliefs, together with the knowledge that CAD risk factors can be identified in the young and that the extreme percentiles ($\leq$5th and $\geq$95) track well into adulthood, serve as the keystone of pediatric preventive cardiology.

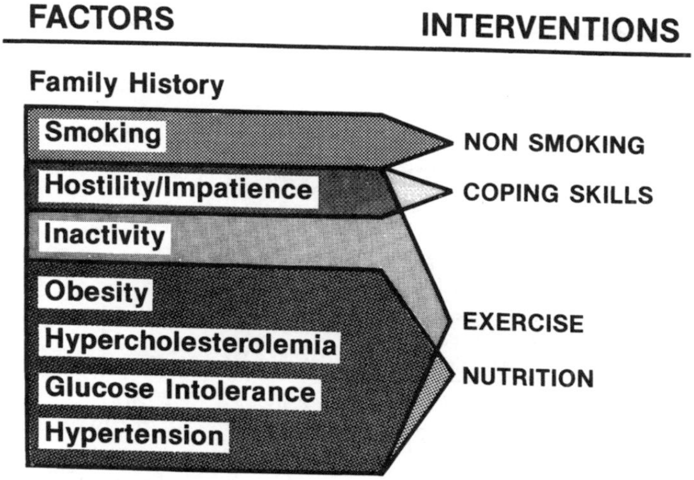

FACTORS   **INTERVENTIONS**

Family History

Factors	Interventions
Smoking	→ NON SMOKING
Hostility/Impatience	→ COPING SKILLS
Inactivity	
Obesity	→ EXERCISE
Hypercholesterolemia	
Glucose Intolerance	→ NUTRITION
Hypertension	

Fig. 17.2. Risk factors and behavioral interventions that may influence the progression of the atherosclerotic process. Risk factors are presented on the left and the behavioral interventions on the right. Exercise (physical activity) and nutrition can influence multiple risk factors.

Identifying children with risk factors and altering their lifestyles (for a lifetime), should reduce the prevalence of adults with these behaviors, and hence reduce prevalence of CAD. The identification of the child with an ''at risk'' profile and subsequent intervention comprise the ''high risk'' strategy. The ''public health'' strategy is the second prevention strategy. Both approaches are illustrated in Figure 17.3 (adapted from Grundy 1986). The adult distribution curve for total cholesterol is presented along with a bar graph showing the fraction of CAD mortality related to the level of cholesterol. The adults with total cholesterol ≥275 mg/dl (7.0 mmol) are at highest individual risk for CAD mortality. However, the majority of deaths occur among those whose values are between 200 mg/dl (5.17 mmol) and 275 mg/dl and thus are at lower individual risk of CAD mortality. Although such individuals are far more difficult to identify in childhood, they contribute the largest number of cases and therefore represent a segment of the population that must be addressed in order to reduce overall mortality.

The first section of this chapter presents evidence that the risk factors for adult disease can be observed in the young. It also discusses the likelihood that these factors will track into later life. Finally, we discuss possible strategies for intervening among the young.

The rationale for such intervention is based primarily on cross-sectional and cross-cultural observations. CAD is multifactorial, and as such, does not currently have a simple solution. The desire to modify the behavior of the young is not only intended to reduce CAD mortality and increase longevity, but to enhance general good health and wellbeing, since these health behaviors, particularly not smoking, maintaining ideal weight, and being active, are beneficial to all children as well as adults. Children should develop healthy eating behaviors not just to make a heart attack less likely 40

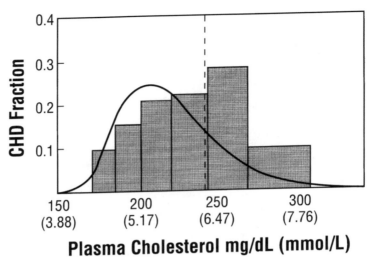

Fig. 17.3. Fraction of total population dying of coronary heart disease (CHD) among Multiple Risk Factor Intervention Trial participants who had different levels of plasma cholesterol at screening. Current distribution of plasma cholesterol values for American adults is superimposed. Approximately 38% of those dying of CHD had cholesterol levels <245 mg/dl (6.34 mmol/l) at screening.

years in the future, but also to reduce the likelihood of obesity and its related problems of glucose intolerance and hypertension, and of cancers related to excess saturated fat intake. Smoking should be eliminated not only to prevent heart disease but also to reduce lung cancer, other related cancers, and chronic lung disease. Preventing smoking among the young is especially important because smoking is a gateway behavior to substance abuse and other high-risk negative behaviors (Miller 1993). A sedentary lifestyle can be related to most of the other risk factors, especially obesity (see Figure 17.2). Anecdotally, it is rare to hear an adult who has begun to be more physically active not volunteer that she or he feels better and is more productive since beginning the activity. The essence of these recommendations is the importance of incorporating heart-healthy programs for the young in a comprehensive package of health behaviors for a lifetime.

Another important aspect of identifying children with risk factors is the fact that they almost universally have at least one parent with a similar or worse risk profile. The child with hypercholesterolemia is likely to have parents who are hypercholesterolemic (Rogers 1990), and the youth who is hypertensive is likely to have parents with hypertension (Treiber 1993). Except for routine gynecologic care, parents of school-age or younger children do not generally receive any ongoing medical care, since they are usually free of overt symptoms of disease. Because of its demographics and psychological profile, this age group does not lend itself readily to professional health interventions. A Center for Disease Control survey demonstrated that only 12% of adults 18 to 34 years of age knew their cholesterol value (CDC 1990). The author's unsubstantiated observations suggest that it is much easier to achieve behavioral change in the young adult (i.e., parents) when the child is the index case, and therefore, the parents alter their own behaviors for the benefit of the child. This is another key rationale for attempting to identify risk factors in children. The payback in young middle-aged adults (where disease is present but not overtly manifest) is potentially high. Looking at risk factor identification and intervention in childhood as an isolated phenomenon, out of context of the family, is not an optimal approach to prevention.

Risk Factor Identification in the Young and Tracking Into Adulthood

Cigarette Smoking

Reducing the prevalence of cigarette smoking is considered to be the single most important factor in reducing premature morbidity and mortality in the United States (Shultz 1991). Smoking, obviously, is not confined to adults. In 1989, 11.2% of American high school seniors were smoking at least one-half pack per day (Johnston 1991). This is a very low estimate because it does not include school dropouts, among whom use of drugs of all sorts is even more prevalent. The peak frequency of smoking onset occurs between 11 and 14 years of age (Pirie 1988). There is a decreasing rate of initiation after high school. The 1991 Youth Risk Behavior Study observed that 15.6% of 11th and 12th graders considered themselves to be frequent cigarette users (MMWR 1992). Females are slightly more likely to smoke than males in high school, but at the college level they are considerably more likely to smoke than males.

Social environment, personality, and behavioral factors are important determinants of future tobacco use, particularly during adolescence, when behavioral choices are complicated by biologic, emotional, cognitive, identity, and social changes (Johnston 1988). Mass media, especially print advertising, create an environment that is tolerant of smoking. Both parental and peer relationships are strong environmental factors. Children of nonsmoking parents smoked at one-half the rate as those with smoking parents. Even more impressive was the peer relationship. The smoking rate was 4% among students with nonsmoking friends, and 38% for those with smoking friends (Lauer 1982). For smoking prevention to be effective there must be educational programs, plus community enforcement of legislation.

Hypercholesterolemia

Numerous studies have demonstrated that hypercholesterolemia can be identified in children. The National Cholesterol Education Program (NCEP), Report of the Expert Panel on Blood Levels in Children and Adolescents (1992), has defined a serum total cholesterol level <170 mg/dl (4.4 mmol/l) as an acceptable level; total cholesterol ≥200 mg/dl (5.17 mmol/l) is considered abnormally elevated. These values correspond approximately to the 75th percentile and 95th percentile in the U.S. population. That same panel of experts has provided an algorithm by which to identify children with lipid abnormalities.

Total cholesterol level in children rises from the neonatal period to a relatively stable level by two years of age (Cresanta 1984). In early adolescence, especially in white males, the total cholesterol tends to decrease modestly until late adolescence when it begins to rise. Figure 17.4 presents the data obtained from the Bogalusa cohort. The childhood level of total cholesterol distributes along a gaussian curve. A child with a total cholesterol level ≥95th percentile or ≤5th percentile tends to maintain similar percentile ranking into adulthood; in some studies being as high as an 80% likelihood. The 95th percentile for total cholesterol in a child is approximately 200 mg/dl (5.17 mmol/l). In an adult the 95th percentile is about 260 mg/dl (6.72 mmol/l) and carries an approximate threefold increased incidence of CAD mortality. Total cholesterol reflects the level of low density lipoprotein (LDL) cholesterol quite well. Of children with a total cholesterol ≥200 mg/dl (5.17 mmol/l), 77% will have an LDL cholesterol ≥130 mg/dl (3.36 mmol/l) (95th percentile) (Garcia 1989).

The NCEP Pediatric Panel recommends targeted screening of children on the basis of a positive family history (first- and second-degree relatives) of premature CAD or elevated total cholesterol level in parents. Others have taken exception to these recommendations (Strong 1988), suggesting that screening of all children should be performed as part of general pediatric care. Such advocates believe that measuring the child's cholesterol in a health care setting is reasonable and is also a means to identify young adults (parents) who do not routinely participate in the preventive health care systems (CDC 1990a). They also assert that measuring the child's total cholesterol. is an effective tool by which to introduce healthy lifestyle behavioral changes. On the other hand, in a small but probably significant number of children and their families, an inappropriate and overzealous, or hyperanxious response of the parent and/or child will be generated by measuring the child's cholesterol (Pugliese 1987). In view of this controversy, it should be recognized that methods designed to avoid this kind of overreactive behavior, or to identify the family at risk for this type of reaction, need to be developed in order to uphold the oath, *nolo non nocere*.

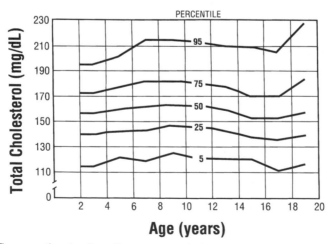

Fig. 17.4. Cross-sectional values for serum total cholesterol for youths 2 to 19 years old. Percentile distribution is shown.

The NCEP Pediatric Panel has recommended that targeted screening for total cholesterol or lipoprotein is indicated in children and adolescents. Newman and colleagues have taken exception to those recommendations, as well as those espoused by many others who suggest that screening of all children should be performed in the setting of general pediatric care. Given all of the controversy, it should be recognized that a reasonably good laboratory procedure is available (i.e., one that will identify 75% of children with an elevated LDL level). The test is inexpensive, valid and reproducible. However, the third leg of the triad of screening criteria, that effective therapy is available, remains less certain. Dietary and other lifestyle interventions are the cornerstone of pediatric hypercholesterolemia therapy, with pharmacologic intervention recommended only for a small percentage of patients, primarily those 10 years of age or older. For dietary therapy to be effective, the family and child must alter their eating patterns, shopping habits, and food preparation. Such changes are never easy, even in the presence of a desire to change.

Hypertension

Hypertension, which contributes significantly to premature morbidity and mortality among adults, has also been recognized in children. The Report of the Second Task Force on Blood Pressure Control in Children (1987) presented normative values for children and defined hypertensive levels. Figures 17.5 to 17.8 shows the percentile distribution by gender and age, as well as presenting the 90th percentile values for height and weight. Table 17.1 classifies hypertension by age group. Longitudinal studies strongly support that systolic pressure tracks quite well into adulthood (Lauer 1989; Berenson 1991). The data are somewhat less convincing for diastolic blood pressure, but that is in large part due to problems inherent in measuring diastolic blood pressure in the young. Moss and Adams (1963), showed that neither the fourth nor the fifth Korotkoff sounds accurately reflected intraarterial diastolic blood pressure in children. They demonstrated that K_4 was too high, while K_5 was too low, often going to zero. The newer oscillometric automated systems reflect diastolic blood pressure more accurately than previous methods and probably should be recommended as the standard.

Using the criteria shown in Table 17.2, the diagnosis of hypertension is made when, on three separate occasions, blood pressure exceeds the 95th percentile. When this criterion is met, approximately two-thirds of the individuals will be hypertensive 3 to 8 years later (Londe 1976). By definition, at any one time 5% of children will have a blood pressure measurement exceeding the 95th percentile. However, in most clinical, as well as epidemiologic studies, when the measurements are repeated on three separate occasions only about 1% of children will be affirmed to be hypertensive. The younger the child, the more likely is the hypertension to be secondary (Jung 1992). A great deal of epidemiologic research has been performed to substantiate the relationship between childhood and subsequent blood pressure levels initially presented by Londe (1966) and Londe and Goldring (1976). More recent research has focused on identifying additional characteristics that will provide a more accurate means of predicting which individual is most likely to become a hypertensive adult. In addition to family history, other predictive factors include ambulatory blood pres-

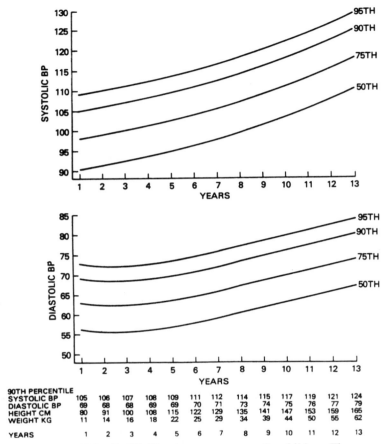

90TH PERCENTILE													
SYSTOLIC BP	105	106	107	108	109	111	112	114	115	117	119	121	124
DIASTOLIC BP	69	68	68	69	69	70	71	73	74	75	76	77	79
HEIGHT CM	80	91	100	108	115	122	129	135	141	147	153	159	165
WEIGHT KG	11	14	16	18	22	25	29	34	39	44	50	55	62
YEARS	1	2	3	4	5	6	7	8	9	10	11	12	13

Fig. 17.5, 17.6, 17.7, 17.8. (A–D) Blood pressure norms for children. These graphs show normal blood pressure ranges for girls (*right*) and boys (*left*). Beneath each designated age is written the 90th percentile for height, weight, and blood pressure. [Task Force on Blood Pressure Control in Children—National Heart, Lung, and Blood Institute, Report of the Second Task Force on Blood Pressure Control in Children. Reproduced by permission of Pediatrics 79:1, Copyright 1987.] *Figure continues.*

sure levels and cardiovascular reactivity to various stressors, for example, exercise, psychological testing, and forehead ice stimulus (Treiber 1993).

Physical Activity

Like smoking, hypercholesterolemia, and hypertension, a sedentary lifestyle is now recognized as an independent risk factor (CDC 1990b) (see Chapter 8). The Center for Disease Control, through its Youth Risk Behavior Survey, demonstrated that only 42% (37% of females and 46% of males) of high-school students participate in physical education classes or sports on a daily basis (CDC 1992b). The National Children

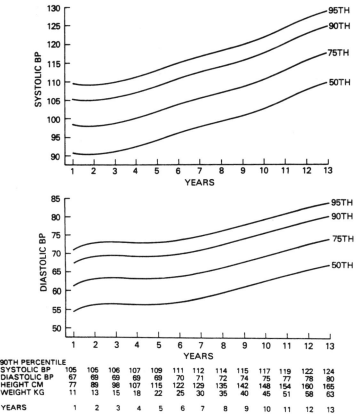

90TH PERCENTILE												
SYSTOLIC BP	105	105	106	107	109	111	112	114	115	117	119	122	124
DIASTOLIC BP	67	69	69	69	69	70	71	72	74	75	77	78	80
HEIGHT CM	77	89	98	107	115	122	129	135	142	148	154	160	165
WEIGHT KG	11	13	15	18	22	25	30	35	40	45	51	58	63
YEARS	1	2	3	4	5	6	7	8	9	10	11	12	13

Fig. 17.6. *Continued.*

and Youth Fitness Studies surveyed fifth- to twelfth-grade students and reported 58.9% engaged in "appropriate physical activity" (Simons-Morton 1988). Baranowski (1987) by observational techniques documented that only 44.9% of third- to fifth-grade students engaged in daily moderate to vigorous physical activity. During recess, Parcel (1989) observed that 70% of the available time involved movement. Oslo boys and girls, 11 to 14 years old, appear to be more active than children in the United States (Tell 1988).

Research has been conducted to determine what conditions promote physical activity in children and what conditions are barriers. A positive attitude toward exercise and sports has a strong positive influence. Environmental factors may have both positive and negative influences (Ferguson 1989). The parents' availability to participate actively or as a means of accessibility to a physical activity has important positive effects. Parental noninvolvement and inaccessibiity of facilities are impediments (Sallis 1992).

It is important for the child's future to learn motor skills at the appropriate age and development. It has been demonstrated that children who do not learn motor skills

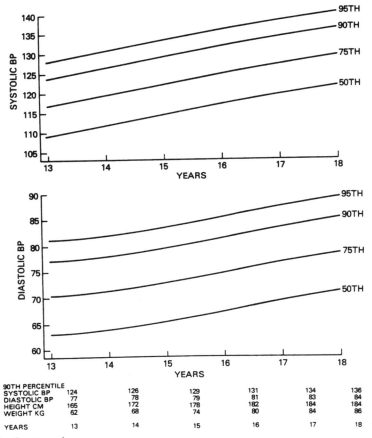

Fig. 17.7. *Continued.*

at the appropriate time during neuromotor maturation are less likely to push themselves to achieve those skills when they are older. As an example, children who do not learn to throw a ball "correctly" at six, seven, or eight years old are unlikely ever to learn that particular skill because the learning process in the presence of their peers would be embarrassing. Therefore, behaviorally, learning motor skills during youth is a critical step in how adult physical activity behavior is determined.

Little tracking data exist for physical activity. Dennison (1988) demonstrated that boys who were more active in high school tended to be more active in their early twenties. Paffenbarger and coworkers (1984) have demonstrated that being physically active in youth, however, does not confer protection from premature morbidity and mortality unless an active lifestyle is maintained as a lifelong behavior.

Obesity

Childhood obesity is prevalent and appears to be increasing in the United States. Depending on the method by which obesity is measured, 25–35% of children and

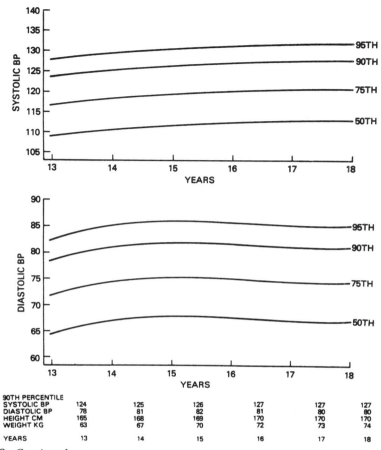

Fig. 17.8. *Continued.*

Table 17.1. Definitions

Normal BP	Systolic and diastolic blood pressures less than the 90th percentile for age and sex
High normal BP[a]	Average systolic and/or average diastolic blood pressure between 90th and 95th percentiles for age and sex
High BP (Hypertension)	Average systolic and/or average diastolic blood pressure greater than or equal to the 95th percentile for age and sex with measurements obtained on at least three occasions.

[a]If the blood pressure reading is high normal for age, but can be accounted for by excess height for age or excess lean body mass for age, such children are considered to have normal blood pressure.

443

Table 17.2. Classification of Hypertension by Age Group

Age Group	Significant Hypertension	Severe Hypertension
Newborn		
7 days	Systolic BP ≥96 mmHg	Systolic BP ≥106 mmHg
8–30 days	Systolic BP ≥104 mmHg	Systolic BP ≥110 mmHg
Infant (<2 years)	Systolic BP ≥112 mmHg	Systolic BP ≥118 mmHg
	Diastolic BP ≥74 mmHg	Diastolic BP ≥82 mmHg
Children (3–5 years)	Systolic BP ≥116 mmHg	Systolic BP ≥124 mmHg
	Diastolic BP ≥76 mmHg	Diastolic BP ≥84 mmHg
Children (6–9 years)	Systolic BP ≥122 mmHg	Systolic BP ≥130 mmHg
	Diastolic BP ≥78 mmHg	Diastolic BP ≥86 mmHg
Children (10–12 years)	Systolic BP ≥126 mmHg	Systolic BP ≥134 mmHg
	Diastolic BP ≥82 mmHg	Diastolic BP ≥90 mmHg
Adolescents (13–15 years)	Systolic BP ≥136 mmHg	Systolic BP ≥144 mmHg
	Diastolic BP ≥86 mmHg	Diastolic BP ≥92 mmHg
Adolescents (16–18 years)	Systolic BP ≥142 mmHg	Systolic BP ≥150 mmHg
	Diastolic BP ≥92 mmHg	Diastolic BP ≥98 mmHg

adolescents may be defined as obese (Gortmaker 1987a) on the basis of either body mass index (BMI)—that is, weight in kilograms divided by the square of height in meters—or triceps skinfold thickness. A BMI in excess of the 85th percentile has been used, arbitrarily, to define obesity. This defines "overweight," which may be due to excess fat or a large frame; 10–15% of youth seen in an obesity clinic are overweight and not overfat (Dietz 1993).

The percentage of fat in the diet of youths in the United States continues to be 20% to 25% greater than recommended (i.e., 36–37% of total energy consumed versus the desired 30%). The daily dietary intake of saturated fat exceeds the recommendations by 40% (i.e., 14% of total daily energy intake versus the desired 10%) (Wright 1991).

In a national survey, 60% of all snacks consumed by eighth to tenth graders were "junk foods" (i.e., high-caloric density for nutritional value), despite widespread knowledge among the students concerning healthful eating patterns. The impact of environment, lack of time to prepare food, lack of personal discipine, and little sense of urgency were all factors that were described as impediments to healthy nutrition patterns. Family patterns of activity and inactivity appear to be significant contributing factors (Kinon 1990). Amount of television viewing, which averages 3–4 hours per day among children and adolescents (Strasburger 1992), has also been shown to reduce energy expenditure among children relative to those engaging in other sedentary activities (Klesges 1993). Eating behavior and energy utilization may also be altered among television viewers.

With approximately three out of four obese adolescents becoming obese adults, tracking from youth to adulthood is highly predictive (Gortmaker 1987b). Longitudinal studies relating childhood obesity to adult morbidity and mortality have uniformly demonstrated deleterious effects of childhood obesity later in life, including both diabetes and elevated systolic and diastolic blood pressure (Mossberg 1989). In a study by Must et al. (1992), mortality in males and morbidity in both elderly males and females was greater when obesity was present during adolescence.

Psychosocial Variables And Children's Cardiovascular Health

A number of psychosocial factors have been associated with cardiovascular diseases in adults (see Chapter 11). Relatively little is known, however, regarding the relationship of these psychosocial factors to CHD risk among the young. However, Type A behavior has been positively related to total cholesterol levels and resting blood pressure in children (Siegel 1981; Hunter 1982). In addition, a recent prospective study found that the aggression/competitiveness and hard driving components of Type A behavior were positively related to subsequent total cholesterol levels and resting systolic and diastolic blood pressures in a six-year follow-up of young Finns (Keltikangah-Jarvinen 1990).

In studies involving children and adolescents, interesting but not entirely consistent findings have emerged concerning associations between anger/hostility and physiologic cardiovascular risk factors. Johnson and coworkers (1987a, 1987b) found that both male and female adolescents who reported suppressing their anger had higher resting systolic and/or diastolic blood pressure. On the other hand, Siegel (1984) found that anger expressed outwardly was associated with elevations in blood pressure in adolescent males. Adolescents' self-reports of hostility levels have been associated with their 24-hour ambulatory systolic and diastolic blood pressures (Southard 1986). Overt hostility has been positively correlated with systolic pressure in a group of normotensive children (Musante 1990) and differentiated a group of adolescents classified as having high blood pressure ($\geq$90th percentile for age and gender) versus normal pressure (Siegel 1981).

Many of the adult psychosocial/cardiovascular disease studies that have been conducted used retrospective or cross-sectional designs and involved individuals with various manifestations of cardiovascular diseases. Thus, whether anger, hostility, and components of Type A behavior pattern play significant causal roles in the development of cardiovascular diseases remains to be explored. To accomplish this, prospective studies with healthy children are needed prior to the establishment of end organ damage and overt evidence of cardiovascular diseases.

Metabolic Factors (Insulin/Glucose)

A metabolic syndrome which often includes hyperinsulinemia, dyslipidemia, and hypertension has been associated with CAD in adults (Ferrannini 1991). Hyperinsulinemia is a marker for insulin resistance (Laakso 1993), and it is a primary factor in the pathogenesis of this metabolic syndrome. Moreover, the fasting insulin level is a significant risk factor for CAD independent of the other risk factors (Ducimetiere 1980). Elevated fasting and glucose-stimulated blood glucose levels are not ordinarily part of this syndrome (Segal 1987), suggesting that the elevated insulin levels are sufficient to maintain normal glucose tolerance.

There are a number of metabolic pathways through which hyperinsulinemia may lead to CAD and hypertension (Weber 1991; Rocchini 1993). These include stimulation of vascular smooth muscle hypertrophy, alteration of ion transport, increased sodium retention, and "inappropriate" sympathetic and/or parasympathetic control of cardiovascular reactivity. Bjorntorp (1993) has summarized the metabolic pathways through which obesity, especially fat stored in the central regions of the body, plays a vital role in this syndrome.

There is evidence that this metabolic syndrome begins in childhood (Burns 1989; Kwiterovich 1993). However, central fatness does not seem to develop as a significant predictor of cardiovascular risk factor levels, independent of total body fatness, until the postpubertal years (Kikuchi 1992). Although fasting glucose values are not highly correlated to fatness, the Bogalusa study showed with a large sample of children that the correlation was statistically significant (Berenson 1981). Deschamps (1977), showed that glucose levels were higher in older obese children during a glucose tolerance test.

A close relationship between percent body fat and fasting insulin level was observed in a study of 7- to 11-year-olds, who ranged widely in percent fat (9–58%) Gutin 1994, in preparation). Adding the waist:hip ratio (an index of central fat deposition) to a multiple regression equation to predict insulin level did not increase the explained variance, supporting the notion that central obesity becomes more of a problem as the children mature. Fatness was also significantly related to an atherogenic index comprised of various lipids, lipoproteins, and apoproteins, but not to blood pressure or fasting glucose.

A preliminary and simplified interpretation of these results is to consider fatness as an environmental factor which leads to early hyperinsulinemia and atherogenesis. Although the risk factors are not yet closely related, perhaps as the person matures the hyperinsulinemia and atherogenesis (and eventually blood pressure and glucose) become related through their mutual association with fatness. The especially close relationship between fatness and insulin in these children supports the suggestion by DeFronzo and Ferrannini (1991) that hyperinsulinemia is a primary factor in the pathogenesis of this metabolic syndrome.

In addition to obesity, physical inactivity is another environmental factor which may influence this syndrome. This is suggested by prospective epidemiologic studies which show activity to be protective against the development of non-insulin-dependent diabetes mellitus (NIDDM) (Manson 1991, 1992). This protection is especially pronounced in those who are at increased risk of NIDDM because of obesity (Helmrich 1991)—that is, physical activity has an effect on the development of NIDDM, which goes beyond its effect in preventing obesity. Thus, two strategies which have been found to be effective in improving glucose metabolism and reducing hyperinsulinemia are weight loss (Knip 1993) and physical training (Tremblay 1990).

Intervention Studies

If a study were begun in 1996 among a youthful population in whom multiple "risk" factors were to be manipulated compared with a free-living control group, it would be at least 2046 before enough hard endpoints were observed to demonstrate effectiveness. Such a study is unlikely given the cost and difficulty in maintaining a cohort for that length of time. Therefore, the rationale for the development of interventions for youth is based upon alternative sources of information.

Obvious acute risk due to an extreme high-risk profile clearly warrants immediate physician intervention. The American Heart Association (AHA) Council on Cardiovascular Disease in the Young, Committee on Atherosclerosis and Hypertension, have developed an integrated approach to preventive cardiology services for children. The AHA has recommended an integrated approach to cardiovascular health promotion in childhood. Rather than focusing on individual risk factors, the AHA through its Committee on Atherosclerosis and Hypertension of the Council on Cardiovascular Disease in the Young, has taken a broad-based approach to the prevention of cardiovascular disease in the young. Table 17.3 lists the committee's recommendations for implementing health promotion in the physician's office.

While treatment and education are fitting and proper in the physician's office, the prevalence of children with an extreme risk profile is relatively low. A much greater

Table 17.3. Cardiovascular Health Schedule

Birth	• Family history for early coronary artery disease, hyperlipidemia if(+), introduce risk factors; parental referral. • Start growth chart. • Parental smoking history → smoking cessation referral.
0–2 Years	• Update family history, growth chart. • With introduction of solids, begin teaching re: healthy diet (nutritionally adequate, low in salt, low in saturated fats) • Recommend "healthy" snacks as finger foods. • Change to whole milk from formula or breast feeding at ~1 year of age.
2–6 Years	• Update family history, growth chart → review growth chart[a] with family (concept of weight for height). • Introduce prudent diet (<30% of calories from fat). • Change to low fat milk. • Start BP chart at ~ 3 years of age[b], review the concept of lower salt intake. • Encourage parent/child play that develops coordination. • Lipid determination in children with (+) family history or with parental cholesterol >240 mg/dl (obtain parental lipids if necessary) → if abnormal, initiate nutritional counseling.

6–10 Years	• Update family history, BP and growth charts
	
	• Complete Cardiovascular Health Profile with Child family history, smoking history
	   BP percentile
	   weight for height
	   measure cholesterol in indicated patients
	   level of activity/fitness
	
	• Reinforce prudent diet.
	  Begin active antismoking counseling.
	• Introduce fitness for health → life sport activities for child/family.
	• Discuss role of TV watching in sedentary lifestyle and obesity.

> 10 Years	• Update family history, BP and growth charts annually. • Review prudent diet, risks of smoking, fitness benefits whenever possible. • Consider lipid profile in indicated patients. • Fitness review of personal cardiovascular health status.

BP, blood pressure.

[a]If weight is > 120 percentile of normal for height, diagnosis of obesity should be considered and subject addressed with child and family.

[b]If 3 consecutive interval BP measurements exceed 95th percentile and BP not explained by height or weight, diagnosis of hypertension should be made and appropriate evaluation considered.

proportion of youth are at moderate risk, and these are the children who eventually account for the majority of CAD cases as adults. The task for CAD prevention then becomes one of improving the health behaviors related to CAD in the general youth population. This type of health promotion has typically focused on the modification of health behaviors such as physical activity, dietary intake, and cigarette smoking.

The major assumptions for the rationale behind this type of youth health promotion for CAD prevention have been as follows:

1. A certain proportion of children and adolescents are at moderate to excess physiologic and behavioral risk (US Congress 1991).
2. The development of physiologic risk factors begins early in life and tracks from childhood into adulthood (Clark 1978; Orchard 1983; Freedman 1985; Lauer 1988; Porkka 1991; Klag 1993).
3. The development of physiologic risk factors depends largely upon the initiation of health-compromising behaviors which also tend to track into adulthood (Kelder 1994).
4. Primary prevention can be achieved through the modification of behaviors known to be related to physiologic risk factors, before behavior patterns are more fully established and resistant to change (Kelder 1995).

Much of the early research in school health education has been focused on knowledge-based classroom programs where it was assumed that providing knowledge (i.e., listing the negative consequence of smoking) would be sufficient for improvement in health behaviors. These early studies typically have reported positive changes in student knowledge and attitudes but have generally failed to demonstrate improvement in health behaviors or positive change in physiologic risk (Saylor 1982; Perry 1992a). Neglected in many of the knowledge-based studies was consideration of the multiple factors in the etiology of health behaviors. Food habits, for example, appear to be influenced by the interaction between individuals and their social and physical environment, not simply on knowledge of the healthfulness of foods.

In the development of youth health promotion programs today, great emphasis is placed on the importance of multicomponent interventions that address not only behavioral change at the individual level but also change within the environment to support behavior modifications (Parcel 1988). A social learning model, derived from social learning theory (Bandura 1986), considers multiple factors in the etiology of human behaviors. Behaviors under this model are believed to be a function of certain psychosocial factors, that is:

1. Behavioral factors (social and behavioral skills, direct reinforcement of health eating)
2. Environmental factors (social support, social norms, opportunities or barriers to healthy eating, parental, and peer role models)
3. Personal factors (knowledge, self-efficacy, values, focus of control)

This model suggests that primary prevention can be achieved through the modification of these three categories of psychosocial risk factors, before behavior patterns are established and become resistant to change. Perry and colleagues (1990a, 1990b) have applied this concept on a school-community level to behaviors related to CAD.

Social learing theory can be applied to the multilevel change strategy because of the inclusion of environmental, personal, and behavioral constructs. The ability of social learning theory to address all three domains can contribute to the design of multicomponent health promotion interventions. In the translation from theory to multiple programmatic components, several intervention strategies for youth health promotion are under research and development. These elements include classroom curriculum, school environment, and inclusion of parents, and mass media (Perry 1988b). The salient features of these components are described below.

Curriculum

Most traditional programs are based on the assumption that if students clearly understand the negative consequences of certain health behaviors, they would make the rational decision not to engage in them. During the 1980s, it became increasingly understood that adolescents' decisions to engage in health related behaviors also involves social influences and normative expectations, not just knowledge (Kelder 1992). It has been hypothesized that resistance to the social pressures to engage in health-compromising behaviors such as tobacco use would be greater if the student had been inoculated or developed specific behavioral skills in advance to counter such pressures. Likewise, students with specific health eating, physical activity skills would be expected to be more likely to eat better and exercise more often.

In addition, several studies have demonstrated that importance of peers in an adolescent's life (Perry 1986, 1988a). Clearly, adolescents are affected by the perceived norms and behaviors of their peers. Some youth, particularly high-risk youth, will respond more favorably to their peers encouraging them to avoid tobacco use, increase physical activity, or eat healthier than to teachers or other adults giving them that same message.

School Environment

Changes in the school organization offer a powerful means of modifying the school environment and culture to support health promotion goals. Research has identified organizational factors such as policy and practices, organizational mission, and human resource development as important instruments for institutional change (Parcel 1988). Specifically, it calls for the creation of local coalitions and planning councils to define, coordinate, and implement health promotion programs. These activities are consistent where the school environment reinforce the norms, skills, and behaviors which are emphasized by the health curriculum.

In addition to organizational and policy level changes, schools can enact specific changes to affect health behaviors. For example, school food service has long been recognized as directly affecting the nutritional intake of children through the provision of breakfast and lunch. A relatively simple environmental intervention would require school food service to prepare foods that adhere to the established U.S. Dietary Guidelines for fat, sodium, and complex carbohydrate consumption (Snyder 1992). Likewise, all students could be required to participate in year-round physical education rather than having the option to select it as an elective.

Parent Education

Parents are perhaps the most potent and significant health role models for their children (Nader 1989). They also provide specific opportunities or barriers to adolescent health behaviors such as determining the foods that are purchased, access to physical activity or tobacco in their homes. Research in youth health promotion supports the inclusion of parents through home-based learning (Perry, Luepker, Murray and Hearn 1989). Parents are usually given activities to complete with their child, typically parenting tip sheets, games, or parent interviews. These activities are designed to increase communication between the parent and child and to reinforce at home the messages learned at school.

Mass Media

The mass media in our society have long been recognized as a powerful influence shaping attitudes, beliefs, norms, and perhaps behaviors of young people. (O'Keefe 1987). The media flood the social environment with images of a range of socially acceptable behaviors for adults, adolescents, and children under various circumstances. These images serve to support or discourage the development of many health-related behaviors, and several public health commentators have criticized the media for their role in promoting tobacco use (Aitkin 1990; Shilling 1990; Dietz 1991). In particular, as children grow older and parental influence over social and health behaviors declines, other environmental components such as peers or the mass media become increasingly more influential (Kandel 1987). Unfortunately, the vast majority of funding for the mass media is obtained from those interested in promoting increased consumption of tobacco and unhealthy products without regard to whether their consumers are children.

Researchers, public health agencies, and local community groups have experimented with the various channels of mass media to counterbalance widespread commercial interests. These groups attempt to present a more accurate depiction of the harmful physical and social consequences of unhealthy behaviors. Public service announcements are most commonly used because they are frequently aired free and their production costs are low. For example, radio announcements have recently been emphasizing the short-term social consequences of cigarette smoking—that is, smelling badly or being unappealing to the opposite sex. Usage of radio is recommended as a low-cost alternative to television. Industry sources report that virtually all youths aged 12–17 listen to radio for an average of about 2.5 hours per day (Radio Advertising Bureau 1987).

Summary of Intervention Effectiveness

It is beyond the scope of this chapter to provide a comprehensive review of the effectiveness of each of these components or of those studies utilizing multiple component strategies. It should be noted, however, that several projects are currently underway to determine intervention effectiveness, and not all questions have been adequately answered. Therefore, only a brief mention of reviews by others will be presented here.

In the area of tobacco prevention, studies over the past 15 years that have applied the social learning models have demonstrated a significant impact on smoking onset rates. Several recent comprehensive reviews of the smoking prevention literature, including two metanalyses, have reported positive findings in the proportion of students who began to smoke when compared with an equivalent or randomly assigned control group (Flay 1985; Tobler 1986; Rundell 1988; Botvin 1989). In these studies, the impact on regular (i.e., weekly) smoking ranged from reductions of 43% to 60%, with maintenance of these effects generally one to three years postintervention. Although in most studies intervention effects diminished over time, several longer term studies have been documented by applying a school plus community multiple-component intervention model. The Class of 1989 study from the Minnesota Heart Health Program found a 40% reduction in smoking onset through 12th grade (Perry 1992b). The North Karalia Project, a school plus community health program, also demonstrated favorable long-term impact on youth smoking rates (Puska 1982; Puska 1984; Vartiainen 1990). Finally, Flynn and colleagues (1992) found significant reductions in smoking onset using a school plus mass media intervention.

Simons-Morton et al. (1988), have reviewed physical activity interventions and they report a variety of short-term (immediate posttest) positive outcomes, including improvements in maximum physical working capacity, performance on long-distance runs, and increases in minutes of elevated heart rates during physical education and during the total day. Sallis and colleagues (1992) have reviewed the literature and concluded that physical education programs have produced short-term improvements in physiologic and behavioral outcomes, while classroom-only health education programs have not. Very few long-term evaluations have been conducted in the area of physical activity, although the Class of 1989 study mentioned above has reported favorable intervention effects through 12th grade (Kelder 1993).

Stone and colleagues (1985, 1989) have reviewed the research efforts, sponsored by the National Heart Lung and Blood Institute during the 1980s, that have tested multiple component programs with children and have reported favorable results for knowledge and attitudes, and modest improvements on nutrition, physical activity, and tobacco use, along with several physiologic measures. The results of these studies have led to the Child and Adolescent Trial for Cardiovascular Health (CATCH), a multisite intervention clinical trial that combines many of the intervention components described above (Perry 1990b). CATCH is currently the largest ($n = 96$ schools) trial for elementary school-aged children designed to test the multiple component intervention hypothesis for physiologic, dietary, physical activity, and smoking outcomes.

In summary, over the past decade, researchers and health education specialists have searched for methods to enhance and sustain school-based intervention effects. Within the school, several innovative strategies have been implemented:

1. Delivering multiple years of behavioral interventions
2. Expanding the interventions to include other types of social skills, such as interpersonal skills, critical thinking, or assertiveness

3. Including same age peer leaders as potent sources of social information
4. Altering school policies, such as changing cafeteria menus to provide healthier foods

There has been a growing recognition, however, that instructing students at school in behavioral skills to promote health and to resist the social influences to behave in unhealthy ways may have limited impact if most of their other sources of socialization (i.e., parents, siblings, of the larger community culture) are delivering a contrasting message. Although schools are efficient and appropriate organizations for implementing prevention programs, reinforcement of these programs outside of schools appears to be necessary for sustained change. Therefore strategies to influence the larger culture have included parental involvement, mass media, and community mobilization.

Summary

Data have been presented that demonstrate that the early pathologic lesions of coronary artery disease are present in the young. Risk factors that predispose adults to CAD are identifiable in children and youth. At least at the extreme ends of the distribution curve (i.e., <5th percentile; >95th percentile) the physiologic risk factors track into or toward adulthood. Since many of the risk factors are related to lifestyle behaviors (smoking, diet, physical activity), it seems prudent to attempt to alter these behaviors in childhood before they become virtually immutable adult behaviors. Intervention programs have been initiated, with the most recent generation of interventions stressing social learning theory and the need for school-based programs to incorporate the family and community into the intervention model.

References

Atkin CK. Effects of televised alcohol messages on teenage drinking patterns. J Adolescent Health Care 1990;11:10–24.

Bandura A. Social learning theory. Englewood Cliffs, NJ: Prentice-Hall, 1977.

Bandura A. Social foundations of thought and action. Englewood Cliffs, NJ: Prentice Hall, 1986.

Baranowski T, Tsong Y, Hooks P, et al. Aerobic physical activity among third to sixth grade children. J Dev Behav Pediatr 1987;8:203–6.

Barefoot J, Dahlstrom W, Williams R. Hostility, coronary heart disease incidence and total mortality: a 25-year follow-up study of 255 physicians. Psychosom Med 1983;45:59–63.

Berenson G, Radhakrishnamurthy B, Srinivasan SR, et al. Plasma glucose and insulin levels in relation to cardiovascular risk factors in children from a biracial population: the Bogalusa Heart Study. J Chron Dis 1981;34:379–91.

Berenson G, Srinivasan SR, Webber LS, et al. Cardiovascular risk in early life: the Bogalusa Heart Study. In: Current concepts. Kalamazoo, MI: Upjohn, 1991.

Biglan A, Glasgow RE, Singer G. The need for a science of larger social units: contextual approach. Behav Ther 1990;21:195–215.

Bjorntorp P. Visceral obesity: a "civilization syndrome." Obesity Res 1993;1:206–22.

Blair SN, Kohl HW, Paffenbarger RS, et al. Physical fitness and all cause mortality: a prospective study of healthy men and women. JAMA 1989;262:2395–401.

Blumenthal J, Williams R, Kong Y, et al. Type A behavior and angiographically documented coronary disease. Circulation 1978;58:634–9.

Booth-Kewley S, Friedman HS. Psychological predictors of heart disease: a quantitative review. Psychol Bull 1987;101:343–62.

Botvin GJ, Dusenbury L. Substance abuse prevention and the promotion of competence. Primary Prev Psychopathol 1989;12:146–78.

Burns T, Moll P, Lauer R. The relation between ponderosity and coronary risk factors in children and their relatives. Am J Epidemiol 1989;129:973–87.

CDC. Factors related to cholesterol screening and cholesterol level awareness: United States, 1989. MMWR 1990a;39:633–7.

CDC. Coronary heart disease attributable to sedentary lifestyle: selected states, 1988. MMWR 1990b;39:541–4.

CDC. Participation in school physical education and selected dietary patterns among high school students: United States, 1991. MMWR 1992b;41:597–601, 607.

CDC. Selected tobacco-use behaviors and dietary patterns among high school students: United States, 1991. MMWR 1992a;41:417–21.

Clark WR, Schott HG, Leaverton PE, et al. Tracking of blood lipids and blood pressure in school age children: the muscatine Study 1978. Circulation 1978;58:626–34.

Cresanta JR, Srinivasan SR, Webber LS, Berenson GS. Serum lipid and lipoprotein cholesterol grids for cardiovascular risk screening of children. Am J Dis Child 1984;138:379–87.

Decklebaum RJ. Cholesterol and prevention of atherosclerosis in children. J Jap Pediatr Soc 1992;96:514–15.

Defronzo R, Ferrannini E. Insulin resistance: a multifaceted syndrome responsible for NIDDM, obesity, hypertension, dyslipidemia, and atherosclerotic cardiovascular disease. Diabetes Care 1991;14:173–94.

Dembroski T, MacDougall J, Williams R, et al. Components of type A, hostility and anger-in: relationship to angiographic findings. Psychosom Med 1985;47:219–33.

Dennison BA, Strauss JH, Mellitis ED, Charney E. Childhood physical fitness tests: predictor of adult physical activity levels? Pediatrics 1988;82:324–30.

Deschamps I, Giron BJ, Lestradet H. Blood glucose, insulin, and free fatty acid levels during oral glucose tolerance tests in 158 obese children. Diabetes 1977;26:89–93.

Diamond EL. The role of anger and hostility in essential hypertension and coronary heart disease. Psychol Bull 1982;92:410–33.

Dietz WH, Strasburger VC. Children, adolescents, and television. Curr Prob Pediatr 1991;21: 8–28.

Dietz WH, Robinson TN. Assessment and treatment of childhood obesity. Pediatr in Rev 1993; 14:337–44.

Dimsdale J, Pierce C, Schoenfeld D, et al. Suppressed anger and blood pressure: the effects of race, sex, social class, obesity, and age. Psychosom Med 1986;48:430–6.

Ducimetiere P, Eschwege E, Papoz L, et al. Relationship of plasma insulin levels to the incidence of myocardial infarction and coronary heart disease mortality in a middle-aged population. Diabetologia 1980;19:205–10.

Enos WF Jr, Beyer JC, Holmes RH. Pathogenesis of coronary disease in American soldiers killed in Korea. JAMA 1955;158:912–14.

Ferguson KJ, Yasalis CE, Pohrehn PR, Kirkpatrick MB. Attitudes, knowledge, and beliefs as predictors of exercise intent and behavior in schoolchildren. J School Health 1989;59: 112–15.

Ferrannini E, Natali A. Essential hypertension, metabolic disorders, and insulin resistance. Am Heart J 1991;121:1274–82.

Flay BR. Psychosocial approaches to smoking prevention: a review of the findings. Health Psychol 1985;4:449–88.

Flynn BS, Worden JK, Secker-Walker RH, et al. Prevention of cigarette smoking through mass media intervention and school programs. Am Public Health 1992;82:827–34.

Freedman DS, Shear CL, Srinivasan SR, et al. Tracking of serum lipids and lipoproteins in children over an 8-year period: the Bogalusa Heart Study. Prev Med 1985;14:203–16.

Friedman M, Rosenman R, Straus R. The relationship of behavior pattern A to the state of coronary vasculature: a study of 51 autopsied subjects. Am J Med 1968;44:525–38.

Garcia RE, Moodie DS. Routine cholesterol surveillance in childhood. Pediatrics 1989;84:751–5.

Glueck CJ, Fallat RW, Tsang R, Buncher CR. Hyperlipidemia in progeny of parents with myocardial infarction before age 50. Am Dis Child 1974;127:70–5.

Gortmaker SL, Dietz WH, Sobol AM, Wehler CA. Increasing pediatric obesity in the United States. Am J Dis Child 1987a;141:535–540.

Gortmaker SL, Dietz WH, Sobol AM, et al. Increasing pediatric obesity in the United States. Pediatrics 1987b;I 41:141–535.

Grundy SM. Cholesterol and coronary heart disease, a new era. JAMA 1986;256:2849–58.

Gutin B, Islam S, Manos T, Smith C, et al. Fatness is a major component of the atherogenic and diabetogenic metabolic syndrome in black and white 7–11 years olds. Manuscript in preparation.

Haynes S, Feinleib M, Levine S, et al. The relationship of psychosocial factors to coronary heart disease in the Framingham study: II. Prevalence of coronary heart disease. Am J Epidemiol 1978;107:384–401.

Haynes S, Feinleib M, Kannel W. The relationship of psychosocial factors to coronary heart disease in the Framingham study: III. Eight-year incidence of coronary heart disease. J Psychosom Res 1980;21:323–31.

Helmrich S, Ragland D, Leung R, Paffenbarger R. Physical activity and reduced occurrence of non-insulin-dependent diabetes mellitus. N Engl J Med 1991;325:147–52.

Holman RL. Atherosclerosis: a pediatric nutrition problem? Am J Clin Nutr 1961;9:565–9.

Hunter S, Wolf T, Sklov M, et al. Type A coronary-prone behavior pattern and cardiovascular risk factor variables in children and adolescents: the Bogalusa Heart Study. J Chron Dis 1982;35:613–21.

Johnson E, Spielberger C, Worden T, Jacobs G. Emotional and familial determinants of elevated blood pressure in black and white adolescent males. J Psychosom Res 1987a;31:287–300.

Johnson E, Schork NJ, Spielberger C. Emotional and familial determinants of elevated blood pressure in black and white adolescent females. J Psychosom Res 1987b;31:731–41.

Johnston LD, O'Mally PM, Bachman JG. Illicit drug use, smoking and drinking by America's high school students, college students and young adults. Rockville, MD: NIDA, 1988.

Johnston LD, O'Mally PM, Bachman JG. Drug use among American high school seniors, college students and young adults. Vol 1: High School Seniors. Rockville, MD: NIDA, 1991.

Jung FF, Ingelfinger JR. Hypertension in childhood and adolescence. Pediatr Rev 1993;14:169–79.

Kandel DB, Andrews K. Processes of adolescent socialization of parents and peers. Int J Addict 1987;22:319–42.

Kelder SH, Perry CL, Klepp KI. Community-wide exercise health promotion: outcomes from the Minnesota Heart Health Program and Class of 1989 Study. J School Health 1989; 63:218–23.

Kelder SH, Perry CL, Klepp KI, Lytle LL. Tracking of adolescent health behaviors. *American Journal of Public Health*, 84 (7),1121–6, 1994.

Kelder SH. Youth cardiovascular disease risk and prevention: the Minnesota Heart Health Program and the Class of 1989 Study. Doctoral Dissertation, University of Minnesota, 1992.

Kelder SH, Perry CL, Trenkner LL, Klepp KI. Community wide youth nutrition education: long-term outcomes from the Minnesota Heart Health Program and the Class of 1989 Study. Health Education Research Theory and Practice 1995;10(2):119–31.

Keltikangas-Jarvinen L, Raikkonen K. Type A factors as predictors of somatic risk factors of coronary heart disease in young Finns: a six-year follow-up study. J Psychosom Res 1990;341:89–97.

Kikuchi D, Srinivasan S, Harsha D, et al. Relation of serum lipoprotein and apolipoproteins to obesity in children: the Bogalusa Heart Study. Prev Med 1992;21:177–90.

Kimm SYS, Gergen PJ, Malloy M, et al. Dietary patterns of U.S. children: implications for disease prevention. J Prev Med 1990;19:432–42.

Klag MJ, Ford DE, Mead LA, et al. Serum cholesterol in young men and subsequent cardiovascular disease. N Engl J Med 1993;328:313–18.

Klepp K, Halper A, Perry CL. The efficacy of peer leaders in drug abuse prevention. J School Health 1986;56:407–11.

Klesges RC, Shelton MS, Klesges LM. Effects of television on metabolic rate: potential implications for childhood obesity. Pediatrics 1993;91:281–6.

Knip M, Nuutinen O. Long-term effects of weight reduction on serum lipids and plasma insulin in obese children. Am J Clin Nutr 1993;57:490–3.

Kwiterovich PO Jr. Pediatric implications of heterozygous familial hypercholesterolemia screening and dietary treatment. Arteriosclerosis 1989;9(Suppl I):I111–20.

Kwiterovich P, Coresh J, Bachorik P. Prevalence of hyperapobetalipoproteinemia and other lipoprotein phenotypes in men (aged <50 years) and women (<60 yrs) with coronary artery disease. Am J Cardiol 1993;71:631–9.

Laakso M. How good a marker is insulin level for insulin resistance? Am J Epidemiol 1993; 137:959–65.

Lauer RM, Connor WE, Leaverton PE, et al. Coronary heart disease risk factors in school children: the Muscatine Study. J Pediatr 1975;86:697–706.

Lauer RM, Skers RL, Massery J, et al. Evaluation of cigarette smoking among adolescents: the Muscatine Study. Prev Med 1982;11:417–28.

Lauer RM, Lee J, Clarke WR. Factors affecting the relationship between childhood and adult cholesterol levels: the Muscatine Study. Pediatrics 1988;82:309–18.

Lauer RM, Clarke WR. Childhood risk factors for high adult blood pressure: the Muscatine Study. Pediatrics 1989;84:633–41.

Londe S. Blood pressure in children as determined under office conditions. Clin Pediatr 1966; 5:71–78, 400–3.

Londe S. Goldring D. High blood pressure in children: problem and guidelines for evaluation and treatment. Am J. Cardiol 1976;37:650–7.

Manson J, Rimm E, Stampfer M, et al. Physical activity and incidence of non-insulin-independent diabetes mellitus in women. Lancet 1991;338:774–8.

Manson J, Nathan D, Krolewski A, et al. A prospective study of exercise and incidence of diabetes among US male physicians. JAMA 1992;268:63–7.

Matthews K. Haynes S. Type A behavior pattern and coronary heart disease risk: update and critical evaluation. Am J Epidemiol 1986;123:923–60.

McAlister A. Population behavior change: a theory-based approach. Public Health Policy 1991; 12:345–61.

McGilll HC Jr, et al. Natural history of coronary atherosclerosis. Am J Pathol 1962;40:37–49.

McNamara JJ, Molot MA, Stremple JF, Cutting RT. Coronary artery disease in combat casualties in Vietnam. JAMA 1971;216:1185–7.

Moss AJ, Adams FH. Index of indirect estimation of diastolic blood pressure: muffling versus complete cessation of vascular sounds. Am J Dis Child 1963;106:364–7.

Mossberg, HO. 40 year follow-up of overweight children. Lancet 1989;2:491–3.

Multiple Risk Factor Intervention Trial Research Group. Mortality rates after 10.5 years for participants in the multiple risk factor intervention trial: findings related to a prior hypothesis of the trial. JAMA 1990;263:1795–801.

Murray DM, Davis-Hearn M, Goldman AE, et al. Four- and five-year follow-up results from four seventh-grade smoking prevention strategies. J Behav Med 1988;11:395–405.

Murray DM, Pirie P, Luepker RV, Pallonen U. Five- and six-year follow-up results from four seventh-grade smoking prevention strategies. J Behav. Med 1989;12:207–18.

Musante L, MacDougall JM, Dembroski TM, Costa PT. Potential for hostility and the dimensions of anger. Health Psychol 1989.

Must A, Jaques PF, Dallal GE, et al. Long-term morbidity and mortality of overweight adolescents: a follow-up of the Harvard growth study of 1922–1935. N Engl J Med 1992; 327:1350–5.

Nader PR, Sallis JF, Patterson TL, et al. A family approach to cardiovascular risk reduction: results from the San Diego Family Heart Project. Health Educ Q 1989;16:229–44.

Namboodiri K, Green P, Martin J, Glueck CJ. Familial aggregation of lipids and lipoproteins: the collaborative family study. JAMA 1983;250:1860–8.

National Cholesterol Education Program: report of the expert panel on blood cholesterol levels in children and adolescents. Pediatrics 1992;89(Suppl 3)Part 2:525–84.

Newman WP III, Freedman DS, Voors AW, et al. Relation of serum lipoprotein levels and systolic blood pressure to early atherosclerosis: the Bogalusa heart study. N Engl J Med 1986;314:138–44.

O'Keefe GJ, Reid-Nash K. Socializing function. In: Berger CR, Chafee SH, eds. Handbook of communication, 1987. Newbury Park, CA: Sage Publications, 1987:419–45.

Orchard TJ, Donahue RP, Kuller LH, et al. Cholesterol screening in childhood: does it predict adult hypercholesterolemia?: the Beaver County experience. J Pediatr 1983;103:687–91.

Paffenbarger RS Jr., Hyde RT, Wing AL, Steinmetz CH. A natural history of athletiscism and cardiovascular health. JAMA 1984;252:491–5.

Parcel GS, Simons-Morton BG, Kilbe LJ. Health promotion: integrating organizational change and student learning strategies. Health Educ Q 1988;15:435–50.

Parcel GS, Simons-Morton B, O'Hara NM, et al. School promotion of healthful diet and physical activity: impact on learning outcomes and self-reported behavior. Health Educ Q 1989;181–99.

PDAY Research Group. Relationship of atherosclerosis in young men to serum lipoprotein cholesterol concentration and smoking: a preliminary report from the pathobiological determinants of atherosclerosis in youth (PDAY) research group. JAMA 1990;264: 3018–24.

Pentz MA, MacKinnon DP, Flay BR, Hansen WB, Johnson CA, Dwyer JH. Primary prevention of chronic diseases in adolescence: Effects of the midwestern prevention project on tobacco use. Am J Epidemiol 1989;130:713–24.

Perry CL, Klepp KI, Halper A, et al. A process evaluation study of peer leader in health education. J School Health 1986;15:62–7.

Perry CL, Klepp KI, Schultz JM. Primary prevention of cardiovascular disease: community-wide strategies for youth. J Consult Clin Psychol 1988a;56:358–64.

Perry CL, Grant M. Comparing peer-led to teacher-led youth alcohol education in four countries. Alcohol Health Res World 19888b;12:322–6.

Perry CL, Klepp KI, Sillers C. Community-wide strategies for cardiovascular health: the Minnesota Heart Health Program Youth Program: Health Ed Res: Theory Prac 1989;4:87–101.

Perry CL, Leupker RV, Murray DM, Hearn MD. Parent involvement with children's health promotion: One-year follow-up of the Minnesota Home Team. *Health Education Quarterly* 1989;16(2):1156–60.

Perry CL, Baranowski T, Parcel G. How individuals, environments, and health behavior interact: social learning theory. In: Glantz K, Lewis FM, Rimer B, eds. Health behavior and health education. San Francisco, CA: Jossey-Bass, 1990a:161–86.

Perry CL, Stone EJ, Parcel GS, Ellison RC, et al. School based cardiovascular health promotion: the child and adolescent trial for cardiovascular health (CATCH). J School Health 1990b; 60:406–13.

Perry CL, Kelder SH. Primary prevention of adolescent substance abuse. In: Nathan PE, Langenbucher JW, McGrady BS, Frankenstein W, eds. Annual review of addictions; research and treatment, Vol. 2. New York: Permagon Press, 1992a.

Perry CL, Kelder SH, Murray DM, Klepp KI. Community-wide smoking prevention: long-term outcomes of the Minnesota Heart Health Program. Am J Public Health 1992;82:1210–16.

Pirie PL, Murry DM, Luepker RV. Smoking prevalence in a cohort of adolescents including absentees, dropouts, and transfers. Am J Public Health 1988;78:176–8.

Porkka KV, Viikari JSA, Akerblom KH. Tracking of serum HDL-cholesterol and other lipids in children and adolescents: the Cardiovascular Risk in Young Finns Study. Prev Med 1991;20:813–824.

Pugliese MJ, Wayman-Daum M, Moses N. Lifshitz F. Parental health beliefs as a cause of non-organic failure to thrive. Pediatrics 1987;80:175–82.

Puska P. Community based prevention of cardiovascular disease: the North Karalia Project. In: Matarazzo JD, Weiss SM, Herd JA, Miller NE, Weiss SM, eds. Behavioral health: a handbook for healthy enhancement and disease prevention. Silver Spring, MD: Wiley, 1984: 1140–8.

Puska P. Vartiainen E, Pallonen U, et al. The North Karalia Youth Project: evaluation of two years of intervention on health behavior and cardiovascular disease risk factors among 15 to 15 year old children. Prev Med 1982;11:550–70.

Radio Advertising Bureau, Radio facts, 27th ed. New York: Author, 1987.

Reisman M. Atherosclerosis and pediatrics. J Pediatr 1965;66:1–7.

Rogers LQ, Fincher RME, Strong WB. Primary prevention of coronary artery disease through a family oriented cardiac risk factor clinic. South Med J 1990;83;1270–2.

Rocchini A. Adolescent obesity and hypertension. Pediat Clin North Am 1990;401:81–92.

Rundell TG, Bruvold WH. A meta-analysis of school-based smoking and alcohol use prevention programs. Health Educ Q 1988;15:317–34.

Sallis JF, Simons-Morton BG, Stone EJ, et al. Determinants of physical activity and interventions in youth. Med Sci Sports Exerc 1992;24(Suppl):S248–57.

Saltykow S. Jugenliche und beginnende Atherosklerose. Hertz 1915;45:1057–89.

Saylor KE, Coates TJ, Killen J, Slinkard LA. Nutrition education research: Feast or famine? In

Coates TJ, Peterson AC, Perry CL, eds. San Francisco, CA: Academic Press, 1982; 355–81.

Schilling RF, McAlister AL. Preventing drug use in adolescents through media interventions. J Consul Clin Psychol 1990;58:416–24.

Schultz JM. Smoking attributable mortality and years of potential life lost. Morbidity and Mortality Weekly Report: United States, 1988. 1991;40:62–71.

Segal K, Dunaif A, Gutin B, et al. Body composition, not body weight is related to cardiovascular disease risk factors and sex hormone levels in men. J Clin Invest 1987a;80: 1050–5.

Shekelle R, Gale M, Ostfeld A, Paul O. Hostility, risk of coronary disease and mortality. Psychosom Med 1983;45:109–14.

Siegel J, Leitch C. Behavioral factors and blood pressure in adolescence: the Tacoma Study. Am J. Epidemioll 1981;113:171–81.

Siegel J. Anger and cardiovascular risk in adolescents. Health Psychol 1984;3:293–313.

Simons-Morton BG, Parcel GS, O'Hara NM, et al. Health-related physical fitness in childhood: status and recommendations. Annu Rev Public Health 1988;9:403–25.

Snyder MP, Story M. Trenkner LL. Reducing fat and sodium in school lunch programs: the "Lunchpower!" intervention study. J Am Diet Assoc 1992;92:1087–91.

Southard D, Coates T, Kolodner K, et al. Relationship between mood and blood pressure in the natural environment: an adolescent population. Health Psychol 1986;5:469–80.

Stone EJ. School-based health research funded by the National Heart, Lung and Blood Institute. J School Health 1985;55:168–74.

Stone EJ, Perry CL, Luepker RV. Synthesis of cardiovascular behavioral research for youth health promotion. Health Educ Q 1989;16:155–69.

Story HC. Evolution and progression of atherosclerotic lesions in coronary arteries of children and young adults. Arteriosclerosis 1989;9(Suppl l):119–32.

Strasburger VC. Children, adolescents and television. Pediatr Rev 1992;13:144–51.

Strong JP, McGill HC, Jr. The natural history of atherosclerosis. Am J Pathol 1962;40:37–49.

Strong WB, Dennison BA. Pediatric preventive cardiology, atherosclerosis and coronary heart disease. Pediatr Rev 1988;303–14.

Strong WB, Deckelbaum RJ, Gidding SS, et al. Integrated cardiovascular health promotion in childhood. Circulation 1992;85:1638–50.

Task Force on Blood Pressure Control in Children. Report of the second task force on blood pressure control in children. Pediatrics 1987;79:1–25.

Tell GS, Vellar OD. Physical fitness, physical activity and cardiovascular disease risk factors in adolescents: the Oslo Youth Study. Prev Med 1988;17:12–24.

Tobler N. Meta-analysis of 143 adolescent drug prevention programs: quantitative outcome results of program participants compared to a control or comparison group. J Drug Issues 1988;16:537–67.

Treiber FA, Musante L, Riley W, et al. The relationship between hostility and blood pressure in children. Behav Med 1989;15:173–8.

Tremblay A, Nadeau A, Despres J-P, et al. Long-term exercise training with constant energy intake. 2: Effect on glucose metabolism and resting energy expenditure. Int J Obesity 1990;14:75–84.

U.S. Congress, Office of Technology Assessment. Adolescent heath, Vol II: background and the effectiveness of selected prevention and treatment services. OTA-H-466. Washington DC: U.S. Government Printing Office, 1991.

Weber M, Smith D, Neutel J, Cheung D. Applications of ambulatory blood pressure monitoring in clinical practice. Clin Chem 1991;3710B:1880–4.

Weight HS, Guthrie HS, Wang MQ, Bernardo V. The 1987–88 nationwide food consumption survey: an update on the nutrient intake of respondents. Nutr Today 1991;May/June: 221–7.

Vartiainen E, Pallonen U, McAlister A, et al. Four year follow-up results of the smoking prevention program in the North Karalia Youth Project. Prev Med 1986;15:692–8.

Vartiainen E, Pallonen U, McAlister A, Puska P. Eight year follow-up results of an adolescent smoking prevention program: the North Karalia Yough Project. Am J Public Health 1990;80:78–9.

V

SECONDARY PREVENTION

18

Strategies for Secondary Prevention

Peter H. Stone and Frank M. Sacks

The last two decades have witnessed dramatic changes in the care of patients with coronary heart disease (CHD). Coronary care units, which developed in the late 1960s, proved to be effective in identifying and treating arrhythmias that complicate acute myocardial infarction (MI), but mortality due to pump failure remained high (Goldman 1982). In the 1980s and early 1990s, early reperfusion strategies using thrombolytic therapy or primary percutaneous transluminal coronary angioplasty (PTCA) to limit infarct size and preserve left ventricular function, further improved survival after MI (Anderson 1993). A simultaneous advance in cardiology has been the appreciation that various post-MI treatment strategies could be implemented routinely to reduce the incidence of recurrent MI, congestive heart failure, and cardiac death following an index MI (i.e., ''secondary'' prevention).

The time course of mortality and cardiac complications following acute MI is characterized by a very high risk period in the first month or so after the index event, followed by a high-risk period for the next 6 months, and then a subsequent period of low and constant risk (Figure 18.1). Prompt initiation of therapies to prevent cardiac complications after MI is therefore essential to provide meaningful protection; most studies of secondary prevention begin within 1 to 3 weeks of MI and maintain therapy for at least one year. This chapter focuses on randomized, placebo-controlled, and blinded studies that use this strategy of secondary prevention. In some studies the investigational therapy begins in the first few hours following MI and continues for the next few weeks or months. The observed effect thus may be due to a reduction in the initial infarct size and not to the effects of more sustained chronic therapy. This therapeutic strategy addresses both reduction of acute infarct size and secondary prevention, so such studies will not be reviewed in this chapter.

Our purpose is to review the underlying pathophysiologic processes responsible for complications following acute MI: the atherosclerotic plaque and the mechanisms of plaque rupture and thrombus formation, ventricular remodeling after MI, and arrhythmogenesis; and then to review the specific agents, interventions, and lifestyle modifications to achieve secondary prevention, that have been studied. Table 18.1 lists

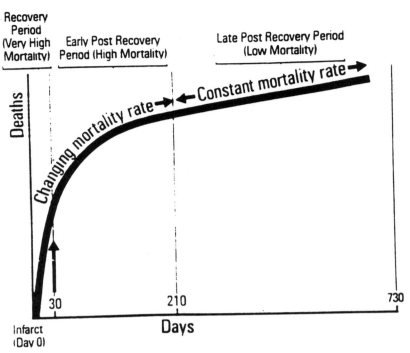

Fig. 18.1. Time course of mortality after an acute myocardial infarction. [From Sherry S. (1980), with permission.]

the potential mechanisms of secondary prevention and the agents and interventions that are included.

Pathophysiologic Processes Responsible for Morbidity and Mortality Following Acute Myocardial Infarction

Nature and Progression of the Atherosclerotic Plaque

The coronary atherosclerotic plaque often starts to develop in the second and third decades of age among individuals in the Western industrialized world. It begins as a fatty streak, which then progresses to smooth muscle proliferation, attraction of macrophages that become laden with lipid (foam cells), formation of an extracellular pool made up of extravasated cholesterol esters and cellular debris (gruel), and formation of an often thin fibrous cap that separates the thrombogenic lipid pool from the circulating bloodstream (Figure 18.2) (Constantinides 1984). Although the luminal encroachment by the atherosclerotic plaque may be due to progressive increases in cellular activity and connective tissue, such growth is often extremely slow. The "growth" or enlargement of an atherosclerotic plaque that brings the patient to clinical attention is usually a stepwise progression from repeated plaque rupture and thrombus

Table 18.1. Potential Mechanisms of Secondary Prevention

I. Prevention of plaque rupture
   A. Reduction of mechanical forces
      1. Beta-blockers
   B. Stabilization of plaque (?)
      1. Lipid-lowering therapy
      2. ACE inhibitors
      3. Antioxidants
      4. Estrogen-replacement therapy
   C. Prevention of vasoconstriction
      1. Ca^{2+} blockers
      2. Estrogen replacement therapy
II. Prevention of superimposed thrombus formation
   A. Aspirin
   B. Coumadin
III. Prevention of left ventricular remodeling and CHF
   A. ACE inhibitors
   B. Hydralazine plus isosorbide dinitrate
IV. Prevention of arrhythmias
   A. Type 1C antiarrhythmic drugs
   B. Beta-blockers
   C. Amiodarone
V. Reduction of myocardial oxygen demands
   A. Beta-blockers
   B. Ca^{2+}-blockers
   C. ACE inhibitors
   D. Cardiac rehabilitation

formation (Falk 1983; Davies 1985; Davies 1990; Fuster 1992). Indeed, the pathophysiologic common denominator that is likely responsible for most acute ischemic coronary syndromes (unstable angina, acute MI, sudden death) is plaque rupture followed by superimposed thrombosis, which may occlude the coronary lumen either partially or completely, and either transiently or permanently (Figure 18.3) (Fuster 1983; Davies 1985).

Plaque rupture occurs when the forces acting on it exceed its tensile strength (MacIsaac 1993). The forces affecting the plaque include mechanical forces, hydrodynamic influences, biochemical stimuli, and physical characteristics of the plaque constituents, and these forces are interwoven in a complex manner that is incompletely understood. Richardson and associates (1989) used computer modeling to show that circumferential stress in an artery is greatest at the intima and that the stresses are maximal at the lateral edge of the plaque cap overlying an extracellular lipid pool. This corresponds to the usual site of plaque rupture (Constantinides 1984). The likelihood of plaque rupture is related both to the magnitude of stresses imposed on the plaque and to the physical properties of the plaque itself. Lee et al. (1991) demonstrated that the plaque becomes stiffer, and perhaps more likely to rupture, as the frequency of applied stress (i.e., heart rate) increases. Beta-blockers may be effective in secondary (and perhaps primary) prevention in part from the reduction in heart rate and the preservation of plaque strength, as well as from the reduction in blood pressure

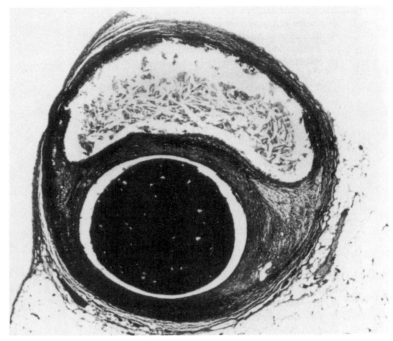

Fig. 18.2. Photomicrograph of a histologic transverse section of an eccentric stenosis. The lumen contains a mass of gelatin/barium used in postmortem angiography. The lipid pool is an apparently open space (*upper portion*) within the intima because cholesterol is dissolved out in the solvents used to prepare histologic slides. The lipid pool does not contain internal collagenous struts. The pool is separated from the lumen by the plaque cap. Elastic/hematoxylin stain, ×20. [From Davies and Thomas (1985), with permission.]

and the force of myocardial contraction factors, which will decrease the mechanical stresses imposed on the plaque. Lipid-lowering therapy may be protective by reducing the size of the extracellular lipid pool (Figure 18.4), thereby reducing the magnitude of circumferential stresses imposed on the plaque cap, and also by reducing the local erosive inflammatory processes affecting the plaque cap. Calcium blockers might be protective by preventing vasospasm that could suddenly increase wall stresses. Cellular infiltrates may also weaken the cap by the effects of macrophage proteases (MacIsaac 1993), and agents that reduce this inflammation may stabilize the plaque. Angiotensin-converting enzyme (ACE) inhibitors may provide a unique vascular benefit by blocking the angiotensin-II effects in the vascular wall and myocardium, and they may prevent the proliferative response to vascular injury (Yusuf 1992).

Once the plaque ruptures, the intensely thrombogenic material within the plaque is exposed to the bloodstream, which leads to rapid thrombosis (Figure 18.5). The amount of thrombus formed, and the likelihood of a clinical event, is dependent on the depth of the rupture and the type and magnitude of the vascular injury (Fuster 1992). The amount of thrombus formed may also be dependent on the degree of

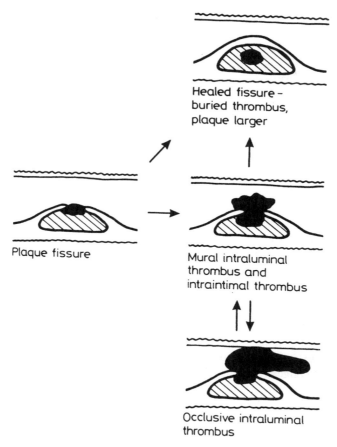

Healed fissure –
buried thrombus,
plaque larger

Plaque fissure

Mural intraluminal
thrombus and
intraintimal thrombus

Occlusive intraluminal
thrombus

Fig. 18.3. "Unstable" coronary plaque and thrombus which may stabilize and undergo reendothelialization or may undergo further thrombosis and totally occlude the artery. [From Davies and Thomas (1985), with permission.]

platelet aggregability and the relative strength of endogenous thrombotic and thrombolytic forces present at the time of plaque rupture (Muller 1989). Platelet-active agents and anticoagulation therapy may reduce the likelihood of forming an occlusive thrombus on a ruptured plaque even if the forces responsible for plaque rupture itself are unaffected (Ridker 1990).

Left Ventricular Remodeling Following Acute MI

The loss of myocardial function following MI initiates a process of ventricular remodeling characterized by progressive enlargement of the left ventricle and a geometric change from an ellipsoid to a more spherical chamber shape, which is associated with progressive increases in wall stress. A vicious cycle is created whereby

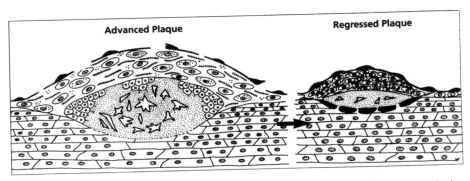

Fig. 18.4. Changes reported to occur during regression of advanced atheromatous lesions in rhesus monkeys and swine models. [From Wissler (1984), with permission.]

an initial compensatory mechanism of ventricular enlargement leads to increased wall stresses, which in turn lead to further increases in ventricular size, which leads to further increases in wall stresses, and so on, culminating in manifestations of congestive heart failure and death. This progressive enlargement begins shortly after MI and continues for the next few months and years. (Figure 18.6) (Gaudron 1993) Those patients most at jeopardy for developing progressive enlargement are those who have experienced an MI that is large in size and anterior in location (Gaudron 1993).

Interventions that reduce intraventricular wall stresses may interrupt the vicious cycle and lead to stabilization of left ventricular size and thus avoid the ultimate complications of congestive heart failure. A number of studies have demonstrated that among patients with long-standing symptomatic congestive heart failure either not related to prior MI (e.g., idiopathic dilated cardiomyopathy) or related to a distant MI, those treated with either enalapril of a combination regimen of hydralazine and iso-

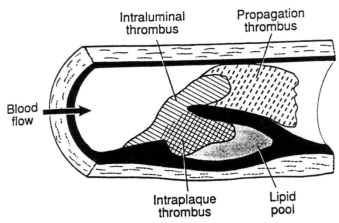

Fig. 18.5. Schematic representation of thrombus forming after rupture of coronary artery plaque. [From Davies (1990), with permission.]

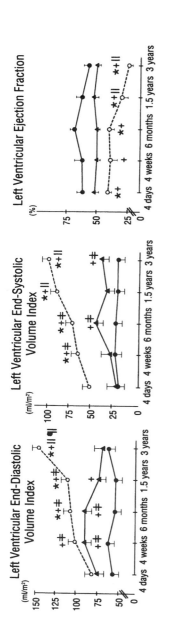

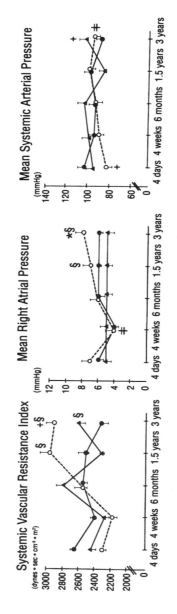

Fig. 18.6. Line graphs indicate course of left ventricular end-diastolic and end-systolic volume indexes, ejection fraction, systemic vascular resistance index, and mean right atrial and systemic arterial pressures in patients with progressive (○), limited (▲), and no (●) left ventricular dilatation from 4 days until 3 years after myocardial infarction. Values are given as mean ±SEM; $p < .05$, * vs limited dilatation; + vs no dilatation; vs 4 days, vs 4 weeks; vs 4 days, 4 weeks, and 6 months; vs 1.5 years. [From Gaudron et al. (1993), with permission.]

469

sorbide dinitrate experience reduced mortality and manifestations of congestive heart failure compared to those receiving conventional therapy plus placebo (CONSENSUS 1987). Since the initiating process of ventricular remodeling is clearly temporally identifiable in those patients with acute MI, the hypothesis of this form of secondary prevention is that early treatment with pre- and afterload reducing agents will limit the impact of the initial loss of myocardial function, and the subsequent ventricular enlargement and remodeling will also be reduced (Pfeffer 1990).

Ventricular Arrhythmias

The arrhythmogenic substrate in a chronic completed MI is generally stable and the predominant mechanism responsible for ventricular tachyarrhythmias is reentry originating in areas of slow conduction in the border zone between normal and infarcted tissue (Weiss 1991). The border zone region is characterized histologically by bundles of viable myocardium interspersed with bands of collagen and connective tissue. Ventricular arrhythmias are particularly prone to occur, and are most ominous, in patients who have had a large infarction (Weiss 1991) and a significantly reduced ejection fraction (Bigger 1986). Slow conduction in the infarct scar provides the substrate for ventricular tachycardia later after MI (Weiss 1991), and the focus of intervention agents has been those drugs that delay conduction (e.g., class IC agents) or prolong refractoriness (e.g., class III agents like amiodarone).

There is a direct and significant relationship between the frequency and complexity of ventricular ectopic activity identified during a predischarge Holter monitor and the risk of death in the subsequent year (Multicenter Postinfarction Research Group [MPRG] 1983). This risk becomes amplified as the degree of left ventricular dysfunction becomes worse (Bigger 1986). Approximately 50% of MI-related deaths are sudden—usually due to ventricular arrhythmias; although many of these sudden deaths occur early after MI, approximately 35 to 50% occur much later (MPRG 1983).

It is unknown whether ventricular ectopic activity is an actual precursor of lethal ventricular arrhythmias or whether it is simply a marker for severe underlying myocardial dysfunction and a proclivity for ventricular arrhythmias. The hypothesis that suppression of ventricular premature beats (VPB) is associated with a reduction in post-MI mortality has led to a number of randomized clinical trials of secondary prevention. Although antiarrhythmic agents reduce ventricular ectopy, they may also be proarrhythmic or may decrease left ventricular function; the net clinical effect will therefore depend on the relative magnitude of the beneficial and detrimental effects in each patient.

Agents Used in Secondary Prevention and Their Proposed Mechanisms of Action

Beta-Adrenergic Blocking Agents

The beta-adrenergic blocking agents exert a number of effects that could be useful in secondary prevention. First, they reduce heart rate, blood pressure, and the force of contractility, and thereby reduce myocardial oxygen demands. These effects may lead to a reduction in infarct size when administered early (Yusuf 1983) or in patients who had been taking a beta-blocker chronically at the time of their infarction (Nidorf 1990). Second, these drugs exert an antiarrhythmic effect, as evidenced by an increase in the threshold for ventricular fibrillation in animals and a reduction in complex ventricular arrhythmias in man (Rossi 1983; Yusuf 1983; Morganroth 1985). Finally, such agents may prevent plaque rupture by reducing the mechanical stresses imposed on the plaque.

A large number of randomized, double-blind, and placebo-controlled trials have shown definitively that routine use of a beta-blocker following an acute MI reduces cardiac morbidity and mortality (Yusuf 1985, 1988; Lau 1992). The most recent up-dated metanalysis, including 17 studies and 20,138 patients, indicated that treatment with a beta-blocker was associated with a cumulative odds ratio of mortality of 0.81 (95% CI: 0.73–0.89, $p < .001$) (Lau 1992). The risk of death was reduced from 10.1% to 8%; that is, the total number of deaths was reduced by 20% (Table 18.2; Figure 18.7) (Yusuf 1985).

A number of studies have classified the mechanism of death into "sudden" and "nonsudden," based on the duration of time from the onset of symptoms to actual death. Sudden death is variably defined as "instantaneous" to "within 2 hours of symptoms" and is presumably due to arrhythmias or cardiac rupture, while nonsudden deaths are those occurring later after the onset of symptoms, and are presumably due

Table 18.2. Total Mortality from Long-Term Trials with Treatments Starting Late, and Mortality from Day 8 Onward in Long-Term Trials That Began Early and Continued After Discharge

Late-Entry Trials (years)	Basic Data from Trials: Deaths/No. Randomized (%)			
	Allocated Beta-Blocker		Allocated Control	
Reynolds (1)	3/38	(8)	3/39	(8)
Wilhelmsson (2)	7/114	(6)	14/116	(12)
Ahlmark (2)	5/69	(7)	11/93	(12)
Multicentre Int. personal communication (1–3)	102/1,533	(7)	127/1,520	(8)
Baber (3–9 months)	28/355	(8)	27/365	(7)
Rehnqvist personal communication (1)	4/59	(7)	6/52	(12)
Norwegian Multicentre (1–3)	98/945	(10)	152/939	(16)
Tavior (mean 4y)	60/632	(9)	48/471	(10)
Hansteen° (1)	25/278	(9)	37/282	(13)
BHAT (median 2)	138/1,916	(7)	188/1,921	(10)
Julian (1)	64/873	(7)	52/583	(9)
Australian/Swedish (2)	45/263	(17)	47/266	(18)
Manger Cats (1)	9/291	(3)	16/293	(5)
EIS (1)	57/858	(7)	45/883	(5)
Rehnqvist (3)	25/154	(16)	31/147	(21)
Subtotal: Late-entry trials	670/8,378	(8)	804/7,970	(10)

Source: Modified from Yusuf et al. (1985), with permission. See original article for citation of specific trials.

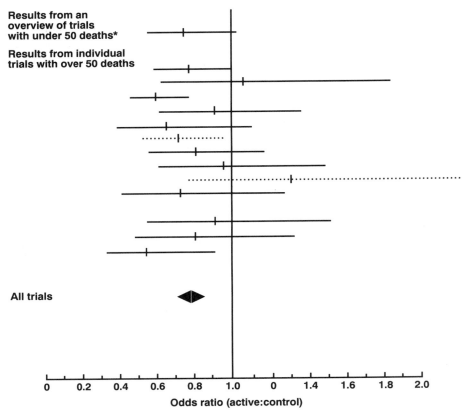

Fig. 18.7. Mortality by allocated treatment in all the randomized trials of long-term beta-blockade following myocardial infarction: odds ratios (active:control), together with approximately 95% or 99% confidence ranges. —, 95% confidence range for trials that ran to scheduled finish. – –, 99% confidence range for trials stopped early due to good/bad trend, ◀▶, 95% confidence range from an overview of all the trials. See original article for citation of specific trials. [From Yusuf et al. (1985), with permission.]

to nonarrhythmic causes, such as reinfarction, and may include a few noncardiac deaths. Tabulation of the results from the available studies indicates a highly significant reduction of approximately 30% in the incidence of sudden death and a nonsignificant reduction of only about 12% in the incidence of nonsudden death (Table 18.3; Figure 18.8) (Yusuf 1985). The fact that beta-blockers were particularly effective in reducing sudden death and in reducing mortality among patients with complex ventricular ectopy at baseline (Friedman 1984) suggests that beta-blockers exert their beneficial effect primarily by reducing the frequency and severity of arrhythmias (Byington 1990).

It is striking that the mortality benefits of the beta-blockers extend to most members of this class of agents (Yusuf 1985). There does not seem to be a significant difference between agents with or without cardioselectivity (i.e., selective $beta_1$-block-

Table 18.3. Sudden Death and Nonsudden Death in Long-term Beta Blocker Trials[a]

Trial	Basic Data from Trials (sudden + other deaths/no. randomized)		Statistical Calculations for Sudden Deaths		Statistical Calculations for Other Deaths	
	Allocated Beta-Blocker	Allocated Control	Observed Minus Expected (O − E)	Variance of O − E	Observed Minus Expected (O − E)	Variance of O − E
Reynolds	3 + 0/39	3 + 0/39	0.0	1.4	0.0	0.0
Wilhelmsson	3 + 4/114	11 + 3/116	−3.9	3.3	+0.5	1.7
Ahlmark	1 + 4/69	9 + 2/93	3.3	2.3	+1.4	1.4
Multicentre Int.	29 + 73/1,533	51 + 76/1,520	−11.2	19.5	−1.8	35.4
Baber	10 + 18/355	6 + 21/365	2.1	3.9	−1.2	9.2
Rehnqvist	3 + 1/59	4 + 2/52	−0.7	1.6	−0.6	0.7
Norwegian Multicentre	66 + 32/945	110 + 42/939	−22.3	39.9	−5.1	17.8
Taylor	33 + 27/632	25 + 23/471	−0.2	13.5	−1.6	11.7
Hansteen	11 + 14/278	23 + 14/282	−5.9	8.0	+0.1	6.7
BHAT	64 + 74/1,916	89 + 99/1,921	−12.4	36.7	−12.4	41.3
Julian	25 + 39/873	14 + 38/583	+1.6	9.1	−7.2	17.5
Australian/Swedish	Not available					
Manger Cats	7 + 2/290	11 + 5/293	−2.0	4.4	−1.5	1.7
EIS	25 + 32/858	24 + 21/883	+0.9	11.9	+5.9	12.9
Rehnqvist	9 + 16/154	21 + 10/147	−6.3	6.8	+2.7	6.0
Ciba-Geigy	2400 patients; not yet available					
Subtotals (excl. 5.5 and 5.13)	289 + 336/8,115	401 + 356/7,704	−63.6	162.3	−20.8	164.0
Percentage and pooled odds ratios ± SE	(3.6 + 4.1%)	(5.2 + 4.6%)	(0.68 ± 0.05)		(0.88 ± 0.07)	

Source: From Yusuf, et al. (1985), with permission. See original article for citation of specific trials.

[a]"Sudden death is defined as death in the shortest period that was reported separately by each author. This varies from "under 1 hour" to "under 24 hours," and unfortunately there is an obvious possibility of investigator-instigated bias in the selection of which interval to report.

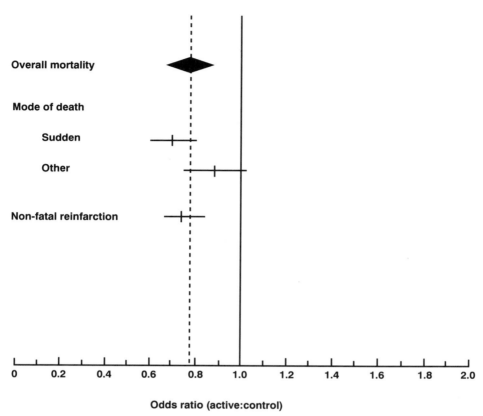

Fig. 18.8. Sudden death, other death, and nonfatal reinfarction in long-term beta-blocker trials that reported these endpoints separately: odds ratios (active:control), together with approximate 95% confidence ranges. See original article for citation of specific trials. [From Yusuf et al. (1985), with permission.]

ers vs nonselective beta-blockers) nor between those with or without membrane-sta- bilizing activity (Figure 18.9). However, the presence of significant intrinsic sym- pathomimetic activity reduced the benefit to nonsignificance (odds ratio: 0.90; 95% CI: 0.77–1.05) (Figure 18.9) (Yusuf 1985). Reduction in heart rate appears to be a critical feature associated with the protective effect of beta-blockers. Indeed, there is a significant relationship between the magnitude of heart rate reduction observed on the active agent and the magnitude of reduction in mortality (Figure 18.10) (Kjekshus 1986).

A substantial number of the large-scale clinical trials have also reported the effect of long-term beta-blocker use on nonfatal reinfarction (Table 18.4). Results from pooled analyses indicate that beta-blocker use is associated with an odds ratio of 0.74 (95% CI: 0.66–0.83; $p < .001$). As observed for mortality, there is also a significant relationship between the magnitude of reduction in heart rate and the reduction in

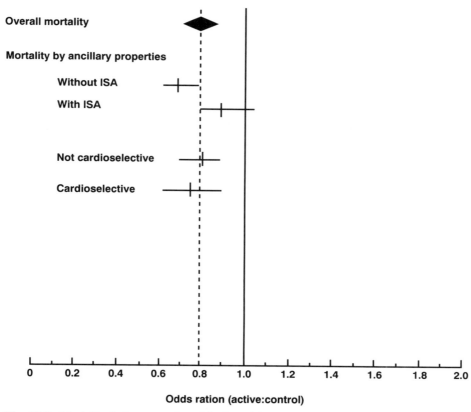

Fig. 18.9. Mortality in long-term beta-blocker trials, by ancillary properties of agent tested: odds ratios (active:control), together with approximate 95% confidence intervals. See original article for citation of specific trials. [From Yusuf et al. (1985), with permission.]

nonfatal recurrent MI ($r = .54$; $p < .05$) (Figure 18.11) (Kjekshus 1986). This observed benefit of reducing nonfatal reinfarction is in addition to the benefit on mortality.

The magnitude of benefit from long-term use of a beta-blocker is also dependent on the patient's risk of mortality following their index MI (Table 18.5). Post hoc analyses of data from the Beta Blocker Heart Attack Trial (BHAT) (Furberg 1984) indicate that those MI patients without electrical or mechanical complications experienced only a 6% relative benefit from the use of propranolol. MI patients with electrical complications experienced a 52% relative benefit, those with mechanical complications experienced a 38% relative benefit, and those with both mechanical and electrical complications experienced a 25% relative benefit. Considering the low cost of routine beta-blocker use, and its substantial benefit, such therapy has a relatively favorable cost-effectiveness ratio: an estimated cost of therapy per year of life saved would be $13,000 in low-risk patients, $3,600 in medium-risk patients, and $2,400 in high-risk patients (Goldman 1988).

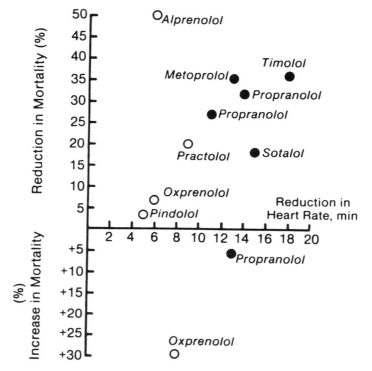

Fig. 18.10. Relation between reduction in heart rate (difference between treatment groups) and percentage of reduction in mortality in large, prospective, double-blind trials with beta-blockers. Open circles, beta-blockers with intrinsic sympathomimetic activity; $r = .6$; $p < .05$. See original article for citation of specific trials. [From Kjekshus (1986), with permission.]

The benefits from routine beta-blocker use seem to persist as long as the active agent is continued (Olsson 1988; Olsson 1991; Yusuf 1993). It is therefore most appropriate after MI to maintain beta-blocker therapy indefinitely in patients who can tolerate it.

The benefits of a beta-blocker in long-term secondary prevention appear to extend to most patient subgroups. The Beta-Blocker Pooling Project (1988) combined the results of nine large trials and found that although high-risk patients were most likely to benefit from beta-blocker therapy, lower risk patients also benefited, even though the absolute and relative benefits were small. The experience using beta-blockers in the elderly is limited, but available data indicate that the benefit may even be greater in patients older than 50 to 60 than in younger patients. Benefit appeared to be similar in both men and women.

The side effects from prolonged beta-blocker use have generally been quite minor, and are quite similar to those seen with placebo (BHAT Research Group 1982). In studies that report it, the incidence of heart failure is slightly but significantly higher

Table 18.4. Nonfatal Reinfarction from Long-Term Trials of Beta Blockers

Trial	Basic Data from Trials (nonfatal reinfarctions/no. randomized)		Ratio of Percentages	Statistical Calculations	
	Allocated Beta-Blocker	Allocated Control		Observed Minus Expected (O − E)	Variance of O − E
Reynolds	3/38 (8%)	2/39 (5%)	1.5	+0.5	1.2
Wilhelmsson	16/114 (14%)	18/116 (16%)	0.9	−0.9	7.3
Ahlmark	3/69 (4%)	14/93 (15%)	0.3	−4.2	3.7
Multicentre Int.	75/1,533 (5%)	97/1,520 (6%)	0.8	−11.4	40.6
Baber	15/355 (4%)	15/365 (4%)	1.0	+0.2	7.2
Rehnqvist	3/59 (5%)	5/52 (10%)	0.5	−1.3	1.9
Norwegian Multicentre	90/945 (10%)	131/939 (14%)	0.7	−20.9	48.8
Taylor	67/632 (11%)	58/471 (12%)	0.9	−4.6	27.1
Hansteen	16/278 (6%)	21/282 (7%)	0.8	−2.4	8.7
BHAT	103/1,916 (5%)	121/1,921 (6%)	0.9	−8.9	52.7
Julian	24/873 (3%)	22/583 (4%)	0.7	−3.6	10.7
Australian/Swedish	25/263 (10%)	28/266 (11%)	0.9	−1.3	11.9
Manger Cats	16/291 (5%)	20/293 (7%)	0.8	−1.9	8.5
EIS	36/858 (4%)	38/883 (4%)	1.0	−0.5	17.7
Rehnqvist	18/154 (12%)	31/147 (21%)	0.6	−7.1	10.3
Ciba-Geigy	2,400 patients; data not yet available				
Barber	9/222 (4%)	21/226 (9%)	0.4	−5.9	7.0
Yusuf	0/11 (0%)	0/11 (0%)	—	0.0	0.0
Wilcox	388 patients; data not available				
Wilcox	1/157 (1%)	5/158 (3%)	0.2	−2.0	1.5
CPRG	3/177 (2%)	7/136 (5%)	0.3	−2.7	2.4
Andersen	427 patients; data not available				
Salathia	800 patients; data not yet available				
Hjalmarson	26/698 (4%)	39/697 (6%)	0.7	−6.5	15.5
Totals available thus far	549/9,643 (5.7%)	693/9,198 (7.5%)	Not calculated	−85.1	284.7

Source: From Yusuf, et al. (1985) with permission. See original article for citation of specific trials.
Pooled odds ratio of 0.74 with 95% confidence intervals of 0.66 to 0.83 ($p < .0001$). Test for heterogeneity: $\chi^2 = 15.5$ on 18 df, NS.

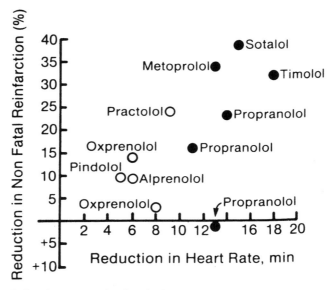

Fig. 18.11. Relation between reduction in heart rate and percentage of reduction in recurrent nonfatal infarctions in large, prospective, double-blind trials with beta-blockers. Open circles, beta-blockers with intrinsic sympathomimetic activity; $r = .59$; $p < .05$. See original article for citation of specific trials. [From Kjekshus (1986), with permission.]

in patients receiving beta-blocker (5.9%) than in patients receiving placebo (5.4%) (pooled odds ratio: 1.16, 95% CI: 1.01–1.34) (Yusuf 1985). However, even patients with a history of mild or moderate congestive heart failure (CHF) also benefited from beta-blocker use; in fact, those patients with CHF actually experienced greater benefit from beta-blockade than did patients without that condition (Byington 1990).

Calcium-Channel Blocking Agents

In contrast to the beneficial effects of the beta-blockers, the Ca^{2+}-blockers have not been effective in routine secondary prevention. The Ca^{2+} blockers differ substantially in their pharmacologic and physiologic actions and thus cannot be considered as a single class of drugs (Stone 1980). Although each of the Ca^{2+}-blockers is a potent agent in vitro to decrease sinoatrial (SA) and atrioventricular (AV) nodal activity (negative chronotropy and dromotropy, respectively), decrease contractility (negative inotropy), and cause arterial vasodilatation, their relative strengths in each of these properties are different. The arterial vasodilation promotes reflex sympathetic activity, which counters each of these direct effects: the reflex activity leads to sinus tachycardia, increased conduction through the AV node, and increased force of contractility. Based on the relative strength of each agent for each direct effect and the strength of the reflex activation, each agent has a different net effect. The dihydropyridines, like

Table 18.5. All-Cause Mortality by Risk and Treatment Groups: BHAT[a]

Risk Group	Placebo Group		Propranolol Group		Absolute Efficacy (100)	Relative Efficacy (%)	Adjusted elative Efficacy[b] (%)
	No. of Pts.	Mortality Rate (%)	No. of Pts.	Mortality Rate (%)			
No electrical or mechanical complications	1,079	6.6	1,047	6.2	0.4	6	-4
Electrical complications only	423	10.9	443	5.2	5.7	-52	-57
Mechanical complications only	202	16.8	201	10.4	6.4	-38	-43
Both electrical and mechanical complications	217	17.1	225	12.9	4.2	-25	-30

Source: From Byington and Furberg (1990), with permission.

[a]Average length of follow-up was 25 months.

[b]Adjusted for 13 variables predictive of mortality.

nifedipine, are relatively more potent vasodilators than negative inotropic, chronotropic, or dromotropic agents, and their net effect therefore is primarily a reduction in arterial pressure associated with reflex increases in heart rate and contractility. The benzothiazepines, like diltiazem, and the phenylalkylamines, like verapamil, are relatively more potent negative chronotropic, dromotropic, and inotropic agents than nifedipine, and their hypotensive effective remains associated with a decrease in heart rate, A-V nodal conduction, and myocardial contractility.

The possible mechanisms of beneficial effect from the Ca^{2+}-blockers might include prevention of coronary vasospasm, if such vasospasm were present, reduction of systemic arterial blood pressure, and prevention of atrial reentrant arrhythmias. Since Ca^{2+}-blockers also reduce the amount of calcium influx associated with MI (Stone 1980), these agents may also be effective by reducing the extent of myocardial damage for a given ischemic insult.

Dihydropyridine Ca^{2+}-Blockers (Nifedipine and Nicardipine). There have been a large number of clinical trials investigating the effect of nifedipine and, to a lesser degree, nicardipine, to prevent morbidity and mortality associated with unstable angina and acute MI (Yusuf 1988, 1991, 1993; Held 1989). Many of these studies may not be methodologically comparable because the doses tested varied, and both the underlying disease manifestation and the timing from onset of the acute ischemic manifestation to initiation of the study drug may have been different. Furthermore, these studies address the concept of reduction in infarct size and prevention of active ischemia rather than the more usual method of secondary prevention, in which therapy is initiated well after the acute ischemic event has resolved, at the time of hospital discharge.

Nevertheless, nifedipine has been uniformly unsuccessful in reducing either mortality or the rate of reinfarction (Figure 18.12). A recent update of a pooled analysis (Yusuf 1991) of stable coronary patients in a coronary regression trial with either nifedipine (Lichtlen 1990) or nicardipine (Waters 1990) showed a trend toward an increase in mortality (7.4% vs 6.5%; odds ratio: 1.16; 95% CI: 0.99–1.35; $p = .07$) and a nonsignificant increase in reinfarction (3.5% vs 3.1%; odds ratio: 1.19; 95% CI: 0.92–1.53) (Table 18.6).

Verapamil and Diltiazem. The calcium channel blockers verapamil and diltiazem can be considered together because their net pharmacologic effect is that of slowing the heart rate and, in some instances, reducing myocardial contractility (Stone 1980), thereby reducing myocardial oxygen demand. These studies are closer to more conventional secondary prevention design, since patients in these studies were treated with the active agent after their index MI was stabilized. Table 18.6 displays a recent pooled analysis performed by Yusuf and colleagues (1991). These results indicate that verapamil and diltiazem had no effect on mortality, but that they exerted a significant effect on reducting the rate of reinfarction (6.0% vs 7.5%; odds ratio: 0.79; 95% CI: 0.67–0.94; $p < .01$). The effect seems similar for both agents.

It should be emphasized that there have not been studies comparing the efficacy of verapamil or diltiazem to a beta-blocker. Beta-blockers more consistently reduce

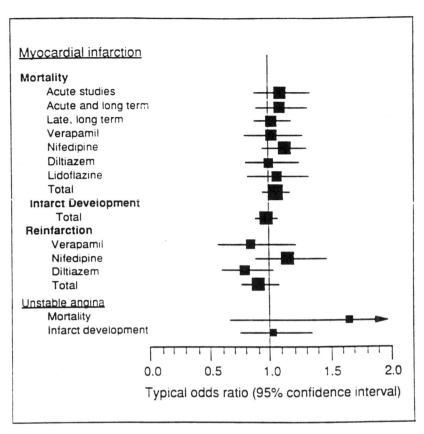

Fig. 18.12. Typical odds of death, infarct development, and reinfarction by disease, type of trials, and drug. Areas of squares are proportional to numbers of patients. *Bars* indicate 95% confidence intervals. *Portions to left* of vertical line (corresponding to odds ratio <1) indicate reduced risk with treatment; *portions to right* of vertical line indicate increased risk with treatment. Upper 95% confidence limit for effect on mortality in unstable angina = 6.2. Note that treatment does not seem to reduce risk of any event. See original article for citation of specific trials. [From Held et al. (1989), with permission.]

both mortality and reinfarction and should be recommended for those patients who can tolerate such medication. Verapamil or diltiazem may be a reasonable alternative for those patients who cannot tolerate a beta-blocker, but who can tolerate one of the Ca^{2+}-blockers, for example, patients with severe COPD or asthma. It should be noted, however, that many patients who cannot tolerate a beta-blocker because of concern of excessive bradycardia or CHF may experience similar complications from diltiazem or verapamil.

At this time we do not have sufficient data to determine whether there are differences in treatment effect based on subgroups such as age and gender.

Table 18.6. Secondary Prevention Trials of Calcium Channel Blocking Agents

Event and Agent	No. Events No. Subjects		Odds Ratio (CI)
	Active	Control	
Mortality			
Dihydropyridine	379/5137	335/5135	1.16 (0.99–1.35)
Verapamil	244/2644	266/2649	0.91 (0.76–1.10)
Diltiazem	180/1574	181/1577	0.99 (0.80–1.24)
Reinfarction			
Dihydropyridine	138/3838	119/3871	1.19 (0.92–1.53)
Verapamil	138/2606	171/2624	0.80 (0.63–1.01)
Diltiazem	113/1557	142/1560	0.79 (0.61–1.02)

Source: From Yusuf et al. (1992), with permission.

CI, confidence interval.

Lipid-Lowering Therapy

There is much evidence from cross-cultural and observational studies that links serum total cholesterol levels with CHD incidence (Keys 1984). Cohort studies also demonstrate the prediction by serum cholesterol not only of initial manifestations of CHD but recurrent CHD events (Rose 1977; Pekkanen 1990). Since, in the general population, LDL cholesterol constitutes most of the serum total cholesterol, the LDL cholesterol level has predictive ability that is similar to total cholesterol. The serum cholesterol-CHD relationship has been found in many populations from diverse ethnic, geographic, and socioeconomic backgrounds. It shows clear "dose-response" properties. LDL cholesterol also has biologic plausibility as a cause of atherosclerosis as demonstrated by genetic and pathophysiologic studies (Gotto 1992).

Clinical trials clearly demonstrate the causal relationship between serum total and LDL cholesterol levels and CHD in populations both with and without clinical CHD (Table 18.7). Most trials have studied patients with established CHD, usually after MI, and constitute "secondary prevention trials." Those that study patients who do not have clinical CHD are termed "primary prevention trials." Since the pathophysiology of atherosclerosis is similar in the development of initial and recurrent clinical CHD, and since the reduction in risk of CHD by serum cholesterol-lowering is similar for initial and recurrent CHD, the distinction between "primary" and "secondary" prevention is probably not relevant when assessing the effect of therapy in terms of relative risk reduction. Therefore, most meta-analyses consider primary and secondary prevention trials together. However, since the likelihood of a CHD event is about five times higher in patients who already have clinical CHD than in those free of clinical disease, more events would be prevented with the same proportional risk reduction in secondary than primary prevention. For this reason, cost-effectiveness analyses favor secondary over primary prevention (Goldman 1992).

Diet, drug, and surgical hypolipidemic therapies have all been employed. The trials described in Table 18.7 used a randomized control group, with an average treatment duration of at least two years. Two years is considered to be a minimum for trials that seek to detect benefit for clinical CHD, since many trials have shown that a

Table 18.7. Controlled Trials of Cholesterol-Lowering and CHD

Name	N	CHD at Entry	Treatment	Duration (yr)	Cholesterol Baseline	Cholesterol Difference (%)	CHD Incidence/yr (%)	CHD Difference (%)	Mortality Incidence (%)	Mortality Difference (%)
Diet Therapy										
Turpienen 1979	676	−	34% Fat p/s 1.5	6	263	−15	1.6	−43	—	—
Leren 1970	206	+	39% Fat p/s 2.4	5	296	−14	7.9	−25	5.3	−24
MRC Low Fat 1965	123-9	+	22% Fat	3	265	−5	11	+4	4.7	−13
MRC Soy Oil 1988	194-9	+	46% Fat p/s 2	4	292	−15	6.6	−14	4.1	−15
Dayton 1989	424-6	+	40% Fat p/s 2	8	233	−13	2.1	−23	5.2	−1
Burr 1989	1015-8	+	Low fat	2	250	−3.5	7.1	−9	5.5	0
	—[a]	+	High fiber	2	?	NC	6.2	+23	5.0	+27
	—[a]	+	Fatty fish	2	?	NC	7.3	−16	6.4	−29
Drug Therapy										
WHO 1978	5331/5296	−	Clofibrate	5	248	−9	0.7	−21	0.3	+46
New-castle 1971	244/253	+	Clofibrate	5	251	−14	6.7	−34	3.8	−42
Scottish 1971	350/367	+	Clofibrate	6	266	−14	3.4	−25	2.3	−7
CDP 1975	1103/2789	+	Clofibrate	5–5.8	251	−7	5	−7	4.2	0
CDP 1975	1119/2789	+	Niacin	5–5.8	251	−10	5	−15	4.2	−4
Dorr 1978	1149/1094	25%	Colestipol	2.1	315	−13	3.1	−23	2.0	−19
Stockholm 1988	279/276	+	Niacin + clofibrate	5	249	−13	7.2	−29	6.8	−26
LRC-CPPT 1984	1906/1900	+	Cholestyramine	7.4	280	−9	1.2	−19	0.5	−7
Helsinki 1988	2051/2030	−	Gemfibrozil	5	289	−10	0.8	−34	0.4	+6
Buchwald 1990	421/417	+	Ileal bypass	9.7	251	−23	3.1	−35	1.5	−22

[a] CHD death + MI.

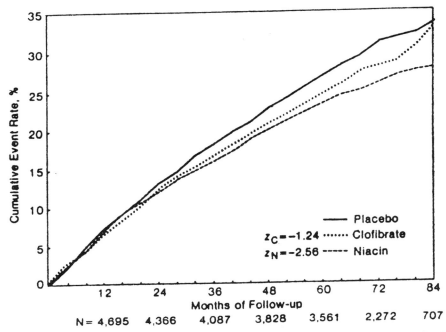

Fig. 18.13. The effect of niacin and clofibrate on recurrent coronary disease in the Coronary Drug Project. [From the Coronary Drug Project Research Group (1975), with permission.]

reduction in CHD rates emerges only after 2 to 3 years (Figure 18.13). As an exception to one of these criteria, the Finnish Mental Hospital trial was included, which did not have random assignment of patients but rather of hospitals (Turpeinen 1979). There are two types of endpoints used in cholesterol-lowering trials; one seeks to determine the effect of lowering serum cholesterol on the traditional endpoint, clinical coronary heart disease (Table 18.7). Another uses coronary arteriography to examine the changes in atherosclerotic vascular narrowing in response to therapy (Table 18.8).

Diet Therapy. Two dietary approaches that lower intake of saturated fat and cholesterol have been studied. One therapeutic diet was relatively high in fat, since it replaced the saturated fat mainly with polyunsaturated fat. The other type of diet was low in fat and high in carbohydrate. The high polyunsaturated fat diets were more successful than the low-fat diets in lowering serum cholesterol, 14% vs 4%, and in lowering CHD, 26% vs 3% (Figure 18.14). Three of the four high polyunsaturated fat trials found a significant reduction in CHD, but the two low-fat trials found no effect. Since controlled feeding studies on metabolic wards demonstrate that the two diets should have lowered serum cholesterol to a similar extent (Mensink 1992), we can only conclude that adherence to the low-fat diet was poor. In this regard, it is notable that an arteriographic trial in which serum cholesterol was significantly lowered by a low-fat diet found less disease progression and the induction of regression

Table 18.8. Coronary Atherosclerosis Regression Trials

Name	N	Treatment	LDL-C Baseline	LDL-C Change (%)	HDL-C Baseline	HDL-C Change (%)	Atherosclerosis	Notes
Duffield 1983	12	Diet + drugs	199	−24	43	+40	Improved	Femoral, QA
Nikkila 1984	20–28	Diet + elofibrate or niacin	214	−19	39	+10	Improved	Visual
Blankenhorn 1987	80–82	Colestipoll and niaacin	170	−38	44	+35	Improved	Visual
Brown 1990	36–46	Niacin + Colestipol	187	−25	37	+38	Improved	QA
		Lovastatin + Colestipol		−39		+10	Improved	
Ornish 1990	17–22	Diet, exercise, weight loss	159	−32	45	0	Improved	
Kane 1990	32–40	Multiple drugs	279	−28	49	+25	Improved	QA
Buchwald 1990	333–362	Intestinal bypass	179	−38	40	+4	Improved	Visual
Schuler 1992	40–52	Diet, exercise	164	−6	35	+3	Improved	QA
Watts 1992	24–26	Diet	194	−13	44	0	Improved	QA
		Diet + cholestyramine	203	−33	48	−3	Improved	
Blankenhorn 1993	123–124	Lovastatin	157	−42			No change	QA
							Improved	Visual
Waters 1994	160	Lovastatin	173	−27	41	+4	Improved	QA
Haskell 1994	150	Diet exercise, drugs, smoking cessation	157	−19	46	+13	Improved	QA
Sacks 1995	39–40	Multiple drugs	137	−41	41	+13	No change	QA

QA, Quantitative Arteriographic Analysis; change, Change in active − change in placebo groups; baseline, mean level for active and placebo groups prior to treatment; if not reported, then mean on trial level for placebo group.

485

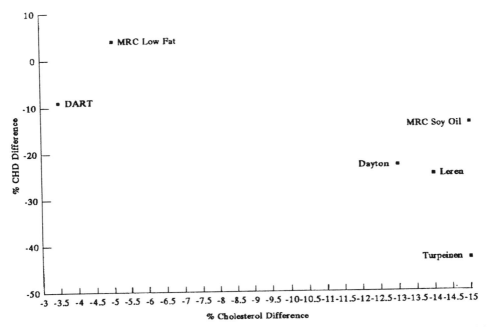

Fig. 18.14. Controlled trials of dietary fat and coronary heart disease.

in coronary artery lesions (Table 18.8) (Watts 1992). Therefore, we believe the evidence is strong for our conclusion: diet therapy that lowers saturated fat and cholesterol, when successfully administered, is capable of improving coronary atherosclerotic disease.

Several trials tested dietary strategies that were alternative to the standard approach of restricting saturated fat and cholesterol intake, and all found a beneficial effect on CHD. The Lyon Diet Heart Study, a small secondary prevention trial, found that a "Mediterranean" diet compared to the standard low-fat diet, reduced CHD events by 73% (de Lorgerli 1994). The specific dietary changes were substitution of animal fat with polyunsaturated vegetable oil rich in alpha-linolenic acid, and replacement of meat with fish, legumes, fruits, and vegetables. Total fat intake did not change. Which of these nutritional changes were responsible for the benefit cannot be determined. A trial from India randomized patients during hospitalization for acute MI into a standard step I diet, or to a dietary program that increased fruits and vegetables and the ratio of polyunsaturated to saturated fat while leaving total fat intake unchanged (Singh 1992). Coronary events were significantly reduced by 40% after 1 year. Finally, the DART trial (Burr 1989), which found that a low-fat diet had no effect on CHD, demonstrated a significant reduction in CHD from a relatively modest intake of fatty fish. Therefore, dietary factors other than saturated fat and cholesterol could have an important influence on CHD.

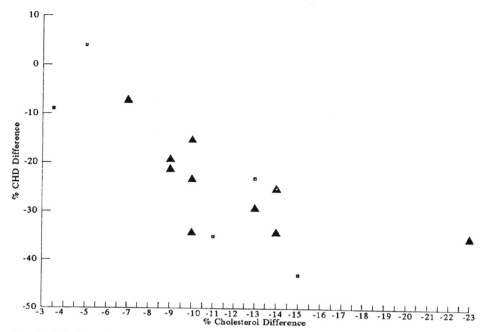

Fig. 18.15. Controlled trials of drug therapy and CHD. Relationship between lowering of serum cholesterol and coronary heart disease.

Drug and Surgical Therapy. Medications are less complicated to administer than diet therapy, and compliance can be considered more predictable. (See Figure 18.15.) Several agents with various mechanisms of action have been shown to lower CHD rates. Clofibrate has a relatively weak hypocholesterolemic effect, but in three of the four trials in which it was used as the single treatment, CHD rates were significantly reduced (Table 18.7). Clofibrate is not used in current practice because of its weak action and results of the WHO trial that indicated adverse effects on cancer and other noncardiovascular diseases (WHO Cooperative Trial 1980). Niacin (nicotinic acid) is a water-soluble vitamin that lowers LDL cholesterol levels when administered in doses 100-fold over that required to prevent pellagra, a nutritional deficiency disease. Niacin also raises HDL cholesterol levels, and lowers serum triglycerides, which may contribute to its beneficial effect on CHD. Niacin, used singly (Coronary Drug Project Research Group 1975) or with clofibrate (Carlson 1988), lowered recurrent CHD rates. Cholestyramine and colestipol are bile acid-sequestering resins that lower serum LDL cholesterol. Since unpleasant gastrointestinal side effects are common, its potential for a substantial hypocholesterolemic response has not been achieved. Nonetheless, CHD rates were lowered in the two trials that used this class of drug (Dorr 1978; LRC-CPPT 1984). Gemfibrozil, like clofibrate, is a fibric acid derivative. Gemfibrozil has a minor action to lower serum LDL cholesterol levels. However, its major action is to lower serum triglycerides, and to raise serum HDL cholesterol levels, particularly in hypertriglyceridemic patients who have low HDL cholesterol levels. Gemfibrozil has been used in one primary prevention trial, and it lowered CHD significantly (Maninen 1988). In contrast to clofibrate in the WHO primary prevention trial (WHO Cooperative Trial 1980), gemfibrozil did not significantly raise noncardiovascular disease rates, although there were adverse trends so that total mortality was not improved. Intestinal bypass surgery was used as an effective hypocholesterolemic treatment before the advent of potent inhibitors of cholesterol synthesis. A secondary prevention trial of this procedure demonstrated substantial lowering of total and LDL cholesterol, and significant reduction in CHD (Buchwald 1990). Viewing the results of cholesterol-lowering trials together, an apparent dose-response effect associates 1% decrease in serum total cholesterol with approximately 2% decrease in CHD rates. In addition to the beneficial effects of lowering total or LDL cholesterol, analyses of the results of several trials suggested that increases in HDL cholesterol caused by the medications also contributed to the decrease in CHD or improvement in coronary lesions (LRC-CPPT 1984; Nikkila 1984; Maninen 1988: Brown 1990). In contrast, increases (LRC-CPPT 1984) or decreases (Maninen 1988) in serum triglyceride levels did not independently benefit CHD.

Trials that employ coronary arteriography to measure change in coronary atherosclerosis are appealing since they require a 10-fold lower sample size and a shorter period of treatment—1 to 2 years vs 5 years—than trials that study clinical CHD events. Improvement in coronary artery narrowing has been demonstrated by many types of therapies, including diet, diet plus exercise, various pharmacologic regimens, and intestinal bypass surgery. Both a decrease in progression of stenosis and mild reversal of disease have been reported. The various nonpharmacologic strategies to reduce atherosclerosis, including the combination of a very low fat diet, vigorous exercise, and yoga (Ornish 1990), the combination of diet plus vigorous exercise (Schuler 1992), and an intensive dietary program as monotherapy (Watts 1992) produced similar amounts of benefit in coronary artery stenosis. Moreover, these nonpharmacologic treatments provided benefits similar to those found with combination drug therapy.

The development of potent inhibitors of hepatic cholesterol synthesis, the HMG CoA reductase inhibitors, greatly improved the efficacy and tolerability of cholesterol-lowering therapy. Standard doses lower LDL cholesterol by 20–30% while producing very few adverse effects. Several large-scale trials (sample size in the thousands) that used these agents in primary (West of Scotland 1992) and secondary prevention (Sacks 1991) are near completion, and one of the large-scale secondary prevention trials was recently reported (Scandinavian Simvastatin Survival Study 1994). In this trial 4,444 patients with clinical coronary disease and a total serum cholesterol 213–310 mg/dl were treated with a lipid-lowering diet and were randomized to receive either simvastatin or placebo. Over the 5.4 years median follow-up period, simvastatin produced mean changes in total cholesterol, LDL and HDL of -25%, -35%, and $+8\%$, respectively, associated with a relative risk of death of 0.70 (95% CI 0.58–0.85, p = 0.0003). Small-scale trials (sample size in the hundreds) that used pravastatin found significant and substantial reductions in myocardial infarction and CHD death (Pitt 1994, Furberg 1994) after surprisingly short durations of therapy, for example, 6 months to 3 years. Results from more large-scale trials of long duration are needed to confirm the potential of these drugs for major benefit without adverse effects that interfere with long-term adherence or cause noncardiovascular disease events. The results from the Scandinavian Simvastatin Survival Study are extremely encouraging.

Previous cholesterol-lowering trials generally enrolled men younger than 60. There is no satisfactory direct information on effects on CHD in women or in the elderly. A coronary disease regression trial found that the women were as likely as the men to receive arteriographically determined benefit from hypocholesterolemic drug therapy (Kane 1990). Nearly all current primary and secondary prevention trials are enrolling women, and they have a higher upper age limit than previous trials. Secondary prevention trials are underway that specifically study various strategies to reduce atherosclerotic disease in women and in the elderly. Particularly since observational epidemiologic studies in women who have CHD found a protective association of postmenopausal estrogen replacement therapy with recurrent CHD (Bush 1987; Sullivan 1990), randomized secondary prevention trials of estrogen are much needed to prove causality. Some are in the early initiation or planning phases at this time.

Virtually all of the serum cholesterol-lowering trials have studied patients with at least moderately elevated levels. Holme (1990) found that the reduction in CHD is proportional to the initial mean cholesterol level. Sacks and colleagues (1991) found a similar result in subgroup analyses of several individual trials. Therefore, at this time, it is not clear whether CHD patients who have average cholesterol levels, for example, <240 mg/dl, will receive benefit from efforts to achieve lower than average levels. In this regard, a recent arteriographic trial conducted in normocholesterolemic patients found no improvement in coronary lesions from intensive combination drug therapy (Table 18.2) (Sacks 1995). The Cholesterol and Recurrent Events trial (CARE), conducted among 4,159 MI survivors, has been designed to test definitively the effect of cholesterol-lowering on CHD in a normocholesterolemic population. The trial is scheduled to end in February 1996.

It is becoming increasingly apparent that many CHD patients have normal or even lower than average total and LDL cholesterol levels. The hypothesis that producing even lower LDL cholesterol reduces CHD is being definitively studied as described in the previous paragraph. This is the approach recommended by the National Cholesterol Education Program (Expert Panel 1993). An alternative approach recognizes that many of these patients have low HDL cholesterol as their sole lipoprotein abnormality. There is no evidence from randomized clinical trials whether therapy to improve HDL levels in such patients will reduce CHD. Although gemfibrozil raises HDL levels in patients with hypertriglyceridemia and low HDL (Manninen 1988), it has a minimal effect on HDL in patients with normal triglyceride levels (Vega 1994). It does, however, substantially lower triglyceride levels regardless of initial level. A secondary prevention trial of gemfibrozil in these "dyslipidemic" patients is in progress (Rubins 1993).

Aspirin and Other Platelet-Active Agents

Inhibition of platelet activation reduces one of the critical pathophysiologic processes responsible for acute coronary events (Table 18.1, Figures 18.3 and 18.5). The processes following plaque rupture, whereby thrombus forms and occludes the coronary artery, are complex and multifaceted; use of aspirin, however, reduces platelet aggregability and thereby may prevent the clinical manifestation of luminal obstruction, even though the plaque rupture is unaffected. Since the process of acute coronary occlusion is often dynamic and characterized by intermittent thrombus formation and dissolution (Falk 1983; Davies 1985), aspirin has been demonstrated to be extremely effective in reducing cardiovascular mortality and infarction even when administered to patients after the onset of acute MI (ISIS-2 Collaboration Group 1988) and unstable angina (Theroux 1988), as well as in secondary prevention initiated after resolution of the acute ischemic event.

The value of aspirin and other antiplatelet agents in secondary prevention has been reviewed by the Antiplatelet Trialists Collaborative Group, initially in 1988 (Antiplatelet 1988) and again in 1994 (Antiplatelet 1994). The trials most recently reviewed include 145 randomized controlled trials: 51,144 patients assigned to antiplatelet therapy and 45,172 patients assigned to control (Antiplatelet 1994). The platelet-active agents included cyclooxygenase inhibitors (aspirin, ibuprofen, sufinpyrazone, etc.), phosphodiesterase inhibitors (e.g., dipyridamole), thromboxane inhibitors, and agents with direct effects on platelet membranes (ticlopidine). The trials of patients treated after MI include approximately 20,000 patients followed for a mean duration of 27 months on study medication. Although each of the studies indicated a substantial magnitude of benefit, few of the individual studies demonstrated a significant effect. The pooled analysis, however, demonstrated that antiplatelet therapy given to patients following MI reduce vascular mortality by 15% (8.1% vs 9.4%, $p < .005$) (Figure 18.16), nonfatal MI by 31% (4.7% vs 6.5%, $p < .00001$) (Figure 18.17), and nonfatal strokes by 39% (1.0% vs 1.5%, $p < .0001$) (Figure 18.18); while having no effect on nonvascular deaths (0.8% vs 0.9%). Combining vascular events (MI, stroke, or death), there was a 25% reduction in patients treated with platelet-active drugs (13.5% vs 17.1%, $p < .00001$) (Figure 18.19). The absolute effects of antiplatelet therapy on various outcomes in the 11 trials in patients with a prior MI are shown in Figure 18.20.

In the trials of high-risk patients, such as those treated for a recent MI, treatment produced similar proportional reductions in middle-aged and elderly patients, in men and women, in hypertensive and normotensive patients, and in diabetic and nondiabetic patients (Antiplatelet 1994). None of these characteristics, therefore, are contraindications to the use of antiplatelet therapy.

Although even the pooled sample sizes are quite small using some of the different specific antiplatelet regimens, there does not appear to be a difference in the incidence of MI, stroke, or death between high-dose aspirin (500–1,500 mg/day) and medium dose aspirin (75–325 mg/day), between aspirin plus dipyridamole and aspirin alone, between sulfinypyrazone and aspirin, or between ticlopidine and aspirin (Antiplatelet 1994). Since aspirin doses higher than 325 mg/day are more gastrotoxic than lower doses, a higher dose is unnecessary for secondary prevention. Recent studies using doses as low as 75–100 mg/day in patients with unstable angina or acute MI indicate that even these low doses may be effective in reducing vascular events (Wallentin 1991; Verheugt 1990). Alternate-day regimens, such as 325 mg every other day as used in the Physicians' Health Study of primary prevention, may also be efficacious.

There is no direct information to indicate how long antiplatelet therapy should be maintained. The pooled analyses from trials of different duration indicate that active

VASCULAR DEATH (or death from unknown cause)

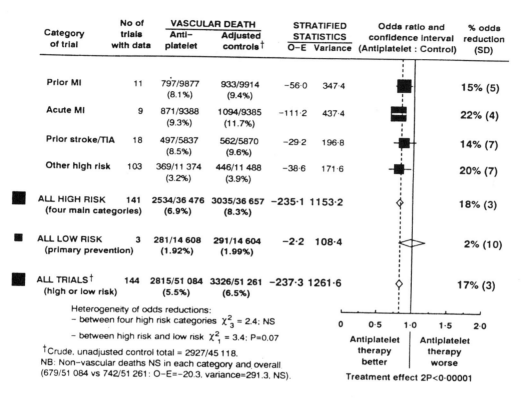

Category of trial	No of trials with data	VASCULAR DEATH		STRATIFIED STATISTICS		Odds ratio and confidence interval (Antiplatelet : Control)	% odds reduction (SD)
		Anti-platelet	Adjusted controls†	O–E	Variance		
Prior MI	11	797/9877 (8.1%)	933/9914 (9.4%)	–56·0	347·4		15% (5)
Acute MI	9	871/9388 (9.3%)	1094/9385 (11.7%)	–111·2	437·4		22% (4)
Prior stroke/TIA	18	497/5837 (8.5%)	562/5870 (9.6%)	–29·2	196·8		14% (7)
Other high risk	103	369/11 374 (3.2%)	446/11 488 (3.9%)	–38·6	171·6		20% (7)
ALL HIGH RISK (four main categories)	141	2534/36 476 (6.9%)	3035/36 657 (8.3%)	–235·1	1153·2		18% (3)
ALL LOW RISK (primary prevention)	3	281/14 608 (1.92%)	291/14 604 (1.99%)	–2·2	108·4		2% (10)
ALL TRIALS† (high or low risk)	144	2815/51 084 (5.5%)	3326/51 261 (6.5%)	–237·3	1261·6		17% (3)

Heterogeneity of odds reductions:
– between four high risk categories χ^2_3 = 2.4: NS
– between high risk and low risk χ^2_1 = 3.4: P=0.07

†Crude, unadjusted control total = 2927/45 118.
NB: Non-vascular deaths NS in each category and overall
(679/51 084 vs 742/51 261: O–E=–20.3, variance=291.3, NS).

0   0·5   1·0   1·5   2·0
Antiplatelet therapy better | Antiplatelet therapy worse
Treatment effect 2P<0·00001

Fig. 18.16. Vascular death (or death from unknown cause). See original article for citation of specific trials. [From Antiplatelet Trialists' Collaboration (1994), with permission.]

therapy is associated with a 28% odds reduction in vascular events in year 1 of treatment, 24% odds reduction in year 2, and 12% in year 3 (Antiplatelet 1994). Since compliance may weaken in the later years of a trial and since a treatment effect early may bias the comparison in later years, it is recommended that antiplatelet therapy be continued indefinitely unless a contraindication develops (Antiplatelet 1994).

Although the decrease in mortality associated with aspirin and coumadin in secondary prevention are similar (see below), the risk of bleeding is far greater with coumadin. Thus, convenience, simplicity, and cost all favor use of aspirin as routine therapy (Verstraete 1991). The use of aspirin is discussed in greater detail in Chapter 12.

Oral Anticoagulants

None of the early individual studies investigating the value of coumadin to prevent recurrent cardiac events achieved statistical significance, although an early meta-anal-

NON–FATAL MYOCARDIAL INFARCTION (with survival to end of study)

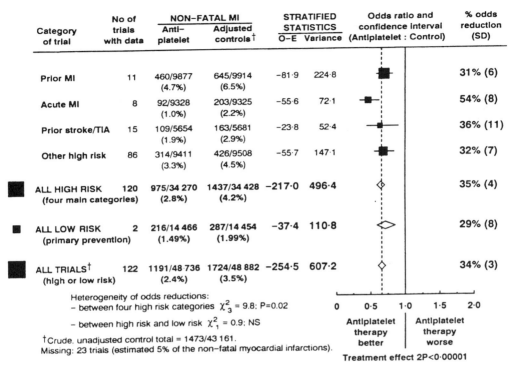

Category of trial	No of trials with data	NON–FATAL MI Anti-platelet	NON–FATAL MI Adjusted controls[†]	STRATIFIED STATISTICS O–E	STRATIFIED STATISTICS Variance	Odds ratio and confidence interval (Antiplatelet : Control)	% odds reduction (SD)
Prior MI	11	460/9877 (4.7%)	645/9914 (6.5%)	−81·9	224·8		31% (6)
Acute MI	8	92/9328 (1.0%)	203/9325 (2.2%)	−55·6	72·1		54% (8)
Prior stroke/TIA	15	109/5654 (1.9%)	163/5681 (2.9%)	−23·8	52·4		36% (11)
Other high risk	86	314/9411 (3.3%)	426/9508 (4.5%)	−55·7	147·1		32% (7)
ALL HIGH RISK (four main categories)	120	975/34 270 (2.8%)	1437/34 428 (4.2%)	−217·0	496·4		35% (4)
ALL LOW RISK (primary prevention)	2	216/14 466 (1.49%)	287/14 454 (1.99%)	−37·4	110·8		29% (8)
ALL TRIALS[†] (high or low risk)	122	1191/48 736 (2.4%)	1724/48 882 (3.5%)	−254·5	607·2		34% (3)

Heterogeneity of odds reductions:
– between four high risk categories χ^2_3 = 9.8; P=0.02
– between high risk and low risk χ^2_1 = 0.9; NS

[†]Crude, unadjusted control total = 1473/43 161.
Missing: 23 trials (estimated 5% of the non–fatal myocardial infarctions).

Scale: 0   0·5   1·0   1·5   2·0
Antiplatelet therapy better | Antiplatelet therapy worse
Treatment effect 2P<0·00001

Fig. 18.17. Nonfatal myocardial infarction (with survival to end of study). See original article for citation of specific trials. [From Antiplatelet Trialists' Collaboration (1994), with permission.]

ysis in 1977 (Chalmers 1977) indicated a 21% reduction in mortality (15.4% vs 20%). These statistical methods using pooling techniques were not well accepted at the time; more recent reanalysis using more rigorous statistical methods confirm that antico-agulation therapy after MI reduces mortality by about 22% (95% CI: -8% to -35%; $p < .0001$) (Peto 1978; Mitchell 1981; Yusuf 1988).

The Dutch Sixty Plus Study (Sixty Plus Reinfarction Study Research Group 1980) randomized patients over the age of 60 who were already receiving anticoagulants for an MI more than six months earlier to either continue on coumadin or to discontinue coumadin and use placebo instead. After two years of follow-up there was a 43% reduction in mortality in the coumadin group (7.5% vs 13.4%, $p = .017$) and a 51% reduction in nonfatal reinfarction (4.1% vs 8.4%; $p = .008$). The anticoagulated group also had fewer intracranial events than the placebo group (3.5% vs 5.6%), although this difference was not statistically significant ($p = .18$). There were more intracranial hemorrhages in the anticoagulated group (1.6%) than in the placebo group (0.2%),

NON–FATAL STROKE (with survival to end of study)

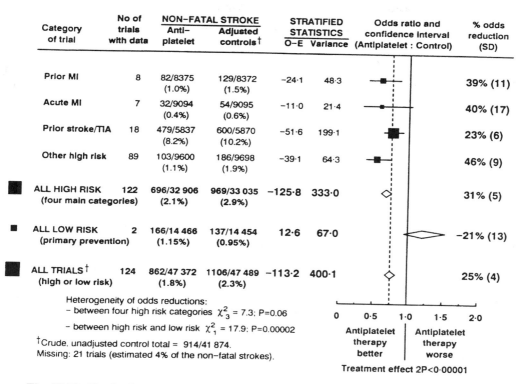

Category of trial	No of trials with data	NON–FATAL STROKE		STRATIFIED STATISTICS		Odds ratio and confidence interval (Antiplatelet : Control)	% odds reduction (SD)
		Anti-platelet	Adjusted controls†	O–E	Variance		
Prior MI	8	82/8375 (1.0%)	129/8372 (1.5%)	−24·1	48·3		39% (11)
Acute MI	7	32/9094 (0.4%)	54/9095 (0.6%)	−11·0	21·4		40% (17)
Prior stroke/TIA	18	479/5837 (8.2%)	600/5870 (10.2%)	−51·6	199·1		23% (6)
Other high risk	89	103/9600 (1.1%)	186/9698 (1.9%)	−39·1	64·3		46% (9)
ALL HIGH RISK (four main categories)	122	696/32 906 (2.1%)	969/33 035 (2.9%)	−125·8	333·0		31% (5)
ALL LOW RISK (primary prevention)	2	166/14 466 (1.15%)	137/14 454 (0.95%)	12·6	67·0		−21% (13)
ALL TRIALS† (high or low risk)	124	862/47 372 (1.8%)	1106/47 489 (2.3%)	−113·2	400·1		25% (4)

Heterogeneity of odds reductions:
- between four high risk categories $\chi^2_3 = 7.3$; P=0.06
- between high risk and low risk $\chi^2_1 = 17.9$; P=0.00002

†Crude, unadjusted control total = 914/41 874.
Missing: 21 trials (estimated 4% of the non-fatal strokes).

Antiplatelet therapy better | Antiplatelet therapy worse

Treatment effect 2P<0·00001

Fig. 18.18. Nonfatal stroke (with survival to end of study). See original article for citation of specific trials. [From Antiplatelet Trialists' Collaboration (1994), with permission.]

but this untoward effect was offset by a beneficial reduction in the incidence of cerebral thrombosis or cerebral emboli. Extracranial hemorrhage was more common in the coumadin group (6.2%) than in the placebo group (0.7%), but there was no fatal extracranial hemorrhages. A recent Norwegian trial confirmed more definitively the value of oral anticoagulation initiated routinely a mean of 27 days post-MI and followed for a mean of 37 months (Smith 1990). In this double-blind trial 1,214 patients were randomly assigned to receive warfarin or placebo. The target International Normalized Ratio (INR) was 2.8 to 4.8 in the treated patients. Among these treated with active therapy there was a 24% reduction in mortality ($p = .027$), 34% reduction in nonfatal MI ($p = .007$), and a 55% reduction in stroke ($p = .0015$). Minor bleeding occurred in 7% of patients treated with warfarin and 4% of patients treated with placebo, although "serious" bleeding occurred in only 0.6% of anticoagulated patients per year compared with 0% in the placebo group.

Earlier studies of anticoagulation therapy have used a target INR of 2.8 to 4.8 to maintain anticoagulation. It is unknown whether lower values of INR would also be

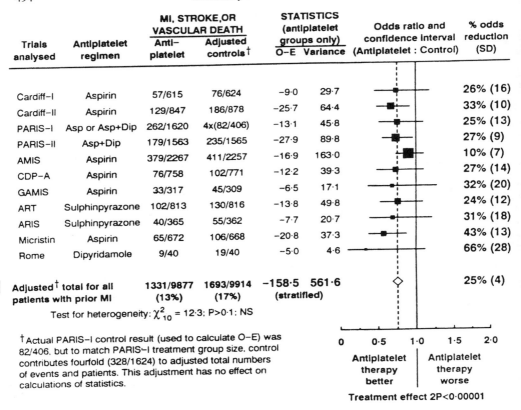

Trials analysed	Antiplatelet regimen	MI, STROKE, OR VASCULAR DEATH		STATISTICS (antiplatelet groups only)		Odds ratio and confidence interval (Antiplatelet : Control)	% odds reduction (SD)
		Anti-platelet	Adjusted controls†	O−E	Variance		
Cardiff−I	Aspirin	57/615	76/624	−9·0	29·7		26% (16)
Cardiff−II	Aspirin	129/847	186/878	−25·7	64·4		33% (10)
PARIS−I	Asp or Asp+Dip	262/1620	4x(82/406)	−13·1	45·8		25% (13)
PARIS−II	Asp+Dip	179/1563	235/1565	−27·9	89·8		27% (9)
AMIS	Aspirin	379/2267	411/2257	−16·9	163·0		10% (7)
CDP−A	Aspirin	76/758	102/771	−12·2	39·3		27% (14)
GAMIS	Aspirin	33/317	45/309	−6·5	17·1		32% (20)
ART	Sulphinpyrazone	102/813	130/816	−13·8	49·8		24% (12)
ARIS	Sulphinpyrazone	40/365	55/362	−7·7	20·7		31% (18)
Micristin	Aspirin	65/672	106/668	−20·8	37·3		43% (13)
Rome	Dipyridamole	9/40	19/40	−5·0	4·6		66% (28)
Adjusted† total for all patients with prior MI		**1331/9877** **(13%)**	**1693/9914** **(17%)**	**−158·5** **(stratified)**	**561·6**		**25% (4)**

Test for heterogeneity: χ^2_{10} = 12·3; P>0·1: NS

† Actual PARIS−I control result (used to calculate O−E) was 82/406, but to match PARIS−I treatment group size, control contributes fourfold (328/1624) to adjusted total numbers of events and patients. This adjustment has no effect on calculations of statistics.

0   0·5   1·0   1·5   2·0

Antiplatelet therapy better   Antiplatelet therapy worse

Treatment effect 2P<0·00001

Fig. 18.19. Proportional effects on vascular events (myocardial infarction, stroke, or vascular death) in 11 randomized trials of prolonged antiplatelet therapy (for 1 month or more) versus control in patients with prior myocardial infarction. *O-E*, observed minus expected; *Asp*, aspirin; *Dip*, dipyridamide; *MI*, myocardial infarction. See original article for citation of specific trials. [From Antiplatelet Trialists' Collaboration (1994), with permission.]

associated with a significant benefit with perhaps lower incidence of bleeding. Lower levels of anticoagulation may also allow for safe and concomitant use of aspirin to provide complementary and perhaps additive mechanisms for secondary prevention. The Coumadin-Aspirin Reinfarction Study (CARS) is now in progress and will determine the safety and efficacy of three regimens: aspirin 160 mg/day, aspirin 80 mg/day plus warfarin 1 mg/day, and aspirin 80 mg/day plus warfarin 3 mg/day.

Angiotensin Converting Enzyme (ACE) Inhibitors

The Cooperative North Scandinavian Enalapril Survival Study (CONSENSUS), Studies of Left Ventricular Dysfunction (SOLVD), and VA Heart Failure Trial (VEHF) studies demonstrated the value of combined afterload and preload reduction therapy

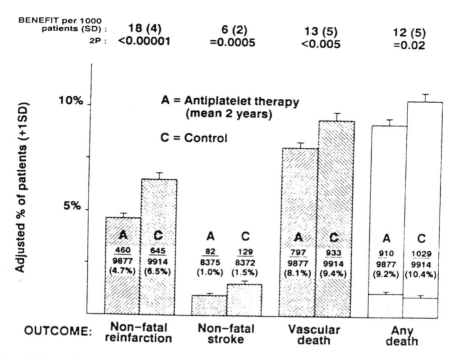

Fig. 18.20. Effects of antiplatelet therapy in patients with prior MI. See original article for citation of specific trials. [From Antiplatelet Trialists' Collaboration (1994), with permission.]

to improve morbidity and mortality in patients with established CHF. Pfeffer and colleagues (Pfeffer 1990) were the first to focus such therapy early after MI at a time when the initial insult of myocardial loss occurred, but before the manifestations of progressive ventricular enlargement, architectural remodeling, and CHF developed. In their studies, the process of progressive enlargement in the rat model did not occur in the setting of small MIs, but were associated only with MIs that were either moderate or large in size. Afterload reduction alone (e.g., with hydralazine) was unable to prevent ventricular remodeling following experimental MI, while combined afterload and preload reduction with an ACE inhibitor (e.g., captopril) was effective. The successful results from their early pilot study in patients with a first anterior MI (Pfeffer 1988) led to a large-scale clinical trial of 2,200 patients with an ejection fraction ≤40%, but without overt CHF, who were randomized to receive either captopril (therapy titrated to 50 mg t.i.d.) or placebo starting 3–14 days after MI in addition to routine post-MI management (Pfeffer 1992). Captopril therapy was associated with a 19% improvement in survival as well as a significant reduction in cardiovascular mortality, and the development and consequences of congestive failure (Figure 18.21). Of note, captopril also significantly reduced the rate of reinfarction,

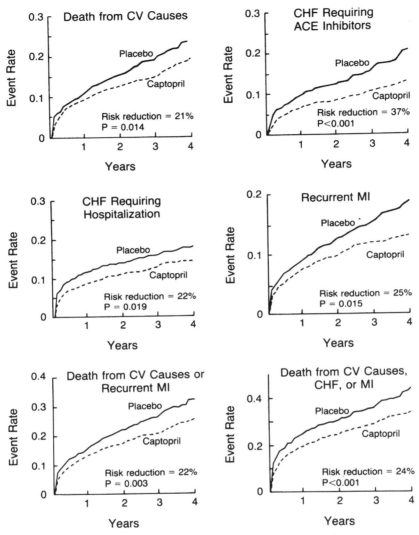

Fig. 18.21. Effect of captopril on morbidity and mortality post-MI. [From Pfeffer et al. (1992), with permission.]

which appeared to be unrelated to the drug's hemodynamic effects and may have been related to the drug's inhibition of growth factors in the vessel wall associated with progressive atherosclerosis. The range of benefits from captopril occurred in addition to the benefits of aspirin, beta-blockade, and thrombolysis. The AIRE study confirmed these findings in post-MI patients who manifested signs of CHF at the time of randomization, Acute Infarction Ramipril Efficacy (AIRE) Study Investigators 1993).

Antiarrhythmic Drugs

Many of the early studies investigating the value of antiarrhythmic drug therapy for post-MI patients were limited by small sample size, concomitant use of other possibly confounding medications, and inconsistent drug adherence (Furberg 1983). Meta-analyses of these combined studies, however, suggested that therapy was associated with a significant increase in mortality (Lau 1992).

The two recently published reports from the CAST (CAST 1989; CAST II 1992) demonstrate definitively that Class I antiarrhythmic therapy to suppress VPBs in a post-MI population actually increases mortality. In this study, large number of antiarrhythmic drugs were screened to identify which agents were most effective in reducing ventricular ectopy, and three agents were selected for study: encainide, flecainide, and moricizine. Patients were enrolled if they had more than six VPBs/hour, which were asymptomatic or mildly symptomatic, a left ventricular ejection fraction $\geq 30\%$, and experienced an MI from six days to two years before enrollment. All patients demonstrated suppression of the VPBs before randomization to drug or placebo. Each of the three active antiarrhythmic agents significantly increased mortality: the groups receiving encainide or flecainide were terminated prematurely because of an excess number of deaths (CAST 1989), and the group receiving moricizine completed the study but were nevertheless found to have an increased mortality (CAST II 1992).

Teo and colleagues (1993) recently completed a meta-analysis evaluating all forms of antiarrhythmic drug therapy used prophylactically following MI. The trials evaluating the specific Class I antiarrhythmic drugs are displayed in Table 18.9 and the effects on mortality in Table 18.10 and Figure 18.22. Except for the CAST studies, none of the individual trials investigating Class I antiarrhythmic agents showed a statistically significant difference in mortality between patients receiving active or placebo treatment. Combining all the patients in these studies, however, there was a significant increase in mortality in those assigned to active antiarrhythmic therapy (odds ratio: 1.14; 95% CI: 1.01–1.28; $p = .03$).

There have been a number of recent studies investigating the efficacy of amiodarone, a highly promising Class III antiarrhythmic agent (Table 18.11). The electrophysiologic properties of this agent are still incompletely understood, but the drug lengthens both the action potential duration and refractory period, it depresses the fast sodium channel, inhibits sympathetic activity, and blocks the L-type calcium channel (Nademanee 1993). Although only one of the trials reported a statistically significant reduction in mortality among patients randomly assigned to receive amiodarone, seven of the nine trials showed a trend toward a reduction in mortality (Teo 1993). When the data from these studies are pooled, the reduction in odds of death associated with amiodarone were significant (odd ratio: 0.71; 95% CI: 0.51–0.97; $p = .03$) (Table 18.11). Ongoing trials involving larger numbers of patients may yield more definitive results.

The conclusion from the CAST trials is that suppression of asymptomatic or minimally symptomatic VPBs in a post-MI population at low risk by the two Class IC and one Class IA agents studied is harmful (CAST and Beyond 1990). It is not clear how these results should be extrapolated to other antiarrhythmic agents or to patients with sustained or symptomatic ventricular tachycardia. Certainly the preliminary re-

Table 18.9. Summary of Trials That Evaluated Class I Antiarrhythmic Agents

| | | No. of Trials[a] | | | | | |
| | | Intervention[b] | | Treatment Duration[c] | | | |
Agent	No. of Patients	Early	Late	Short	Medium	Long	Total
Class IA							
Quinidine	207	1	1	2	—[d]	—	2
Procainamide hydrochloride	364	2	3	2	1	2	5
Disopyramide	2,912	6	1	5	2	—	7
Imipramine hydrochloride	202	—	1	—	—	1	1
Moncizine	2,897	—	3	1	—	2	3
Class IB							
Lidocaine (intravenous)	2,640	10	—	10	—	—	10
Lidocaine intramuscular	7,475	7	—	7	—	—	7
Tocainide	1,446	5	1	4	—	2	6
Phenytoin	718	1	1	—	—	2	2
Mexiletine hydrochloride	1,734	6	1	3	2	2	7
Class IC							
Aprindine	513	—	3	—	1	2	3
Encainide hydrochloride	1,181	—	3	1	—	2	3
Flecainide	844	—	2	—	—	2	2
Quin/ids/mex[e]	96	—	1	—	—	1	1
Total	23,229	38	21	35	6	18	59

Source: From Teo KK et al. (1993), with permission. See original article for citation of specific trials.

[a]In all trials, patients were randomized to active or control treatment. Study design was open label or unblinded in eight trials, single blind in one trial, and double blind in the rest.

[b]Early intervention indicates treatment allocation was assigned within 72 hours of onset of symptoms or as soon as possible after hospital admissionn; late intervention indicates patients enrolled at least 4 days after myocardial infarction.

[c]Durations of treatment: short indicates 2 weeks or less; medium, longer than 2 weeks, but shorter than 3 months; long, 3 months or longer.

[d]Ellipses indicate not available.

[e]Quin/dis/mex indicates the combination of quinidine, disopyramide, and mexileteine hydrochloride vs placebo.

498

Table 18.10. Summary of Mortality in Randomized Trials of Class I Antiarrhythmic Agents[a]

Agent (No. of Trials)	Allocation: No. Deaths/No. Randomized		Odds Ratio (95% CI)	p
	Active Treatment	Control		
Class IA				
Quinidine (2)	10/94	6/113	2.05 (0.73–5.78)	.17
Procainamide hydrochloride (5)	15/182	19/182	0.77 (0.38–1.56)	.46
Disopyramide (7)	104/1,460	98/1,452	1.06 (0.80–1.41)	.68
Imipramine hydrochloride (1)	7/102	6/100	1.15 (0.38–3.54)	.80
Moricizine (3)	117/1,454	88/1,443	1.39 (1.04–1.87)	.02
Subtotal (18)	253/3,292	217/3,290	1.19 (0.99–1.44)	.07
Class IB				
Lidocaine (Intravenous) (10)	103/1,379	76/1,261	1.23 (0.91–1.68)	.18
Lidocaine (Intramuscular) (7)	53/3,737	47/3,738	1.02 (0.68–1.53)	.94
Tocainide (6)	20/721	23/725	0.87 (0.47–1.60)	.66
Phenytoin (2)	41/359	40/359	1.04 (0.65–1.65)	.88
Mexiletine hydrochloride (7)	89/872	89/862	0.99 (0.72–1.36)	.94
Subtotal (32)	306/7,068	275/6,945	1.06 (0.89–1.26)	.50
Class IC				
Aprindine (3)	28/258	37/255	0.72 (0.53–1.22)	.22
Encainide hydrochloride (3)	45/619	24/562	1.82 (1.12–2.97)	.02
Flecainide (2)	24/426	13/418	1.82 (0.94–3.53)	.07
Subtotal (8)	97/1,313	74/1,235	1.31 (0.95–1.79)	.10
Quin/dis/mex (1)	4/49	5/47	0.75 (0.19–1.79)	.68
Total (59)	660/11,712 (5.6%)	571/11,517 (5.0%)	1.14 (1.01–1.28)	.03

Source: From Teo et al. (1993), with permission. See original article for citation of specific trials.

[a]CI indicates confidence interval; Quin/dis/mex, the combination of quinidine, disopyramide, and mexiletine hydrochloride vs placebo.

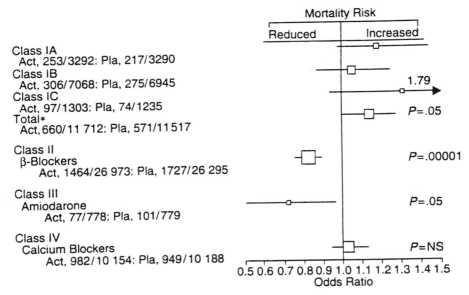

Fig. 18.22. Effects of antiarrhythmic agents on mortality. Typical odds ratio (*OR*) by classes (I, II, III, and IV) and subclasses IA, IB, and IC. Areas of squares are proportional to the variance for each trial or group of trials. *Bars* indicate 95% confidence intervals. *Portions to left* of vertical line (corresponding to OR < 1.0) indicate reduced risk with treatment; *portions to right* of vertical line indicated increased risk with treatment. Mortality data (number of deaths/number allocated treatment) are provided for active treatment (*ACT*) and placebo or control (*Pla*). Note that in the trials of class I agents there was an overall increased risk (with excesses observed in classes IA, IB, and IC). The use of classes II and III significantly reduced risk, and with class IV there was a nonsignificant trend toward excess risk. *Asterisk* indicates that data from a small trial of three class I agents (quinidine, disopyramide, and mexiletine), excluded from data for the individual subclasses, have been included in overall class I data. Please see original article for citation of specific trials. [From Teo et al. (1993), with permission.]

sults with amiodarone are encouraging. As discussed earlier, the beta-blockers have also been remarkably effective in secondary prevention and, in particular, in preventing sudden death due presumably to arrhythmias. One of the major mechanisms of beta-blocker action appears to be an antiarrhythmic effect, and, quite uniquely, these drugs have not been known to be proarrhythmic. Trials are now in progress investigating a variety of intervention modelities such as antiarrhythmic drugs and antitachycardia devices, and their results are awaited with great interest.

Estrogen Replacement Therapy

Estrogen replacement therapy (ERT) for postmenopausal women exerts important effects of improving the lipid risk factors (lowering serum LDL and raising serum HDL), improving vascular endothelial function, and may exert an independent antiathero-

Table 18.11. Summary of Mortality in Randomized Trials of Amiodarone

Trial	Allocation, No. Deaths/ No. Randomized		Odds Ratio (95% CI)	p
	Active Treatment	Control		
Hockings et al.	16/100	11/100	1.53 (0.68–3.44)	.30
Burkart et al.	5/98	15/114	0.39 (0.16–0.98)	.05
Cairns et al.	5/48	6/29	0.43 (0.10–1.77)	.22
Nicholas et al.	8/26	8/24	0.89 (0.27–2.89)	.84
Ceremuzynski et al.	21/304	33/308	0.62 (0.36–1.09)	.10
Hamer et al.	6/19	6/15	0.70 (0.17–2.82)	.62
Garguichevich et al.	6/56	12/51	0.40 (0.15–1.11)	.08
Spanish trial				
EF 0.20–0.25	4/115	9/123	0.48 (0.16–1.46)	.20
EF <0.20	6/11	1/15	10.37 (1.86–76.28)	.02
Total	77/778	101/779	0.71 (0.51–0.97)	.03

Source: From Teo KK et al. (1993), with permission. See original article for citation of specific studies.

sclerotic effect on the arterial wall itself (Grady 1992; Belchetz 1994). See Chapter 16 for a more detailed review of the cardioprotective effects of estrogen.

The relationship between ERT and coronary disease has been studied in many clinical trials, although randomized secondary prevention trials of estrogen therapy in postmenopausal women with CHD have not been conducted. The majority of published cohort studies and cross-sectional angiographic studies demonstrate a significant reduction in the risk of coronary disease. A number of case-control studies have reported less consistent results. Metanalyses indicate highly significant risk reductions for CHD of 35% to 45%, and pooled analyses of internally controlled prospective studies and cross-sectional angiographic trials indicate risk reduction of 50% (Grady 1992). Some studies have demonstrated significant risk reduction for nonfatal and fatal CHD, as well as all-cause mortality. Some studies indicate that the risk reduction associated with ERT is even more substantial in women with existing vascular disease, and the American College of Physicians has recently published guidelines indicating that postmenopausal women with coronary disease constitute a group most likely to benefit from hormone replacement therapy and recommend its use in these patients.

Although the observational studies have generally concluded that hormone replacement therapy exerts an independent protective effect against coronary, one cannot adjust entirely for possible confounding effects and other sources of bias in observational studies. The NHLBI has now initiated prosective, double-blind, randomized, and placebo-controlled studies, such as the Women's Health Initiative and the Angiographic Trial in Women, to test reliably the effects of hormone replacement therapy on postmenopausal women with coronary disease; the results are awaited with great interest.

Cardiac Rehabilitation and Exercise Training

The long-term benefits of cardiac rehabilitation are controversial. It has been difficult to demonstrate mortality benefits for exercise training in individual trials due to small

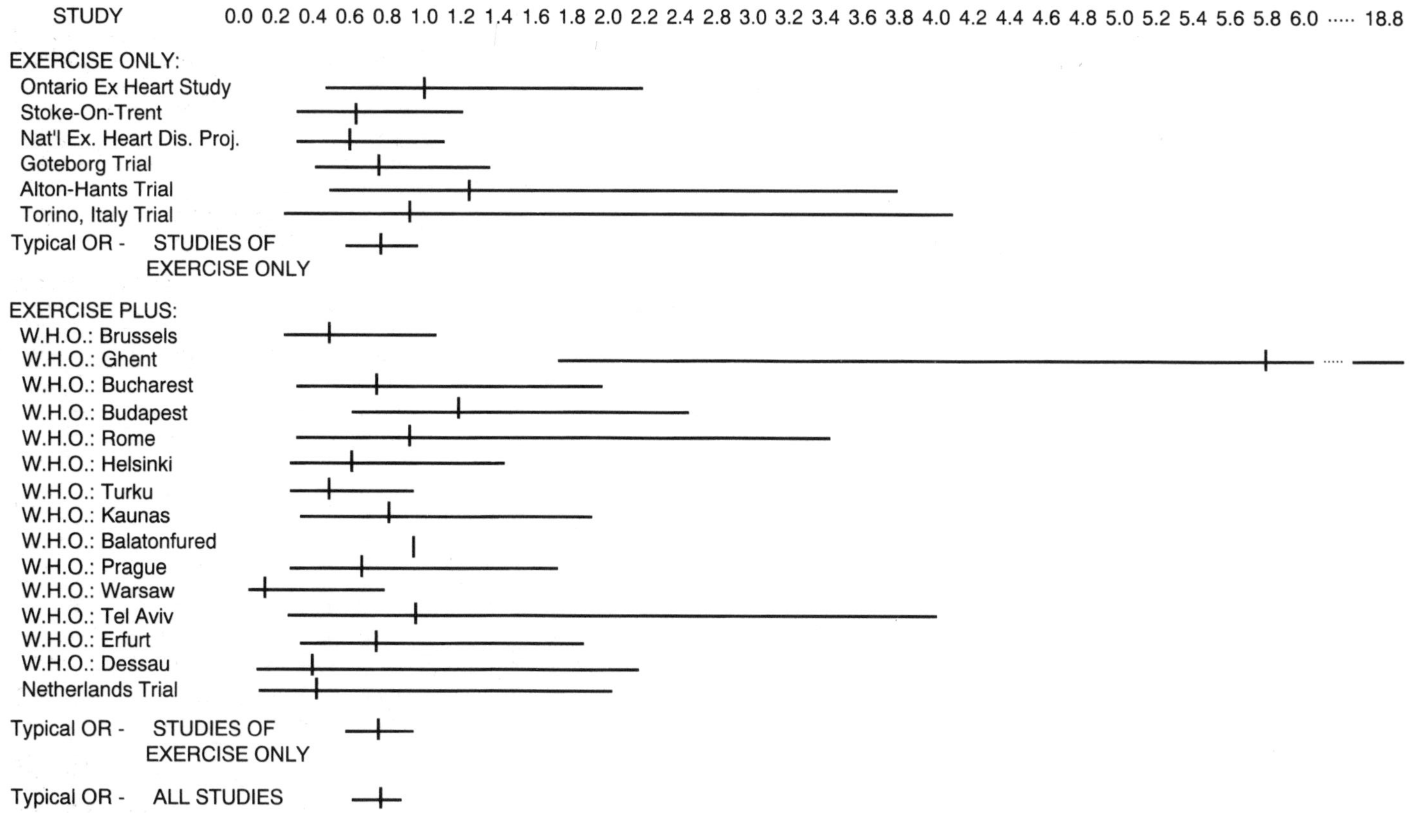

Fig. 18.23. Chart of effects of pooling from randomized trials of cardiac rehabilitation on the estimate of mortality 3 years after randomization. *Short vertical lines* indicate the point estimates; *horizontal lines* depict the 95% confidence intervals. See original article for citation of specific trials. [From O'Connor et al. (1989), with permission.]

Table 18.12. Cumulative Metanalyses of Secondary Prevention Treatment

Treatment	Trials (No.)	Patient (No.)	Cumulative Odds Ratio (95% CI)	Cumulative p Value
Anticoagulants	12	4,975	0.78 (0.67–0.90)	<.001
Rehabilitation regiman	23	5,022	0.80 (0.76–0.95)	.012
Beta-blockers	17	20,138	0.81 (0.73–0.89)	<.001
Cholesterol reduction	8	10,775	0.86 (0.79–0.94)	<.001
Antiplatelet agents	10	18,411	0.90 (0.82–1.00)	.051
	9	13,917	0.83 (0.74–0.93)	.002
Ca^{2+} channel blockers	6	13,114	1.01 (0.09–1.12)	.91
Class 1 antiarrhythmics	11	4,336	1.28 (1.02–1.61)	.03

Source: From Lau et al. (1992), with permission⟩

sample size and inadequate compliance. In the United States, the National Exercise and Heart Disease Project (Shaw 1980) was one of the most closely controlled and well-executed randomized studies of the effects of exercise in post-MI patients. The study was a three-year multicenter trial that randomized men to a supervised exercise program or to routine post-MI care. In the intervention group, overall mortality was reduced by 37%, cardiovascular deaths by 29%, nonsudden cardiovascular deaths 56%, and all MIs by 24%. Despite enrollment of 651 subjects, however, none of the differences in the study achieved statistical significance. O'Connor and colleagues (1989) have calculated that a trial would require at least 4,000 patients to reliably detect a 20% reduction in cardiovascular mortality. Prohibitive costs may prevent the performance of such a study.

Table 18.13. Recommendations for Routine Secondary Prevention Management

Treatment	Recommended	Comment
1. Beta-blockers	Yes	For all patients, especially those whose MI was complicated by electrical or mechanical disturbances
2. Aspirin	Yes	For all patients without contraindications. Optimal dose probably ≤325 mg q.d. or q.o.d.
3. Anticoagulants	Yes	Unless anticoagulants are specifically indicated (i.e., presence of LV mural thrombus or prior stroke), aspirin is a more convenient and safe intervention than coumadin
4. ACE inhibitors	Yes	For patients with LVEF < 40%
5. Cholesterol-lowering strategies	Yes	Especially in patients with an elevated baseline serum cholesterol level.
6. Ca^{2+}-channel blockers	Possibly	Diltiazem or verapamil may be indicated if the patient cannot tolerate a beta-blocker
7. Antiarrhythmic Agents		
Class 1	No	
Class 3 (Amiodarone)	Possibly	More definitive studies are in progress.
8. Habitual exercise	Yes	For all patients

A meta-analysis of all randomized trials of cardiac rehabilitation after acute MI was recently reported, which accumulated a large enough "sample size" to form statistically meaningful conclusions (O'Connor 1989). Although none of the individual studies was large enough to demonstrate a statistically significant difference in outcome, the combined cohort of 4,554 patients indicated that exercise training significantly reduced the risk of death by 20% and fatal reinfarction by 25% (Figure 18.23). The reduced risk of cardiovascular mortality and fatal MI persisted for at least three years after the index event, while a reduction in sudden death was noted for the first year after MI. No benefit was observed for nonfatal recurrent MI. The benefits of habitual exercise are further supported by data from the Determinants of Myocardial Infarction Onset Study (Mittleman 1993). Interviews were conducted with patients soon after their MI to assess the relationship of heavy exercise with the incidence of MI. Among patients who usually exercised less than once/week, heavy exertion was associated with a relative risk of 107 for MI (95% CI: 67–117). However, patients who exercised five or more times/week had a 50-fold less relative risk (2.4; 95% CI: 1.5–3.7). Thus, frequent exercise may actually be protective from MIs associated with exertion.

Summary and Conclusions

Patients remain at increased risk of death and recurrent MI following an index MI. Secondary prevention efforts are directed at reducing the likelihood and consequences of plaque rupture in a coronary artery and subsequent thrombus formation, preventing left ventricular enlargement and remodeling, and preventing the development of fatal ventricular arrhythmias. Table 18.12 summarizes the meta-analysis results from the large number of studies attempting to accomplish these goals. In many instances the specific mechanism of action of the intervention cannot be determined precisely, but can only be surmised. The sample sizes utilized by many of the individual studies have been inadequate to achieve definitive statistically significant results, but the meta-analyses provide a technique whereby the "pooled" study cohorts provide adequate sample size. The results of these individual and pooled analyses indicate that beta-blockers, antiplatelet agents, anticoagulants, ACE inhibitors, and most likely cholesterol-lowering agents are beneficial and should be recommended routinely for most patients after MI unless contraindicated (Table 18.13). Participation in a program of exercise training is also of significant value. In contrast, Ca^{2+}-blockers and Class 1 antiarrhythmic drugs are not useful when employed routinely and may even increase mortality.

The results of these carefully controlled clinical trials, and of the pooled analyses when individual studies were of inadequate statistical power, now enable physicians to select carefully among the many interventions currently available (Table 18.13) to provide optimal and routine protection to patients post-MI.

Acknowledgment

We are grateful to Mr. John A. Loring for help in the preparation of this manuscript.

References

Acute Infarction Ramipril Efficacy (AIRE) Study Investigators. Effect of ramipril on mortality and morbidity of survivors of acute myocardial infarction with clinical evidence of heart failure. Lancet 1993;342:821–8.

Anderson HV, Willerson JT. Thrombolysis in acute myocardial infarction. N Engl J Med 1993; 329:703–9.

Antiplatelet Trialists' Collaboration. Secondary prevention of vascular disease by prolonged antiplatelet treatment. Br Med J 1988;296:320–31.

Antiplatelet Trialists' Collaboration. Collaborative overview of randomized trials of antiplatelet treatment. Part I: Prevention of death, myocardial infarction, and stroke by prolonged antiplatelet therapy in different categories of patient. Br Med J 1994;308:81–106.

Becker RC. Antiplatelet therapy in coronary heart disease. Emerging strategies for the treatment and prevention of acute myocardial infarction. Arch Pathol Lab Med 1993;117:89–96.

Belchetz PE. Hormonal treatment of post-menopausal women. N Engl J Med 1994;330:1062–71.

Beta-Blocker Heart Attack Trial Research Group. A randomized trial of propranolol in patients with acute myocardial infarction. I. Mortality results. JAMA 1982;247:1707–14.

Beta-Blocker Pooling Project Research Group. The Beta-Blocker Pooling Project (BBPP): Sub-group findings from randomized trials in post-infarction patients. Eur Heart J 1988;9:8.

Bigger JT, et al. Prevalence, characteristics, and significance of ventricular tachycardia detected by 24-hour continuous electrocardiographic recordings in the late hospital phase of acute myocardial infarction. Am J Cardiol 1986;58:1151–60.

Brown G, Albers JJ, Fisher LD, et al. Regression of coronary artery disease as a result of intensive lipid-lowering therapy in men with high levels of apolipoprotein B. N Engl J Med 1990;323:1289–98.

Buchwald H, Varco RL, Matts JP, et al. Effect of partial ileal bypass surgery on mortality and morbidity from coronary heart disease in patients with hypercholesterolemia: report of the Program of the Surgical Control of Hyperlipidemias (POSCH). N Engl J Med 1990; 323:946–55.

Burr ML, Gilbert JF, Holliday RM, et al. Effects of changes in fat, fish, and fibre intakes on death and myocardial reinfarction: diet and reinfarction trial (DART). Lancet 1989;2: 757–61.

Bush TL, Barrett-Connor E, Cowan LD, et al. Cardiovascular mortality and noncontraceptive use of estrogen in women: results from the Lipid Research Clinics Program Follow-up Study. Circulation 1987;5:1102–9.

Byington RP, Furberg CD. Beta blockers during and after acute myocardial infarction. In: Francis, Aplert, eds. Modern coronary care. Boston, MA: Little, Brown, 1990:511–39.

Cairns JA, Gent M, Singer J, et al. Aspirin, sufinpyrazone, or both in unstable angina: results of a Canadian multicenter trial. N Engl J Med 1985;313:1369–75.

Cardiac Arrhythmia Suppression Trial (CAST) Investigators. Preliminary report: effect of encainide and flecainide on mortality in a randomized trial of arrhythmia suppression after myocardial infarction. N Engl J Med 1989;321:406–12.

Cardiac Arrhythmia Suppression Trial II Investigators. Effect of the antiarrhythmia agent moricizine on survival after myocardial infarction. N Engl J Med 1992;327:227–33.

Carlson LA, Rosenhamer G. Reduction of mortality in the Stockholm Ischaemic Heart Disease Secondary Prevention Study by combined treatment with clofibrate and nicotinic acid. Acta Med Scand 1988;233:405–18.

CAST and Beyond: implications of the Cardiac Arrhythmia Suppression Trial. Circulation 1990; 81:1123–7.

Chalmers TC, Matta RJ, Smith H, Kunzler AM. Evidence favoring the use of anticoagulants in the hospital phase of acute myocardial infarction. N Engl J Med 1977;297:1091–6.

Cohn JN, Archibald DO, Zeische S, et al. Effect of vasodilator therapy on mortality in chronic congestive heart failure: results of a Veterans' Administration Cooperative Study. N Engl J Med 1986;314:1547–52.

CONSENSUS Trial Study Group. Effects of enalapril on mortality in severe congestive heart failure: results of the Cooperative North Scandinavian Enalapril Survival Study (CONSENSUS). N Engl J Med 1987;316:1429–35.

Constantinides P. Atherosclerosis: a general survey and synthesis. Surv Synth Pathol Res 1984; 3:477–98.

Coronary Drug Project Research Group. Clotibrate and niacin in coronary heart disease. JAMA 1975;231:360.

Davies MJ, Thomas AC. Plaque fissuring: the cause of acute myocardial infarction, sudden death, and crescendo angina. Br Heart J 1985;53:363–73.

Davies MJ. A macro and micro view of coronary vascular insult in ischemic heart disease. Circulation 1990;82(Suppl II):II-38–46.

De Lorgerli M, Renaud S, Mamelle N, et al. Mediterranean alphs-linolenic acid-rich diet in secondary prevention of coronary heart disease. Lancet 1994;343:1454–9.

Dorr AE, Gunderson K, Schneider JC Jr, et al. Colestipol hydrochloride in hypercholesterolemic patients: effect on serum cholesterol and mortality. J Chron Dis 1978;31:5–14.

Expert Panel. Report of the National Cholesterol Education Panel on detection, evaluation, and treatment of high blood cholesterol in adults. Arch Intern Med 1988;148:36–69.

Expert Panel on Detection, Evaluation, and Treatment of High Blood Cholesterol in Adults. Summary of the second report of the National Cholesterol Education Program (NCEP) expert panel on detection, evaluation, and treatment of high blood cholesterol in adults (Adult Treatment Panel II). JAMA 1993;269:3015–23.

Falk E. Plaque rupture with severe pre-existing stenosis precipitating coronary thrombosis: characteristics of coronary atherosclerotic plaques underlying fatal occlusive thrombi. Br Heart J 1983;50:127–34.

Friedman LM, Byington RP, Capone RJ, et al. Effect of propranol in post-infarction patients with mechanical or electrical complications. Circulation 1984;69:761.

Furberg CD. Effect of antiarrhythmic drugs on mortality after myocardial infarction. Am J Cardiol 1983;52:32C–6C.

Furberg CD, Hawkins CM, Lichstein E, for the Beta-Blocker Heart Attack Trial Study Group. Circulation 1984;69:761–765.

Furberg CD, Byington RP, Crouse JR, Espeland MA. Pravastatin, lipids, and major coronary events. Am J Cardiol 1994;73:1133–4.

Fuster V, Badimon L, Badimon JJ, Chesebro JH. The pathogenesis of coronary artery disease and the acute coronary syndromes. N Engl J Med 1992;326:242–50, 310–18.

Gaudron P, Eilles C, Kugler I, Ertl G. Progressive left ventricular dysfunction and remodeling after myocardial infarction. Circulation 1993;87:755–63.

Goldman L, Cook F, Hashimoto B, et al. Evidence that hospital care for acute myocardial infarction has not contributed to the decline in coronary mortality between 1973–1974 and 1978–1979. Circulation 1982;65:936–42.

Goldman L, Sia BST, Cook EF, et al. Cost and effectiveness of routine therapy with long-term beta-adrenergic antagonists after acute myocardial infarction. N Engl J Med 1988;319:152–7.

Goldman L, Gordon DJ, Rifkind BM, et al. Cost and health implications of cholesterol lowering. Circulation 1992;85:1960-8.

Gotto AM, Farmer JA. Risk factors for coronary artery disease. In: Braunwald E. Heart disease, 4th ed. Philadelphia: WB Saunders, 1992:1125–60.

Grady D, Rubin SM, Petitti B, et al. Hormone therapy to prevent disease and prolong life in postmenopausal women. Ann Intern Med 1992;117:1016–36.

Held PH, Yusuf S, Furberg CD. Calcium channel blockers in acute myocardial infarction and unstable angina: an overview. Br Med J 1989;299:1187–92.

Holme I. An analysis of randomized trials evaluating the effect of cholesterol reduction on total mortality and coronary heart disease incidence. Circulation 1990;82:1916–24.

ISIS-2 Collaboration Group. Randomized trial of intravenous streptokinase, oral aspirin, both, or neither among 17,187 cases of suspected acute myocardial infarction: ISIS-2. Lancet 1988;2:349.

Kane JP, Malloy MJ, Port TA, et al. Regression of coronary atherosclerosis during treatment of familial hypercholesterolemia with combined drug regimens. JAMA 1990;269:3007–12.

Keys A, Menotti A, Aravanis C, et al. The seven countries study: 2,289 deaths in 15 years. Prev Med 1984;13:141–154.

Kjekshus JK. Importance of heart rate in determining beta-blocker efficacy in acute and long-term acute myocardial infarction intervention trials. Am J Cardiol 1986;57:43F–9F.

Lau J, Antman EM, Jimenez-Silva J, et al. Cumulative meta-analysis of the therapeutic trials for myocardial infarction. N Engl J Med 1992;327:248–54.

Lee RT, Grodzinsky AJ, Frank EH, et al. Structure-dependent dynamic mechanical behavior of fibrous caps from human atherosclerotic plaques. Circulation 1991;83:1764–70.

Lewis H, Davis J, Archibald D. Protective effects of aspirin against acute myocardial infarction and death in men with unstable angina: results of a Veterans Administration cooperative study. N Engl J Med 1983;309:396–403.

Lichtlen PR, Hugenholtz PG, Rafflenbenl W, et al. , on behalf of the INTACT group. Retardation of angiographic progression of coronary artery disease by nifedipine: results of the International Nifedipine Trial on Antiatherosclerotic Therapy (INTACT). Lancet 1990;335:1109–13.

MacIsaac AI, Thomas JD, Topol EJ. Toward the quiescent coronary plaque. J Am Coll Cardiol 1993;22:1228–41.

Manninen V, Elo O, Frick H, et al. Lipid alterations and decline in the incidence of coronary heart disease in the Helsinki Heart Study. JAMA 1988;260:641–51.

Mensink RP, Katan MB. Effect of dietary fatty acids on serum lipids and lipoproteins: a meta-analysis of 27 trials. Arterioscler Thromb 1992;12:911–19.

Mitchell JRA. Anticoagulants in coronary heart disease: retrospect and prospect. Lancet 1981;2:1014–17.

Mittleman MA, Maclure M, Tofler GH, et al., for the Determinants of Myocardial Infarction Onset Study Investigators. Triggering of acute myocardial infarction by heavy physical exertion: protection against triggering by regular exertion. N Engl J Med 1993;329:1677–83.

Morganroth J, Lichstein E, Byington R, et al. Beta-blocker heart attack trial: impact of propranol therapy on ventricular arrhythmias. Prev Med 1985;14:346.

Muller JE, Tofler G, Stone PH. Circadian variation and triggers of onset of acute cardiovascular disease. Circulation 1989;79:733–43.

Multicenter Postinfarction Research Group. Risk stratification and survival after myocardial infarction. N Engl J Med 1983;309:331–6.

Nademanee K, Singh BN, Stevenson WG, Weiss JN. Amiodarone and post-MI patients. Circulation 1993;88:764–74.

Nidorf S, Parsons RW, Thompson PL, et al. Reduced risk of death at 28 days in patients taking a beta-blocker before admission to hospital with myocardial infarction. Br Med J 1990;300:71–4.

Nikkila EA, Viikinkoski P, Valle M, Frick MH. Prevention of progression of coronary athero-sclerosis by treatment of hyperlipidaemia: a seven year prospective angiographic study. Br Med J 1984;289:220–3.

O'Connor GT, Buring JE, Yusuf S, et al. An overview of randomized trials of rehabilitation with exercise after myocardial infarction. Circulation 1989;80:234–44.

Olsson G, Oden A, Johansson L, et al. Prognosis after withdrawal of chronic postinfarction metoprolol treatment: a 2–7 year follow-up. Eur Heart J 1988;9:365–72.

Olsson G. How long should post MI β-blocker therapy be continued? Primary Cardiol 1991; 17:44–9.

Ornish D, Brown SE, Scherwitz LW, et al. Can lifestyle changes reverse coronary heart disease? Lancet 1990;336:129–33.

Peto R. Clinical trial methodology. Biomed Pharmacother 1978;28(Special Issue):24–36.

Pekkanen J, Linn S, Heiss G, et al. Ten-year mortality from cardiovascular disease in relation to cholesterol level among men with and without pre-existing cardiovascular disease. N Engl J Med 1990;322:1700–7.

Pfeffer MA, Lamas GA, Vaughan DE, Parisi AF, Braunwald E. Effect of captopril on progres-sive ventricular dilatation after anterior myocardial infarction. N Engl J Med 1988;319: 80–6.

Pfeffer MA, Braunwald E. Ventricular remodeling after myocardial infarction. Experimental observations and clinical implications. Circulation 1990;81:1161–72.

Pfeffer MA, Braunwald E, Moye LA, et al. Effect of captopril on mortality and morbidity in patients with left ventricular dysfunction after myocardial infarction: results of the Sur-vival and Ventricular Enlargement Trial: The SAVE Investigators. N Engl J Med 1992; 327:669–77.

Pitt B, Mancini GBJ, Ellis SG, et al., for the PLAC I Investigators. Pravastatin limitation of atherosclerosis in the coronary arteries (PLAC I). J Am Coll Cardiol 1994;131A [Abstract].

Randomised trial of cholesterol lowering in 4444 patients with coronary heart disease: the Scandinavian Simvastatin Survival Study (4S). Lancet 1994;344:1383–9.

Richardson PD, Davies MJ, Born GV. Influence of plaque configuration and stress distribution on fissuring of coronary atherosclerotic plaques. Lancet 1989;2:941–4.

Ridker PM, Manson JE, Burning JE, et al. Circadian variation of acute myocardial infarction and the effect of low-dose aspirin in a randomized trial of physicians. Circulation 1990; 82:897–902.

Rose G, Reid DD, Hamilton PJ, et al. Myocardial ischemia risk factors and death from coronary heart disease. Lancet 1977;1:105–9.

Rossi PRF, Yusuf S, Ramsdale D, et al. Reduction of ventricular arrhythmias by early intra-venous atenolol in suspected acute myocardial infarction. Br Med J 1983;286:506–10.

Rubins HB, Robins SJ, Iwane MK, et al. Rationale and design of the Department of Veterans Affairs High-Density Lipoprotein Cholesterol Intervention Trial (HIT) for secondary prevention of coronary artery disease in men with low high-density lipoprotein choles-terol and desirable low-density lipoprotein cholesterol. Am J Cardiol 1993;71:45–52.

Sacks FM, Pfeffer MA, Moye L, et al. Rationale and design of a secondary prevention trial of lowering normal plasma cholesterol levels after acute myocardial infarction: the Cho-lesterol and Recurrent Events Trial (CARE). Am J Cardiol 1991;68:1436–46.

Sacks FM, Pasternak RC, Gibson CM, et al., for the Harvard Atherosclerosis Reversibility Project (HARP) Group. The effect on coronary atherosclerosis of improving plasma cholesterol levels in normocholesterolemic patients. Lancet 1994;344:1182–6.

Scandinavian Simvastatin Survival Study Group. Design and baseline results of patients with stable angina and/or previous myocardial infarction. Am J Cardiol 1993;71:393–400.

Schuler G, Hambrecht R, Schlierf G, et al. Regular physical exercise and low-fat diet. Effects on progression of coronary artery disease. Circulation 1992;86:1–11.

Shaw LW. Effects of a prescribed supervised exercise program on mortality and cardiovascular morbidity in patients after a myocardial infarction: the National Exercise and Heart Disease Project. Am J Cardiol 1980;48:39.

Sherry S. The anturane reinfarction trial. Circulation 1980;62(Suppl V):V-73–V-78.

Singh RB, Rostogi SS, Verma R, et al. Randomized controlled trial of cardioprotective diet in patients with recent acute myocardial infarction: results of one year follow-up. Br Med J 1992;304:1015–19.

Sixty Plus Reinfarction Study Research Group. A double-blind trial to assess long-term anticoagulant therapy in elderly patients after myocardial infarction. Lancet 1980;2:989–93.

Smith P, Arnesen H, Holme I. The effect of warfarin on mortality and reinfarction after myocardial infarction. N Engl Med 1990;323:147–52.

SOLVD Investigators. Effect of enalapril on survival in patients with reduced left ventricular ejection fractions and congestive heart failure. N Engl J Med 1991;325:293–302.

Stone PH, Antman EM, Muller JE, Braunwald E. Calcium channel blocking agents in the treatment of cardiovascular disorders. II. Hemodynamic effects and clinical applications. Ann Intern Med 1980;93:886–904.

Sullivan JM, Zqaag RV, Hughes JP, et al. Estrogen replacement and coronary artery disease: effect on survival in postmenopausal women. Arch Intern Med 1990;150:2557–662.

Teo KK, Yusuf S, Furburg CD. Effects of prophylactic antiarrhythmic drug therapy in acute myocardial infarction: an overview of results from randomized controlled trials. JAMA 1993;270:1589–95.

Theroux P, Ouimet H, McCans J, et al. Aspirin, heparin, or both to treat acute unstable angina. N Engl J Med 1988;319:1105–11.

Turpeinen O, Karvonen MJ, Pekkarinen M, et al. Dietary prevention of coronary heart disease: the Finnish Mental Hospital Study. Int J Epidemiol 1979;8:99–118.

Verheugt FWA, van der Laarse A, Funke-Kupper AJ, et al. Effects of early intervention with low-dose aspirin (100 mg) on infarct size, reinfarction and mortality in anterior wall acute myocardial infarction. Am J Cardiol 1990;66:267–70.

Verstraete M. Risk factors, interventions and therapeutic agents in the prevention of atherosclerosis-related ischemic diseases. Drugs 1991;42(Suppl. 5):22–38.

Vega GL, Grundy SM. Lipoprotein responses to treatment with lovastatin gemfibrozil, and nicotinic acid in normolipidemic patients with hypoalphalipoproteinemia. Arch Intern Med 1994;154:73–82.

Wallentin LC and the Research Group in Instability in Coronary Artery Disease in Southeast Sweden. Aspirin (75 mg/day) after an episode of unstable coronary artery disease: long-term effects on the risk for myocardial infarction, occurrence of severe angina, and the need for revascularization. J Am Coll Cardial 1991;18:1587–93.

Waters D, Lesperance J, Francetich M, et al. A controlled clinical trial to assess the effect of a calcium channel blocker upon the progression of coronary atherosclerosis. Circulation 1990;82:1940–53.

Watts GF, Lewis B, Brunt JN, et al. Effects on coronary artery disease of lipid-lowering diet, or diet plus cholestyramine. In: St. Thomas' Atherosclerosis Regression Study (STARS). Lancet 1992;339:563–9.

Weiss JN, Nademanee K, Stevenson WG, Singh B. Ventricular arrhythmias in ischemic heart disease. Ann Intern Med 1991;114:784–97.

West of Scotland Coronary Prevention Study Group. A coronary primary prevention study of Scottish men aged 45–64 years; trial design. J Clin Epidemiol 1992;45:849–60.

Wissler RW. Principles of the pathogenesis of atherosclerosis. In: Braunwald E, ed. Heart disease: a textbook of cardiovascular medicine, 2nd ed. Philadelphia: WB Saunders, 1984.

WHO cooperative trial on primary prevention of ischaemic heart disease using clofibrate to lower serum cholesterol: mortality follow-up. Report of the Committee of Principal Investigators. Lancet 1980;2:379–85.

Yusuf S, Sleight P, Rossi PRF, et al. Reduction in infarct size, arrhythmias, chest pain and morbidity by early intravenous beta-blockade in suspected acute myocardial infarction. Circulation 1983;67(Pt 2):32–41.

Yusuf S, Peto R, Lewis J, et al. Beta blockade during and after myocardial infarction: an overview of the randomized trials. Prog Cardiovasc Dis 1985;27:335–71.

Yusuf S, Held P, Furberg C. Update of effects of calcium antagonists in myocardial infarction or angina in light of the second Danish Verapamil Infarction Trial (DAVIT-II) and other recent studies. Am J Cardiol 1991;67:1295–7.

Yusuf S, Pepine CJ, Garces C, et al. Effect of enalapril on myocardial infarction and unstable angina in patients with low ejection fractions. Lancet 1992;340:1173–8.

Yusuf S, Lessem J, Jha P, Lonn E. Primary and secondary prevention of myocardial infarction and strokes: an update of randomly allocated, controlled trials. J Hypertens 1993; 11(Suppl 4):S61–S73.

VI

FUTURE DIRECTIONS AND CONCLUSIONS

19

Future Directions in Coronary Disease Prevention

Paul M. Ridker, J. Michael Gaziano, and JoAnn E. Manson

This book has focused predominantly on available methods for cardiovascular disease prevention. Wherever possible, data supporting the use of a particular intervention have been explicitly provided so that clinicians and their patients can weigh the net benefits and risks that are likely to be associated with smoking cessation, cholesterol reduction, blood pressure control, and other prudent changes. If successfully implemented on a population basis, these measures will lead to large reductions in morbidity and mortality from coronary heart disease (CHD). For clinicians, such patient-oriented interventions form the cornerstones of current practice (Manson 1992).

In the near future, a wide variety of prevention-oriented interventions will become available, greatly expanding the tools for primary and secondary prevention. In this chapter, we provide a brief discussion of the scientific and clinical agendas that may determine future directions in cardiovascular disease prevention.

The Scientific Agenda

The primary scientific goal over the next decade will be to obtain more high-quality information concerning several promising but unproven preventive measures, particularly for interventions which carry the possibility of risk. Much of this information will need to come from large-scale randomized trials so that the true benefit:risk ratio associated with a given intervention can best be judged. Two potentially important preventive strategies—postmenopausal estrogen replacement therapy and prophylactic antioxidant vitamin use—illustrate the importance of these issues. With regard to estrogen replacement therapy, prospective randomized trials of adequate sample size must be completed so that the postulated benefits of these hormones on CHD and osteoporosis can be accurately weighed against the potential for increased risks of cancer of the endometrium and breast, as well as probable increases in disease of the gallbladder (Goldman 1991). With respect to antioxidant vitamin use, the hypothesized benefits of vitamin E, beta-carotene, and vitamin C found in several observational studies (Manson 1993) must be tested in prospective randomized clinical trials, particularly as recent findings provide little evidence of efficacy for this prevalent preventive practice (Alpha-Tocopherol 1994; Greenberg 1994).

Recognizing the need to resolve these issues, the National Institutes of Health have funded the nationwide Women's Health Initiative (WHI), which includes a large-scale trial of estrogen replacement therapy (Cotton 1992). The WHI involves 40 clinical centers and plans to enroll 160,000 women, 60,000 of whom will participate in one or more of the randomized trial components, which include hormone replacement therapy, low-fat diet modification, and/or calcium and vitamin D supplementation. Other large-scale initiatives currently underway include the Women's Health Study (WHS), a prospective randomized trial of aspirin, vitamin E, and beta-carotene being conducted among a cohort of over 40,000 postmenopausal women (Womens' Health Study Research Group 1992a, 1992b), and the Women's Antioxidant Cardiovascular Study (WACS), a trial evaluating vitamins C and E and beta-carotene in the secondary prevention of CHD in women (Manson 1994). By design, these trials include very large numbers of women, a group generally not enrolled in earlier randomized trials and for whom little information is currently available on prevention (Wenger 1993). A similar secondary prevention trial of vitamin E is being planned by the GISSI Prevention Group (GISSI Prevention Study Group 1993). This latter trial is also designed to assess possible benefits of polyunsaturated fatty acids in secondary prevention of CHD.

Aggressive pharmacologic and lifestyle interventions designed to reduce low density lipoprotein cholesterol will also be evaluated in future trials to ascertain whether the costs and potential risks of this approach are acceptably balanced by a reduction in cardiovascular events. Subgroups of particular interest include individuals without CHD as well as those with known atherosclerosis but free from prior clinical events. In this regard, it is important to recall that among subjects with average cholesterol levels, it is not yet clear that net benefits will accrue from pharmacologic interventions to lower cholesterol (Rossouw 1990; Law 1994). Here again, large-scale randomized trials will be necessary to describe clearly the true risks associated with this approach as well as how large (and costly) any true benefits will be. Several such trials evaluating this issue are currently underway, including the Cholesterol and Recurrent Events (CARE) secondary prevention trial (Sacks 1991), and the Oxford University trials of primary prevention among subjects at moderate risk. The independent and combined effects of antihypertensive agents and cholesterol-reducing drugs are also being prospectively evaluated in the National Heart Lung and Blood Institute supported ALLHAT (Antihypertensive and Lipid-Lowering Treatment to Prevent Heart Attack Trial) study, which will include 40,000 high risk subjects. This trial will also provide important information for African-American individuals, who are to constitute over half of the randomized cohort.

In the important area of prevention among subjects with known CHD, other promising interventions are under evaluation. For example, data from the Studies of Left Ventricular Dysfunction (SOLVD)(SOLVD Investigators 1991, 1992) and Survival and Ventricular Enlargement (SAVE)(Pfeffer 1992) trial have led to the hypothesis that angiotensin-converting enzyme (ACE) inhibitors may play an important role in preventing myocardial infarction (MI) as well as reducing overall cardiovascular mortality. Indeed, based on the observation that recurrent rates of MI appear lower among subjects taking ACE inhibitors and upon laboratory evidence suggesting that the renin-angiotensin system may adversely effect fibrinolytic capacity (Ridker 1993a, 1995; Wright 1994), trials are now being planned to assess the efficacy of ACE-inhibiting agents for both primary and secondary prevention.

Rapid advances are also being made in the area of thrombus prevention. Specifically, a series of agents appear to have potential efficacy against several different aspects of thrombus formation. Most promising among such agents are direct thrombin inhibitors such as hirudin and hirulog (which are pharmacologically similar to hirudins isolated from medicinal leeches), as well as platelet antagonists such as the glycoprotein IIb/IIIa receptor inhibitor, and the integralins (Heras 1990; Badimon 1991). As clinical experience with these agents accumulates, randomized trials will be required to assess whether these new approaches to thrombus prevention are both efficacious and safe. If properly designed, such trials will compare the newer agents to aspirin alone, a low-cost therapy which has generally been effective and well tolerated. Recognizing that more anticoagulation is not necessarily better, other investigations are underway evaluating less aggressive antithrombotic regimens. For example, the ongoing Coumadin Aspirin Reinfarction Study (CARS) is designed to determine the safety and efficacy of very low dose aspirin either alone or in combination with low dose coumadin in the secondary prevention of MI.

In addition to obtaining further information regarding cardiovascular interventions, a second major scientific goal will be the systematic evaluation of new screening techniques designed to identify high-risk patients. In current practice, the National Cholesterol Education Program has been highly successful in increasing cholesterol awareness and screening. However, for new and potentially expensive tests such as plasma fibrinogen (Wilhelmsel 1984; Meade 1986; Kannel 1987; Yarnell 1991), factor VII (Meade 1986), D-dimer (Fowkes 1993; Ridker 1994a), lipoprotein(a) (Ridker 1993b; Schaefer 1994), and endogenous fibrinolytic activity (Hamsten 1985; Meade 1993; Ridker 1993c, 1994b), it is not yet clear whether assessing potential abnormalities of hemostasis and thrombosis adds substantially to our ability to detect individuals at risk for future cardiovascular disease. Toward this end, several prospective studies of screening are currently underway, including the Atherosclerotic Risk in Communities (ARIC) study (ARIC Investigators 1989), the Italian Progetto Lombardo Aterotrombosi (PLAT) study (Cortellaro 1991), and the European Cooperative Action on Thrombosis (ECAT) trial (Haverkate 1993). Prospective studies are critically important in evaluating the predictive role of hemostatic and thrombotic markers, since levels may change after a vascular event, making retrospective studies unreliable. For example, lipoprotein(a)—a unique lipoprotein with putative atherogenic properties—has often been considered an independent risk factor for CHD because of the finding in several retrospective studies of a positive association between this factor and risk of MI. However, in two recently published studies evaluating baseline levels of Lp(a) and the risk of future MI, the positive predictive value of measure Lp(a) was found to be poor (Ridker 1993b; Schaefer 1994). Indeed, one study found no association at all between Lp(a) and future vascular risk whereas the other found only a small positive association (Ridker 1993b, 1994c; Schaefer 1994).

Prevention research in the areas of endothelial dysfunction and silent ischemia may also lead to new interventional strategies (Meridith 1993). In particular, recent evidence from the Asymptomatic Cardiac Ischemia Pilot study suggests that low or moderate doses of anti-anginal medication can effectively suppress asymptomatic ischemia (Knatterud 1994; Pepine 1994). Based on this finding, a large-scale clinical trial is now underway to assess whether this medically aggressive approach translates into reduced rates of future cardiovascular events.

The Clinical Agenda

The second major direction cardiovascular disease prevention should take in the future is to greatly expand community-based intervention and surveillance programs. While direct physician contact will continue to be a major focus for cardiovascular prevention, it is widely recognized that successful efforts must start with healthy individuals, most of whom are outside the medical care system. Recent pathologic studies confirming that the precursors of CHD are present in many individuals at the age of 10 to 15 years strongly indicate that prevention efforts need to begin early in life (PDAY Research Group 1990).

At this time, a number of successful community-based cardiovascular prevention programs are underway. In general, the goals of these programs are to increase awareness of heart-healthy lifestyles as early as possible during elementary level education, and then reinforce these lifestyle patterns during vulnerable teenage years. Although many programs stress dietary moderation and early attention to establishing lifelong exercise habits, the most critical component of all early intervention programs must be to reduce the numbers of individuals starting a cigarette habit. This strategy is effective largely because few individuals completing their teenage years as nonsmokers ultimately become habitual nicotine consumers. Community-based initiatives to establish smoke-free worksites, public buildings, and entertainment establishments have proven successful in countering aggressive marketing to members of this vulnerable group by the tobacco industry (Breo 1993; Pertman 1994). The wider recognition of passive smoking as an important cause of CHD should also help to achieve this goal. Current data support the conclusion that environmental tobacco smoke appears to increase CHD mortality among nonsmokers by 20–70% (Wells 1994) and is responsible for as many as 40,000 ischemic heart disease deaths in the United States each year (Steenland 1992). For individuals already smoking, clinic-based strategies using proven smoking cessation techniques need to be aggressively implemented (Silagy 1994; Tang 1994).

Other outreach programs will focus specifically on case findings for very high risk individuals. For example, the MED-PED (Make Early Diagnosis to Prevent Early Deaths) program in Salt Lake City has been established to aggressively identify and bring under medical care individuals who are relatives of patients with known familial hypercholesterolemia. For subjects identified in such programs, early detection of coronary risk has proven successful in reducing rates of premature coronary events. While this approach to cardiovascular prevention is useful for individuals at very high genetic risk, the majority of cardiovascular events will occur in subjects not considered eligible for aggressive early intervention programs. Thus, broad-based approaches will remain the primary means of altering risk for the population at large.

Fortunately, programs based at the worksite focusing on cardiovascular risk reduction will likely grow in the future as the potential benefits of such programs become evident to large numbers of employers. When viewed simply in terms of improved productivity and reduced insurance premiums, the advantages of jobsite programs offering incentives for employees to begin regular exercise, undergo cholesterol testing, and attend smoking cessation classes should rapidly become apparent. In the current climate of health care reform and insurance restructuring, primary prevention programs can be expected to receive substantial federal and industry support (Fries 1993; Russell 1993). While potentially effective, jobsite programs must be seen as but one component of a broad prevention initiative directed toward implementing strategies based on currently available scientific knowledge. Such strategies will require an integrated team approach employing the skills of physicians, nurse practitioners, and health counselors, coupled with education programs and media campaigns directed at both children and adults.

Finally, successful integration of the scientific and clinical agendas for future cardiovascular prevention will also lead to changes in the process of medical education itself. Medical school and postgraduate training programs focusing on primary prevention will increase in the future as mandated shifts from subspecialty training to primary care training evolve. The recent establishment of Departments of Preventive Medicine at many medical schools and of residency training programs in cardiovascular prevention signals the widespread recognition that physician education also needs to change if cardiovascular risk reduction programs are to succeed fully.

References

Alpha-Tocopherol, Beta Corotene Cancer Prevention Study Group. The effect of vitamin E and beta carotene on the incidence of lung cancer and other cancers in male smokers. N Engl J Med 1994;330:1029–35.

ARIC Investigators. The Atherosclerosis Risk In Communities (ARIC) Study: design and objectives. Am J Epidemiol 1989;129:687–702.

Badimon L, Merino A, Badimon J, et al. Hirudin and other thrombin inhibitors: experimental results and potential clinical applications. Trends Cardiovasc Med 1991;1:261–7.

Breo DL. Kicking butts: AMA, Joe Camel, and the ''black-flag'' war on tobacco. JAMA 1993; 270:1978–84.

Cortellaro M, Boschetti C, Cofrancesco E, et al., and the PLAT Study Group. The PLAT Study: a multidisciplinary study of hemostatic function and conventional risk factors in vascular disease patients. Atherosclerosis 1991;90:109–18.

Cotton P. Women's Health Initiative leads way as research begins to fill gender gaps. JAMA 1992;267:469–70.

Fowkes FGR, Lowe GDO, Housley E, et al. Cross-linked fibrin degradation products, progression of peripheral arterial disease, and risk of coronary heart disease. Lancet 1993;342:84–6.

Fries JF, Koop CE, Beadle CE, et al., and the Health Project Consortium. Reducing health care costs by reducing the need and demand for medical services. N Engl J Med 1993;329: 321–5.

GISSI Prevention Study Group. Preventive intervention study on the atherosclerotic and thrombotic component of post acute myocardial infarction risk. GISSI Prevention Protocol, 1993.

Goldman L, Tosteson AN. Uncertainty about post-menopausal estrogen: time for action, not debate. N Engl J Med 1991;325:800–2.

Greenberg ER, Baron JA, Tosteson TD, et al. A clinical trial of antioxidant vitamins to prevent colorectal adenoma. N Engl J Med 1994;331:141–7.

Hamsten A, Wilman B, de Fai, Blomback M. Increased plasma levels of a rapid inhibitor of tissue plasminogen activator in young survivors of myocardial infarction. N Engl J Med 1985 313:1557–63.

Haverkate F, van de Loo JCW, Thompson SG, on behalf of the ECAT Angina Pectoris Study Group. Hemostasis risk markers, inflammatory and endothelial reactions in angina pectoris: results of the ECAT Angina Pectoris Study. Thromb Hemos 1993;69:1537(A).

Heras M, Chesebro JH, Webster MWI, et al. Hirudin, heparin, and placebo during deep arterial injury in the pig: the in vivo role of thrombin in platelet-mediated thrombosis. Circulation 1990;82:1476–84.

Kannel WB, Wolf PA, Castelli WP, D'Agostino RB. Fibrinogen and risk of cardiovascular disease: the Framingham Study. JAMA 1987;258:1183–6.

Knatterud G, Bourassa MG, Pepine CJ, et al. Effects of treatment strategies to suppress ischemia in patients with coronary artery disease: 12-week results of the asymptomatic cardiac ischemia pilot (ACIP) study. J Am Coll Cardiol 1994;24:11–20.

Law MR, Thompson SG, Wald NJ. Assessing possible hazards of reducing serum cholesterol. Br Med J 1994;308:373–9.

Manson JE, Tosteson H, Ridker PM, et al. Current concepts: primary prevention of myocardial infarction. N Engl J Med 1992;326:1406–16.

Manson JE, Gaziano JM, Jonas MA, Hennekens CH. Antioxidants and cardiovascular disease: a review. J Am Coll Nutr 1993;4:426–32.

Manson JE, Gaziano JM, Spelsberg A, et al. A secondary prevention trial of antioxidant vitamins and cardiovascular disease in women: rationale, research design, and methods. Ann Epidemiol 1995;5:261–9.

Meade TW, Mellows S, Brozovic M, et al. Haemostatic function and ischaemic heart disease: Principal results of the Northwick Park Heart Study. Lancet 1986;2:533–7.

Meade TW, Ruddock V, Stirling Y, et al. Fibrinolytic activity, clotting factors, and long-term incidence of ischaemic heart disease in the Northwick Park Heart Study. Lancet 1993; 324:1076–9.

Meridith IT, Yeung AC, Weidinger FF, et al. Role of impaired endothelium-dependent vasodilation in ischemic manifestations of coronary artery disease. Circulation 1993;87(Suppl V):V56–V66.

PDAY Research Group. Relationship of atherosclerosis in young men to serum lipoprotein cholesterol concentrations and smoking: a preliminary report from the Pathobiological Determinants of Atherosclerosis in Youth (PDAY) Research Group. JAMA 1990;264: 3018–24.

Pepine CJ, Geller NL, Knatterud, et al. The symptomatic cardiac ischemia pilot (ACIP) study: design of a randomized clinical trial, baseline data and implications for a long-term outcome trial. J Am Coll Cardiol 1994;24:1–10.

Pertman A. After slow start, antismoking engine is roaring. The Boston Globe, Sunday April 10, 1994, page 1.

Pfeffer MA, Braunwald E, Moye LA, et al., on behalf of the SAVE Investigators. Effect of captopril on mortality and morbidity in patients with left ventricular dysfunction after myocardial infarction. N Engl J Med 1992;327:669–77.

Ridker PM, Gaboury CL, Conlin PR, et al. Stimulation of plasminogen activator inhibitor in vivo by infusion of angiotensin II: evidence of a potential interaction between the renin angiotensin system and fibrinolytic function. Circulation 1993a;87:1969–73.

Ridker PM, Hennekens CH, Stampfer MJ. A prospective study of lipoprotein(a) and the risk of myocardial infarction. JAMA 1993b;270:2195–9.

Ridker PM, Vaughan DE, Stampfer MJ, et al. Endogenous tissue-type plasminogen activator and risk of myocardial infarction. Lancet 1993c;341:1165–8.

Ridker PM, Hennekens CH, Cerskus A, Stampfer MJ. Plasma concentration of cross linked fibrin degradation product (D-dimer) and the risk of future myocardial infarction. Circulation 1994a;90:2236–40.

Ridker PM, Hennekens CH, Stampfer MJ, et al. Prospective study of endogenous tissue plasminogen activator and risk of stroke. Lancet 1994b;343:940–3.

Ridker PM, Hennekens CH. Lipoprotein(a) and risks of cardiovascular disease. Ann Epidemiol 1994c;4:360–2.

Ridker PM, Vaughan DE. Potential antithrombotic and fibrinolytic properties of the angiotensin converting enzyme inhibitors. J Thromb Thrombol 1995;1:251–7.

Rossouw JE, Lewis B, Rifkind BM. The value of lowering cholesterol after myocardial infarction. N Engl J Med 1990;323:1112–9.

Russell LB. The role of prevention in health reform. N Engl J Med 1993;329:352–4.

Sacks FM, Pfeffer MA, Moye L, et al. Rationale and design of a secondary prevention trial of lowering normal plasma cholesterol levels after acute myocardial infarction: the Cholesterol and Recurrent Events Trial (CARE). Am J Cardiol 1991;68:1436–46.

Schaefer EJ, Lamon-Fava S, Jenner JL, et al. Lipoprotein(a) levels and risk of coronary heart disease in men: the Lipid Research Clinics Coronary Primary Prevention Trial. JAMA 1994;271:999–1003.

Silagy C, Mant D, Fowler G, Lodge M. Meta-analysis on efficacy of nicotine replacement therapies in smoking cessation. Lancet 1994;343:139–42.

SOLVD Investigators. Effect of enalapril on survival in patients with reduced left ventricular ejection fractions and congestive heart failure. N Engl J Med 1991;325:293–301.

SOLVD Investigators. Effect of enalapril on mortality and the development of heart failure in asymptomatic patients with reduced left ventricular ejection fraction. N Engl J Med 1992;327:685–91.

Steenland K. Passive smoking and risk of heart disease. JAMA 1992;267:94–9.

Tang JL, Law M, Wald N. How effective is nicotine replacement therapy in helping people to stop smoking? Br Med J 1994;308:21–6.

Wells AJ. Passive smoking as a cause of heart disease. J Am Coll Cardiol 1994;24:546–54.

Wenger NK, Speroff L, Packard B. Cardiovascular health and disease in women. N Engl J Med 1993;329:247–56.

Wilhelmsen L, Svardsudd K, Korsan-Bengtsen K, et al. Fibrinogen as a risk factor for stroke and myocardial infarction. N Engl J Med 1984;311:501–5.

Women's Health Study Research Group. The Women's Health Study: summary of the study design. J Myocard Ischemia 1992a;4:27–29.

Women's Health Study Research Group. The Women's Health Study: rationale and background. J Myocard Ischemia 1992b;4:30–40.

Wright RA, Flapan AD, Alberti GMM, et al. Effects of captopril therapy on endogenous fibrinolysis in men with recent, uncomplicated myocardial infarction. J Am Coll Cardiol 1994;24:67–73.

Yarnell JWG, Baker IA, Sweetnam PM, et al. Fibrinogen, viscosity, and white blood cell count are major risk factors for ischemic heart disease: the Caerphilly and Speedwell Collaborative Heart Disease Studies. Circulation 1991;83:836–44.

20

Summary and Conclusions

JoAnn E. Manson, J. Michael Gaziano, Paul M. Ridker, and Charles H. Hennekens

The public health importance of the primary prevention of myocardial infarction (MI) is indisputable. During the past few decades, researchers have made great strides in identifying both lifestyle and genetic factors affecting the risk of developing coronary heart disease (CHD), as discussed throughout this book. The process of disease prevention involves not only understanding disease mechanisms and identifying risk factors but also establishing intervention strategies that will reduce risk, weighing the benefits of any given intervention against the risks and costs, establishing guidelines for health providers and the general public, and finally, implementing these guidelines. The current epidemiologic data, outlined in previous chapters, strongly support a role of risk factor modification for the prevention of CHD. In this chapter we summarize data on the strength of the association with CHD and the size of the effect for each risk factor, as well as the anticipated reduction in risk attributable to intervention.

The strength of evidence for an association of cardiovascular disease with each risk factor is summarized in Table 20.1. The quality of evidence for each risk factor, the estimated magnitude of the risk reduction that could be achieved through modification of that factor, and the type(s) of intervention strategies available to reduce risk are presented. There are three risk factors for which the strength and consistency of the association with atherosclerotic disease indicate a clear causal relationship and the benefits of intervention are well documented: cigarette smoking, elevated serum cholesterol, and hypertension. Public policy measures as well as individual counseling are clearly warranted for all three.

There is little doubt that smoking cessation will reduce risks of myocardial infarction as well as other cardiovascular diseases and cancer. There are clear benefits of smoking cessation even among those with established coronary artery disease. Half of the estimated 60% reduction in risk of MI occurs within the first few months of stopping. The vast majority of those who give up smoking do not use an organized cessation program. The efficacy of smoking intervention programs range from 6% one-year success rate for physician counseling, to 18% for self-help programs, and 20 to 26% for pharmacologic interventions with nicotine gum or patch.

The totality of evidence indicates a clear causal link between elevated serum cholesterol and CHD. Specifically, a 10% increase in serum cholesterol is associated with a 20–30% increase in risk of CHD, and elevations earlier in life may be associated with higher increases in risk. Treatment to lower cholesterol by 10% has been shown to reduce risks of CHD death by 10% and CHD events by 18%, and treatment for more than five years yields a 25% reduction in CHD events. Results from recent overviews are consistent with a slight reduction in total mortality associated with cholesterol reduction. The effects of cholesterol lowering on specific nonvascular causes of death, such as cancer or trauma, are not significantly different from the null. Although it remains possible that cholesterol lowering may not affect total mortality, and it may increase the risk of some nonvascular causes of mortality, there is currently a lack of statistical power to address these issues in either individual trials or in an overview. Existing data support nonpharmacologic public health measures to lower the serum cholesterol of the population. While open debate should continue on who should be aggressively treated with lipid-lowering drugs, there is little debate over those at highest risk, particularly those with existing disease.

Elevation of systolic or diastolic blood pressure has consistently been associated with an increased risk of CHD. A 7-mmHg increase in diastolic blood pressure from any baseline blood pressure was associated with a 27% increase in CHD. Pooled data from randomized trials indicate that a decrease in diastolic blood pressure of 5 to 6 mmHg results in a 14% to 16% reduction in risk of CHD events. The JNC V (Joint National Committee on the Detection, Evaluation, and Treatment of High Blood Pressure [Fifth Report]) recommendations of nonpharmacologic modifications in lifestyle alone for mild hypertensives and as an adjunct to pharmacologic intervention in moderate-to-severe hypertensives are justified and warranted. The optimal strategy to reduce systolic blood pressure below 140 and diastolic blood pressure below 90 mmHg will depend on the other risk factors present. Nonpharmacologic therapies that have been shown to be effective in the management of hypertension and are recommended in the JNC V report include weight loss, limitation of alcohol intake to no more than 1 oz of ethanol per day, aerobic exercise, and reduction of sodium intake. The efficacy of pharmacologic therapy has been well documented and appears to be cost effective.

With regard to obesity and physical inactivity there is little doubt that these factors are associated with substantial increases in the risk of CHD. There are scant randomized trial data suggesting a benefit of exercise or weight reduction in lowering risks of CHD, and it is unlikely that such randomized trial data will be available in the near future. Evidence from observational studies suggest that maintenance of an ideal body weight and a physically active lifestyle will likely reduce the risk of myocardial infarction by 35–55%. In addition, it is clear that regular exercise and maintenance of ideal body weight improve other cardiovascular risk factors, and therefore justify their importance as part of a preventive program. Efforts at reducing prevalence of physical inactivity and obesity, however, have been disappointing.

Mounting evidence suggests that maintaining normoglycemia among insulin-dependent diabetics may translate into reduced risk of microvascular disease, but data are insufficient to provide estimates of the reduction of CHD risks. While oral hypoglycemic agents and insulin can improve glycemic control, their role in the reduction of risk from macrovascular complications of non–insulin-dependent diabetes re-

Table 20.1. Quality of Evidence Concerning Modifiable Risk Factors, Types of Interventions, and Likely Risk Reductions for MI

Risk Factor	Quality of Evidence	Type(s) of Intervention[a]	Likely Risk Reduction[b]
Smoking cessation	Excellent	Lifestyle/pharmacologic	50–70% within 5 years of smoking cessation
Cholesterol reduction	Excellent	Lifestyle/pharmacologic	A 2–3% reduction in risk of MI for each 1% reduction in serum cholesterol level; on average, dietary interventions result in about 10% reductions in cholesterol, while reductions with pharmacologic therapy often exceed 20%
Hypertension prevention	Excellent	Lifestyle/pharmacologic	A 2–3% decline in risk for each 1 mmHg reduction in diastolic BP, which average 5–6 mmHg with a combination of dietary and pharmacologic therapies; in clinical practice, decreases of 20 mmHg or more are often achieved. Comparable reductions in MI risk can be achieved by treating patients with isolated systolic hypertension
Physical activity	Good	Lifestyle	35–55% reduction in risk associated with maintenance of an active lifestyle, as compared with a sedentary lifestyle; data are not available on the role of interventions to increase physical activity in reducing risk of MI
Obesity	Good	Lifestyle/pharmacologic	A 35–55% lower risk associated with maintaining ideal body weight as compared with being 20% or more above desirable weight; data are not available on the role of sustained weight loss in the prevention of MI
Diabetes	Fair/poor for glycemic control. Good for medication of traditional CHD risk factors.	Lifestyle/pharmacologic	Risk reduction associated with maintenance of normal glycemia is unknown; available evidence strongly supports modification of traditional CHD risk factors in this extremely high-risk group

		Lifestyle/pharmacologic	
Psychosocial factors	Fair/poor	Lifestyle/pharmacologic	While the role of modification of psychosocial factors on MI risk is unclear, some epidemiologic evidence supports an association between these variables and traditional coronary risk factors, including serum lipids and blood pressure
Diet	Varies with specific dietary component	Lifestyle	Available evidence generally supports a reduced risk of MI with increased consumption of fruits and vegetables, fiber, monounsaturated fatty acids, and moderate amounts of alcohol; in contrast, increased dietary intakes of saturated fats and *trans*-fatty acids appear to increase risk of MI
Antioxidant vitamins	Poor	Pharmacologic	Not known
Aspirin	Excellent	Pharmacologic	Low-dose aspirin is associated with a 30–35% reduction in risk of a first MI in men
Estrogen replacement	Good	Pharmacologic	40–50% reduction of MI risk among current vs never users of ERT; randomized trials of hormone replacement therapy are currently ongoing

MI denotes myocardial injection. CHD denotes coronary heart disease.

[a]The efficacy of current strategies to modify risk varies by intervention, ranging from good to excellent for treatment of hypertension, reduction of serum cholesterol, prophylactic low-dose aspirin; fair for smoking cessation, dietary modification, exercise, and estrogen replacement therapy (ERT); and fair to poor for weight loss and maintenance of normal glycemia in diabetes. Data are not available for alcohol or antioxidant vitamins.

[b]Estimated reductions in risk refer to the independent contribution of each risk factor for MI and do not address the wide range of known or hypothesized interactions between them.

mains unclear. Treatment of non–insulin-dependent diabetes with insulin often results in weight gain. In contrast to well-controlled IDDM, those with NIDDM are much more likely to have multiple coronary risk factors than are the general population. Thus, of paramount importance in reducing risks of CHD in the diabetic patient is the favorable modification of associated risk factors, including treatment of hypertension, reduction of serum cholesterol, weight reduction, and increased physical activity.

Recent evidence also suggests that hormone replacement therapy in postmenopausal women may reduce the risk of CHD by an estimated 40–50%. An additional benefit of estrogen replacement may be reduced risk of osteoporosis related fractures. These apparent benefits in terms of cardiovascular disease must be weighed against the known or potential risks of hormone replacement therapy including increased risks of endometrial and possibly breast cancer. The increased risk of endometrial cancer can be attenuated by progestin; however, it is unclear whether or not progestins will attenuate the cardiovascular benefits as well. Large-scale, randomized trial data are not yet available to assess fully the risks and benefits of postmenopausal hormone replacement. The ongoing Women's Health Initiative will address the risks and benefits of treatment of postmenopausal women with estrogen alone, as well as the use of estrogen and progestin in combination, compared to placebo. Currently available observational data suggest that the benefits of treatment outweigh the risks particularly for those who are at high risk for myocardial infarction.

The totality of evidence suggests inverse association between moderate alcohol consumption and myocardial infarction, which is mediated, in large part, by changes in HDL levels. Consumption of one drink per day appears to reduce the risk of MI by 30–50%, and there appears to be no additional benefit at higher drinking levels. Any individual or public health recommendations must consider the complexity of alcohol's metabolic, physiologic, and psychological effects. The risk:benefit ratio for moderate alcohol consumption may vary widely from individual to individual and between the sexes. A discussion of drinking habits should be undertaken by the health care provider in the context of dietary counseling. One to two drinks per day appears to be safe for most people, but recommendations must be individualized. Other conditions such as hypertension, diabetes, liver disease, tendency toward excess, family history of alcoholism and possibly breast and colon cancer should be taken into account when discussing alcohol consumption.

Diet represents an important aspect of any myocardial prevention program. Dietary habits will greatly impact other risk factors including weight, dyslipidemia, hypertension, and diabetes. Low fat diets have been shown to reduce the risk of MI and even cause regression of coronary artery disease. While there is a general consensus that reduction in saturated fat intake reduces the risk of coronary heart disease, whether to replace these fats with carbohydrates or mono- or polyunsaturated fats remains controversial. Replacement of saturated fats with carbohydrates reduces not only LDL cholesterol but also HDL cholesterol, while replacement with monounsaturated fats reduces LDL and may raise HDL. Recent data suggest that *trans*-fatty acids found in hydrogenated vegetable oils may increase risk of CHD possibly by increasing LDL and lowering HDL cholesterol. Foods high in these *trans*-fatty acids include margarine, vegetable shortening, and processed foods such as cookies, crackers, and candies. One of the most consistent findings in dietary research is that those who consume higher amounts of fresh fruits and vegetables have lower rates of heart disease and stroke as well as cancer. Possible explanations for these associations include high fiber content, vitamin content, particularly antioxidant vitamins, or replacement of fats. Regardless of the precise mechanism, most researchers agree that consumption of fresh fruits and vegetables is an important part of a healthy diet. The USDA recommends 2 to 4 serving of fresh fruit and 3 to 5 servings of fresh vegetables per day.

Combined data from two randomized trials suggest that prophylactic aspirin use in healthy males reduces the risk of myocardial infarction by 33%. This benefit appears to be greatest among those older than 50 years of age. There was an apparent, through not statistically significant, increased risk of stroke in the largest of the two studies, the Physicians' Health Study. There are observational data in women, but randomized trial data among women are not yet available. The ongoing Women's Health Study will address the risk:benefit ratio of treatment with aspirin in healthy women.

The impact of psychological factors such as depression and stress appear to contribute to increasing risk of CHD; further data are needed to confirm the relationship and to establish efficacy of interventional strategies. Therapeutic interventions, while not blinded, suggest a role as part of a prevention program, particularly for those with known CHD.

Hemostatic factors, such as fibrinogen, Lp(a), tPA, von Willebrand factor, and factor VII, represent a promising area for future research. Whether or not these hemostatic parameters represent independent risk factors for atherosclerotic disease or are in the causal pathway for other risk factors is not entirely clear. Other risk factors, such as cigarette smoking, alcohol consumption, and dyslipidemia, appear to alter the levels of various hemostatic risk factors and may enhance platelet aggregability. Additional observational data and interventional trials aimed at altering these hemostatic factors will provide valuable information on the role of these factors in the treatment and prevention of atherosclerotic disease. At this point, recommendations specifically targeted at modifying these factors are premature.

While mounting basic and human data suggest a role for lipid oxidation in the development of atherosclerotic disease, the efficacy as well as the risk of supplementation with antioxidants remains unclear. Randomized trial data will become available from ongoing trials upon which rational decisions can be based.

Reduction of risk during or immediately following myocardial infarction has been demonstrated for beta-blockers, thrombolytic agents, and aspirin, and in the secondary prevention of subsequent events for beta-blockers, aspirin, and ACE inhibitors (among those with low ejection fraction). Particular attention given to the modification of traditional coronary risk factors following myocardial infarction and known atherosclerotic disease generally provides substantial benefits in reduced morbidity and mortality. Aggressive risk factor modification for secondary prevention is cost effective for those individuals at high risk for subsequent MI.

In summary, primary and secondary prevention have contributed substantially to the reduction in CHD mortality rates over the last few decades. In addition to developing a better understanding of mechanistic and epidemiologic determinants of atherosclerotic disease, considerably more attention must be given to effective strategies for the implementation of existing guidelines for risk factor modification. Many lifestyle changes are difficult to achieve and even harder to maintain over the long term.

Interventions need to involve not only the affected individuals, but often families, workplaces, schools and even whole communities. For clinicians, identification of the strategy most likely to be successful for each individual is key. Further research on the cost:benefit and risk:benefit ratios will enable better targeting of interventions for maximal individual and societal benefit. More widespread use of multifaceted self-help and health professional-directed prevention programs should help sustain the decline in cardiovascular disease mortality rates in the United States.

ADDITIONAL
APPENDICES AND
PATIENT EDUCATION MATERIALS

Appendix A

Nutrition Guidelines for Reducing Coronary Risk

In the past 25 years, major progress has been made in our understanding of the role of diet in the development of coronary heart disease. It is now clearly established that lowering elevated blood cholesterol levels decreases the risks of developing heart disease. Several dietary factors are known to influence the levels of blood lipids—some more strongly than others. Also, dietary changes may lower the risk of heart disease through other mechanisms. Currently, modifications in the American dietary lifestyle are recommended for prevention as well as treatment of coronary artery disease.

The average American male consumes about 335 mg of cholesterol per day; the average woman about 200 mg/day. Between 34% and 38% of the calorie content of the typical American diet comes from all types of fat. Many Americans eat about 12% to 16% of their calories as saturated fat. Varying levels of total fat as well as type of fat can be recommended according to an individual's coronary risk profile or treatment goal. (Please refer to glossary for definition of cholesterol and fat terms).

The degree of aggressiveness with regard to dietary fat modification continues to be a topic of debate. A stepped approach is recommended by the American Heart Association and the National Cholesterol Education Program's (NCEP) Expert Panel on Detection, Evaluation and Treatment of High Blood Cholesterol in Adults. Table A1 illustrates the NCEP dietary recommendations.

The Step-One Diet is recommended for all healthy Americans above the age of 2. For those with blood lipid (fat) levels that are elevated or for those who have coronary disease, a more restrictive saturated fat and cholesterol diet (Step-Two Diet) is recommended.

Some researchers believe that an even more aggressive fat restriction (no more than 10% of calories) is necessary to stop or reverse the progression of existing cor-

Table A1.

Nutrient	Percent of Calories	
	Step-One Diet	Step-Two Diet
Total fat	<30%	<30%
Saturated fatty acids	<10%	<7%
Polyunsaturated fatty acids	Up to 10%	Up to 10%
Monounsaturated fatty acids	10%–15%	10%–15%
Carbohydrates	50%–60%	50%–60%
Protein	10%–20%	10%–20%
Cholesterol (mg)	<300 mg/day	<200 mg/day

onary artery disease (CAD). Other researchers speculate that the focus needs to be on strict management of the *types* of fat while permitting fairly liberal amounts of total fat (35%–40% of calories). A third approach is a vegetarian lifestyle. Although researchers continue to debate the level of total fat recommended in the diet, there is general agreement that *saturated* fat should be restricted.

Guide for Total Fat and Saturated Fat

The recommended amounts of total and saturated fat are based on total caloric intake per day. (To determine calorie needs, refer to Table A3.)

Table A2 translates varying daily calorie levels into suggested *maximum* daily grams of fat and saturated fat based on two levels. The 30% fat with 10% saturated fat is a guide for currently healthy consumers interested in modifying their intake. The 20% total fat with 5% saturated fat can be used for individuals interested in further reducing their total and saturated fat intake.

A rough rule for estimating grams of fat based on 30% of calories is to divide your desirable body weight in pounds by 2, assuming moderate activity and weight-stable diet. A guide to choosing low-fat foods is provided in Table A4.

Table A2.

Daily Calorie Level	Grams of Total Fat[a] Based on 30% of Calories	Grams of Saturated[a] Fat Based on 10% of Calories	Grams of Total Fat[a] Based on 20% of Calories	Grams of Saturated[a] Fat Based on 5% of Calories
1,200	40	13	27	7
1,300	43	14	29	7
1,400	47	16	31	8
1,500	50	17	33	8
1,600	53	18	36	9
1,800	60	20	40	10
2,000	67	22	44	11
2,200	73	24	49	12
2,400	80	27	53	13
2,800	93	31	62	15

[a] Rounded to the nearest whole number.

Table A3. Guidelines for Determining Desirable Weight and Caloric Needs

To Estimate Desirable Body Weight:

Build	Women	Men
Medium	Allow 100 lb for first 5 ft of height, plus 5 lb for each additional inch	Allow 106 lb for first 5 ft of height, plus 6 lb for each additional inch
Small	Subtract 10%	Subtract 10%
Large	Add 10%	Add 10%

To Calculate Daily Caloric Needs*

1 **Select a Desired Weight** (DW) in pounds. **DW** = _____

2 Determine Daily Basal Calorie Requirements (from above). (amount of calories needed daily to maintain the body's functions when a person is inactive) Multiply **DW** × **10** = _____

3 **Add Daily Activity Calories** (Those needed for various levels of exercise - <u>choose only one</u>)

For sedentary people: (almost no exercise) Multiply **DW** × **3** = _____

For moderate exerciser: (20 minutes, 3–5 times/week) Multiply **DW** × **5** = _____

For strenuous exercisers: (1 hour, 5–7 times/week) Multiply **DW** × **10** = _____

Total Daily Requirements: (Basal Calories + Activity Calories) [#2 plus #3 above] = _____

4 **Subtract Daily Calories for Weight Loss.** To lose 1 pound a week, subtract 500 calories from Total Daily Requirements. To lose 2 pounds, subtract 1,000 calories. − _____

Daily Calories Needed for Weight Plan = _____

*Note: This table uses average numbers. Caloric needs will vary depending on frame size, metabolic needs, and levels of activity.

Source: From American Diabetes Association and the American Dietetic Association, 1977, with permission.

Determination of Calorie Needs

Secrets of Success Even though no specific weight-loss strategy can be identified as the most likely to succeed, a recent National Institutes of Health Technology Assessment Conference outlines some of the features that are particularly effective. First and foremost, programs should be based upon realistic goals and include a low-calorie diet aimed at producing slow, steady weight loss. Most weight-loss experts recommend that dieters shed no more than 1–2 pounds a week. Losses exceeding 2 pounds per week may promote loss of lean muscle tissue. While the diet must provide fewer

Table A4. Heart-Smart Substitutions: A Guide to Choosing Low-Fat, Low-Saturated Fat Foods

Higher Fat	Lower Fat
Whole milk, 2% milk	Skim milk
Condensed milk	Non-fat or low-fat condensed milk
Regular evaporated milk	Evaporated skim milk
Cream	Evaporated skim milk
Coffee creamer	Non-fat (skim) powdered milk
Non-dairy creamer	Non-fat, non-dairy creamer
Ice cream	Sorbet, water ice, nonfat ice milk or non-fat frozen yogurt
Sour cream	Nonfat sour cream or nonfat plain yogurt
Whipping cream	Evaporated skim milk whipped with vanilla and sugar Nonfat vanilla yogurt as a topping
Cream cheese	Nonfat cream cheese
Whole-milk cheeses	Nonfat cheeses, low-fat cheeses with <2 g fat per oz
Egg	Cholesterol-free egg substitute Egg whites
Cold cuts	Turkey breast Lunch meats with <2 g fat per oz Bean spreads (humus, etc.) Tuna fish
Hot dogs, frankfurters, sausage	Low-fat hot dogs (beef, turkey, chicken) with <2 g fat per link
Croissants, donuts, sweet rolls	Raisin bread, bagel, English muffin, whole wheat or rye breads
Potato chips	Pretzels, breadsticks, flavored rice cakes
Corn chips	Baked tortilla chips
Regular microwave popcorn	Air-popped popcorn, fat free caramel corn
Fudge sauce	Chocolate syrup
One square bakers unsweetened chocolate	3 T cocoa powder and 1 T canola oil
Milk chocolate candy	Hard candy, jelly beans
Coconut	Small portion chopped walnuts, coconut abstract
Commercial baked products	Angel cake, nonfat baked products, nonfat cookies, home-baked items with appropriate ingredients

calories than the individual burns every day, it must be tasty enough so that the person can sustain the regimen. (See Table A3 to determine calorie needs.)

The initial weight-reduction diet should allow a smooth transition into a new regimen aimed at long-term weight control and cardiovascular risk-factor reduction. In addition, at least 100 minutes of exercise a week can encourage early weight loss and help sustain the improvement.

Alternative Approaches to the Step-One and Step-Two Diets

High Monounsaturated Fatty-Acid Diet (Mediterranean-Style Diet)　An alternative approach suggested for cholesterol lowering is the replacement of saturated fatty acids with monounsaturated fatty acids (MFA) to make up about 20% of the fat calories. This Mediterranean style diet is still low in saturated fatty acids (5% to 9% of calories) and maintains a total fat intake of 35% to 40%. Studies have shown that MFAs are as effective as polyunsaturated fatty acids (PFAs) in lowering plasma cholesterol when replacing saturated fatty acids in the diet. Polyunsaturated fatty acids, however, often lower HDL cholesterol levels. MFAs do not have the same effect on HDL cholesterol levels and this diet may result in improved LDL and HDL levels. Mediterranean style diets emphasize the inclusion of generous servings of vegetables, fruits, and grains as the carbohydrate sources. Simple sugars are at a minimum. For some patients, diets high in MFAs may be more palatable and therefore compliance may be increased. (See Table A5 for example.)

Low-Fat, High-Carbohydrate Diet (Asian-Style Diet)　Low to very-low-fat, high-carbohydrate diets may be effective cholesterol-lowering alternatives for some individuals. Some researchers suggest a diet providing no more than 20% of calories as total fat with saturated fatty acids limited to 5% to 6% of calories and less than 100 mg of dietary cholesterol per day. Carbohydrates supply at least 65% of calories. (See Table A5 for examples.) This diet results in lower LDL levels but also reduces HDL levels. Diets even lower in total fat, saturated fatty acids, and cholesterol have been advocated by Pritikin and Ornish. These diets limit total fat to about 10% of calories. Major dietary changes make adherence to these plans more difficult. However, with highly motivated individuals this dietary approach can prove effective.

Vegetarian Diet　A considerable body of scientific evidence suggests benefits of vegetarian lifestyles in prevention of several chronic diseases, such as coronary heart disease, obesity, and diabetes mellitus. Vegetarian diets are healthful and nutritionally adequate when appropriately planned. Vegetarian diets differ in the extent to which they avoid animal products. Veganism completely excludes meat, fish, fowl, eggs, and dairy products. Lacto-vegetarianism is the avoidance of meat, fish, fowl, and eggs, whereas lacto-ovo-vegetarianism involves avoidance of only meat, fish, and fowl.

Studies of vegetarians indicate that this population generally has lower death rates from several chronic diseases than do nonvegetarians. Death rates from coronary heart disease is lower in vegetarians than in nonvegetarians. Total serum cholesterol and LDL cholesterol levels are usually lower, while HDL cholesterol and triglyceride levels vary, depending on the type of vegetarian diet that is consumed. Vegetarians generally have

Menu Example	kcal	Fat (gm)	Saturated Fat (gm)
Breakfast			
1 doughnut	104	5.7	1.2
12 oz coffee	7	0	0
1 T cream (half & half)	20	1.7	1.0
1 T sugar	45	0	0
Lunch			
2 slices deli ham	104	6	1.9
1 oz Swiss cheese	107	7.7	5.4
2 slices white bread	134	2.0	0.4
1 small bag potato chips	140	8.0	1.8
1 apple	81	0.5	0.1
16 fluid oz cola	202	0	0
1/2 cup tomatoes	24	0.3	0
3 pieces lettuce	8	0.1	0
Dinner			
4 oz roast beef (lean)	396	30.5	12.6
1 baked potato	115	0	0
1/2 cup carrots, boiled	35	0.1	0
1/2 cup green beans, canned	13	0	0
1 cup 2% milk	121	4.6	2.9
1 T margarine (stick)	101	11.3	2.2
Dessert			
1 cup frozen low-fat vanilla yogurt with 2 tbsp chocolate syrup	280	2.5	1.6
Totals	2,037	81	31.1

% calories from fat = 36%
% calories from saturated fat = 14%

Mediterranean Style Diet

Menu Example	kcal	Fat (gm)	Saturated Fat (gm)
Breakfast			
1 medium peach	75	0.2	0
1 cup yogurt, plain, nonfat	127	0.4	0.3
1 tsp olive oil	40	4.5	0.6
3/4 cup diced tomatoes	35	0.4	0.1
1 slice cracked wheat bread	66	0.9	0.1
Lunch			
1 whole pita bread	165	0.7	0.1
2 servings green salad	64	0.3	0
2 T olive oil	239	27.0	3.6
1/2 cup hummus	211	10.4	1.5
2 T balsamic vinegar	30	0	0
2 oz olives (black)	95	12.6	1.2
1 cup skim milk	86	0.4	0.3
1 apple	81	0.5	0

Table continues

	kcal	Fat (gm)	Saturated Fat (gm)
Dinner			
4 oz fish (bass)	110	2.6	0.5
1 cup brown rice	216	1.8	0.4
1 cup spinach	41	0.5	0
1/2 cup eggplant	14	0.1	0
1 whole pita bread	165	0.7	0.1
2 T olive oil	239	27.0	3.6
Totals	2,099	91.0	12.4

% calories from fat = 39%
% calories from saturated fat = 5%

Asian Style Diet

Menu Example	kcal	Fat (gm)	Saturated Fat (gm)
Breakfast			
1 cup white rice	264	0.6	0.2
1 cup chicken broth	39	1.4	0.4
1/2 cup broccoli	22	0.3	0
1/2 cup grape juice	64	0.1	0
1 orange	62	0.2	0
3 oz tofu	123	7.4	1
Lunch			
3 oz pork loin	259	18.4	6.6
1 cup white rice	264	0.6	0.2
1/2 cup pea pods	34	0.2	0
1/2 T sesame oil	60	6.8	1
1 cup apple juice	112	0.2	0
Snack			
1 cup tea	2	0	0
1 pear	118	0.8	0
Dinner			
3 oz fish (bass)	82	1.9	0.4
1/2 cup bean sprouts	13	0	0
2 1/2 cups cooked cellophane noodles	416	0.5	0
1/4 cup onions, cooked	23	0.1	0
1/4 cup mushrooms	4	0	0
1/4 cup green snap beans	11	0	0
1/2 cup mustard greens	11	0.2	0
1/2 T sesame oil	60	6.8	1
Dessert			
1/4 cup melon, fresh	14	0.1	0
1/4 cup strawberries, fresh	11	0.1	0
1/4 cup grapes, fresh	15	0	0
Totals	2,083	46.7	10.8

% calories from fat = 20%
% calories from saturated fat = 5%

lower blood pressure and lower rates of adult-onset diabetes than do nonvegetarians, which may decrease the risk of coronary heart disease in the vegetarian population.

Vegetarian diets that are low in animal foods (including avoidance of whole-milk dairy sources) are typically lower in total fat, saturated fat, and cholesterol than non-vegetarian diets. Attention may be needed to ensure adequate intake of iron, vitamin B_{12}, vitamin D, and calcium through dietary or supplemental means.

Fresh Fruits and Vegetables One of the most consistent findings in dietary research is that those who consume higher amounts of fresh fruits and vegetables have lower rates of heart disease and stroke. Some have even speculated that the declining heart disease and stroke rates in the United States are due, at least in part, to increased consumption of fresh fruits and vegetables. In addition, cancer rates are also lower among those who have higher intake of fresh fruits and vegetables.

The exact mechanisms of these apparent protective effects are unclear. Possible explanations include high content of vitamins, particularly antioxidant vitamins, such as vitamins C, E, and beta-carotene, as well as high-fiber content. It is also possible that consumption of these very-low-fat foods may translate into lower total fat intake. Regardless of the precise mechanism, most researchers agree that consumption of fruits and vegetables is an important part of a healthy diet. The USDA recommends two to four servings of fresh fruit as well as three to five servings of vegetables per day. A serving is generally defined as one piece (an apple or potato) or one-half cup of prepared fruit or vegetable.

Other Diet-Related Issues

Fish Oil and Shellfish Studies in Greenland Eskimos and in the Zutphen, Netherlands suggest an inverse association between the consumption of both fish and omega-3 fatty acids and coronary heart disease. The mechanism by which omega-3s affect CHD is not known. In addition, the amount of omega-3 fatty acids required to reduce risk is unknown. Eskimos consume 4–5 g of omega-3s daily, an amount present in 1.5–2 lb of fish rich in omega-3 fatty acids. Fish highest in omega-3s include salmon, mackerel, trout, and tuna. It is prudent to recommend increased consumption of all types of fish. Although some shellfish are considered a relatively high source of dietary cholesterol (such as shrimp, crab, and squid), shellfish are extremely low in both total and saturated fat (3 oz shrimp has 1 g of total fat and 0.1 g of saturated fat). Therefore, in moderation, shellfish can be a part of a heart-healthy diet. At this time, fish oil capsule supplementation is not recommended, since safety, proper dosages, effectiveness, duration, and side effects of long-term ingestion have not been established.

Trans-*Fatty Acids* *Trans*-fatty acids are found in margarines and vegetable shortenings. Such products begin as a *liquid* vegetable oil, but are changed into a soft *solid* form in the manufacturing process.

The amount of *trans*-fatty acids in the American diet has progressively risen as the food industry has responded to consumer demands for products with less saturated fat. The amount of *trans*-fatty acids in margarines ranges from 10% to 30% of total fat and often exceeds 25% in cookies, crackers, pastries, and deep-fried foods such as french fries and doughnuts.

Research shows that *trans*-fatty acids are not a heart-healthy replacement for saturated fats. These *trans*-fatty acids are found to raise the LDL cholesterol and lower the HDL cholesterol in the blood. Concern about *trans*-fatty acids has intensified, as newer research found that women who ate large amounts of margarine and shortening in cookies, white bread, and other baked goods have a 70% higher risk of heart disease than women who consumed little or none of them.

Even "modest" consumption of *trans*-fatty acids can have a detrimental effect on heart health. Women who ate 4 or more teaspoons of margarine a day (1–4 g of *trans*-fatty acids) had a 66% higher risk of heart disease than those who ate margarine less than once a month. (Refer to Table A6 for *trans*-fatty acid content of some foods. Consumers should keep in mind that food labels do not show the amount of *trans*-fatty acids.)

Fiber There are two types of fiber—soluble and insoluble—and they play different roles in the body. The fiber content of a food is a combination of both types of fiber. Table A7 shows the amount of total fiber and soluble fiber in selected foods.

Insoluble fiber is not soluble in the intestinal tract. It does not appear to help lower blood cholesterol, but does aid in normal bowel function. Insoluble fibers are found in the skin, peels, and husks of fruits, vegetables, and whole-grain products.

Table A6. *Trans*-Fatty Acid Content of Some Foods

Food	*Trans*-Fatty Acids (grams)
Animal products	
Beef (5 oz)	0.9
Butter (1 tsp)	0.1
Chicken (5 oz)	0.1
Pork (5 oz)	0.1
Vegetable fats	
Reduced-calorie mayonnaise (1 tsp)	0.01
Soft margarine (1 tsp)	0.27[a]
Stick margarine (1 tsp)	0.62[a]
Vegetable oil (1 tsp)	0.02[a]
Vegetable shortening	0.63
Commercial and fast-food products	
Cake (1 piece)	1.04[a]
Cookie (1)	0.86[a]
Corn chips (1 oz)	1.42[a]
Cracker (1)	0.12[a]
Danish pastry (1)	3.03[a]
Doughnut (1)	3.19
Deep-fat french fries,	
Large order (4 oz)	5.5
Small order (2.5 oz)	3.6
Muffin	0.09[a]
Pie (1 piece)	1.00[a]
Pizza (1 slice)	0.13[a]
Potato chips (1 oz)	0.11[a]

Source: From N Engl J Med 1993;329:1969–70; with permission.

[a] The grams listed represent the average of several brands.

Table A7. Dietary Fiber Content of Selected Foods

Food	Total Dietary Fiber (gm)	Water-Soluble Fiber (gm)	Percentage Soluble Fiber
Oatmeal, dry, 1/3 cup	2.6	1.3	52%
Oat bran, dry, 1/3 cup	4.0	2.0	50%
All-bran, 1/3 cup	8.6	1.4	17%
Corn flakes, 1 cup	0.4	0.1	29%
Brown rice, 1/2 cup	2.4	0.5	20%
Spaghetti, 1/2 cup	0.8	0.3	40%
White bread, 1 slice	0.5	0.3	49%
Whole-wheat bread, 1 slice	1.4	0.3	22%
Carrots, raw, 1/2 cup	1.3	0.6	48%
Broccoli, frozen, 1/2 cup	2.8	1.3	45%
Kidney beans, canned, 1/2 cup	7.9	2.0	25%
Pinto beans, canned, 1/2 cup	4.3	1.0	23%
White beans, canned, 1/2 cup	5.0	1.5	30%
Apple, raw, 1 small	2.7	1.0	35%
Orange, 1 small	1.1	0.6	58%
Purple plums, canned, 1/3 cup	2.9	1.0	33%
Blueberries, 1/2 cup	2.5	0.3	40%

Source: Adapted with permission from Anderson JW, Bridges SA. Fiber. Am J Clin Nutr 1988;47:440; and from Anderson JW, Plant Fiber in foods. HCF Nutrition Research Foundation, Inc, PO Box 22114, Lexington, KY 40522, 1986. A more extensive list can be purchased from Dr. James Anderson, HCF Nutrition Research Foundation, Inc, PO Box 22124, Lexington, KY 40522.

Water-soluble fibers are found in fruit pectins, dried beans, guar gum, legumes, oat grains, barley, and psyllium. Like water-insoluble fibers, they are useful in increasing bulk and easing bowel movements. However, water-soluble fibers have an additional property: they can lower blood cholesterol level.

Not all water-soluble fibers perform the same way. For example, one researcher found that oat bran increased the removal of bile acids from the body, whereas the addition of beans to the diet had the opposite effect. Yet, both these water-soluble fibers lowered the total body cholesterol by about the same amount. The effect of water-soluble fibers also depends upon how much dietary fat an individual consumes. To be effective in cholesterol lowering, a diet rich in soluble fiber should be a part of a diet low in saturated fatty acids, *trans*-fatty acids, and dietary cholesterol. To date, there is no evidence that the addition of fiber alone to a diet already high in fat, saturated fat, and cholesterol is an effective cholesterol-lowering mechanism.

The average American consumes only 10–20 g of dietary fiber per day. The recommended level of total fiber for adults is 20–35 g/day. Any increases in fiber intake must be accomplished gradually to avoid discomfort and intestinal gas. Fluid intake should be liberal and adequate (6–10 8-oz cups/day).

Some practical hints to increase the fiber in the diet include:

1. Increase consumption of whole beans, such as kidney beans, chick peas, navy beans, and pinto beans. Use in salads, soups, dips, and as a "meat extender" in casseroles.

2. Use whole-grain rather than white breads.
3. Use oat bran or oatmeal for part of the flour called for in baked products like muffins or as a "meat-extender" in preparation of meatloaf, etc.
4. Leave on and eat the skin on fruits and vegetables.

Glossary

Cholesterol

A soft, waxy substance. Essential to life, it is made in sufficient quantity by the body for normal body function, including the manufacture of hormones, bile acid, and vitamin D. It is present in all parts of the body, including the nervous system, muscle, skin, liver, intestines, and heart.

- **Blood cholesterol**—Cholesterol that is manufactured in the body's liver and absorbed from the food you eat and is carried in the blood for use by all parts of the body. A high level of blood cholesterol leads to atherosclerosis (hardening of the arteries) and coronary heart disease.
- **Dietary cholesterol**—Cholesterol that is in the food you eat. It is present only in foods of animal origin, not in foods of plant origin. Dietary cholesterol, like dietary saturated fat, tends to raise blood cholesterol, which increases the risk for heart disease.

Fat

One of the three nutrients that supply calories to the body. Fat provides kcal/g; more than twice the number provided by carbohydrate or protein. In addition to providing calories, fat helps in the absorption of certain vitamins. Small amounts of fat are necessary for normal body function.

- **Total fat**—The sum of the saturated, monounsaturated, and polyunsaturated fats present in food. A mixture of all three in varying amounts is found in most foods.
- **Saturated fat**—A type of fat found in greatest amounts in foods from animals such as meat, poultry, and whole-milk dairy products like cream, milk, ice cream, and cheese. Other examples of saturated fat include butter, the marbling and fat along the edges of meat, and lard. The saturated fat content is high in some vegetable oils like coconut, palm kernel, and palm oils. Saturated fat raises blood cholesterol more than anything else in the diet.
- **Unsaturated fat**—A type of fat that is usually liquid at refrigerator temperature. Monounsaturated fat and polyunsaturated fat are two kinds of unsaturated fat.

Monounsaturated fat—A slightly unsaturated fat that is found in greatest amounts in foods from plants, including olive and canola (rapeseed) oil and most nuts. When substituted for saturated fat, monounsaturated fat helps reduce LDL cholesterol and increase HDL cholesterol.

Polyunsaturated fat—A highly unsaturated fat that is found is greatest amounts in foods from plants, including safflower, corn, sesame, and soybean oils. When substituted for saturated fat, polyunsaturated fat helps reduce blood cholesterol.

Hydrogenation

A chemical process that changes liquid vegetable oils (unsaturated fat) into a more solid saturated fat. This process improves the shelf life of the product, but also increases the saturated fat content. Many commercial food products contain hydrogenated vegetable oil. Although the original fat source may be a heart-healthy unsaturated oil, the process of hydrogenation results in increasing the saturated fat content.

Lipids

Fatty substances, including cholesterol and triglycerides, that are present in blood and body tissues.

Lipoproteins

Protein-coated packages that carry fat and cholesterol through the blood. Lipoproteins are classified according to their density.

- **High-density lipoproteins (HDL)**—Lipoproteins that contain a small amount of cholesterol and carry cholesterol away from body cells and tissues to the liver for excretion from the body. Low levels of HDL are associated with an increased risk of coronary heart disease. Therefore, the higher the HDL level, the better. Referred to as "good" cholesterol.
- **Low-density lipoproteins (LDL)**—Lipoproteins that contain the largest amount of cholesterol in the blood. LDL is responsible for depositing cholesterol in the artery walls. High levels of LDL are associated with an increased risk of coronary heart disease and are therefore referred to as "bad" cholesterol.

Saturation

Saturation refers to the way molecules are structured in fat. All fats contain atoms of carbon and hydrogen; the more saturated the fat, the fewer spaces it has for extra hydrogen atoms.

Triglycerides

Lipids (fat-like substances) carried through the bloodstream to the tissues. The bulk of the body's fat tissue is in the form of triglycerides, stored for later use as energy. We get triglycerides primarily from the fat in our diet.

Prepared by Katherine McManus, RD, Connie Roberts, RD, and JoAnn E. Manson, MD.

Appendix B

Lipid-Lowering Agents

(DOSAGE, BENEFITS/RISKS, RELATIVE COSTS)

Drug Type	Usual Dosage and Frequency	Effect on Lipid Subtypes			Selected Adverse Effects[a]	Relative Cost[b]
		LDL	HDL	TG		
Bile-acid binding resins					Constipation; other gastrointestinal complaints	
Cholestyramine	4–12 gm bid	↓↓	↔↑	↔↑		$$–$$$
Colestipol	5–10 gm bid	↓↓	↑	↑		$$$
Nicotinic acid					Flushing; pruritus; gout; hepatic toxicity; gastrointestinal complaints; postural hypotension; glucose intolerance; blurred vision	
Niacin	1–2 gm tid	↓	↑	↓		$
HMG-CoA reductase inhibitors					Gastrointestinal complaints; headache; fatigue; myalgia; rash; myositis; rhabdomyolysis; hepatic toxicity	
Lovastatin	10–80 mg qd	↓↓	↔↑	↔↓		$$$$
Fluvastatin	10–40 mg qd	↓↓	↑	↔↓		Unavailable
Pravastatin	10–40 mg qd	↓↓	↑	↔↓		$$$$
Simvastatin	10–40 mg qd	↓↓	↑	↔↓		$$$$
Fibric acid derivatives					Gastrointestinal complaints; cholesterol gallstones	
Gemfibrozil	600 mg bid	↓	↑	↓		$$$
Clofibrate	500–1,000 mg bid					$
Other					Gastrointestinal complaints; increased QT interval on EKG	
Probucol	500 mg bid	↓	↓↓	↔		$$$
Fish oil						
Omega-3 fatty acids	1 gm qd	↔	↔	↓↓		$

Source: Adapted from Choice of cholesterol-lowering drugs. Med Lett 1993; 35:19–22.

[a]Partial list of adverse effects. See package insert for complete listing.

[b]Scale is based on average wholesale price for 30 days' treatment (1994 Blue Book, First Data Bank, San Bruno, CA). Scale: $ for under $25, $$ for $25–49,99, $$$ for $50–74,99, $$$$ for $75 or over. Relative differences between agents may vary for retail prices, which tend to be substantially higher. Further variations in prices may occur for other reasons including individual patient factors as well as individual arrangements between drug suppliers and patient care organizations.

Prepared by Christopher O'Donnell, MD and JoAnn E. Manson, MD.

Appendix C

Oral Antihypertensive Agents

(DOSAGE, BENEFITS/RISKS, RELATIVE COSTS)

First-Line Agents

Adrenergic Inhibitors

Drug Type	Usual Dosage and Frequency	Conditions in Which There May Be Additional Risk	Conditions in Which There May Be Additional Benefit	Selected Adverse Effects[a]	Relative Cost[c]
Beta-adrenergic blocking drugs		Bradycardia/heart block; congestive heart failure; asthma/COPD; severe peripheral vascular disease; diabetes mellitus (type I or II); dyslipidemia	Angina pectoris; hypertrophic cardiomyopathy; vascular headache; postmyocardial infarction	Fatigue; depression; decreased exercise tolerance; gastrointestinal complaints; bradycardia; bronchospasm; insomnia; increased triglycerides; decreased HDL cholesterol	
Atenolol	25–100 mg qd				\$–\$\$
Betaxolol	5–40 mg qd				\$\$
Bisoprolol	5–20 mg qd				\$–\$\$
Metoprolol[b]	50–200 mg qd or bid				\$\$–\$\$\$
Nadolol	20–240 mg qd				\$\$–\$\$\$
Propranolol[b]	60–240 mg qd or bid				\$–\$\$
Timolol	10–40 mg bid				\$\$–\$\$\$
Beta-adrenergic blocking drugs with intrinsic sympathomimetic activity		Bradycardia/heart block; congestive heart failure; asthma/COPD; severe peripheral vascular disease; diabetes mellitus (type I or II); dyslipidemia	Angina pectoris; hypertrophic cardiomyopathy; vascular headache	Similar to other beta-blockers, but with less bradycardia and lipid alterations; rare drug-induced lupus (acebutolol)	
Acebutolol	200–1,200 mg bid				\$\$\$
Carteolol	2.5–10 mg qd				\$\$
Penbutolol	20–80 mg qd				\$\$\$
Pindolol	10–60 mg bid				\$\$–\$\$\$
Mixed alpha-beta–adrenergic blocking drugs		Bradycardia/heart block, congestive heart failure, asthma/COPD, liver disease	Cyclosporine-associated hypertension	Similar to other beta-blocking drugs; also, orthostatic hypotension; fever; hepatic toxicity	
Labetolol	200–1,200 mg bid				\$\$

544

Drug	Dosage	Indications	Side effects	Cost
Alpha-adrenergic blocking drugs		Hypertrophic cardiomyopathy	Orthostatic hypotension and syncope with first dose; palpitations; headache	
Doxazasin	1.0–16 mg qd			$$
Prazosin	1.0–20 mg bid or tid			$–$$
Terazosin	1.0–20 mg qd			$$
Angiotensin Converting Enzyme (ACE) inhibitors		Hypertrophic cardiomyopathy; severe renal artery disease; pre-eclampsia; advanced renal insufficiency	Cough; rash; hyperkalemia; dysgeusia; angioedema; should not be used during second or third trimester of pregnancy	
Benazapril	10–40 mg qd or bid			$$
Captopril	12.5–150 mg bid			$$$
Cilazapril	2.5–5 mg qd or bid			Unavailable
Enalapril	2.5–40 mg qd or bid			$$$$
Fosinopril	10–40 mg qd or bid			$$
Lisinopril	5–40 mg qd or bid	Congestive heart failure; postmyocardial infarction		$–$$
Perindopril	1–16 mg qd or bid			Unavailable
Quinapril	5–80 mg qd or bid			$$
Ramipril	1.25–20 mg qd or bid			$$
Spirapril	12.5–50 mg qd or bid			Unavailable
Calcium Channel Blocking Drugs		Angina pectoris; hypertrophic cardiomyopathy (diltiazem and verapamil)	Headache; dizziness; peripheral edema (especially dihydropyridines); gingival hyperplasia; constipation (especially verapamil); other gastrointestinal complaints; heart block and bradycardia (diltiazem and verapamil)	
		Congestive heart failure		
Diltiazem[b]	90–360 tid			$$$–$$$$
Verapamil[b]	80–480 mg bid or tid			$–$$$
Amlodipine	2.5–10 mg qd			$$–$$$

Table continues

Oral Antihypertensive Agents *Continued*

Drug Type	Usual Dosage and Frequency	Conditions in Which There May Be Additional Risk	Conditions in Which There May Be Additional Benefit	Selected Adverse Effects[a]	Relative Cost[c]
Felodipine	5–20 mg qd				$$
Isradipine	2.5–10 mg qd or bid				$$
Nicardipine	60–120 mg tid		Cyclosporine-associated hypertension		$$$$
Nifedipine[b]	30–120 mg tid				$$$–$$$$
Diuretics					
Thiazide-type diuretics		Hypertrophic cardiomyopathy; pre-eclampsia; dyslipidemia; type II diabetes mellitus		Hypokalemia; hypomagnesemia; hyponatremia; hyperuricemia; hypercalcemia; rash; increased cholesterol; increased triglycerides; weakness	
Bendroflumethiazide	2.5–5 mg qd				$$
Benzthiazide	12.5–50 mg qd				$
Chlorothiazide	125–500 mg qd or bid				$
Chlorthalidone	12.5–50 mg qd				$
Cyclothiazide	1–2 mg qd				Unavailable
Hydrochlorothiazide	12.5–50 mg qd				$
Hydroflumethiazide	12.5–50 mg qd				$
Indapamide	2.5–5 mg qd				$
Methyclothiazide	2.5–5 mg qd				Unavailable
Metolazone	0.5–5 mg qd				$
Polythiazide	1–4 mg qd				$
Quinethazone	25–100 mg qd				$$
Trichlormethiazide	1–4 mg qd				$
Loop diuretics		As for thiazides		As for thiazides, except no hypercalcemia	
Bumetanide	0.5–5 mg qd or bid				$
Ethacrynic acid	25–100 mg qd or bid				$
Furosemide	20–320 mg qd or bid				$

Potassium sparing diuretics		As for thiazides; renal insufficiency	Hyperkalemia; gynecomastia (spironolactone); gastrointestinal complaints; rash; irregular menses (spironolactone)	
Amiloride	5–10 mg qd or bid			$$
Spironolactone	25–100 mg qd or bid			$
Triamterene	50–150 mg qd or bid			$
Diuretic combinations		Similar to those for individual components	Similar to individual components	
HCTZ/spironolactone	1 tab qd (aldactazide)			$
HCTZ/triamterene	1 tab qd (dyazide, maxzide)			$
HCTZ/amiloride	1 tab qd (moduretic)			$
Alternative (usually Second-Line) Agents				
Central alpha-2 agonists			Drowsiness; sedation; dry mouth/fatigue; orthostatic hypotension; rebound hypertension; blood dyscrasias	
Clonidine	0.1–1.2 mg bid			$–$$
Clonidine patch	0.1–0.3 mg weekly			$$
Guanabenz	4–64 mg bid			$$$
Guanfacine	1–3 mg qd			$$
Methyldopa	250–2,000 mg bid	Pre-eclampsia or HTN in pregnancy		$–$$
Direct vasodilators		Angina pectoris	Tachycardia; fluid retention; headache; lupus-like syndrome (hydralazine); pleural or pericardial effusion (minoxidil); hirsutism (minoxidil)	
Hydralazine	50–300 mg bid, tid or qid	Pre-eclampsia		$$

Table continues

547

Oral Antihypertensive Agents *Continued*

Drug Type	Usual Dosage and Frequency	Conditions in Which There May Be Additional Risk	Conditions in Which There May Be Additional Benefit	Selected Adverse Effects[a]	Relative Cost[c]
Minoxidil	2.5–80 mg qd or bid				$–$$
Peripheral adrenergic agonists				Orthostatic hypotension; gastrointestinal complaints (especially diarrhea); lethargy and depression (reserpine and *Rauwolfia*)	
Guanedrel	10–75 mg bid	Asthma			$$$
Guanethidine	10–100 mg qd	Asthma			$
Rauwolfia serpentina	50–200 mg qd				$
Reserpine	0.05–0.25 mg qd				$

Source: Adapted from (1) Joint National Committee on Detection, Evaluation, and Treatment of High Blood Pressure. The fifth report of the joint national committee on detection, evaluation, and treatment of high blood pressure (JNC V). Arch Intern Med 1993;153:154–83. (2) Drugs for hypertension. Med Lett 1993;35:55–60.

[a]Partial list of adverse effects. See package insert for complete listing.

[b]Longer acting forms ("sustained release," "extended release," etc.) also available; see package insert for dose information.

[c]Scale is based on average wholesale price for 30 days' treatment (1994 Blue Book, First Data Bank, San Bruno, CA). Scale: $ for under $24, $$ for $25–49.99, $$$ for $50–74.99, $$$$ for $75 or over. Relative differences between agents may vary for retail prices, which tend to be substantially higher. Further variations in prices may occur for other reasons including individual patient factors as well as individual arrangements between drug suppliers and patient care organizations.

Prepared by Christopher O'Donnell, MD and JoAnn E. Manson, MD.

Appendix D

Postmenopausal Hormone Replacement Therapy (Patient Counseling on Indications and Potential Benefits and Risks)

Why is the hormone estrogen important to a woman's health?
During a woman's reproductive years, her ovaries produce a class of hormones called estrogens. Their primary role is to prepare the uterine lining for possible pregnancy. However, estrogens also help maintain strong, dense bones and protect women from cardiovascular disease (heart attacks).

During her 40s, a women's estrogen levels gradually decline. Eventually, usually around age 50, she will cease ovulating and stop having periods. Menopause is technically defined as 1 year without any periods. The average age at menopause for U.S. women is 51 years. After menopause the ovaries no longer produce estrogens. Menopause most often occurs as part of the normal aging process. However, a woman who has had her ovaries surgically removed will also experience menopause.

Lack of estrogens can cause many physical changes. Some of these are obvious, such as hot flashes. Others are more subtle. Bones become progressively less dense and more prone to fracture, a condition known as osteoporosis. Also, a woman's risk of heart disease begins to rise. Some women are more likely to develop osteoporosis or cardiovascular disease than others. While family history, diet, and exercise can affect your chances of getting these diseases, the absence of estrogens after menopause always plays an important role.

What is hormone replacement therapy (HRT) and why is it prescribed?
The purpose of hormone replacement therapy is to substitute replacement or synthetic forms of estrogen for the estrogens normally produced by the ovaries. By taking low-

dose estrogen tablets, women may be able to relieve some bothersome menopausal symptoms. Doing so can also help prevent some of the effects of low estrogen levels that may be harmful to a woman's health.

Taking estrogen on a short-term basis (2–3 years) can alleviate common discomforts such as hot flashes, hot sweats, vaginal dryness, and mood swings. Most women find this treatment very effective.

Estrogen can also be given on a more long-term basis (more than 5 years). Studies suggest that long-term therapy may reduce the risk of hip fracture by 25% and cardiovascular disease by 35%. Risk of breast cancer, however, may be increased by about 25% with long-term use of HRT.

What are the risks of these health outcomes in women?

A postmenopausal woman is 6–10 times more likely to die of cardiovascular disease than of breast cancer or osteoporosis. Overall mortality rates of women taking estrogen have been shown to be 20% to 40% lower than the mortality rates of other women the same age, but results from randomized trials are not yet available.

Synthetic forms of the hormone progesterone, called progestins, are often prescribed along with estrogen to reduce some of the risk associated with estrogen use.

What are the risks of taking estrogen alone or combined with progestins?

Studies have shown that estrogen, given alone, markedly increases the risk of endometrial cancer (cancer of the uterine lining). However, endometrial cancer is relatively rare. For a 50-year-old woman, endometrial cancer causes death one-fourth as often as hip fractures. Endometrial cancer that does arise in patients taking estrogen is usually detected much earlier and is often less malignant than non–estrogen-related cases. The increased risk can be eliminated if progestins are taken in addition to estrogens. Unfortunately, adding progestins may somewhat decrease the cardiovascular benefits of estrogen. If a woman has had her uterus removed, she does not need progestins in addition to estrogen.

Estrogen's relationship to breast cancer risk has also received much attention. Studies show that at the low doses most frequently prescribed, there is probably little if any increased risk of breast cancer during the first 10–15 years of therapy. Longer periods of treatment may somewhat increase the risk of breast cancer. Also, a woman whose sister or mother has had breast cancer is at slightly increased risk. Therapy that combines estrogen and progestins is less well studied. It is uncertain whether combined therapy raises the risk of breast cancer, and studies have suggested that both increased and reduced risks compared with estrogen alone.

Finally, women taking estrogens are somewhat more likely to get gallstones. Table D1 summarizes the information we have on the possible benefits and risks of estrogen alone and a combined estrogen/progestin regimen. This information is not conclusive, however, because it is not based on randomized clinical trials; rather it represents "best estimates" from the evidence that is currently available.

Who should consider HRT?

All women should receive information and counseling about the potential benefits and risks of hormone replacement therapy. Although it is a complex and personal decision,

Table D1. Possible Benefits and Risks of Hormone Replacement Therapy

	Hormone Therapy Regimen	
	Estrogen Alone	Estrogen Plus Progestin
Possible Benefits		
Coronary heart disease	May decrease risk of heart disease by 35%	May decrease risk of heart disease 20–35%, but less information than for estrogen alone
Fractures due to osteoporosis	May decrease risk of hip fracture by 25%	May decrease risk of hip fractures by 25%, but less information than for estrogen alone
Menopausal symptoms	Less "hot flashes" and other menopausal systems	Less "hot flashes" and other menopausal symptoms
Bladder function	Fewer bladder problems	Fewer bladder problems
Possible Risks		
Breast cancer	May increase risk of breast cancer by 25%	May increase risk of breast cancer by 25%, but less information than for estrogen alone
Uterine cancer	May increase risk of uterine cancer	No known increase in risk of uterine cancer
Blood clots	May increase risk of blood clots in legs or lungs	May increase risk of blood clots in legs or lungs
Side effects and vaginal bleeding	More period-like symptoms (see text for information on vaginal bleeding)	More period-like symptoms (see text for information on vaginal bleeding)

Source: Modified from Grady D, et al. Ann Intern Med, 1992, with permission.

a woman should consider hormone replacement therapy unless she has one of the following conditions: unexplained vaginal bleeding, chronic liver failure, a personal history of breast cancer, a recent heart attack or stroke, or a history of blood clots caused by estrogen use (e.g., birth control pills). Women with a family history of breast cancer should be cautious about HRT use. Women with risk factors for, or a history of, osteoporosis or cardiovascular disease should strongly consider HRT. Women who have had hysterectomies, surgical removal of ovaries, or early menopause are also particularly good candidates for HRT.

Remember that some women are more susceptible to osteoporosis and cardiovascular disease than others. Women who are thin, short, white or Asian, or know that their mothers or grandmothers had osteoporosis are at greater risk for osteoporosis and associated fractures. Smoking and sedentary lifestyle are other risk factors for osteoporosis. Any woman who has had her ovaries surgically removed is also at higher risk. Because bone loss is most rapid in the first few years of menopause, those whose treatment begins at that time are benefitted the most. Risk factors for cardiovascular disease include smoking, high cholesterol, high blood pressure, diabetes, obesity, sedentary lifestyle, and family history of heart disease or strokes. A group of researchers has estimated the increase in life expectancy that may occur among women who are

Table D2. Estimated Net Change in Life Expectancy (on Average)

	Estrogen	Estrogen Plus Progestin
No risk factors	+0.9 years	+0.1 years
Hysterectomy	+1.1 years	
History of heart disease	+2.1 years	+0.9–2.2 years
At risk for heart disease	+1.5 years	+0.6–1.6 years
At risk for breast cancer	+0.7 years	−0.5–+0.8 years
At risk for hip fracture	+1.0 years	+0.2–1.1 years

Source: From Grady D, et al. Ann Intern Med, 1992, with permission.

treated with long-term hormone replacement therapy (10–20 years). Although there is a lot of uncertainty in these estimates, they conclude that the women who are most likely to benefit are those with a history of heart disease or who are at increased risk of heart disease, those at increased risk of hip fracture, and women who have had a hysterectomy. Women least likely to benefit are those at increased risk of breast cancer (e.g., family history of breast cancer). Table D2 shows the estimated changes in life expectancy for a 50-year-old woman treated with long-term hormone therapy, based upon her risk factor status.

How is HRT given?

A combination of estrogen and progestin can be given either cyclically or continuously. Two regimens that are common in clinical use are:

1. Estrogen plus cyclic progestin. Estrogen (generally a dose of 0.625 mg of oral conjugated or the equivalent) is taken on days 1 through 25 of the month and a progestin (such as medroxyprogesterone acetate at a dose of 5–10 mg orally) is added for 10–14 days per month (often taken on days 15 through 25 of the cycle). On days 26 through 30, no hormones are taken and vaginal bleeding will usually occur. This is a traditional approach that imitates the normal menstrual cycle. The estrogen patch is an alternative method of treatment, but this route may not provide the lipid and heart disease benefits.
2. Continuous combined estrogen and progestin. With continuous therapy, women take estrogen (generally at a dose of 0.625 mg/day orally) with a daily low dose of progestin (often medroxyprogesterone acetate, 2.5 mg/day orally, or the equivalent). These hormones are taken throughout the month without interruption.

If a woman has had a hysterectomy, estrogen is given alone without the addition of progestin.

What are the side effects of HRT?

Side effects depend upon the dosage and kind (cyclic or continuous) of therapy. Cyclic therapy usually causes vaginal bleeding similar to menstruation. Most often, this bleeding is lighter and lasts for a shorter time than a normal menstrual period. Some women will stop having this bleeding after several months of therapy. Women who experienced severe PMS before menopause are unlikely to have similar problems when taking HRT. Cyclic therapy with estrogen and progestins may cause bloating and breast tenderness or heaviness. These symptoms can usually be alleviated by lowering or eliminating the progestins.

With continuous therapy, women usually experience some unpredictible spotting and breakthrough bleeding during the first 4–6 months of therapy. Over 80% of women will have no more bleeding after 6 months of continuous therapy. Because women on continuous therapy receive lower doses of progestins, bloating and breast tenderness are much less common.

Also see Table D1 for summary of health risks associated with HRT.

Will screening tests of the uterus be required?
When estrogen is taken together with a progestin, no special screening tests of the uterus are generally required before starting therapy. During therapy, if bleeding occurs other than at the times expected (during the interval off hormones for the cyclic regimen) or persisting more than 6–9 months for the continuous regimen, an evaluation of the lining of the uterus (endometrium) may be required. Also, if bleeding is unusually heavy (heavier than normal menstrual period) or prolonged (longer than 10 days at a time), evaluation of the uterus may be necessary.

How do I know if HRT is right for me?
The decision to start hormone replacement therapy is complicated. There are still many unanswered questions about HRT and long-term studies are ongoing. You must weigh the risks and benefits based on your health status, risk factors, and personal preference. You must also consider HRT's possible side effects as well as the current understanding of its potential complications.

HRT is not right for everyone. If you feel you might be a good candidate for HRT or would like to know more about it, please contact your clinician. She or he can answer your questions and help you determine if HRT is right for you.

Modified, with permission, from patient education materials prepared by the Clinical Publications Program at Harvard Community Health Plan, Brookline, MA and Grady D, et al: Ann Intern Med 1992;117:1016–37.

Index